Manual for Research Ethics Committees

The sixth edition of the *Manual for Research Ethics Committees* is a unique compilation of legal and ethical guidance which will prove invaluable for members of research ethics committees, researchers involved in research with humans, members of the pharmaceutical industry and students of law, medicine, ethics and philosophy. Presented in a clear and authoritative form, it incorporates the key legal and ethical guidelines and specially written chapters on major topics in bioethics by leading academic authors and practitioners, pharmaceutical industry associations and professional bodies. In the sixth edition there are 15 new chapters covering key issues from participation in clinical trials to cloning, and for the first time the manual has been produced in one easy-to-search hardback volume.

Sue Eckstein is Research Fellow at the Centre of Medical Law and Ethics, King's College London, and the organiser of the Centre's short courses on the ethics of research on humans.

Editorial Committee

Dr Calliope (Bobbie) Farsides
Senior Lecturer, Centre of Medical Law and Ethics, King's College London

Professor Jonathan Glover
Director, Centre of Medical Law and Ethics, King's College London

Dr John Lamberty
Chairman, South East Multi-Centre Research Ethics Committee and former Chairman, Brighton Local Research Ethics Committee

Baroness O'Neill
Principal, Newnham College, Cambridge

Professor Daniel Wikler
Professor of Bioethics and Professor of Philosophy, University of Wisconsin, and Consultant in Ethics to WHO

Manual for Research Ethics Committees

6th edition

Centre of Medical Law and Ethics, King's College London

EDITED BY

Sue Eckstein

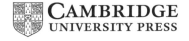

PUBLISHED BY THE PRESS SYNDICATE OF THE UNIVERSITY OF CAMBRIDGE
The Pitt Building, Trumpington Street, Cambridge, United Kingdom

CAMBRIDGE UNIVERSITY PRESS
The Edinburgh Building, Cambridge CB2 2RU, UK
40 West 20th Street, New York, NY 10011-4211, USA
477 Williamstown Road, Port Melbourne, VIC 3207, Australia
Ruiz de Alarcón 13, 28014 Madrid, Spain
Dock House, The Waterfront, Cape Town 8001, South Africa

http://www.cambridge.org

First published 1992
Second – Fifth editions published 1994–97: ISBN 1 898 484 007
Sixth edition published 2003
Third printing 2006

Printed in the United Kingdom at the University Press, Cambridge

Typefaces Utopia 8.5/12 pt and Dax   *System* LATEX 2$_\varepsilon$ [TB]

A catalogue record for this book is available from the British Library

Library of Congress Cataloguing in Publication data

ISBN 0 521 81004 3 hardback

Every effort has been made in preparing this book to provide accurate and
up-to-date information which is in accord with accepted standards and
practice at the time of publication. Nevertheless, the authors, editors and
publisher can make no warranties that the information contained herein
is totally free from error, not least because clinical standards are constantly
changing through research and regulation. The authors, editors and
publisher therefore disclaim all liability for direct or consequential
damages resulting from the use of material contained in this book. Readers
are strongly advised to pay careful attention to information provided by
the manufacturer of any drugs or equipment that they plan to use.

The publisher has used its best endeavours to ensure that the URLs for
external websites referred to in this book are correct and active at the time
of going to press. However, the publisher has no responsibility for the
websites and can make no guarantee that a site will remain live or that the
content is or will remain appropriate.

Contents

Editorial board

The editor is most grateful to Jane Peek for her assistance in the obtaining of copyright permissions.

Finally, particular thanks to Bobbie Farsides for her on-going encouragement and advice.

Acknowledgements

The Editor of this Manual, on behalf of the Centre of Medical Law and Ethics, would like to thank all those who have so kindly contributed to the contents of the Manual.

The following authors and organisations have kindly given their permission for the Centre of Medical Law and Ethics to include or reprint their work in the Manual:

Richard Ashcroft
Alzheimer's Society
Association of the British Pharmaceutical Industry
Phil Bates
Jennifer Blunt
BMJ Publishing Group
The British Psychological Society
British Sociological Association
Keith Britton
Kenneth Calman
Central Office for Research Ethics Committees
Ruth Chadwick
Pamela Charnley Nickols
The Council of Europe
The Council for International Organisations of
    Medical Sciences
Alan Cribb
The Department of Health
Nick Dunn
Philippa Easterbrook
European Forum for Good Clinical Practice
Office for the Official Publications of The European
    Communities, the European Parliament and the
    Council of the European Union
Calliope (Bobbie) Farsides
Tom Farsides
Sev Fluss
Rosemary Foley

Gene Therapy Advisory Committee
General Medical Council
Andrew Grubb
Joan Houghton
Human Fertilisation and Embryology Authority
The Information Commissioner
Hazel Inskip
International Conference on Harmonisation
Janet Jeffs
Crispin Jenkinson
Joint United Nations Programme on HIV/AIDS (UNAIDS)
Ian Kennedy
Penney Lewis
Anthony Madden
Richard Mayon-White
The Medical Devices Agency
Medical Research Council
Elizabeth Mellor
Sabine Michalowski
Niall Moore
Richard Morris
National Commission for the Protection of Human
    Subjects of Biomedical and Behavioral Research
National Council for Hospice and Specialist Palliative Care
    Services
National Union of Students
Richard H. Nicholson
Nuffield Council on Bioethics

Office for Human Research Protections
Michael Parker
Royal College of Nursing
The Royal College of Paediatrics and Child Health:
    Ethics Advisory Committee
The Royal College of Pathologists
The Royal College of Psychiatrists
David K. Raynor
Elizabeth Ryan
Rosamund Scott
Jonathan Silcock
The Stationery Office
Julie Stone
United Nations Development Programme
Frank Wells
WHO Special Programme for Research and Training
    in Tropical Diseases (TDR)
World Bank
World Medical Association

Contributors

Part I

Richard Ashcroft
Department of Primary Health Care and General Practice, ICSM
Charing Cross Campus, Reynolds Building, St Dunstan's Road,
London W6 8RP, UK

Phil Bates
School of Law, King's College London, Strand, London
WC2R 2LS, UK

Jennifer Blunt
North West MREC, Gateway House, Piccadilly South, Manchester
M60 7LP, UK

Keith Britton
Department of Nuclear Medicine, St Bartholomew's Hospital,
London EC1A 7BE, UK

Sir Kenneth Calman
University of Durham, Old Shire Hall, Durham DH1 3HP, UK

Ruth Chadwick
Institute for Environment, Philosophy and Public Policy,
Lancaster University, Furness College, Lancaster LA1 4YG, UK

Pamela Charnley Nickols
Charnley Nickols Associates Ltd., 6 Dove Lane, Long Eaton, Notts
NG10 4LP, UK

Alan Cribb
Centre for Public Policy Research, King's College London,
Franklin-Wilkins Building, Waterloo Road, London SE1 8WA, UK

Nick Dunn
Primary Medical Care, University of Southampton, Aldermoor
Health Centre, Aldermoor Close, Southampton SO16 5ST, UK

Philippa Easterbrook
Division of Medicine, Guy's, King's and St Thomas' School of Medicine, Weston Education Centre, Cutcombe Road, London SE5 9RT, UK

Sue Eckstein
Centre of Medical Law and Ethics, King's College London, Strand, London WC2R 2LS, UK

Calliope (Bobbie) Farsides
Centre of Medical Law and Ethics, King's College London, Strand, London WC2R 2LS, UK

Tom Farsides
Department of Social Psychology, University of Sussex, Falmer, Brighton, Sussex BN1 9RH, UK

Rosemary R. Foley
Department of Clinical Physics, St Bartholomew's Hospital, London EC1A 7BE, UK

Andrew Grubb
Cardiff Law School, Cardiff University, Law Building, Museum Avenue, PO Box 427, Cardiff CF10 3XJ, UK

Joan Houghton
CRC Trials' Centre, Rayne Institute, 123 Coldharbour Lane, London SE5 9NU, UK

Hazel Inskip
MRC Environmental Epidemiology Unit, Southampton General Hospital, Southampton SO16 6YD, UK

Janet Jeffs
Oxford Radcliffe Hospitals, Legal Services Department, Stable Block, Osler Road, Headington, Oxford OX3 9RP, UK

Crispin Jenkinson
Health Services Research Unit, University of Oxford, Institute of Health Sciences, Headington, Oxford OX3 7LF, UK

Ian Kennedy
School of Public Policy, University College London, 29/30 Tavistock Square, London WC1H 9EZ, UK

Penney Lewis
School of Law, King's College London, Strand, London WC2R 2LS, UK

Anthony Madden
Department of Anaesthesia, Southmead Hospital, Westbury on Trym, Bristol BS10 5NB, UK

Richard Mayon-White
Oxfordshire Health Authority, Richards Building, Old Road, Headington, Oxford OX3 7LG, UK

Elizabeth Mellor
Pharmacy Services, The Leeds Teaching Hospitals NHS Trust, St James's University Hospital, Beckett Street, Leeds LS9 7TF, UK

Sabine Michalowski
Department of Law, University of Essex, Wivenhoe Park, Colchester CO4 3SQ, UK

Niall Moore
The MRI Centre, The John Radcliffe, Headley Way, Headington, Oxford OX3 9DU, UK

Richard Morris
Department of Primary Care and Population Sciences, Royal Free and University College Medical School, Royal Free Campus, Rowland Hill Street, London NW3 2PF, UK

Richard H. Nicholson
Bulletin of Medical Ethics, 8 Rose Cottage, Aberdeen Centre, 22–24 Highbury Grove, London N5 2EA, UK

Nuffield Council on Bioethics
28 Bedford Square, London WC1B 3JS, UK

Michael Parker
The ETHOX Centre, University of Oxford, Old Road, Oxford OX3 7LF, UK

David K. Raynor
Pharmacy Practice and Medicines Management, School of Healthcare Studies, Baines Wing, PO Box 214, University of Leeds, Leeds LS2 9UT, UK

Rosamund Scott
School of Law, King's College London, Strand, London WC2R 2LS, UK

Jonathan Silcock
Pharmacy Practice and Medicines Management, School of Healthcare Studies, Baines Wing, PO Box 214, University of Leeds, Leeds LS2 9UT, UK

Julie Stone
Department of Ethics and Law Applied to Medicine, Barts and The London, Queen Mary's School of Medicine and Dentistry, Turner Street, London E1 2AD, UK

Frank Wells

MedicoLegal Investigations Ltd, Old Hadleigh, London Road, Capel St Mary, Ipswich IP9 2JJ, UK

Part II

Alzheimer's Society

Gordon House, 10 Greencoat Place, London SW1P 1PH, UK

Association of the British Pharmaceutical Industry (ABPI)

12 Whitehall, London SW1A 2DY, UK

The British Psychological Society

St Andrews House, 48 Princess Road East, Leicester LE1 7DR, UK

British Sociological Association

Unit 3F/G, Mountjoy Research Centre, Stockton Road, Durham DH1 3UR, UK

The Caldicott Committee

Department of Health, Richmond House, 79 Whitehall, London SWIA 2NS, UK

Central Office for Research Ethics Committees (COREC)

Room 76, B Block, 40 Eastbourne Terrace, London W2 3QR, UK

Council for International Organisations of Medical Sciences (CIOMS)

c/o WHO, CH-1211 Geneva 27, Switzerland

Council of Europe

Directorate General, Legal Affairs, Treaty Office, F-67075 Strasbourg, Cedex, France

Department of Health

Complaints and Clinical Negligence, Policy Unit, Quarry House, Quarry Hill, Leeds LS2 7UE, UK

Department of Health

Richmond House, 79 Whitehall, London SWIA 2NS, UK

European Forum for Good Clinical Practice

EFGCP Secretariat, Schoolbergenstraat 47, B-3010 Kessel-Lo, Belgium

The European Parliament and the Council of the European Union

Office for Official Publications of the European Communities, 2 Rue Mercier, L-2985 Luxembourg

General Medical Council (GMC)

178 Great Portland Street, London W1W 5JE, UK

Gene Therapy Advisory Committee

Department of Health, Richmond House, 79 Whitehall, London SWIA 2NS, UK

Human Fertilisation and Embryology Authority

Paxton House, 30 Artillery Lane, London E1 7LS, UK

The Information Commissioner

The Information Commissioner's Office, Wycliffe House, Water Lane, Wilmslow, Cheshire SK9 5AF, UK

International Conference on Harmonisation of Technical Requirements for Registration of Pharmaceuticals for Human Use (ICH)

ICH Secretariat, c/o IFPMA, 30, Rue de St Jean, PO Box 758, 1211 Geneva 13, Switzerland

Joint United Nations Programme on HIV/AIDS (UNAIDS)

20 Avenue Appia, 1211 Geneva 27, Switzerland

Medical Devices Agency

Hannibal House, Elephant and Castle, London SE1 6TQ, UK

Medical Research Council (MRC)

20 Park Crescent, London W1B 1AL, UK

National Commission for the Protection of Human Subjects of Biomedical and Behavioral Research

Office for Human Research Protection (OHRP), The Tower Building, 1101 Wootton Parkway, Suite 200, Rockville, MD 20852, USA

The National Council for Hospice and Specialist Palliative Care Services

First Floor, 34–44 Britannia Street, London WC1X 9JG, UK

National Union of Students

Nelson Mandela House, 461 Holloway Road, London N7 6LJ, UK

Office for Human Research Protections

The Tower Building, 1101 Wootton Parkway, Suite 200, Rockville, MD 20852, USA

Royal College of Nursing

20 Cavendish Square, London W1M OAB, UK

Royal College of Paediatrics and Child Health: Ethics Advisory Committee

BMJ Publishing Group, BMA House, Tavistock Square, London WC1H 9JR, UK

Royal College of Pathologists

2 Carlton House Terrace, London SW1Y 5AF, UK

The Royal College of Psychiatrists
17 Belgrave Square, London SW1X 8PG, UK

The Stationery Office
HMSO, St Clements House, 2–16 Colegate, Norwich NR3 1BQ, UK

UNDP/World Bank/WHO Special Programme for Research and Training in Tropical Disease (TDR)
WHO, CH-1211 Geneva 27, Switzerland

World Medical Association
Boite Postale 63, 01212 Ferney-Voltaire Cedex, France

Introduction

Where is the Life we have lost in living?
Where is the wisdom we have lost in knowledge?
Where is the knowledge we have lost in information?
  T.S. Eliot   From *The Rock* (1934) pt. 1

Members of Research Ethics Committees have the responsibility of ensuring that medical research on humans is conducted in an ethical manner. In order to fulfil this function, Research Ethics Committees must engage in reasonable discussion and consideration of the ethical issues in each of the research proposals they have to review. This is demanding and time-consuming work, and the responsibilities entailed are considerable. On the one hand there is the need to contribute to the evidence base upon which modern medicine is based, on the other is the need to protect those who participate in the research process.

To assist in this process of review, the Centre of Medical Law and Ethics began producing the Manual for Research Ethics Committees. Under the editorship of Claire Foster, the Manual grew from the slim ring binder of 1992 to the two very large and very heavy black volumes of the 1997 5th edition.

The Manual has had a loyal readership over the past decade, with orders increasingly coming not only from Local Research Ethics Committees and Multi-centre Research Ethics Committees but also from research institutes, hospitals, universities and pharmaceutical companies in the UK, North America, India, Africa and Australia.

Ethics in medical research is no longer an issue to which a passing nod can be given in order to fulfil minimum requirements. Public outcry over research scandals in the UK and the USA, and increasing controversy about research carried out in developing countries, has forced ethics towards its proper place at the top of the research agenda. In the light of these developments, this seems to be an appropriate time to produce a new edition of the manual which offers a radical reorganisation and rewriting of much of the material contained in earlier editions.

The 6th edition of the *Manual for Research Ethics Committees* is divided into two distinct parts which are designed to complement each other.

Part I contains 24 chapters on various aspects of research on humans. Fifteen of these have been especially commissioned for the 6th edition and the nine chapters that appeared in the 5th edition have been revised and updated, where appropriate, by the original authors. Part I has been divided into four main sections.

Section I contains three chapters on fundamental ethical and legal considerations which will be key reading for all members of Research Ethics Committees.

Section II contains 15 chapters on various aspects of the research process, including new chapters on areas that appear to be of increasing interest or concern for members of RECs such as student research, genetic research, qualitative research and research in complementary and alternative medicine.

Section III comprises four chapters on protecting the interests of research participants which concentrate on consent, confidentiality and information, and a subsection on protecting the interests of vulnerable research participants.

Section IV deals with research in an international context, particularly the issues that can arise when medical research is carried out by Western researchers in developing countries.

Part II of the Manual contains 45 key guidelines from international and national organisations, government departments, Royal Colleges, professional bodies and research institutions. These have been ordered under the same headings as the chapters in the first part of the Manual. This is intended to help readers find the guidelines that inform a particular issue. However, the index at the back of the Manual should be used as a comprehensive search tool for guidelines and information.

Readers should not expect to find *all* relevant guidelines in this Manual. Over the past 10 years, there has been a proliferation of guidelines which could fill a volume several times the size of this one. To cite just one example, over 350 international guidelines on bioethics are included in the European Forum for Good Clinical Practice's listing.

A significant amount of thought and consultation has gone into deciding which current guidelines should be included in full, which guidelines to use summaries of, which to simply refer to and which to omit.

Readers familiar with previous editions of the Manual will note that the Royal College of Physicians of London's advice 'Guidelines on the practice of ethics committees in medical research involving human subjects (1996)' has been omitted from this edition of the Manual as permission was not granted to reproduce the full version. Readers should check the RCP's website for details of their guidelines.

Since the publication of the 5th edition of the Manual, a number of key guidelines, such as the Declaration of Helsinki, have been revised. The latest versions of the guidelines are reproduced in the Manual, though the nature of information is such that it is inevitable that between the writing of this introduction and the production of the Manual, a number of guidelines may already be out of date.

Websites which are particularly important to check regularly include:

The Association of Research Ethics Committees (AREC)
http://www.arec.net/

British Medical Association (BMA)
http://bma.org.uk/

Central Office for Research Ethics Committees (COREC)
http://www.corec.org.uk

Centre of Medical Law and Ethics, King's College London (CMLE)
http://www.kcl.ac.uk/depsta/law/research/cmle/

Department of Health
http://www.doh.gov.uk/

Ethics Research Information Catalogue (ERIC)
http://www.eric-on-line.co.uk

The General Medical Council (GMC)
http://www.gmc-uk.org/standards/guidance.htm

Medical Research Council (MRC)
http://www.mrc.ac.uk/

Nuffield Council on Bioethics
http://www.nuffieldbioethics.org/home/

Royal College of Physicians of London (RCP)
http://www.rcplondon.ac.uk/

Where relevant, some useful websites are listed at the end of chapters in the first section of the Manual. Readers should be aware that although websites were correct at the time of publication, addresses may have changed in the meantime.

Periodicals such as the *Bulletin of Medical Ethics* (http://www.bullmedeth.info/) and the *Journal of Medical Ethics* (http://jme.bmjjournals.com/) will also alert readers to the publication of new guidelines and to key ethical debates.

Because of space constraints, copies of relevant Government Acts have not been include in the Manual. However, there is a list of references at the end of the chapter on The Law Relating to Consent.

Finally, it is important to take note of the words of T.S. Eliot above. Written guidelines, with all the information they contain, are no substitute for either knowledge or wisdom. Guidelines are simply a tool and should be used in the correct circumstance and with care, as any tool would be used.

Those involved in the ethical review of research proposals should be aware that guidelines in isolation do not contain the answers to the complex issues that are debated in every meeting of research ethics committees. Similarly, those involved in the funding, design and implementation of research should be aware that the guidelines cannot be used as a substitute for the careful consideration of ethical issues at all stages of the research process.

Sue Eckstein
Centre of Medical Law and Ethics
King's College London

Fundamental ethical and legal considerations

The ethics of clinical research

Calliope (Bobbie) Farsides

Centre of Medical Law and Ethics, King's College London, UK

History is unfortunately peppered with stories of abuse carried out in the context of medical research. No one can remain unaware of the dreadful medical atrocities of the Nazi period, some of which were carried out by doctors motivated as much by scientific curiosity as by Nazi ideology.[1] In the late 1990s, the US President, Bill Clinton, offered an apology to the families of those men involved in the infamous Tuskegee project,[2] and in the opening years of the new millennium there has been international concern over the conduct of clinical trials in the developing world. In an attempt to protect individuals from abuse, international and national guidelines now govern this area of science, and in the United Kingdom research is carefully monitored through the work of funding bodies, peer review systems, Local Research Ethics Committees (LRECs) and Multi-Centre Research Ethics Committees (MRECs). However, at ground level, the moral responsibilities primarily lie with those who design and carry out the research, and then publicise the findings. It is therefore crucially important that these individuals understand the ethical issues that arise when human beings come under the scientific gaze.

The benefits of good medical research speak for themselves. In our own lifetime, killer diseases have been eradicated, death sentences have been lifted from a number of diseases, and incredible advances have been made in such areas as reproductive technology and transplant surgery. However, there are still important battles to be won, and discoveries we yearn to make. If research is to continue to bring about the benefits we hope for, we have to accept that there will be costs involved. The moral question is what type of benefits ought we to pursue and at what cost to individuals and society?

Research passes through various phases, so over time one individual might be involved in different types of research intervention, be it as a researcher or volunteer participant. In the past, researchers have been keen to make the distinction between therapeutic and non-therapeutic research, where therapeutic research permits the hope of a direct health-related benefit to the participant, whilst non-therapeutic research means that the participant might be a healthy volunteer, or a patient who is asked to contribute to some work unrelated to their particular problem, or to participate in very early research which will not be at a stage to benefit them. In these cases the potential benefits are of a different type, possibly financial. Whilst the specific issues raised may differ, the fundamental questions remain the same: ought we to do this research, and if so how ought we to do it? The distinction between therapeutic and non-therapeutic is thus becoming increasingly blurred. It is tempting to think that the clear presence of quantifiable costs and benefits means that the ethical status of medical research could, and should, be judged through consequentialist means. However, this assumption needs to be explored.

Consequentialism

In the simplest terms a consequentialist believes that the morality of an action should be judged in terms of the consequences that follow from it. If the consequences are on balance good, then so is the action; if the consequences are bad, then the action must be seen in the same way. This means that a proposed course of action need not be seen as intrinsically good or bad, but rather must be judged

---

[1] Annas, G. and Grodin, M. (eds.) (1992). *The Nazi Doctors and the Nuremberg Code.* New York: Oxford University Press.

[2] Jones J.H. (1981). *Bad Blood: The Tuskegee Syphilis Experiment.* New York: The Free Press.

in terms of what is predicted to follow on from it. To coin a cliché, for the consequentialist, the ends justify the means.[3]

The most famous variant of consequentialism is utilitarianism, the theory developed by Jeremy Bentham in the mid-nineteenth century.[4] Bentham had a reductionist view of human nature in which he claimed that all human beings were fundamentally concerned primarily with the pursuit of pleasure and the avoidance of pain. He believed that a moral theory should acknowledge this fact, and thus to be moral is to be concerned with the maximisation of pleasure and the minimisation of pain. Human nature inclines one to be concerned about one's personal pain and pleasure; morality requires that we be equally concerned with the pain and pleasure of all sentient beings.

Should we be doing this?

In the context of clinical research we can see that a consequentialist could support a piece of research as morally acceptable if we minimised the harms and maximised the benefits resulting from the intervention, and on balance created more good than harm. This sounds intuitively appealing and certainly offers a starting point for ethical analysis. However, clinical experimentation also highlights the problems with the consequentialist approach when applied to real life.

First, we have to ascertain what counts as a benefit in this context, and how the value of different types of benefit compare. Defining and calculating happiness was a difficult problem for Bentham and his followers; defining and calculating benefits in this context is also challenging. How do we compare the benefit of curing a disease with the benefits of preventing it in the first place? How do you compare the benefits of palliating symptoms with increasing patient satisfaction through other means? Is reducing the cost of health care a significant benefit compared with improving treatment? How does one weight 'hope' and 'worth' as benefits of involvement? All these questions might be relevant when deciding how to allocate a pool of money between different types of research, but they might also have an impact

on the types of risks (if any) you would allow people to run in pursuit of the types of benefits on offer.

Having looked at the type of benefits available, we also have to identify to whom the benefits attach and ask whether this further weights their significance. Utilitarianism demands that we treat each individual as one and no more than one. However, when there are a wide range of potential beneficiaries as in the case of clinical trials – participants in the trials (healthy or unhealthy), other sufferers of the same condition, future sufferers (some as yet unborn), researchers and student researchers, society as a whole, health-care professionals, and drug companies – there are still complex calculations to be made. Knowing to whom benefits attach might help us to decide how to allocate resources to research, and it could also help us decide what costs it would be acceptable to attach to whom.

One might assume that the consequentialist ideal would be to conduct a piece of research which imposed minimum costs upon the smallest possible number of people, but secured substantial benefits for a significantly higher number of people (particularly those who participated). However, this ideal type model is not always possible, nor indeed is the consequentialist necessarily committed to it above all else. As we shall see, the consequentialist can justify some rather different outcomes, some of which are less intuitively appealing. Furthermore, what the consequentialist would see as morally desirable might not fit comfortably with the realities of a commercially driven pharmaceutical industry, or western dominated models of health-care delivery. Furthermore, the globalism inherent in consequentialism might sometimes be at odds with the localised concerns of those deliberating upon research protocols, a dilemma reflected in the sometimes difficult relationship between Local Research Ethics Committees (LRECs) and Multi-Centre Research Ethics Committees (MRECs).

Some examples

- One can see that research that is directed at the alleviation of widespread and significant suffering should easily pass the consequentialist test, even if quite significant risks are posed to a relatively small amount of research participants. It is worth bearing in mind that allowing the costs to be too high might undermine public support for clinical research with dire consequences, and the consequentialist would wish to avoid this risk. On this basis, research to alleviate the HIV epidemic in Africa should gain significant support because of the scale of the problem and the consequent degree of suffering entailed. However, we know that, in the past, such work was not given high

[3] For a more detailed examination of consequentialist positions see the following: Glover, J. (ed.) (1990). *Utilitarianism and Its Critics.* Macmillan.

Samual, S. (ed.) (1988). *Consequentialism and its Critics.* Oxford: Oxford Readings in Philosophy.

Smart J.J.C. and Williams B. (1973). *Utilitarianism: For and Against.* Cambridge: Cambridge University Press.

[4] Bentham, J. (1970). *Introduction to the Theory of Morals and Legislation.* Ed. J.H. Burns and H.L.A. Hart. London: Athlone Press.

priority due to the financial realities of the regions involved, which meant that the benefits would not be purchasable at the prices dictated by market forces. In consequentialist terms the sums worked out; in commercial terms they did not.

- At a local level one sometimes encounters proposals advocating trivial but commercially motivated research; for example, post-licensing drug comparisons that have more to do with marketing than with useful clinical comparison. The benefits to drug companies of usurping a market leader might be great, but the benefits to patients will be negligible if the treatment is already known to have nothing new to offer. Here, the consequentialist sums do not add up, but the commercial ones do.
- A difficult problem is posed by student research. The benefits to the particular student and the benefits to society and future patients of having well-trained professionals will speak in favour of supporting student research. However, the costs borne by the participants in student research projects might be higher and the benefits to be gained by the research itself may be small or non-existent. Here, the benefits and costs might, to some extent, appear incommensurate.

Distinguishing between types of benefit and looking at the potential quantity of benefits on offer, and assessing who gains the benefits as opposed to bearing the costs of research can offer the basis for a searing critique of current practice. By evaluating the moral costs and benefits, one can decide what ought to be done, but it is often the case that other types of accounting are shown to determine what is done.

How should we do research?

A key to proceeding appropriately in consequentialist terms must be the provision of adequate information to facilitate the evaluation of costs and benefits and allow for a rational decision to be made. An initial problem arises from the fact that the ideal starting point for a piece of clinical research is a position of equipoise.[5] This is a scientific or methodological as well as an ethical issue. Put simply, being in equipoise means that, when attempting to compare two approaches, be it a new drug with an established drug, or the use of a new procedure where none was previously attempted, the researcher should not proceed if he or she has any fixed assumptions about how the new option will be better. Only the results of

the comparison will show which is the more beneficial approach. Until the results are available, the researcher cannot promise any benefits to those who enrol in the trial, she or he can only explain what is hoped for. Admittedly, all consequentialist calculations are based on potentially unreliable calculations about future benefits, but one could argue that in this case the problem is heightened by the fact that the trial is only going ahead because the benefits are as yet unknown. This must be highlighted when providing a potential participant with the information upon which they will base their own consequentialist calculation when deciding whether or not to participate.

A consequentialist approach will necessarily impact upon who are recruited as participants in research projects. This will, in part, be determined by the preceding question of what research should be done, but once that has been decided recruitment will be effected by the requirement to secure 'the greatest good of the greatest number'. As a maximising theory, consequentialism is more concerned with the total quantity of benefits and costs than with their distribution. This can cause problems when considering how to evaluate the moral acceptability of the distribution of costs and benefits in a particular case. In some cases we might allow that a small number of participants might risk a very severe harm in the interests of securing a benefit for a much larger number of people, but in other cases this might be deemed unacceptable. Those charged with the ethical monitoring of research ought surely to be troubled if they discover over time that the same type of people are always bearing the costs and different types of people are deriving the benefits. An example of this is where research is carried out in the developing world in order to create products that will realistically only be available in richer countries.

Theoretically, a consequentialist could consider any distribution of costs and benefits, subject to the greatest happiness of the greatest number being secured. Certainly, early versions of utilitarianism were criticised in this regard despite the pragmatic constraints that would usually operate. However, it should be possible for consequentialism to tackle the problem of distribution by allowing multiple criteria for evaluating consequences, including distributive ones. A consequentialist could thereby address not only how much benefit would follow a proposed intervention, but also how those benefits are to be distributed – the sort of questions that need to be raised in cases such as these:

- A small number of people are paid a large amount of money to risk significant harm in the interests of a very large number of people enjoying a small increase in their quality of life.

---

[5] Freedman, B. (1987). Equipoise and the ethics of clinical research. *New England Journal of Medicine*, **317**, 141–5.

- A large number of people suffer a minor inconvenience in the interests of a very small number of people benefiting significantly
- One person loses his/her life in the course of a trial that will benefit other sufferers of a rare disease
- No money is given to fund research into rare diseases affecting small numbers of people

In some cases such decisions might be challenged by others as morally unacceptable on grounds of justice and fairness. The fear is that consequentialism leaves little room for judging the impact of research upon the individual participant due to its focus upon the group as a whole. As a maximising theory, it does not pay due regard as to how costs and benefits are distributed.

Consequentialist goals might also impact upon the preference that scientists show for particular methodologies. Clinical research is a form of scientific endeavour, and one could argue that the first step towards ensuring the ethical validity of a piece of research is to ensure the scientific validity of the proposed project. Thus the means must be fitting to the ends. If there are to be any benefits gained (which there must be for the consequentialist), then the scientific approach must be suitable to the task, the methodology must be appropriate, and the investigator should have the ability and resources necessary for the task. Consequentialism therefore requires scientists to make a valid assessment of their ability to attain the potential benefits by the means proposed before proceeding. This can only be of benefit to society, and to those whose time would otherwise be wasted in the course of badly designed or under-resourced research.

However, the consequentialist will also want to know that research will have a beneficial impact (it is not enough to establish a truth; one needs to persuade others of it in order to secure the benefits), and, on occasion, this goal could conflict with the interests of participants. Different scientific questions will demand different approaches, but in this age of evidence-based medicine the fact is that, in terms of impact, the most benefits will probably be derived from the research that produces the most widely accepted form of evidence that something works. In practice, this means that a large randomised controlled trial (be it with or without placebo, blinded or not) will usually be seen as the gold standard, and the benefits to be derived from other forms of research might immediately be assumed inferior. This is, in part, due to the inherent power of the results acquired through such means, but might also be due in part to lingering prejudices against other forms of methodology, notably small-scale qualitative studies. Thus the consequentialist might have to commit wherever possible to a form of experimentation that is

acknowledged to entail specific costs for participants and complex ethical problems. It could therefore be argued that the maximising nature of consequentialism immediately increases the potential for a large number of participants being involved in what has been seen as ethically challenging research.

In some contexts, for example where patient numbers will always be small, where drug companies are not interested in funding large-scale trials, or where the ethical problems posed by this particular approach are considered insurmountable, other research approaches will have to be adopted. It is possible, therefore, that on occasion ethics will dictate that maximum benefits in terms of impact are forfeited because of the costs entailed for individual participants by using the most effective means of pursuing them. There is always the need to balance the value of scientific knowledge and proof against the costs of acquiring it, and it is no coincidence that research has proceeded more slowly in the contexts where potential research participants are viewed as particularly vulnerable.

Clinical experimentation can provide numerous examples where the utility calculation could still work in favour of proceeding, but the moral problems should be apparent. The problem with such cases is that, in the interests of an undeniably significant good, certain individuals are required to bear an unusually high risk of significant harm. In the early stages of research (Phase One and Phase Two trials) they are asked to do so with no hope of direct personal benefit in terms of cure or improved health. The fact that we accept the need for such trials suggests that, in part at least, we adopt a consequentialist approach to our evaluation of clinical trials.

Consequentialism

- Seeks to maximise benefits and minimise harms
- Pays less attention to the way in which harms and benefits are distributed than to how they balance out
- Need not place limits on the level of acceptable harm if it is outweighed by a significant benefit
- Allows that beneficial ends might be pursued by potentially harmful means.

Consequentialism provides us with the means to critique the allocation of funds, researchers' time and participants' time/commitment to medical research on a global level, but offers us little scope to concentrate upon the impact of research upon individual participants once that individual has been counted in as one part of the whole picture. One is left with the sense that one needs to temper the potential excesses that could result from a purely consequentialist approach. It is not enough to know that, at the end of the exercise, the benefits will substantially outweigh the harms, we need to monitor how those costs and benefits are distributed, and where necessary we need to ensure that they are limited. It is therefore prudent to look to another type of ethical theory for guidance.

Deontological approaches

Unlike consequentialism which is forward looking, deontological theories judge the morality of a choice or action by looking back at the intentions or motivations behind it, and the duties or obligations it seeks to fulfil or honour.[6] Whilst one might hope for good consequences to follow, this is irrelevant to the moral judgement of the action. *Logically I can do the right thing with disastrous consequences, or bring about a good outcome by immoral (and therefore unacceptable) means.* The deontologist will not allow the ends to justify the means and must therefore be concerned with the details of how research is conducted and what is done to whom, irrespective of the benefits on offer.

Whereas Bentham has come to epitomise the consequentialist approach, the figurehead of deontology is the eighteenth century German philosopher Immanuel Kant. Whilst one must be careful not to oversimplify Kant's elegant theorising, his most useful idea in this context is that no one should treat another person merely as a means to an end but rather as an end in themselves.[7] Thus we should acknowledge our duties towards others, and seek only to do unto them as we would have done unto us. The individual research participant is thus protected from having his or her own rights or interests overlooked in the interests of pursuing a substantial communal good. Deontological theories and theorists tend to vary much more than those who follow the consequentialist model; thus it is somewhat misleading to make general claims about 'deontology'. However, for the sake of simplicity one can make some claims about how such theories differ from consequentialist approaches.

Consequentialism and good medical science could be seen as having similar goals and being in step when the science in question seeks to alleviate suffering and promote well being. Moral concerns of a deontological type might well work in opposition to scientific goals, and will undoubtedly increase some of the costs of clinical research in the interests of minimising the toll on those involved as participants. Thus there is always the potential for conflict. Deontological theories are restrictive by nature, in contrast to the permissiveness of consequentialism. It is sometimes claimed that Kant was much better at telling people what not to do, as opposed to helping them decide what they ought to do when faced with a number of options. There is a risk of this happening when deontological considerations are brought to bear in the context of clinical research. It is therefore important to remember that it is possible to prescribe as well as prohibit, to require as well as disallow. It is also important to acknowledge that, on occasion, it might be impossible to reconcile the competing rights and duties that can be shown to be relevant in a particular case. The important thing is to explore how both the basic and particular rights people can claim, and the fundamental duties we have towards others, translate within the research setting. As reflected in the later sections of this book, the deontologist can appeal to law and to professional guidance, but ultimately the individual researcher might be left to decide which are the most important moral rights and duties in a particular case.

The deontological approach:
- Concentrates attention upon the individual researcher or participant
- Outlines the duties and rights of the respective parties
- Seeks to prioritise particular moral duties or rights as appropriate to the situation
- Permits or prohibits actions on the basis of their relationship to the relevant moral responsibilities
- Can pronounce some rights and duties absolute and non-negotiable whilst giving others only *prima facie* status.

Researchers as moral agents

Those conducting health-related research often have to combine the roles of scientist and carer, roles which, though related, might entail different types of duty that might at times conflict. The situation might be further complicated by the perception of the research subject as to which role should, or does, take primacy, and the assumptions they make on the basis of this. If someone has been in the long-term care of a physician, he or she might assume that the physician would have the same attitude towards them when acting as a research scientist as when offering care on an ordinary basis. However, scientific demands might, at times, require the scientist/physician to pursue the interests of the project as opposed to that of an individual patient who might, for example, be randomised into a placebo group where their preference was for the new drug. There

[6] Davis, N. (1991). Contemporary deontology. In *A Companion to Ethics*, ed. P. Singer, pp. 205–218. Oxford: Blackwell.

O'Neill, O. (1991). Kantian ethics. In *A Companion to Ethics*, ed. P. Singer, pp. 175–185. Oxford: Blackwell.

[7] Kant, E. (1949). *The Critique of Practical Reason and Other Writings in Moral Philosophy* trans. L.W. Beck. Chicago: University of Chicago Press.

Foundations of the Metaphysics of Morals (1959). trans. L.W. Beck, Indianapolis: Bobbs-Merrill. 1959.

would therefore appear to be a fundamental duty for potential researchers to consider the extent to which they can combine the roles of carer and scientist without compromising either.

The right to be included vs. the right to be protected

Traditionally, a significant moral duty in the context of clinical research has been the duty to protect the vulnerable from inappropriate inclusion in trials. We commonly refer to 'vulnerable groups' and the expectation is that they will be spared the risks and costs involved with being a research participant whatever the benefits on offer.[8] However, we now realise that members of these groups might actually want to participate and that they should have the right to do so. We might also feel that having lost out on the benefits of research in the past, we need to find more sophisticated ways of protecting their interests rather than simply excluding them from the practice. The challenge facing committee members is to decide when the right to be included trumps the very real concern with protecting the individual from the costs of doing so. Furthermore, the committee needs to decide what additional duties might attach to those wishing to engage members of vulnerable groups in their research.[9]

Recruitment

It is easy to see why clinical research needs to rely on the participation of volunteers as opposed to conscripts. It is important to ensure that those who become involved in research understand themselves as having done so voluntarily. Indeed, one could take this further and say that it is important for researchers to prioritise voluntariness, even when a level of false consciousness prevents potential participants from realising the extent to which they are subject to coercive elements.

[8] Jonas, H. (1972). Philosophical reflections on experimenting with human subjects. In *Experiments with Human Subjects*, ed. P. Freund, pp. 1–31. Allen Unwin, **and in** *Daedalus* 1969 98:219–247.

[9] Alderson, P. and Montgomery J. (1996). *Health Care Choices: making decisions with children*, London: Institute for Public Policy Research.

Fulford, K.W.M. and Howse, K. (1993). Ethics of research with psychiatric patients: principles, problems and the primary responsibility of researchers. *Journal of Medical Ethics*, **19**, 85–91.

Nicholson, R.H. (1986). *Medical Research with Children: Ethics Law and Practice*, Oxford: Oxford University Press. Mental Health Act Commission (1997). *Research Involving Detained Patients*. Position Paper 1 Nottingham: Mental Health Act Commission.

The primary moral duties when recruiting to research are:

(i) to ensure that the participation is voluntary and uncoerced

(ii) to recruit a sample appropriate to the research question/hypothesis and scientific methodology

(iii) to ensure that recruits are chosen in a non-discriminatory manner.

The first point relates to the process of recruitment. Whilst few, if any, practitioners could be accused of forcing their patients to become research participants, it is important to recognise the forces that work against voluntariness in this context. The fact of being a patient is often enough to make an individual feel disempowered, dependent and certainly apprehensive. Practical realities, such as long waiting times for appointments or procedures, might make a patient unwilling to rock the boat, once they have been seen. Despite several high profile cases of misconduct in the late 1990s, doctors still command respect in our society, and individual patients might take the fact that an invitation has come from their doctor as an endorsement. This might be particularly true in the context of a long-term caring relationship where the patient might assume that anything the doctor proposes is bound to be in the patient's interest.

In the context of non-therapeutic research, the issue of payment sometimes arises and with it the potential for inducement or manipulation. This subject reappears in its own right below, but suffice to say that, in terms of permitting the appropriate recruitment of volunteers, it is important to ensure that the level of financial reward available is not so high as to lead people to unreasonably discount the risks they might run by participating.

The second requirement – a demand for appropriate sampling – is generated by the pre-existing duty to produce scientifically valid work that has a chance of producing valuable results. Sometimes the inclusion criteria are determined by the subject under study and the methodology employed. So, an interview-based study looking at pregnant women's views on, or experience of, midwifery care would justifiably exclude all men and non-pregnant women. However, the same study might seek to exclude non-English speaking women. The reason given might be the lack of resources for translation. In another case there might be an age limit or an exclusion of women of childbearing age. In all cases the important issue is the reason given and whether or not it should be seen as scientifically and morally relevant. In practice, many exclusions are based on financial or pragmatic considerations and there would be a much better scientific result if a wider group were recruited. In some cases the result of excluding people on the basis of race, class or gender is plainly discriminatory and should be challenged.

The third point relates to the inclusion and exclusion criteria that might be morally acceptable or unacceptable in clinical research. In the past we have largely accepted the idea that one protects vulnerable groups by excluding them from research. However, we now realise that this can lead to those groups becoming even more vulnerable because they are rendered therapeutic orphans due to the lack of research involving people like them. The obvious cases are children, the elderly, and people with cognitive impairment. A right to equal treatment means that the members of vulnerable groups should be able to access treatments that have been appropriately tested, and this must involve the recruitment of members of the group to clinical trials. However, where their extra vulnerability is proven (rather than wrongly assumed), steps must be taken to offer them appropriate protections.

In evaluating a research protocol one needs to address:

(i) the suitability of the inclusion/exclusion criteria given the scientific methodology
(ii) in the absence of valid scientific reasons, the moral reasons for excluding potential participants
(iii) the manner in which recruitment is managed and the context within which it occurs.

Participants not subjects

One of the most significant implications of a deontological approach is that the person involved in research can, and should, be characterised as something other than a mere subject or object of scientific curiosity. One way of underlining this is to use the term, research participant, as opposed to research subject. By adopting the title participant one highlights the importance of avoiding the use of people as means to ends, and instead acknowledges their independent status, their rights, and the duties we have towards them. Furthermore, by incorporating the idea of participation, one suggests the scope for active involvement in research design, conduct and dissemination which many see to be of both scientific and moral value. Admittedly, in some contexts full participation is not possible, and the term might seem inappropriate. In other situations individuals might be happier with the passive role of subject. Even so, the symbolic value of the term is significant, and should be preferred in the majority of cases. One of the potential advantages of engaging people as participants rather than subjects is that they might more easily recognise and embrace some of the duties that they need to acknowledge

in order to secure a valid and ethical outcome from the research.

Whilst the deontologists will not wish to unquestioningly sacrifice the interests of research participants to a greater good such as significant scientific advance, they must reconcile the duties of researchers and the rights of participants in such a way as to ensure maximum protection and scientific viability. A participant will be given significant rights, which enable them to withdraw from any trial should they wish to do so, but whilst participating they will be bound by certain duties which are seen as necessary for the scientific validity of the trial and the ethical protection of participants. So, whilst consent remains valid, the participant is bound to a duty of concordance with the requirements of the protocol being followed; this might in turn entail a duty of openness and veracity in the reporting of experiences relevant to the trial.

Consent

One of the most fundamental ways in which we demonstrate our respect for others is by gaining their consent to actions that will impact upon them. In medical treatment generally and in clinical research specifically there is a moral and legal duty upon health-care professionals to acquire the consent of participants. Raanon Gillon tells us that consent in a health-care setting entails:

...a voluntary un-coerced decision made by a sufficiently autonomous person on the basis of adequate information to accept or reject some proposed course of action that will affect him or her.[10]

It is important to stress that consent is a process, not a single event, and that the ethical standards which must be met to ensure the validity of the consent might be far more stringent than the legal ones. A signature on a consent form means very little in the absence of a full account of how it was acquired. This subject could fill a book in its own right,[11] but it is possible to sketch in the major issues that arise in relation to acquiring a research participant's consent.

• Concerns about voluntariness and coercion re-emerge, as outlined above in relation to recruitment. It is important not to approach those whose autonomy is known to be too compromised to allow them to consent, but it is

[10] Gillon, R. (1986). *Philosophical Medical Ethics*, p. 113. Chichester: John Wiley.

[11] Doyal, L. and Tobias, J.S. (eds.) (2001). *Informed Consent in Medical Research*, London: BMJ Books.

also important to support those who might be vulnerable to coercion despite their competence and autonomy in other contexts.

- Information giving is key to the successful consent process, just as it is crucial to a valid consequentialist evaluation of pros and cons. Information must be sufficiently detailed to allow for an informed choice between the various options; it must be appropriately aligned to what the patient already knows about their condition and their prognosis.[12] It must be provided in clear and non-patronising language, and, where necessary, in the language of the non-English speaking participant. The way in which information is given should be appropriate to the context and to the individuals involved, wherever possible combining verbal and written information and, if necessary, as in the case of children or cognitively impaired adults, visual aids. As experienced committee members will know, there is an art to producing a good patient information sheet, and sometimes practitioners find themselves on a steep learning curve.

- Ideally, a participant should be given time to deliberate upon the information they have been given before deciding whether or not to consent. This should usually be possible through the appropriate timing of information giving and through the careful staging of the consent process. However, in some contexts an immediate decision is required,[13] and we are well aware that these are the contexts in which issues of consent can become very problematic. Where there is no time for measured deliberation, it is particularly important that information is given as clearly and as fully as possible and that those giving consent (sometimes on behalf of children or incompetent adults) are encouraged to ask as many questions as they want.

- Consent should be seen as an on-going requirement rather than as a one-off event at the start of a project. This raises questions about how informed a participant should be kept, given that information collected in the course of the trial might, if known, affect their willingness to continue. Good scientific practice might require that a participant continues in a trial until definitive results can be produced, even if early results suggest that a trial drug shows promising results. This would be the case if the drug was being compared to an acceptable, though possibly slightly inferior, alternative, and in such a case it might be acceptable to keep participants in the dark until the trial is complete. However, where information relating to significant harms becomes available, there would be a moral duty to ensure that consent was re-negotiated in the knowledge of this. In some extreme cases a practitioner could decide to withdraw patients from a trial, despite their willingness to continue, if she thought that the risks had become too high. Thus there might be a duty to revisit consent in the face of reported adverse events, but if there is a suggestion in the data that a trial drug is significantly better than a standard treatment, this information could be withheld until the data is sufficiently robust. (The situation would probably look different if one was looking at a new treatment for a life-threatening disease for which there was no effective treatment at present.)

- All LREC and MREC committee members will be familiar with the need to reassure participants of their right to withdraw at any time without needing to provide reasons for doing so, and in the knowledge that their care will not suffer as a result. This is an important right which must be underlined given the worries about coercion and non-voluntariness outlined above. Without the right to refuse or withdraw, the right to consent is meaningless, a difficult issue in English law as it relates to consent of minors.

Confidentiality and anonymity

Medical data is highly sensitive, and health-care professionals have always acknowledged an explicit duty of confidentiality to their patients. More so than ever with the growth of genetics, we have an interest in keeping tight control over information about our bodies. Other changes are also having an impact, with the growth of multi-agency involvement in patient care; research problems can arise in the context of multi-disciplinary research if the professional groups involved do not share the same attitude and commitment to preserving the confidentiality of patients. The growing importance of qualitative research heightens the need to address the ethical issues relating to the collection, storage and analysis of potentially sensitive data. Particularly where samples, data or records are going to be stored over a long period of time, or where there is the potential for their being used for multiple purposes, the initial assurance of confidentiality and anonymity must be honoured.[14]

[12] Tobias, J.S. and Souhami, R.L. (1993). Fully informed consent may be needlessly cruel. BMJ **307**, *British Medical Journal*, 199–201.

[13] Biros, M.H., Lewis, R.J., Olson, C.M., Runge, J.W., Cummins, R.O. and Fost, N. (1995). Informed consent in emergency research: consensus statement from the coalition conference on acute resuscitation and critical care researchers. *Journal of the American Medical Association*, **272**, 1283–7.

[14] Gostin, L. (1991). Ethical principles for the conduct of human subject research: population based research and ethics, *Law Medicine and Health Care*, **19**, 191–202.

This is an area in which duties of research participants might also need to be made explicit. For example, in the context of qualitative research involving group discussions, participants need to understand that they also have a duty of confidentiality towards their fellow participants. Or, where participants have been brought together in a common location for treatment or testing, they should understand that any other people attending have the right for this to remain confidential.

Dissemination

At the beginning of this piece, it was argued that the scientific integrity of a piece of research is a necessary component of its ethical value. This issue extends beyond the design and the management of the research to its completion and dissemination. It is increasingly stressed that there is strong duty to publish and publicise research findings. One can see that there would be consequentialist support for this idea where the results would clearly benefit society, but the consequentialist could theoretically decide that publication of some research finding would not be in the public interest. Publication of results needs to be handled delicately in order to preserve anonymity and confidentiality but also to minimise the harms associated with publication.

Recompense or compensation

As mentioned above, deontologists care about moral motivation and distinguish between good and bad motives. A consequentialist, on the other hand, believes that securing the appropriate outcome is the priority, and that we should motivate people to contribute towards good ends. This difference comes to the fore when discussing the possibility of offering financial reward to those who participate in research. The deontologist might face difficulties with this issue, wishing on the one hand to protect participants from exploitation, but also preferring that they participate for the 'right sort of reasons' for example, altruism as opposed to financial need. This preference is not simply born of a desire to promote the moral welfare of the participant, but might also be linked to worries about inducement and indirect coercion. Thus consent which is given when the only rewards are the rewards of being a good person might be seen as more robust than consent which is given on the promise of financial or other benefit. Having said this, the financial reality might be that the person conducting the research is being handsomely rewarded, and it could

be seen as unfair not to pass some of the benefit on to the participants.

Conclusion: tempered consequentialism

Anyone who has studied moral philosophy will know how difficult it is to give a fair account of differing approaches to moral reasoning without devoting far more space than is available here. They will also know that there are other ways of thinking about moral questions that have not even been given a mention. It is rare these days for people not to be aware of the work of the American theorists, Beauchamp and Childress, who propose a form of moral principalism which has gained widespread support amongst health care professionals.[15] Similarly, much has been done in recent years to revive the tradition of virtue ethics which traces its roots back to the work of Aristotle.[16] Feminist ethics now has a rich and varied literature, which has contributed usefully to many debates. All these approaches have something to offer, but the priority here has been to present an introductory guide to two ways of thinking which intuitively appeal at some level to most people. A further aim has been to show some of the incompatibilities between these approaches, in the interests of de-personalising some of the disputes that might emerge during committee deliberations.

With this in mind, we invite you to use the many forms of guidance available in this manual to help decide whether a piece of work offers significant enough benefits to appropriate parties to justify the predicted costs involved. Having decided this, one then has to decide whether the participants upon whom the success of the venture depends can be safely and appropriately recruited and adequately protected during their participation. If that is possible, then practical mechanisms need to be put into place to secure these ends, and the research needs to be monitored to ensure that the safeguards remain in place. Thus a combination of approaches is required, borrowing the larger perspective from the consequentialist, and the specific detail from the deontologist. The goal of an ethics committee is to facilitate ethically sound practice, and to encourage researchers to honour their moral responsibilities towards participants. This is not an easy task, but society should be grateful to those who accept the responsibility and who give time and effort to ensuring that health-care practice is

[15] Beauchamp, T. and Childress, J. (2001). *Principles of Biomedical Ethics.* 5th edn. Oxford: Oxford University Press.
[16] Crisp, R. and Slote, M. (1997). *Virtue Ethics.* Oxford: Oxford Readings in Philosophy.

informed by evidence based on scientifically and ethically acceptable research.

SUGGESTED READING

BMA (1993). *Medical Ethics Today: its Practice and Philosophy*. London: BMJ Publishing Group.

Davis, N. (1991). Contemporary deontology. In *Companion to Ethics*, ed. P. Singer, pp. 205–218. Oxford: Blackwell.

Doyal, L. and Tobias, J.S. (eds.) (2001). *Informed Consent in Medical Research*. London: BMJ Books.

Foot, P. (1978). *Virtues and Vices and Other Essays in Moral Philosophy*. Oxford: Blackwell.

Freeman, B. (1987). Equipoise and the ethics of clinical research. *N Eng J Med*, **317**, 141–145.

Glover, J. (ed) (1990). *Utilitarianism and Its Critics*. Macmillan.

Jonas, H. (1972). Philosophical reflections on experimenting with human subjects. In *Experiments with Human Subjects*, ed. P. Freund, pp. 1–31. Allen Unwin. **and in** *Daedalus* 1969 98:219–247.

O'Neill, O. (1991). Kantian ethics. In *Companion to Ethics*, ed. P. Singer, pp. 175–185. Oxford: Blackwell.

Oakley, A. (1990). Who's afraid of the randomized controlled trial? In *Women's Health Counts*, ed. H. Roberts, pp. 167–194. Routledge.

Scheffler, S. (ed). (1988). *Consequentialism and its Critics*. Oxford: Oxford Readings in Philosophy.

Smart, J.J.C. and Williams, B. (1973). *Utilitarianism: For and Against*. Cambridge: Cambridge University Press.

Smith, T. (1999). *Ethics in Medical Research: A Handbook of Good Practice*. Cambridge University Press.

USEFUL WEBSITES

Alder Hey (Royal Liverpool Children's Inquiry)
http://www.rlcinquiry.org.uk/download/index.htm

The American Journal of Bioethics
http://ajobonline.com/

The Bristol Royal Infirmary Inquiry
http://www.bristol-inquiry. org.uk/

British Medical Association
http://www.bma.org.uk/

Bulletin of Medical Ethics
http://www.bullmedeth.info/

Centre of Medical Law and Ethics
http://www.kcl.ac.uk/depsta/law/research/cmle/

Committee on Publication Ethics
http://www.publicationethics.org.uk

Ethical issues in research – bibliography
http://www.nlm.nih.gov/pubs/cbm/hum_exp.html

The Hastings Center
http://www.thehastingscenter.org/

Informed Consent in Medical Research
http://www.informedconsent.bmjbooks.com/

Journal of Medical Ethics
http://jme.bmjjournals.com/

Kant and Kantian ethics
http://ethics.acusd.edu/kant.html

Kennedy Institute of Ethics Journal
http://muse.jhu.edu/journals/
kennedy_institute_of_ethics_journal/

Medical Research Council
http://www.mrc.ac.uk/index/public_interest/
ethics_and_best_practice.htm

Royal College of Physicians of London
http://www.rcplondon.ac.uk

Stanford Encyclopaedia of Philosophy
http://plato.stanford.edu/contents.html

Utilitarian ethics
http://ethics.acusd.edu/utilitarianism.html

Research ethics committees and the law

Ian Kennedy[1] and Phil Bates[2]

[1]School of Public Policy, University College London, UK
[2]Centre of Medical Law and Ethics, School of Law, King's College London, UK

The legal framework for the regulation of medical research on human beings has not been set out in legislation. As a result, many developments have taken place through the publication of official circulars and guidance. For example, the current framework for the functions and operation of Research Ethics Committees is described in the Department of Health document *Governance Arrangements for NHS Research Ethics Committees* (July 2001). This document replaces the Department of Health circular HSG(91)5 which required District Health Authorities to set up local Research Ethics Committees (LRECs) in 1991, and circular HSG(97)23 which dealt with the establishment of Multi-centre Research Ethics Committees (MRECs) in 1997. (These documents apply to England and Wales, but there are equivalent documents for Scotland.) These official publications do not have the same legal force as legislation. Therefore, Research Ethics Committees do not have the legal status of a statutory body, with clearly defined legal powers and duties. Thus, any authority that an Ethics Committee wields is informal and extralegal. Such authority should not, however, be underestimated. Within the National Health Service, the *Governance Arrangements for NHS Research Ethics Committees* places a clear responsibility upon Health Authorities to set up, support and monitor NHS Local Research Ethics Committees, and the Department of Health's document, *The Research Governance Framework for Health and Social Care* (2001), states: 'The Department of Health requires that all research involving patients, service users, care professionals or volunteers, or their organs, tissue or data, is reviewed independently to ensure it meets ethical standards.'

The original version of this article was written by Ian Kennedy in 1994. The article was revised and updated by Phil Bates of The School of Law, King's College London in 2001, who takes responsibility for its current accuracy.

(para 2.2.2) Therefore, although there is no clear legal obligation on a potential researcher to submit a protocol to an Ethics Committee for approval, researchers within the NHS will be denied access to patients and data without such approval. Furthermore, those who fund research ordinarily stipulate that research must be approved by a Research Ethics Committee if it is to be funded. In relation to the publication of research, it is standard practice, at least in English journals, for editors not to publish research results if proper approval was not sought or given.

European Law has also had an impact upon the legal framework for medical research. On November 29, 1993, there came into force the Medicines (Applications for Grant of Product Licences – Products for Human Use) Regulations 1993 (SI 1993 No. 2583). This gives effect to the 1991 Directive 91/507/EEC of the European Union, which requires 'all phases of clinical investigation' to be in accordance with 'good clinical practice'. It has sometimes been argued that this reference to 'good clinical practice' is a reference to the European Community's *Guidelines on Good Clinical Practice for Trials on Medicinal Products in the European Community*, issued in 1991, and that these guidelines have legal force as a result. However, these guidelines have been replaced by the *ICH Good Clinical Practice Guidelines*, which have not been incorporated into English law, and the better view may be that the 1991 guidelines did not have legal force in any case. Further developments in the European Law relating to clinical trials are likely as a result of the implementation of the Clinical Trials Directive 2001/20/EC. This directive was agreed in 2001, and implementation is due to take place during 2003/4.

Finally, as a matter of Human Rights Law, a Research Ethics Committee is likely to be recognised as a 'public authority', which is defined by the Human Rights Act 1998 to include 'any person certain of whose functions are functions of a public nature'. Under the Human Rights Act, it is unlawful for a public authority to act in a way that is incompatible with the 'Convention rights'. These are the rights in the European Convention on Human Rights that are incorporated into English law by the Human Rights Act. Therefore, Research Ethics Committees may need to consider Article 3 of the European Convention, which states that: 'No one shall be subjected to torture or to inhuman or degrading treatment or punishment.' In *X v Denmark*, Application No 9974/82, the European Commission of Human Rights stated that 'medical treatment of an experimental character and without the consent of the person involved may under certain circumstances be regarded as prohibited by Article 3.' Another important Convention right, is the right to respect for private and family life, under Article 8 of the European Convention. Although the right to privacy and family life is not absolute, interference with this right should be 'proportionate' to achieve a legitimate purpose, as defined in Article 8.2.

The role of the Research Ethics Committee is to advise. It does not itself authorise research. This is the responsibility of the NHS or other body under whose auspices the research will take place. That said, once a Research Ethics Committee constitutes itself and reviews research proposals, it takes on legal duties. These duties derive from the central purposes of the Committee: to protect the dignity, rights, safety and well-being of all actual or potential research participants, while ensuring that valid and worthwhile research is carried out. According to *Governance Arrangements for NHS Research Ethics Committees:* 'RECs are responsible for acting primarily in the interest of potential research participants and concerned communities, but they should also take into account the interests, needs and safety of researchers who are trying to undertake research of good quality. However, the goals of research and researchers, while important, should always be secondary to the dignity, rights, safety, and well-being of the research participants.' (para 2.3)

Research Ethics Committees are not courts or legal advisors. Therefore, it is not the function of Research Ethics Committees to provide legal advice, or to provide authoritative resolution of legal issues, even if the committee has members with legal expertise. The Department of Health's *Research Governance Framework* states: 'It is not the role or responsibility of the research ethics committees described above to give legal advice, nor are they liable for any of their decisions in this respect. Irrespective of the decision of a research ethics committee on a particular application, it is the researcher and the NHS or social care organisation who have the responsibility not to break the law. If a research ethics committee is of the opinion that implementation of a research proposal might contravene the law, it should

advise both researcher and the appropriate authority of its concerns. The researcher and the organisation will need then to seek legal advice.' (para 3.12.7)

The *Research Governance Framework* states that 'research ethics committees and their members must act in good faith and provide impartial and independent advice within their remits and terms of reference.' (para 3.12.2). In order to provide such advice, the single most important legal duty imposed on the members of the Committee is to address those issues that are relevant to any decision about a research proposal before deciding whether or not to approve it. To comply with this duty, Committee members must satisfy themselves on a number of matters, and in particular, those listed in paragraphs 9.13–9.18 of the *Governance Arrangements for NHS Research Ethics Committees*, which relate to:

- scientific design and conduct of the study
- recruitment of research participants
- care and protection of research participants
- protection of research participants' confidentiality
- informed consent process
- community considerations.

The duties described above are imposed on Committee members as individuals, since the Committee has no separate legal identity. It follows from what has already been said that Committee members have onerous responsibilities, and it is necessary to consider the circumstances in which members may incur legal liability for breach of their duties. It could be said that, since the role of the Committee is solely advisory, no question of liability arises, as the final decision to authorise a research project is made elsewhere. Since, however, the Committee exists to provide expert advice and can assume its advice will be relied upon, it is doubtful that this argument would prevail. On this basis, it is likely that Committee members have a duty of care towards those who might be harmed by their involvement in research. However, a successful claim would need to show that there had been a breach of this duty, because the Committee member has not acted reasonably. It is a matter for debate what the law would require of a reasonable Committee member. However, a failure on the part of a Committee member to satisfy him or herself on any of the issues referred to above might render him or her liable to a legal claim in negligence by a research participant if the research participant suffers harm as a consequence. (Obviously, the Committee member will not be in breach of his or her duty if a participant is harmed through the carelessness of the researcher.) Note, however, that the law does not require the Committee member to get things right. Rather, as has been said, the obligation is to behave reasonably. Clearly, the expertise of the member may limit what he or she can do, but the law is likely to require that any reasonable member finding a matter on which he or she is unsure, should seek advice, (subject to the constraints of confidentiality), and may not simply remain in a state of ignorance. Further attempts to particularise what is reasonable may not be helpful, since much will depend on the facts of any particular case, and the resources and backgrounds of the particular Committee (subject, of course, to the proviso that a certain basic minimum of resources must be available). For example, the obligation to satisfy themselves that proper arrangements exist for compensation in the event of injury may appear onerous to many members who would argue that they are not specialists in insurance and finance. The response may be that their duty is to make reasonable enquiry, to ascertain, in other words, that the investigator is aware of the need to arrange indemnity and that he or she is making provision for it. To expect more of members may be unreasonable.

Finally, even if a Committee member can be shown to have acted unreasonably, it will be necessary to show that this breach of duty has caused harm to the research subject. It will also be possible to argue that the allocation of damages should reflect the relative responsibilities of others, such as those carrying out the research itself. As has been said, if a Committee member were found liable, this liability would be personal. Thus, each Committee member must, if he or she is to serve on a Committee, make all reasonable efforts to comply with these various duties. If unable to do so, despite reasonable efforts, the wise course would be to resign so as to avoid incurring liability. In addition, members would be well advised to ensure that they are indemnified against the possibility of legal proceedings. The *Governance Arrangements for NHS Research Ethics Committees* acknowledges the possibility of legal actions against members of RECs, when it states: 'The appointing Authority will take full responsibility for all the actions of a member in the course of their performance of his or her duties as a member of the REC other than those involving bad faith, wilful default or gross negligence. A member should, however, notify the appointing Authority if any action or claim is threatened or made, and in such an event be ready to assist the Authority as required.' (para 4.14)

As well as the possibility of legal actions for negligence against Committee members, there is a further cluster of duties imposed on Research Ethics Committees, which might be the subject of applications to the courts for judicial review, seeking to have the decision of the Committee declared invalid. (In another context, a judicial review action was brought against an Ethical Committee decision in *R v Ethical Committee of St Mary's Hospital (Manchester) ex parte H* [1988] 1 FLR 512.) Judicial review actions are likely to focus upon whether the decision of the Committee is within its terms of reference, has been made fairly, and in accordance with Human Rights law, or whether the decision is so unreasonable that no reasonable Committee would have made such a decision. It is conceivable that actions of this sort might be brought by a researcher who has been denied approval. Finally, there are a range of administrative obligations placed upon Committees, particularly those listed in the *Governance Arrangements for NHS Research Ethics Committees,* which relate to the composition of the Committee, its working procedures, and documentation of its decisions.

REFERENCES

Department of Health circular HSG(91)5.

Department of Health circular HSG(97)23.

European Clinical Trials Directive 2001/20/EC.

European Community's *Guidelines on Good Clinical Practice for Trials on Medicinal Products in the European Community* (1991).

European Directive 91/507/EEC.

Governance Arrangements for NHS Research Ethics Committees (July 2001).

Human Rights Act 1998.

ICH Good Clinical Practice Guidelines.

Medicines (Applications for Grant of Product Licences – Products for Human Use) Regulations 1993 (SI 1993 No. 2583).

R v Ethical Committee of St Mary's Hospital (Manchester) ex parte H [1988] 1 FLR 512.

The Research Governance Framework for Health and Social Care (2001).

X v Denmark, European Commission of Human Rights, Application No 9974/82.

3

The regulation of medical research: a historical overview

Richard H. Nicholson

Bulletin of Medical Ethics

Attempts to regulate the conduct of medical research have a surprisingly long history. The first regulations were made just over 100 years ago. Since 1970, however, there has been exponential growth in writing regulations, laws, codes of practice and guidelines. Such activity would suggest that they are an effective way of ensuring high standards of ethical conduct in research involving human participants, but there is little evidence to show this to be true.

Many regulations, including the earliest, have been written in response to various scandals in medical research. Public outcry at the abuse of human rights in medical experiments in the Nazi concentration camps, or in the Tuskegee syphilis study, for instance, led to the writing of the Nuremberg Code and the US National Research Act. Yet a review of the development of research ethics in the twentieth century suggests that such scandals may have made little difference. What seems to be making some difference is the commercial pressure exerted by the pharmaceutical industry to ensure that Good Clinical Practice standards are applied wherever pharmaceutical research is undertaken, to satisfy regulatory agencies. This has been mediated through various transnational guidelines, which individual countries have subsumed as laws or regulations.

Early German scandals

Another perception needing to be challenged is that informed consent was somehow an American invention, after the Second World War, or perhaps even more recently. In fact, a legal requirement for the informed consent of the subject of human experimentation was first made in a ministerial directive issued in Berlin in 1900. The need for such a directive arose from the work of Professor Neisser – remembered now by the organisms that cause gonorrhoea and

meningitis – neisseria gonorrhoea and neisseria meningitidis. In 1898, at the University of Breslau, he tried to develop an anti-syphilis serum. He injected cell-free serum from syphilitic patients into other patients – mostly prostitutes – without their full knowledge or consent: some developed syphilis as a result. In 1900 the Royal Disciplinary Court (of Prussia) fined him and levied costs, together representing two-thirds of his annual income.

The Prussian parliament discussed the case, and the Minister for Religious, Educational and Medical Affairs issued a regulation in 1900, of which the following is the first clause:

Directive to all medical directors of university hospitals, polyclinics, and other hospitals
I I advise the medical directors of university hospitals, polyclinics, and all other hospitals that all medical interventions for other than diagnostic, healing, and immunisation purposes, regardless of other legal or moral authorisation, are excluded under all circumstances, if
(1) the human subject is a minor or not competent due to other reasons;
(2) the human subject has not given his unambiguous consent;
(3) the consent is not preceded by a proper explanation of the possible negative consequences of the intervention...

Berlin, 29 December 1900.[1]

The rest of the directive required that any such intervention be approved in advance by the director of the institution and be properly recorded.

Not only was that first regulation of research on human subjects more restrictive than most rules today, but it specifically required consent to be obtained after relevant information had been given. What is not clear is how much effect it had in practice. By the late 1920s there was frequent criticism in the German press of unethical research undertaken by the medical profession, in collaboration with a creative chemical industry that was soon to produce the first sulphonamides. As a result, there was further debate in the German parliament, and in February 1931 the German Minister of the Interior issued 'guidelines for innovative therapy and scientific experiments on man'. Although only guidelines, they were given some force by the introductory statement[2] that the Reich Health Council 'has agreed that all physicians in open or closed health care institutions should sign a commitment to these guidelines when entering their employment'.

Grodin rightly calls these guidelines 'visionary in their depth and scope'.[3] They start by acknowledging the need both for 'innovative therapy' and 'human experimentation' – which today we usually call 'therapeutic' and 'nontherapeutic' research – and at the same time remind the physician of his '... major responsibility for the life and health of any person ... ' on whom he performs research. They stress the importance of keeping to the principles of medical ethics, of prior assessment of risks and benefits, of obtaining consent, of giving extra protection to subjects under 18 years of age, of not exploiting social hardship, of having a senior physician in charge of all research, of training physicians about their special duties when acting as researcher, and of writing up thorough reports of the research. However, although these guidelines may have been visionary, and even though they remained valid until 1945[4], they were no match for the Nazi ideology that permitted and encouraged horrendously inhumane 'experiments' in the concentration camps, without any semblance of volunteering or of consent.

The other great totalitarian state of the 1930s also developed legal regulation of medical research. In Russia dissemination of news and views was too tightly controlled for any public outcry about unethical medical research to have been possible. But a number of cases of 'medical experimentation' by doctors produced adverse effects in patients and caused disquiet. The work of 'legal and investigatory institutions was complicated by the absence of official rules regulating the conditions of medical experimentation'.[5] So the Scientific Medical Council of the People's Commissariat of Health Care set up a commission to develop rules, which were published as a decree in 1936.[6] Like the German directive of 1931, many of the decree's concepts are similar to those later found in the Declaration of Helsinki: there must, for instance, be prior animal experiments, there must be

informed consent, and the results of the research must be reported.

None of these three regulations was well known outside Germany and Russia, whereas the responses to the Nazi concentration camp experiments became very well known. The first response was the 'Doctors' Trial', starting in Nuremberg in 1946, in which 23 physicians were put on trial for crimes against humanity. Part of the judgement[7] delivered by the entirely American tribunal in 1947 became known as the Nuremberg Code: it sets out ten fundamental principles for the ethical conduct of medical research, and starts with the blunt statement that 'The voluntary consent of the human subject is absolutely essential'.

The second response was the setting up of the World Medical Association. By having a global organisation of physicians it was hoped that ethical standards of behaviour could be agreed, in which doctors around the world could be supported by a sense of global solidarity. At an early stage it became clear that the WMA would have to set down ethical principles for medical research, not least because the Nuremberg Code was almost totally ignored. Physicians and researchers outside Germany regarded it as something that applied just to nasty Nazis: as Jay Katz put it 'It was a good code for barbarians but an unnecessary code for ordinary physician–scientists'.[8] The WMA agreed some brief principles in 1954, and worked on them for a decade before the first Declaration of Helsinki was agreed at its meeting in Helsinki in 1964.[9]

The need for clear guidance was becoming apparent. In 1966, Henry Beecher in the US,[10] and a year later Maurice Pappworth in the UK,[11] created immense public and professional debate with their publications demonstrating how much flagrantly unethical research was going on in each country. One of the unethical studies cited by Beecher was the injecting of cancer cells into elderly, debilitated patients at the Jewish Chronic Disease Hospital in New York in 1963. Since it had been funded by the US National Institutes of Health, an enquiry was held which resulted in an order to all institutions receiving funding from them to set up ethics review committees. This led to the earliest European research ethics committees being established. Pappworth's book, scandalous though its contents may have been, was either ignored or vilified in the UK. Both publications demonstrated that, even if there were awareness of the existence of the Nuremberg Code among researchers, it had no influence on ethical standards in research in the US or UK.

It was another major scandal that led to the first modern law regulating medical research to be passed, in the United States. The scandal was the revelation of the Tuskegee syphilis study. It started in 1932, to study the natural history of syphilis in about 400 black men, mostly poor and uneducated, in Alabama. They were not told of the study, but were told they had 'bad blood' and were followed up regularly, along with about 200 controls. Their co-operation was relatively easily obtained, with promises of free transport and free hot lunches on study days, and of free medical care and burial, after autopsy. The researchers went to considerable lengths to try to ensure that they did not receive specific treatment: by the time the study was halted in 1972, however, as many as one-third of the men may have had curative treatment for their syphilis.

The study was run by the US Public Health Service. A PHS physician, on hearing of the study in the 1960s had tried hard to have it stopped, but an *ad hoc* committee decided in 1969 to continue it. It was only when *The New York Times* broke the story in July, 1972[12] that the study was halted. Another, external, committee concluded that the research had been unethical from the beginning, and recommended setting up a national board to regulate federally funded research with human participants.[13]

There was a dual response to this scandal. The US Congress passed the National Research Act in 1974, which established the National Commission for the Protection of Human Subjects of Biomedical and Behavioral Research. Over the next few years it issued valuable reports on several aspects of research ethics, including the document that came to be known as the *Belmont Report*.[14] Also in 1974, a new chapter was added to the Code of Federal Regulations (CFR), requiring that federally funded research should have prior review by an Institutional Review Board (IRB), and laying down minimum standards for obtaining informed consent for research interventions. The work of the National Commission was reflected in a series of amendments to the CFR, which reached something close to its present state in 1981.

How effective the American regulations have been is a matter for conjecture. Many IRB members confess that their time is spent on assessing whether research proposals meet the regulatory requirements, rather than on discussing whether they are ethical. In recent years there have been several high-profile, but temporary, shutdowns of some of the largest medical research programmes in the US,[15] because of their failure to follow the regulations. The US is now moving beyond regulations to certification of IRB administrators, accreditation of programmes of protection for human research participants, and mandatory training in research ethics for researchers.

In the UK, the making of regulations on the conduct of medical research has also depended on having a scandal but, although several examples of unethical research in recent years could be cited, it was not until the late 1990s that the necessary scandal arose. Parental complaints, that their premature infants in North Staffordshire had been put into a study of an alternative sort of ventilator without their knowledge or consent, led to the setting up of the Griffiths' inquiry.[16] While the full story may yet take some time to emerge, the inquiry's recommendations have developed into the framework for research governance, and the governance arrangements for research ethics committees. Their effectiveness, or lack of it, will take a while to demonstrate, but there is one hopeful sign. Unlike the other regulations discussed, the authorities have promised that the money necessary to make the new UK scheme work will be provided.

The financial element may be crucial, because the regulations that seem to have been most effective are the Good Clinical Practice (GCP) arrangements for research sponsored by the pharmaceutical industry. In July 1990, GCP guidelines prepared by the Committee for Proprietary Medicinal Products of the European Commission were finally approved.[17] Although the guidelines lacked legal force, European drug regulatory authorities expected the pharmaceutical industry to keep to them if the results of their clinical trials were to be considered by the regulators for drug licensing. They were extended in May 1996 by the International Conference on Harmonisation of Technical Requirements for Registration of Pharmaceuticals for Human Use Harmonised Tripartite Guideline for Good Clinical Practice[18] – otherwise known as ICHGCP. Tripartite in the title reflects the agreement to this guideline of the regulatory authorities in Europe, Japan and the United States, which require clinical trials for licensing purposes to conform to it. The ICH guidelines specify a minimum data set to be included on patient information sheets, which has helped to improve the level of information given to potential participants, and also require auditing of research data, which has led to most of the discoveries of data fabrication that have occurred in the UK. Under the terms of the EU clinical trials directive, most features of the guidelines will be subsumed into British law by mid-2003.

Just as successive British governments over the last 50 years have felt the need to pass ever-increasing numbers of laws, so an ever-increasing number of health-care organisations have written more and more guidelines on the conduct of research. The answers to ensuring that medical research involving human participants is conducted ethically may, however, lie elsewhere: in ensuring that researchers understand their ethical obligations when undertaking research, and in ensuring that ethics review committees are adequately supported to provide the necessary oversight.

REFERENCES

1 Vollmann, J. & Winau, R. (1996). The Prussian regulation of 1900: early ethical standards for human experimentation in Germany. *IRB: A Review of Human Subjects Research*, **18(4)**, 9–11.

2 *Reichsgesundheitsblatt*, 11 March 1931; 10:174–5. In English translation in *International Digest of Health Legislation* 1980; 31; 408–11.

3 Annas, G.J. & Grodin, M.A. (eds.) (1992). *The Nazi Doctors and the Nuremberg Code*, p. 131. Oxford: Oxford University Press.

4 Fischer F.W. & Breuer, H. (1979). Influences of ethical guidance committees on medical research – a critical reappraisal. In: Howard-Jones N, Bankowski Z. (eds.). *Medical Experimentation and the Protection of Human Rights*. Geneva: CIOMS.

5 Bychkov, I.Y. (1939). On the question of legal regulation of medical experiments on human subjects. *Soviet Med J*, **1**, 61–68.

6 On the conduct of study of new medicines and medical methods associated with risk for the life and health of patients. Resolution of the Bureau of the Scientific Medical Council of April 23, 1936. In *Book of Resolutions – People's Commissariat of Health Care of the RSFSR*. Moscow, Scientific Medical Council. No 1–4, pp. 37–38.

7 *Trials of war criminals before the Nuremberg Military Tribunals under Control Council Law 10*. Washington DC: US Govt. Printing Office, 1950; Military Tribunal Case 1, *US v. Karl Brandt et al.*, at pp. 171–184.

8 Katz, J. (1992). The consent principle of the Nuremberg Code: Its significance then and now. In: Annas, G.J. & Grodin, M.A. (eds.). *The Nazi Doctors and the Nuremberg Code*, p. 228 Oxford: Oxford University Press.

9 World Medical Association (1999). *Declaration of Helsinki*. 1964, 1975, 1996 versions reprinted in *Bull Med Eth*, No. 150, 13–17.

10 Beecher, H.K. (1966). Ethics and clinical research. *N Engl J Med*, **274**, 1354–1360.

11 Pappworth, M.H. (1967). *Human Guinea Pigs*. London: Routledge & Kegan Paul.

12 Heller, J. (1972). Syphilis victims in US study went untreated for 40 years *NY Times*, 26 July at pp. A1, A8.

13 *Final Report of the Tuskegee Syphilis Study Ad Hoc Advisory Panel* (1973). Washington, DC: US Government Printing Office.

14 National Commission for the Protection of Human Subjects of Biomedical and Behavioral Research. *The Belmont Report: Ethical Principles and Guidelines for the Protection of Human Subjects of Research*. Washington, DC, Dept. of Health, Education and Welfare, 1979.

15 See, for instance, *Bull Med Eth* 1999; No. 153, 3–6, and *Bull Med Eth* 2001; No. 171, 3–7.

16 *Report of the review into the research framework in North Staffordshire* (2000). Birmingham: NHS Executive West Midlands.

17 Committee for Proprietary Medicinal Products (1990). *Good Clinical Practice for Trials on Medicinal Products in the European Community*. Brussels: European Commission.

18 *ICH Guideline for Good Clinical Practice* (1996). Paris: International Federation of Pharmaceutical Manufacturers Associations.

The research process

The regulation of medical research in the UK

Pamela Charnley Nickols

Charnley Nickols Associates Ltd

Regulatory responsibilities

Clinical research is controlled in the UK, in Europe and in most of the world by three different and parallel systems:

1. Legislation: a matter of what the law requires in terms of actions and responsibilities. The first European Directive intended to address the subject of Good Clinical Practice was 91/507/EEC[1]. The European Commission has recently reported that a second directive, the Directive on GCP in Clinical Trials, has been adopted. It was signed off by the European Parliament and Council on 4 April 2001[2].

2. Regulatory or competent authority overview: the issue of licences to conduct research, manufacture products and market medicines for human use. This also involves the supervision of compliance with legal standards and accepted guidelines and the provision of expert ongoing safety review.

3. Ethics committee activities: providing pre-study opinion, ongoing review, safety review, termination reports and acting as an independent referee on behalf of the subject and society.

Legislation: history

The process of regulation in most areas began with international codes of practice such as the Nuremberg Code[3], the Declaration of Helsinki[4] (original version 1964) and national guidelines for the conduct of clinical trials, which subsequently evolved into legislation.

In terms of legislation the United States took the lead with a series of measures through the 1960s to 1980s which evolved into the Code of Regulations of the Food and Drug Administration 21 CFR[5]. Individual European national governments together with the European Community[6] then produced their own legislation.

Common themes emerged from the various approaches to GCP and resulted in harmonisation of standards within Europe[7] during the late 1980s and early 1990s and Directive 91/507/EEC.

During the 1990s a major international initiative, the International Conference on Harmonisation of the Technical Requirements for Registration of Pharmaceuticals for Human Use took up the momentum and produced agreement on the harmonisation of requirements in Europe, the United States and Japan.

Globally, nations not originally part of the ICH initiative are joining in and adopting these standards and requirements.

Current legislation

The recent European Directive on clinical trials requires Member States to bring in legislation by 1 May 2003 and implement that legislation by 1 May 2004.

The Directive proposes technical procedures to harmonise the conduct of clinical studies throughout Europe. Supplementary implementing texts (guidelines) in line with the principles of GCP will be introduced under new comitology procedures. Some work has already been carried out in this context by European Union (EU) GCP inspectors. Until these are available, the Commission's precise intentions with regard to the detailed interpretation of the provisions of the Directive cannot be stated.

However, some matters are clearly covered in the text of the Directive itself. Particularly relevant here is that it makes compliance with the principles of good clinical practice a legal requirement. It requires all Member States to put into place inspection procedures to assess this compliance and it addresses a range of other specific issues.

It is important to note that the statement that the principles of good clinical practice (GCP) shall be adopted and, if necessary, revised to take account of technical and scientific progress, is equally relevant to non-industry sponsored research and industry sponsored research.

The scope of the Directive

Under the Directive, a clinical trial is defined as any investigation in human subjects:
* to discover or verify the clinical, pharmacological and/or other pharmacodynamic effects,

and/or
* to identify any adverse reactions of one or more investigational medicinal products

and/or
* to study absorption, distribution, metabolism and excretion of one or more investigational medicinal products with the object of ascertaining its (their) safety and/or efficacy.

What will be the consequences of the Directive?

The most significant implication is that all those involved in the conduct of clinical trials will have their responsibilities, duties and functions governed by law. These responsibilities will include adherence to GCP principles.

Thus, non-industry sponsors and charitable sponsors and investigators and the volunteers who make up the membership of independent ethics committees (IECs) will become bound to adhere to the same standards to which those in industry-sponsored research already aspire. Harmonisation is, in fact, one of the key themes of the proposed Directive.

Ethics Committees

The Directive states that Research Ethics Committees (RECs) will give an opinion on 'any subject requested before a clinical trial commences'. In particular they are to consider:
* the relevance of the trial and the trial design
* the protocol
* the suitability of the investigator and supporting staff
* the investigator's brochure
* the quality of the facilities
* the adequacy and completeness of the written information to be given

* the procedure to be used for obtaining informed consent
* recruitment arrangements
* the compensation provisions and insurance or indemnity arrangements
* the proposed remuneration for investigators and subjects.

The REC is required to give its reasoned opinion to the applicant and the relevant competent authority.

The time limits envisaged by the Directive require RECs to supply an initial opinion within 60 days of receipt of a valid submission. During that period they may make a single request for supplementary information and the 'clock stops' while the information is provided.

Regulation by the Regulatory Authority in the UK

The Licensing Authority

The Licensing Authority for human medicines in the UK consists of Government Ministers comprising the Minister of Health, the Minister of Agriculture, Fisheries and Food and Ministers in government health departments in Scotland and Northern Ireland. The Secretary of State for Health acts on behalf of the Licensing Authority and is responsible for the control of medicines for human use in the UK. The Secretary of State receives advice from a Departmental Supervisory Board on the Medicines Control Agency's plans and performance.

The UK Medicines Control Agency

The United Kingdom Medicines Control Agency is the executive arm of Government that regulates the pharmaceutical sector and implements policy in this area. It operates as an Executive Agency of the Department of Health and its primary function is to safeguard public health by ensuring that medicines on the UK market meet appropriate standards of:
* safety
* quality
* efficacy.

The Medicines Control Agency (MCA) is an Executive Agency of the UK Department of Health and its Chief Executive is responsible to the Secretary of State for its operation.

The MCA Mission Statement is:

To promote and safeguard public health through ensuring appropriate standards of safety, quality and efficacy for all medicines on the UK market. Also, to apply other relevant controls and provide information which will contribute to the safe and effective use of medicines[8].

Additionally, the Agency is required to advise Ministers on policy relating to pharmaceuticals and regulatory systems and assist Ministers in achieving their high level objectives on health.

Aims and objectives

The MCA's primary objective is to safeguard public health by ensuring that all medicines on the UK market meet appropriate standards of safety, quality and efficacy. Safety aspects cover potential or actual harmful effects; quality relates to development and manufacture; and efficacy is a measure of the beneficial effect of the medicine on patients. The Agency achieves its objective through:

- a system of licensing before the marketing of medicines
- monitoring of medicines and acting on safety concerns after they have been placed on the market
- checking standards of pharmaceutical manufacture and wholesaling
- enforcement of requirements
- responsibility for medicines control policy
- representing UK pharmaceutical regulatory interests internationally
- publishing quality standards for drug substances through the *British Pharmacopoeia*.

Structure

The MCA is divided into seven divisions, of which three are particularly relevant to clinical research:

1 Licensing Division

This Division carries out the pre-marketing assessment of the medicine's safety, quality and efficacy, examining all the research and test results in detail, before a decision is made on whether the product should be granted a marketing authorisation. The Division is also responsible for the approval and monitoring of all clinical trials undertaken on patients in the UK. It is responsible for the licensing of new drugs, abridged applications, European licensing, homoeopathic registrations, parallel imports and the approval of, and monitoring of, safety in clinical trials.

The assessments are undertaken by multi-disciplinary teams of physicians, pharmacists, toxicologists, scientists and statisticians. In fulfilling this function the Division works closely with the Committee on the Safety of Medicines and the Medicines Commission.

2 Post-Licensing Division

After medicines have been authorised, this Division monitors them as used in everyday practice to identify previously unrecognised or changes in the patterns of their adverse effects. Changes, if necessary, are then made to the marketing authorisation. This Division evaluates over 10 000 variations made each year to marketing authorisations and the renewal applications made every five years. The Division is also responsible for any changes to the legal classification and supply of medicines, product information and ensuring advertisements are not false, misleading or suggest indications for use other than those permitted by the marketing authorisation.

The Post-Licensing Division is also responsible for pharmacovigilance, which is the process of:

(a) monitoring medicines as used in everyday practice to identify previously unrecognised or changes in the patterns of their adverse effects

(b) assessing the risks and benefits of medicines in order to determine what action, if any, is necessary to improve their safe use

(c) providing information to users to optimise safe and effective use of medicines

(d) monitoring the impact of any action taken.

Information from many different sources is used for pharmacovigilance including spontaneous adverse drug reaction (ADR) reporting schemes, clinical and epidemiological studies, the world literature, morbidity and mortality databases. The Division runs the UK's spontaneous adverse drug reaction reporting scheme (called the Yellow Card Reporting Scheme) which receives reports of suspected adverse drug reactions from doctors, dentists, pharmacists and coroners. All suspected adverse reactions should be reported for new medicines; these are labelled with a ▼ symbol on product information and advertisements. For established medicines, health professionals are requested to report only serious adverse reactions.

3 Inspection and Enforcement Division

All UK manufacturers, wholesalers and importers of medicines must also be licensed. This Division carries out regular inspections of these premises to ensure that the required standards of quality assurance are maintained. The Division also investigates suspected illegal activities and may prosecute if appropriate. The *British Pharmacopoeia* is also produced by staff within the Division, in collaboration with the British Pharmacopoeia Commission.

The GCP Compliance Unit is part of the Inspection Group within the Inspection and Enforcement Division. The ICH *Note for Guidance on Good Clinical Practice* (CPMP/ICH/135/95)[9], defines GCP as 'a standard for the design, conduct, performance, monitoring, auditing, recording, analyses, and reporting of clinical trials that provides assurance that the data and reported results are credible and accurate, and that the rights, integrity, and confidentiality of trial subjects are protected'.

GCP inspectors assess compliance with the requirements of GCP guidelines and applicable regulations, and this involves conducting on-site inspections at pharmaceutical sponsor companies, contract research organisations, investigational sites and other facilities involved in clinical trial research. At present, these inspections are conducted on a voluntary basis.

Changes in the UK legislative requirements for clinical trials on medicinal products are anticipated now that the EU Directive relating to the implementation of Good Clinical Practice in the conduct of clinical trials has been adopted. The Directive requires Member States to appoint inspectors to evaluate compliance with GCP. Inspections will no longer be voluntary. The GCP Compliance Unit also works with other EU Member States on GCP inspections associated with centralised EU marketing applications; these inspections are co-ordinated by the EMEA (The European Agency for the Evaluation of Medicinal Products) and the Unit also provides a service to address GCP queries.

Advisory bodies set up under the Medicines Act[10]

The Medicines Commission

The Medicines Commission was established in 1968 with functions assigned to it by, or under, the Medicines Act 1968. Members are appointed by Ministers. Its most important roles are to advise Ministers on matters relating to medicinal products including the membership and functioning of such committees as the Committee on Safety of Medicines and to consider appeals against potential decisions of the Licensing Authority.

Committee on Safety of Medicines (CSM)

The CSM is one of the independent advisory committees established under the Medicines Act (Section 4) which advises the UK Licensing Authority (Government Health Ministers) on the quality, efficacy and safety of medicines in order to ensure that appropriate public health standards are met and maintained.

The Committee's responsibilities are, broadly, twofold:
- To provide advice to the Licensing Authority on whether new products (new active substances) submitted to the UK Medicines Control Agency (MCA) should be granted

a marketing authorisation. These responsibilities require close collaboration with the MCA's Licensing Division.
- To monitor the safety of marketed medicines, in close association with the MCA's Post-Licensing Division to ensure that medicines meet acceptable standards of safety and efficacy.

Regulatory approval[11]

A clinical trial is usually arranged by the supplier of the medicinal product who will ask a practitioner to conduct a trial using his product. In these cases it is for the supplier to make an application for a product licence, clinical trial certificate of supplier's exemption, submitting detailed information on the product and, where necessary, the protocol for the trial. If appropriate, the Licensing Authority will then grant the licence, issue the certificate, or approve the exemption, and the practitioner may proceed with the trial. Approval, if given, is usually subject to certain conditions; the holder of the licence, certificate, or exemption is responsible for bringing these conditions to the attention of the practitioner.

Clinical trial certificate – CTC

During the first 10 years of control of medicines (1971 to 1981) a CTC was required for trials evaluating new active substances and some established substances for new indications.

Obtaining a CTC required application to the MCA with large volumes of supporting data on quality and relevant safety in addition to any clinical data.

Applications for CTCs were assessed as for marketing authorisation and this was a long process, sometimes as long as 18 months. There was a right of appeal to the CSM in the case of refusals.

The final approval covered a range of trials using the same product and was valid for 2 years.

Clinical trial exemption – CTX

Under the Medicines (Exemption from Licences) Order 1981, the exemption scheme was introduced. This expedited the response process.

Applicants must submit an outline of the research proposal with a summary of data obtained so far to support the proposal. They must provide details of the drug, indication, and project to be undertaken. The scheme supports electronic submissions.

A registered medical practitioner must certify the accuracy of the summary provided and assessment by MCA must be within the statutory time of 35 days (plus optional extension of 28 days in complex cases).

The CTX is valid for 3 years and may be renewed or varied.

Apart from the requirement for certification by a registered medical practitioner, other conditions of the exemption are that the Company undertakes to inform MCA of:

• any serious unexpected adverse reaction
• any refusal by an ethics committee
• any data or reports which affect product safety
• changes in manufacturer or importer
• changes in manufacture affecting bioavailability or shelf-life
• information in usage guideline.

There is no right of appeal against refusal to grant a CTX.

Doctor's and Dentist's Exemptions

If a practitioner wishes to conduct a clinical trial using one or more unlicensed products, he or she must notify the Licensing Authority by making use of the Doctors and Dentists Exemption Scheme (the DDX Scheme) giving:

(i) his or her name and address
(ii) the name and address of the supplier
(iii) the name and structure of the product, its pharmaceutical form, the product licence number if applicable, route, dose and duration of administration
(iv) details of the proposed trial, its aim, design, indication, patient details, duration of trial.

The practitioner (consultant in charge for hospital-based studies) must sign a declaration that the trial is not to be carried out under the arrangements made by or on behalf of:

• the person who manufactured the product
• the person responsible for its composition
• the person selling or supplying it.

unless such person is the doctor by whom, or under whose direction, the product is to be administered in the trial.

If the product is to be supplied from within the UK, Form MLA 163 should be completed by the supplier and forwarded together with the completed MLA 162. Using this form the supplier certifies that the study is not being undertaken at the initiative of the supplier.

These clinical trial certificate exemptions are allowed on condition that the practitioner agrees that all serious or unexpected adverse reactions occurring during the course of the trial will be notified to the Licensing Authority immediately.

Thus, in summary, a DDX is not appropriate for sponsored initiated studies. The trial must be undertaken on the initiative of the doctor or dentist and without instigation of manufacturer.

It appears that the product may be supplied free or on a chargeable basis by the manufacturer or supplier and results may be given to the manufacturer or supplier by the practitioner.

CTC/CTX/DDX/MA or PL numbering system

Each licence, authorisation or exemption is numbered uniquely and contains a code identifying the nature of the licence, authorisation or exemption, a company specific number and an incremental number relating to that company. DDXs, where there will be no company involved, are prefixed MF8000 followed by an incremental number from the DDX register.

Possible grounds for refusal/termination of exemption (CTX and/or DDX)

The product is no longer safe or of satisfactory quality
Changes in trial conduct have adverse effect on safety of patients
There was a deficient or incorrect original notification
There has been a breach of the conditions for exemption.

Trials that do not require notification or application for certificate or exemption

In certain circumstances a practitioner may carry out a trial without such an authority and without submitting a notification or application of his own. These are:

• studies in healthy volunteers
• clinical trials using licensed products in exact dose form covered by current product licences (but used in a manner or for an indication outside the terms of the licence, notification is required in the form of a CTX or DDX)
• clinical trials involving placebo or licensed comparitor in the manner and indication covered by current product licences.
• clinical trails using only products specially prepared under the supervision of a pharmacist in a registered pharmacy, hospital or health centre.

Named patient supplies

No authorisation is required for a doctor or dentist to prescribe an unlicensed medicine to a particular patient. This is because this does not represent a clinical trial. There is a therapeutic intention and no research is being conducted.

Ethics Committee Approval

It is one of the basic principles of the Declaration of Helsinki that all studies on human subjects should be approved by an independent ethics committee.

Phases of product development

Discovery/synthesis

Modern drugs are rarely discovered by chance. Molecular biology and computer simulation techniques permit the systematic screening of molecules and prediction of their likely therapeutic activities. A variety of formulations may be developed and assessed for their pharmacological activity. An essential aspect of this initial phase of development is the establishment of analytical techniques for the detection and quantification of levels of the compound, its intermediate and degradation products.

Animal/laboratory work

The International Conference on Harmonisation has developed a number of detailed guidelines[12] which describe the pre-clinical laboratory testing required as part of the drug development process. The standards of Good Laboratory Practice[13] apply and in the UK, pre-clinical research is subject to inspection and membership of the GLP Monitoring Authority Scheme. The type and duration of tests required are specified to justify single and multiple dose administration to humans in clinical research and also the pre-clinical research required to support eventual regulatory submission. The experiments to be carried out investigate genotoxicity (toxic effect on genetic material), toxicity, oncogenicity (causing the development of tumours) and reproductive toxicology, covering fertility and reproduction, teratogenicity (producing congenital malformations) and perinatal and post-natal studies.

Phase I – First/early administration to humans

Phase I studies must be based on information obtained from previous pre-clinical and laboratory work. They are performed in order to assess tolerability and to study pharmacokinetics and pharmacodynamics in healthy volunteers.

Payments are made to volunteers, which should be in proportion to the time and inconvenience suffered. They should not represent an incentive and, as with all clinical research, there should be no coercion to participate. Because of the level of payments and the usually residential nature of such studies, careful screening is performed to reduce risk to the subjects themselves and to avoid confounding effects. In particular, it is important that the primary health-care provider be contacted with the prior approval of the potential subject in order to check for possible reasons for exclusion.

Dose escalation studies may be performed in healthy or patient volunteers to investigate both tolerability and dose response.

Particular patient groups may be recruited into Phase I studies in order to assess the effects of the product in people with hepatic or renal impairment or in the elderly population.

Later in the drug development process there may be a return to Phase I – like studies in order to investigate drug interactions and to perform pharmacokinetic studies of new formulations.

The Association of the British Pharmaceutical Industry offers guidelines for the conduct of studies in non-patient volunteers.[14]

In the UK at present regulatory notification/approval is not required for this type of study. The provisions of the Directive will require all such studies to be notified in future. Ethics Committee approval is required. If the information is intended to form part of a subsequent regulatory submission, standards of good clinical practice pertain and the Directive will mandate these standards for all Phase I studies in the future.

Phase II – First/early administration to patients

In Phase II there is usually the first exposure of the product to patients with the target disease. A small number of patient volunteers take part in short term, usually placebo controlled, studies. As the pharmacokinetics of the drug in patients may be different from healthy volunteers they are re-evaluated.

Dose ranging studies may be performed and risk-benefit ratios must be assessed to assist the decision as to whether it is appropriate to proceed to Phase III and with what formulations and doses.

Phase II studies require Ethics Committee approval, regulatory approval and application of GCP standards.

Phase III – Confirmation of efficacy and safety in patients

Phase III studies are typically larger-scale studies than any carried out before and frequently more costly. They may be of longer duration, involving many patients and are conducted in a range of situations including hospital clinics and general practice. Such studies should be statistically based to permit valid inferential techniques to be used to evaluate safety and efficacy in a larger population.

Intention to treat studies attempt to mimic the realities of the future prescribing situation.

Phase III studies are usually comparator studies with an established product or, where none exists and/or there are no ethical issues, a placebo. They may involve adult patients and also include paediatric and geriatric studies. Increasingly, Phase III studies involve a quality of life element as well as risk/benefit analysis from efficacy and safety data. This may be important because it may be taken into account by those who regulate health service resource allocation.

Phase III studies require Ethics Committee approval and regulatory approval. Adherence to GCP standards is essential if results are to be meaningful and the safety profile is to be interpreted correctly.

Marketing authorisation

Application for a marketing authorisation is based on information from the pre-clinical testing phase and studies performed during Phases I to III. The UK Medicines Control Agency is the licensing authority which provides the expert assessors for non-biotechnological products. The products of biotechnology are assessed by the European Medicines Evaluation Agency.

Phase IV – Further studies after marketing authorisation

Phase IV studies may be run by, or in collaboration with, the company's marketing department. They are usually comparative studies and are conducted in a much wider range of patient populations than is possible prior to marketing authorisation.

There are a number of types of Phase IV study including case control studies, Post-Marketing Surveillance Studies (PMS studies) or studies for the safety assessment of marketed medicines (SAMM) studies, to evaluate safety and detect previously unreported adverse events which have a low incidence rate. The Association of the British Pharmaceutical Industry provides guidelines for the conduct of such studies[15].

Studies within the marketing authorisation, in the same indication and at the same dose, do not require regulatory notification/authorisation. Under the Directive, if such studies are non-interventional in terms of the definition provided, they may fall outside the mandatory scope of the Directive.

However, studies of range extensions (new indications) and new formulations will not be non-interventional and will require full adherence to the Directive's provisions, including regulatory notification/approval, Ethics Committee approval and adherence to GCP standards.

What is a clinical trial?

An investigation by a doctor or dentist involving administration of a medicinal product to a patient to assess the product's safety and efficacy.

UK Medicines Act 1968
Chapter 67 Section 31

(1) 'In this Act "clinical trial" means an investigation or series of investigations consisting of the administration of one or more medicinal products of a particular description –

  (a) by, or under the direction of, a doctor or dentist to one or more patients of his, or

   by, or under the direction of two or more doctors or dentists, each product being administered by or under the direction of one or other of those doctors or dentists to one or more patients of his,

  where (in any case) there is evidence that medicinal products of that description have effects which may be beneficial to the patient or patients in question and the administration of the product or products is for the purpose of ascertaining whether, or to what extent, the product has, or the products have, those or any other effects, whether beneficial or harmful.'

Under the Clinical Trial Directive, the definition of a clinical trial is wider (see the section Current Legislation of this article).

What is a medicinal product?

'A substance which is administered to human beings ... for a medicinal purpose' (Medicines Act 1968)

Medicinal purposes are listed as:
• treating or preventing disease
• diagnosing
• contraception
• anaesthesia.

NB This definition does not include products when there is no evidence of benefit, i.e. healthy volunteer studies.

In European legislation, the definition is somewhat wider. A human medicine is defined as a product for the treatment and prevention of disease; for administration to make medical diagnosis; or for restoring, correcting or modifying physiological functions in human beings.

Borderline products

Substances such as cosmetics, foods, dietary supplements, vitamins, amino acids, minerals and toothpastes are not generally subject to the regulations concerning medicinal products.

However, ingredients, function, presentation, labelling and promotion may affect the status of a product.

As this is an area where the classifications are not always entirely clear, the MCA will offer advice on the status of a product in cases of doubt.

Manufacture, handling, storage and use of investigational products

It is one of the 13 principles of GCP, that investigational products should be manufactured, handled and stored in accordance with the applicable good manufacturing practice (GMP) and that they should be used in accordance with the protocol.

The ICH GCP Guidelines require clear documentation of responsibilities and delegations in relation to the investigational product, maintenance of complete records of despatch, shipment, receipt, dispensing, compliance, return and eventual destruction, documentation of appropriate shipping, storage and use and provision of training to the subject or person responsible for administration of the product.

Marketing authorisations (formerly product licences)

There are three categories of marketing authorisation for prescription or sale in the UK and these determine the access route for the public to the product:

1 General Sale List *GSL*

   GSL products can be sold 'over the counter' or 'off the shelf' without the supervision of a pharmacist or medically qualified person.

2 Pharmacy – *P*

   Pharmacy only products can only be purchased from a pharmacy, under pharmacist supervision

3 Prescription Only Medicines – *POM*

   POM products must be prescribed by a doctor or dentist and cannot be purchased directly without prescription from a pharmacy or other retail outlet.

Relevant abbreviations

ABPI   Association of British Pharmaceutical Industry
ADE   Adverse drug event
ADR   Adverse drug reaction
AE   Adverse event
AR   Adverse reaction
CFR   Code of Federal Regulations
CTC   Clinical Trial Certificate
CTX   Clinical Trial Exemption

Competent authority – regulatory authority – licensing authority

CPMP   Committee for Proprietary Medicinal Products
CRF   Case report (record) form
CV   Curriculum vitae
DDX   Doctor's and Dentist's Exemption
EEC   European Economic Community
EU   European Union
EFPIA   European Federation of Pharmaceutical Industries' Associations
EMEA   European Medicines Evaluation Agency
FDA   Food and Drug Administration (USA)
GCP   An international ethical and scientific quality standard for the design, conduct, performance, monitoring, auditing, recording, analysis and reporting of clinical trials that provides assurance that the data and reported results are credible and accurate, and that the rights, integrity and confidentiality of the subjects are protected.
GSL   General Sale List – sale without pharmacy or medical supervision
GLP   Good laboratory practice
GMP   Good manufacturing practice
ICH   International conference on harmonisation of technical requirements for registration of pharmaceuticals for human use
IEC   Independent Ethics Committee
IB   Investigator Brochure
JPMA   Japan Pharmaceutical Manufacturers Association
MA   Marketing Authorisation
MCA   Medicines Control Agency (UK)
MHW   Ministry of Health and Welfare Japan (or JMHW)
MS   Member State (EU)
P   Pharmacy only – obtainable from a pharmacy, under pharmacist supervision
Phase I   First administration to man
Phase II   First administration to patients
Phase III   Confirmation of efficacy and safety in patients
Phase IV   Further studies after marketing authorisation
PhRMA   Pharmaceutical Research and Manufacturers of America
Pre Clinical Animal/Laboratory work

POM   Prescription Only – must be prescribed by
a doctor or dentist

SAE   Serious adverse event

SAR   Serious adverse reaction

REFERENCES

1 Commission Directive 91/507/EEC of 19 July 1991 modifying the Annex to Council Directive 75/318/EEC of 20 May 1975 on the approximation of the laws of Member States relating to the analytical, pharmatoxicological and clinical standards and protocols in respect of the testing of medicinal products (OJ No L 270 of 26.9.1991).

2 Directive 2001/20/EC of the European Parliament and of the Council of 4 April 2001 on the approximation of the laws, regulations and administrative provisions of the Member States relating to the implementation of good clinical practice in the conduct of clinical trials on medicinal products for human use.

3 Nuremberg Code: Trials of War Criminals before the Nuremberg Military Tribunals under Control Council Law No.10, Vol.2, Nuremberg, October 1946–April 1949, US Government Printing Office, Washington DC, pp. 181–182.

4 Declaration of Helsinki, World Medical Association 'Ethical Principles for Medical Research involving Human Subjects' Adopted by the 18th WMA General Assembly Helsinki, Finland, June 1964 and amended. Most recent amendment 52nd WMA General Assembly, Edinburgh, Scotland, October 2000.

5 Code of Federal Regulations. Good Clinical Practice Parts 50, 54, 56, 312 and 314. US Federal Register – revised April 1, 2000 and subsequent revisions.

6 Council Directive 75/318/EEC of 20 May 1975 on the approximation of the laws of Member States relating to the analytical, pharmatoxicological and clinical standards and protocols in respect of the testing of medicinal products (OJ No L 147 of 9.6.1975).

7 The Rules Governing Medicinal Products for Human Use in the European Union (Vol. I of the series 'The rules governing medicinal products in the European Community'), Commission of the European Communities: Luxembourg, revised July 1995.

8 Towards Safe Medicines – A Guide to the Control of Safety, Quality and Efficacy of Human Medicines in the United Kingdom, Medicines Control Agency, revised 1997.

9 Good Clinical Practice: Harmonised Tripartite Guidelines, ICH E6 1996, updated September 1997 with post-Step 4 errata included.

10 Medicines Act 1968. London: HMSO.

11 Medicines Act 1968 – Guidance Notes on Applications for Clinical Trial Exemptions and Clinical Trial Certificates, Medicines Control Agency, revised December 1995.

12 ICH Safety Guidelines – Series S.

13 UK GLP Regulations (1999). UK Good Laboratory Practice Monitoring Authority.

UK GLPMA Guide to UK GLP Regulations, UK Good Laboratory Practice Monitoring Authority, 1999.

OECD Principles of Good Laboratory Practice, revised 1997, Environment Directorate, OECD, Paris 1998.

14 ABPI Clinical Guidelines for Medical Experiments in Non-patient Volunteers 421/88/6600M – March 1988, amended May 1990 and ABPI Clinical Guidelines for Facilities for Non-patient Volunteer Studies 422/89/ 6600M – 1989.

15 ABPI Guidelines for Phase IV Clinical Trials 416/93/ 6600M – September 1993. ABPI Guidelines for Company Sponsored Safety Assessment of Marketed Medicines (SAMM) 420/94/6600M – January 1994.

Observational and epidemiological research

Nick Dunn

Department of Primary Medical Care, University of Southampton, UK

The scope of epidemiology

Epidemiology has been usefully defined as the study of the distribution and determinants of disease in human populations.

Most epidemiologists would regard the randomised controlled trial (RCT) as the 'gold standard' of experimental design, which produces the most reliable of results in the pursuit of the aims of epidemiology. Unfortunately, there are many situations in which the RCT is not feasible: either it is too expensive to run, or it is impossible to recruit enough patients, or it is ethically unjustifiable. In such circumstances, observational research methods are needed.

Types of epidemiological study

These can be either descriptive or analytic.

'Descriptive' encompasses quantitative studies, e.g. censuses and surveys, and qualitative studies, e.g. focus groups, and supply essential data for many analytic studies.

Analytic studies seek to establish relationships between diseases and their causes, and deal with quantitative data. There are four main categories of analytic studies:

 (i) Cohort
 (ii) Case-control
 (iii) Cross-sectional
 (iv) Ecological

All these types of study are known as observational: that is, they involve observing what is happening, without interfering with the 'natural' situation. Randomisation in such a study means the selection of a random sample of the population for observation, and has nothing to do with random allocation of treatment, which is seen in an RCT.

Cohort study

As can be seen from the diagram, the design of the study is prospective – i.e. moves forward in time from identification of the 'exposure' (the putative causal factor) to measurement of the occurrence of disease ('outcome'). The rate of occurrence of disease, per unit time, in the exposed cohort is calculated and expressed as a ratio of the rate in the non-exposed cohort, giving the rate ratio, which is the usual statistical measure.

Cohort studies are arguably the best observational design, which resemble an RCT most closely. They are not always possible, however, since they are often expensive and require time for the follow-up period, which may be several years. Cohort studies are particularly appropriate for the situation where the exposure is rather rare (e.g. a chemical pollutant only produced by specialised industries), and when there may a number of outcomes to be studied (e.g. this pollutant may cause several diseases). They have the advantage of allowing the study of temporal sequences in disease development (e.g. how soon does cancer develop, after exposure to this pollutant, and is this feasible in view of our knowledge of this cancer?). Their principal disadvantages are expense, and the potential for patients to become lost to follow-up over the passage of time.

Case-control study

In the case-control study, case and controls are identified first, and then enquiries made (either by interview, or through case notes) as to the history of exposure in the past. A 'case' is someone who has the disease under study and a 'control' someone who has not. This is a retrospective design, which has some inherent problems (see below), and is perhaps not as strong a design as the cohort is. However, it is often cheaper, and is usually quicker.

Design of a cohort study

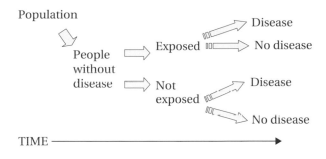

Design of a case-control study

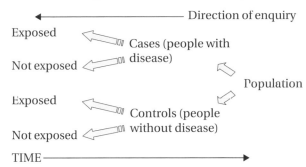

Case-control studies are good for studying outcomes that are rare, since all the cases can be gathered together into the study from a wide geographical area. They are not good for rare exposures, and are particularly prone to biases, since the exposure is recorded after the development of the outcome, and patients' memories are prone to inaccuracies.

A particularly important feature of these studies is the selection of controls. This is not as simple a task as it sounds! The controls must be representative of the population from which the cases are drawn, and must be eligible to become a case, should they develop the disease. If cases are drawn only from a tertiary, specialist, hospital, then the controls must not simply come from GP surgeries in the surrounding district, but should be drawn from those patients attending the hospital for other diseases.

Cross-sectional study

This is a design that represents a 'snapshot' in time, where a sample of the population is studied by enquiring about the exposure and outcome at the same time. For example, we might stop the first 100 people that pass in the street, and enquire whether they were smokers, and also whether they suffered from asthma. We might then draw conclusions as to the causation of asthma from the smoking habits of asthmatics, compared to non-asthmatics. Such studies are quick, relatively easy to do and inexpensive. They are also fraught with difficulties, since it may be difficult to establish the chronological relationship between the exposure and outcome (the classic chicken and egg situation). They are also not suitable for studies of rare diseases or exposures, unless using very big sample sizes.

Ecological study

In this design, comparison is made between whole populations, as opposed to between individuals in populations.

For example, we know that there are large differences between countries in the incidence of certain cancers, such as stomach and oesophageal. One clue as to the causation might lie in diet, and it is possible to find the average intakes of certain foodstuffs per person in individual countries. This allows a plot to be made of incidence of cancer versus foodstuff intake in several countries, and thus a search for correlation can be made.

It is obvious that such studies are rather crude, but they may point the way to further, more refined, studies in the future, and thus ecological studies are useful as a building block to the elucidation of disease causation. It should be pointed out that it is not possible to draw conclusions about *an individual's* risk of developing disease, from an ecological study result; this is known as the 'ecological fallacy'.

What are the pitfalls common to all observational studies?

Because these studies are observing natural situations, they are prone to difficulties. These difficulties need to be anticipated in any research protocol, and suitable methods of dealing with them elucidated, otherwise the research may produce misleading results.

Confounding

Smokers often have yellow fingers, and smokers often die from lung cancer. Thus, we might conclude that the yellow fingers cause the cancer. This is obviously incorrect: yellow fingers are a confounding factor to the relationship between smoking and cancer. Confounders are an alternative explanation, a different route between cause and effect. A confounder must have an association with the exposure under question, and also be a risk factor for the outcome. They may give a completely false result, or they may simply modify the strength of a genuine relationship between an exposure and an outcome. Researchers need to take the effect of confounding into account, either by appropriate design, or else in the analysis, or a combination of both. Therefore, potential confounders need to be identified in the protocol, and either data collected on them, to allow the process of statistical adjustment, or else dealt with in some other way (e.g. matching or exclusion).

Bias

Bias can operate at many stages of a study. Selection bias means that the persons included in the study are not truly representative of all those available (e.g. patients taken from one hospital, but not another. There may be subtle differences in the admissions policies of the two hospitals.) Information bias means that the data collected is incomplete and/or influenced by some extraneous factor, such as media coverage of the issue under investigation. Observer bias operates if the research assistant who is carrying out the interviews in some way influences the way in which the questions are answered (they may do this, even subconsciously, if they are aware of the research question under investigation). Such bias may also occur if the specialist checking medical diagnostic information is aware of the status of the patient, with regard to the exposure of interest. There are many other possible biases, but all have the same effect of producing information that is 'weighted' towards one camp or the other, and produces a false impression of the real situation. Unlike confounding, bias cannot be adjusted for during statistical analysis, and therefore needs to be acknowledged and dealt with in the design stage of a study. Measures must be taken to minimise the effect of bias (e.g. careful training of research staff, 'blinding' of investigators where possible), and these measures should be delineated in the protocol.

Sample size

As with any study, there must be calculations to estimate the number of people to include in the cohorts, or as cases/controls, in order to have a reasonable chance of obtaining a result that is not simply the result of chance. The power of a study, that is its ability to avoid a false-negative result, is usually set at 80% or 90%, and the significance, the ability to avoid a false positive result, at 95%.

There are other influences on the necessary sample size:
(a) how subtle an association is between exposure and outcome needs to be shown. This is a matter for judgement by the researchers, e.g. should the study be able to show an odds, or rate, ratio of two (in which case large numbers will be needed) or of five (smaller numbers needed).
(b) studies of rare outcomes or exposures need relatively large numbers.

Although the numbers produced by the formulae, or computer packages, for sample size, are approximate only, they should be shown clearly in the protocol.

How good a research tool is epidemiology?

This is of relevance to ethics committees, since what is the point of expending great time, effort and money on such research if it cannot produce worthwhile results? Observational studies are important because:

- Many situations do not lend themselves to clinical trials or laboratory research, either because it is practically impossible, or because it is ethically unjustifiable to randomise patients.
- It is frequently the building block on which RCTs, or other studies, are based.
- It is impossible to say that any single observational study reveals 'the truth'. However, when several studies all point in the same direction, or when the measure of association is particularly strong (e.g. a rate ratio, or odds ratio, of 10), and when there has been proper allowance for confounding and/or bias, then the chances of a true result are increased.
- Many important breakthroughs have resulted from observational studies: e.g. Doll's study on smoking and lung cancer (Doll & Hill,1950), various studies on rubella and congenital malformations (e.g. Sheridan, 1964).

REFERENCES

Doll, R & Bradford Hill, A. (1950). Smoking and carcinoma of the lung: preliminary report. *Br Med J*, **30**; 739–748.

Sheridan, M. (1964). Final report of a prospective study of children whose mothers had rubella in early pregnancy. *Br Med J*, **2**; 536–539.

Social survey research

Crispin Jenkinson

Health Services Research Unit, University of Oxford, UK

What is social survey research?

Social researchers have available to them a wide variety of research methods. They may send questionnaires through the post to elicit information, they may interview individuals on the doorstep or they may conduct interviews over the telephone. All of these methods of information gathering can be used to gain a structured and systematic set of data, and, this, in essence, is the major feature of the social survey. Quite simply, social surveys are characterised by information on the same variables (such as attitudes and beliefs) being collected from at least two (and usually far more) individuals.

This document outlines the purpose of surveys, how they are undertaken, and potential problems in the gaining of survey data.

Why undertake social surveys?

The major purpose of social surveys is to describe the characteristics of a sample of people, or to attempt to gain some insight into the possible causes of certain phenomena. However, the social survey is, unlike randomised controlled trials, a non-experimental design. Social survey research does not attempt to influence medical interventions. Instead social survey researchers attempt to find patterns in data that are consistent and systematic. Such data can be used to inform policy decision making. Thus, for example, surveys have been conducted in which respondents were asked about their health and their behaviour. From such data it has been found that, for example, those who smoke and drink heavily are more likely to report certain illnesses. Such information can be used to inform campaigns aimed at improving people's behaviour.

How are surveys conducted?

Select a population

To begin with, the population under study is defined. A population may be large, and very heterogeneous (such as everybody in the country), or smaller, and more defined, such as 'all people in Oxford attending rheumatology clinics'. Once the population has been defined, the survey researchers must decide whether they have the time and resources to survey everybody in the defined population. If not they must sample from the population. The number of people who can be surveyed will be influenced by the survey method adopted, as some methods are more time consuming and expensive than others.

Decide on a survey method

A number of methods of social survey research exist. By far the most common that are used in survey research are face-to-face interviewing, telephone interviewing and postal survey.

Face-to-face interviews

Face-to-face interviewing has been found to be the most likely method of gaining high levels of response. Furthermore, it is a method that can provide data as to why respondents do not wish, or are unable, to complete a questionnaire. Interviewing is, however, costly, especially if interviewers continue to call back at addresses where they have been unsuccessful in gaining responses at early attempts.

Telephone interviews

Respondents may be randomly selected from telephone books or registers, and rung at home. It is highly desirable that possible respondents are informed by post that they will be rung at home. Possible dates and times should be suggested. This is desirable as respondents are more likely to be in at the time of the call and less likely to believe the call to be malicious. Providing the respondent with a telephone number to call back is also desirable. Furthermore, it should be stressed both in the original contact letter and the call itself that the respondent can terminate the call at any time. If respondents choose to end the interview prematurely they should not be called back. Telephone interviews are costly and time consuming. Furthermore, they are restricted to those who own telephones and as such a random sample may not be truly representative of the population it intends to survey.

Postal surveys

Postal surveys are perhaps the most commonly adopted survey method used by social scientists, especially in instances where large sample sizes are required. The census is an example of this sort of research. However, the census is sent to every household in the country. It is rare for an entire population to be surveyed, and generally surveys are sent out to randomly selected sub-samples. Whilst this method of research is popular due, in large measure, to the fact that it is relatively inexpensive, it does have its limitations. To begin with it is difficult, if not impossible, to ascertain why certain people do not respond. Secondly, any misunderstanding of questions that a respondent may experience can rarely be explained. This may lead to inaccurate or misleading answers.

If necessary, gain a sample of the population

For the most part, the purpose of survey research is to make claims at the population level, whatever the population may be. It is therefore imperative that surveys that do not include all members of a given population do contain a representative sample. Thus, if 70% of a certain population is female, then in a random sample of the population we would expect approximately 70% of responses to come from women. If samples are not representative, it is not possible to extrapolate to the population (i.e. to make claims about the population on the basis of the data gained from the sample). It is vital that any survey research makes it clear how the sample will be gained. A sample collected in, for example, an airport would not be representative of the UK population. It may, if collected with due care, be representative of air travellers.

In order for samples to be accurate representations of the population, researchers must ensure that everybody in the population has an equal chance of inclusion in the survey.

Random sampling is, however, not always possible. In instances where it is unlikely that random sampling would gain a high response rate then researchers may select a technique known as 'snowball sampling', whereby respondents are asked to inform people they know that the survey is being undertaken. Such a technique is often adopted where research is being conducted on sensitive topics. Thus, if one wishes to know the sexual practices of the gay community a snowball sample is more likely to gain a good response rate than simple random sampling. Whatever method of sampling is used, it is imperative that the method to be adopted is clearly outlined and explained.

What questions are to be asked?

It is imperative that questionnaires used for survey research are reliable and valid. A reliable questionnaire is one that provides the same responses when administered to the same individuals at different times, providing, of course, that they have experienced no changes in their life, health state etc. in-between administrations of the questionnaire. A valid questionnaire is one that measures what it purports to measure.

Questionnaire design and question formulation are not straightforward tasks. Even apparently simple questions can lead to ambiguities. Thus, for example, a question such as 'Do you own a car?' to which the possible responses are 'yes' or 'no' may at a superficial glance seem to cover all the options. However, it can lead to difficulty. The question may be answered by someone who has just sold his or her car, but is in the process of buying another one, or others who own a car, but not in England (they may have one in the country where they own their holiday home!), or others who own a car (their parents have given it to them) but have not yet passed their driving test, or perhaps even someone who owns a car sales garage and all the cars for sale in it, but is not a car driver. Questionnaire designers must think about the exact data they are collecting. Affirmation of the question 'Do you own a car?' does not necessarily imply that individuals can drive, or use a car in the UK. Careful phrasing of questions is vital, and pilot studies should be undertaken to ensure that questions can be easily understood by the respondents to whom they are being directed.

There exist a large number of established questionnaires that can be used to assess just about everything from personality type to quality of life. However, selection of an established measure, or measures, should not be undertaken lightly. For example, there are a large number of questionnaires that purport to measure 'health status'. These measures differ in important respects. Most seek information on mobility, emotional state, social functioning, pain, etc. However, the way in which questions are phrased, the time scale addressed, and the length and complexity of measures differ enormously. Researchers must clearly state why they have chosen a particular measure in preference to others. Inappropriate measures may produce incorrect or, at the very least, misleading data. For example, questionnaires that ask respondents about the past month of their life are inappropriate for a follow up study where the question is repeated with a gap of only a few days between.

Furthermore, researchers should ensure that any established questionnaire they use is appropriate for the mode of administration they intend to adopt. For example, many questionnaires have not been designed for use in telephone interviewing. Indeed, even those that have been designed with the intention that they may be administered by different methods can produce somewhat different results in different settings. This problem should be borne in mind when analysing data. Finally, it is desirable that the same mode of administration is used throughout a study.

Limitations and criticisms of surveys

It is important to realise that surveys are not able to establish causal links. Research undertaken using survey data may provide support for an association which may be causal, but for such a claim to be made a more experimental research method is required. Within health research the classic 'experimental design' is the randomised controlled trial (RCT). Survey research may indicate areas where RCTs may be appropriately undertaken.

Some social researchers argue that surveys cannot gain access to meaningful aspects of social action. Thus, by requiring individuals to complete a pre-determined set of questions, and undertaking statistical analysis on such data, the real feelings and motives of individuals may be overlooked. Some argue that to gain insight into human behaviour a more 'in-depth' unstructured approach is required, such as participant observation, or in-depth interviewing. Often such approaches are used to inform the design of questionnaires which are then sent out in social surveys. However, such statistical analysis of data can cloud important individual variations. As such it is important to realise that large scale survey research can provide data on samples or populations. To attempt to apply such data at an individual level may be quite inappropriate.

USEFUL WEBSITES

The Centre for Applied Social Surveys
http://www.socstats.soton.ac.uk/cass/intro.html

The National Centre for Social Research
http://www.natcen.ac.uk/

Approaching qualitative research

Alan Cribb

Centre for Public Policy Research, King's College London

Qualitative research poses a series of challenges for Research Ethics Committees. This chapter elucidates the nature of qualitative research, discusses its appraisal, and rehearses the ethical issues it raises. In the process implications for Research Ethics Committees are indicated. These implications are summarised at the end of the chapter.

Introducing qualitative research

What is qualitative research?

Qualitative research is a label for a family of methods and, just as with quantitative research methods, there are differences and disagreements within the family. However the common denominator of the qualitative approach to social research is a focus on *meaning*, and on the social world as made up of systems of meaning. For example, one good account of qualitative methods, which highlights their distinctiveness, is that they embody '... *an approach to the study of the social world which seeks to describe and analyse the culture and behaviour of humans and their groups from the point of view of those being studied.*' (Bryman, 1988, p. 46) It is essential to qualitative research methods that they get 'inside' the social world, in particular into the *cultures* of groups and the *subjectivities* of individuals. Most qualitative researchers will want to move beyond this 'first person' point of view, and to incorporate more theoretical or technical analyses that derive from their disciplinary interests and which help them and us to understand the social world. But they will certainly want to ensure that however abstract or theoretical their work becomes, it somehow takes into account, and remains connected to, the cultures and subjectivities of those they are studying.

The fundamental distinctiveness of qualitative research

Should qualitative research be seen as competing with, or complementary to, quantitative research? This is a debate that will run and run. At a practical level it often makes sense to see the two approaches as complementary, and the two can be combined to good effect within research projects. At this level the approaches differ mainly in the kind of data they use, and hence in the ways of handling these data (see later sections). But the two sets of approaches derive from different, and sometimes conflicting, theoretical foundations. *The rationale of qualitative research is, at a fundamental level, different from that of quantitative research.* It is essential to stress this distinctiveness, and for that reason we will say a little more about the foundations of qualitative research. (Indeed, in the account offered here we have, if anything, erred on the side of over-stressing the differences between qualitative and quantitative approaches.)

Whereas quantitative researchers can be seen as methodological cousins of physical scientists such as physicists and chemists, qualitative researchers are better viewed as methodological cousins of humanities scholars such as historians and biographers. Just as it would be foolish to try to evaluate the work of a historian by the criteria of a physicist, it is foolish to evaluate purely qualitative research by quantitative criteria. Of course this is not to say that criteria of rigour do not apply to history, or to qualitative research, merely that in each case the appropriate criteria have to be applied. Research Ethics Committees should give this matter serious consideration. Ideally, they should have members who are knowledgeable about qualitative research and have a 'feel' for it. If not, they should have ready access to a group of experienced qualitative assessors.

The distinctiveness of qualitative research stems from its orientation towards the 'first person' point of view and its historical association with an *interpretative* research tradition. This tradition is based upon the recognition that the social world is constituted (to some degree) by *meanings*. A few moments, thought reveals that many things which are central to people's lives – their hopes and fears, commitments and identities – are products of cultural systems. If Martians landed in an Islington party and were introduced to a Roman Catholic, opera loving, Labour voting, member of Amnesty International they would have to investigate these cultural movements before they could get close to understanding the person. Similarly if they landed in other countries and settings they would have to investigate other cultural forms and products. People are made up of culture in just as real a sense as they are made of cells and organs.

The cultural construction of the social world is a problem for all social research because cultures continuously change across space and time – there are no fixed or universal points. In dealing with cultural forms, researchers face extraordinary diversity and complexity. Consequently it is extremely difficult to make successful generalisations about the social world. Quantitative researchers seek to manage this complexity by using experimental and statistical methods to work towards some defensible generalisations. Qualitative researchers tend to be more sceptical about the possibility of, and the value of, these kinds of statistical generalisations. They place their emphasis upon capturing specific cultural fields and first person points of view. Instead of attempting to 'control for' differences between cultural groups and fields, they seek to get inside them.

Ethnography: an archetype for qualitative research

A more practical way to get a feel for the nature of qualitative research is to reflect on the work of an anthropologist who goes to study the lives of a distant community. This is only one example of qualitative research but is, in some respects, archetypal. Here we can imagine that the anthropologist might live and work in the community they are studying for months or years. He or she will immerse themselves in all the facets of society including the domestic and the public, the sacred and the profane. Although anthropologists may always remain 'outsiders' in certain ways, they will also strive towards understanding an 'insiders' point of view. Their analyses and theories about the community under study will be grounded in this process of immersion, and they will strive to communicate their

understandings so as to 'open up' and illuminate the community for others.

Further consideration of this example illustrates the methodological flavour of qualitative research:

(a) The kinds of data involved are many and varied – they might include tape-recordings of conversations, video footage, notes on observations, copies of documents, physical artefacts.

(b) The research process is exploratory, inductive and, at least for a time, open-ended – the contours of the investigation are not clear in advance but emerge over time.

(c) Although an element of quantification may prove useful in handling and presenting the data, the whole data set cannot be translated into measurements and correlations without sacrificing the rich holistic 'picture' which the researcher is attempting to draw. Rather the goal of analysis is to pull the different facets of the picture together into a framework which somehow captures, conveys and helps us to understand the complex whole.

(d) The researcher as the interpretative agent is, quite explicitly, the main research instrument – his or her identity and point of view is implicated in the precise way the data is collected and analysed. For this reason the qualitative researcher must be as reflexive as possible about the ways in which they are constructing the accounts they present. (Of course, quantitative researchers also construct their research accounts but this is less often acknowledged in methodological accounts.)

Not all qualitative research involves such a broad focus or a process of wholesale immersion. Some qualitative research is only partly analogous to ethnography and shares only certain features and techniques in common with it. But the characteristics highlighted above – rich and complex data sets, emergent research designs, holistic analyses and researcher reflexivity – are quite typical of a qualitative approach to research. Together they mean that qualitative research proposals often look strange to those coming from different styles of inquiry.

Examples of qualitative research strategies

Participant observation

This is the archetypal strategy of the anthropologist mentioned above. The process of immersion can be used – to different degrees – to study a wide range of more or less circumscribed fields and roles, e.g. a hospital, a clinical directorate, a clinic, the role of a ward sister. This approach can be extended beyond actual physical settings to explore more diffuse or metaphorical 'settings' or fields, e.g. homelessness, chronic illness. This entails a range of different data collection and handling techniques.

Non-participant observation

This is similar to above except the fieldwork is conducted predominantly in the role of 'researcher' and not significantly through the adoption of insider roles.

Unstructured or semi-structured interviews

Many of the research techniques of qualitative research can be used independently of the archetypal process of researcher immersion. Unstructured or semi-structured interviews are the most common data collection technique of the qualitative researcher and are often used as the main means of data collection. Rather than have a defined series of questions for which they are seeking clear-cut answers, interviewers simply indicate the general domains of interest and encourage the respondent to talk freely about whatever they choose within these domains. The interview resembles a natural conversation in some respects. Over time (over the course of a research project or even over a single interview) the researcher may well define a sharper focus and probe for more specific information. But the emphasis will remain upon eliciting the respondent's own perspective and words. This same technique of relatively unstructured, or loosely structured interviews, is sometimes used with groups rather than with single individuals only.

Documentary analysis

Another technique which can be abstracted from participant observation and used on its own, or in combination with others, is the collection and qualitative analysis of existing texts. Institutions, for example, are usually 'drowning' in texts such as policy statements, records, memos, minutes, leaflets and pamphlets – these provide a valuable data source for anyone wishing to analyse the official and less formal discourses of the institution.

As we have noted, qualitative research covers a broad range of research approaches and techniques. Furthermore these techniques can be deployed within different styles of research. For example, in research traditions where the gap between 'the researcher' and 'the researched' is narrowed ('collaborative research'), or where the research-practice split is broken down ('action research'), or as a complementary component within more quantitative approaches such as surveys.

Examples of qualitative research uses

Qualitative research has an extensive set of uses. As we have seen, it has a particular use in studying what might be labelled as 'tribes', cultures, settings or fields, and 'voices'. For example:

1 Understanding institutional and professional groups – in order to understand change (or its absence) within health services or health care and medical education, it is essential to understand the cultures and identities of professional groups and sub-groups, and the institutional climates and frameworks in which they work.

2 Understanding lay (and professional) beliefs and cultures with regard to health and illness. This is necessary to understand such matters as uptake of services, adherence, and the possibilities of health promotion.

3 Needs assessment and quality of life research. Although both of these lines of inquiry tend to rely heavily on measurement they both also depend heavily on qualitative research (both as a preliminary to, and as a complement to, the use of measurement).

4 Biography and health. The study of individual and collective life history is central to understanding the relationship between lifestyle and health, and the experience of chronic illness.

5 The evaluation of policies and services. Once again it is difficult to accomplish health-related evaluation in a meaningful way without incorporating at least a component of qualitative research into the research design.

These are only illustrations but are hopefully sufficient to show the potential importance of health-related qualitative research.

Appraising qualitative research

'It's not proper research' – Prejudices against qualitative research

But how can qualitative research be useful if it does not conform to the canons of 'proper' quantitative research? If it is bad research, then talk of its relevance and usefulness is surely misplaced. This is certainly true. However, it is wrong to automatically label all qualitative research as somehow 'falling short', and those who do so are either ignorant about qualitative research or, in some cases, simply prejudiced against it. The most common complaints about qualitative research proposals are that they (a) use numbers too small to be useful and (b) are 'subjective'. In the next section we will say something more about rigour in qualitative research, but we begin by acknowledging, and responding to, these widespread perceptions.

Small numbers

Qualitative research often uses comparatively small numbers of respondents. But these numbers are not too small to be useful except in one specific and irrelevant respect. Quantitative research aims to achieve statistical generalisability, but qualitative research does not. It is vital to understand this distinction. The ideal for quantitative research is to say that the measures and correlations which apply in the study sample are a reasonable indicator of those which pertain across the population which the sample represents. Consequently much effort goes into trying to ensure that quantitative research samples are statistically representative of the relevant population.

The emphasis in qualitative research studies is quite different. Here the emphasis is: (a) to capture the particular cases studied (individuals, settings, policies etc.) in all of their complexity as richly, vividly and accurately as possible; and (b) to construct descriptions and analyses which may have some more general relevance and value. In other words, qualitative research does not make specific empirical claims which extend beyond the cases studied but it can generate ideas which have wider relevance at a theoretical level. (The need for 'accuracy' is about achieving what is sometimes labelled 'internal validity' as opposed to 'external validity' or generalisability, but some qualitative researchers choose to avoid the term 'validity' – not because accuracy is unimportant but because of some of the misleading quantitative associations of the term.)

An example may help to illustrate the point. An in-depth qualitative study of the lives of a comparatively small number of medical students in one medical school can shed light on a broad range of factors which affect their learning, their attitudes to medicine and medical specialities, their relationships with others, including their tutors and patients. Now the lives of other medical students – even within the same school – will, of course, all be different. For instance perhaps the study does not happen to include any students over 30, or any students living at the parental home, or any Muslim students etc. It would be plain foolish for anyone to think that they could predict the attitudes of the whole student population on the basis of the small sample studied. But this particular shortcoming does not mean that the study is useless. It may be of considerable practical benefit to the medical school in question. It could, for example: (i) show quite vividly how – in the case of the students in question – aspects of the school's climate, curriculum organisation, practices, etc. – support or undermine certain important skills and attitudes (ii) thereby suggest, perhaps neglected, issues and domains of concern which managers and medical educators should focus on. Indeed if the study is sufficiently rich and imaginative it is quite likely to have some relevance to medical education as a whole and to very different medical schools. For example the analysis may produce new ways

of conceptualising the relationships between formal and informal curricula. And these conceptualisations may prove to be valuable to many other settings even though, of course, the substance of these relationships will be different from setting to setting.

This example also makes it clear that sampling is not irrelevant in qualitative research. It would be sensible in this case for the researchers to make some effort to reflect some of the diversity of the student population rather than none of it. But the rationale for sampling is different. Qualitative researchers want their analyses to be as rich and accurate as possible – this contributes to the power, plausibility and hence influence of their work – and this entails taking into account, as far as possible within the constraints of their study, the diversity and complexity of the field. In practice this means that qualitative sampling can seem odd to those unfamiliar with the tradition. It is quite normal for a qualitative researcher to carefully select their research participants (known as *purposive sampling*) to reflect the needs of their research agenda. For example, a qualitative researcher may well search for some highly unusual or 'discrepant' cases to include in their sample, because these shed alternative light on the field and provide a challenge to more reductionist and sweeping analyses.

Subjectivity

Qualitative research is sometimes dismissed as being subjective or 'purely subjective'. Again this dismissal is merely a product of a certain restricted conception of knowledge. In order to respond to this concern it is necessary to distinguish between different senses of subjectivity and objectivity. In some senses qualitative research is, of course, openly 'subjective'. It is concerned with subjectivities and it is produced by researchers who are ready to own the influence that their own subjectivity has on its production – this latter is the 'reflexivity' discussed above. Furthermore qualitative research does not aim for a position of 'objectivity' in the sense of a neutral position outside of a cultural vantage point. Even if this is a possible model for the physical sciences, qualitative researchers would not take it seriously as a model for social research – given that both researched and researchers are necessarily within culture. However qualitative research is perfectly capable of 'objectivity' in other senses. Indeed in all of the important respects in which this idea can be meaningfully applied to social research there is no clear-cut distinction to be made between qualitative and quantitative research:

First, all aspects of qualitative research can be *open to scrutiny* – the aims, design, conduct, data, and processes of analysis should be available (as far as confidentiality will allow) to inspection and critique by others.

Second, qualitative researchers can seek to reduce partiality and *increase impartiality* in their research – they can do this not by striving for an illusory neutrality but by striving to represent and balance a range of perspectives in their analyses, and by acknowledging their own limitations.

Third, qualitative research can aim to produce research results which have *general applicability* – although, as explained above, here this does not mean making specific empirical claims about wider populations but producing theoretical results which can be applied, and 'tested out', in other contexts.

There are some qualitative researchers who would want to resist the value or relevance of this preoccupation with 'objectivity'. But for all those people for whom 'objectivity' is at the heart of research appraisal, qualitative research is simply not – as is often assumed – at some intrinsic disadvantage.

Assessing rigour

The quality and potential value of qualitative research, as with all research, depends crucially upon a thorough and open assessment of the rigour of its design, conduct and publication. It is essential that lower technical or ethical standards are not applied to the assessment of qualitative research. However, as we have stressed throughout, it is also essential that the standards applied are the appropriate ones. In the remainder of this chapter we will concentrate on some of the distinctive challenges posed by qualitative research to those interested in assessing its rigour and its other ethical implications.

Qualitative research proposals, for example, will often not include a definitive account of the proposed project's sampling, research instruments or research trajectory. This is because much qualitative research is exploratory, or at least relatively open-ended, with the definitive focus only emerging through the research process. Assessors must understand and respect this fact. However, researchers cannot expect assessors to endorse a vague, undifferentiated and purely open-ended proposal. Assessors who have a responsibility for funding, access, or the protection of well-being can reasonably expect the research team to clearly specify (a) the fixed elements of the project design (b) a detailed indication of the shape the research is likely to take and (c) any areas of uncertainty involved and the parameters of the proposed research. Assessors will then be able to make informed judgements about the scope and conditions of permissions to be sought and when, and under what circumstances, the research team would need to seek further permissions. As a minimum, assessors should expect to see an account of:

(i) The aims and expected outcomes of the study
(ii) An explicit discussion of, and some justification of, (a) sampling (b) methods of data collection (c) methods of data analysis
(iii) A consideration of the potential methodological and ethical problems associated with the proposed project.

Some of the more specific things an experienced qualitative research assessor is likely to look for are:

(i) Evidence of reflexivity
(ii) The use of different kinds and sources of data so that the same field is viewed (and compared) from different angles – this is known as 'triangulation'
(iii) Attention to the complexity of the field and to 'discrepant cases'
(iv) A readiness to include an element of quantification if and where it is appropriate.

Qualitative researchers can explain and justify their techniques of rigour by reference to a substantial body of theoretical, methodological and argumentative literature. However they should also be able to provide an accessible and thoughtful account of their purposes and practices. It is quite likely that despite the merits of the technical literature available the latter will inspire more confidence in others.

Of course the major reasons for Research Ethics Committees to monitor and regulate the design and rigour of proposed research is to protect the well-being of research subjects and to ensure that the autonomy and choices of potential research subjects are respected. These are the themes of the next two sections.

Assessing the impact on well-being

The relationship between the qualitative researcher and their research subjects tends to be closer than that associated with other styles of research. The researcher often spends a good deal of time interacting with the research participants, often in their actual or professional 'homes', talking fairly freely with them, developing relations of trust and sometimes reciprocal involvement. For this reason qualitative research can represent particular threats to the well-being of research participants.

Although not physically invasive qualitative research is, in many ways, the most socially and emotionally invasive form of research. As we have seen, it aims to get 'inside' social situations and individual subjectivity. In most instances the possibilities of harm are very slight, and it is most common for research participants to enjoy taking part in the research and sharing their experiences and lives with an interested researcher. However, it is easy to see that in other instances the risks are real – for example, in a research project exploring the experience of life-threatening illness, or bereavement. Some areas are more sensitive than others, and some participants are in more vulnerable positions than others. As usual, the more invasive the proposed research and the higher the risks of harm, the more the researcher needs to provide a justification for their study and to set out convincing safeguards for the participants' well-being.

The procedures and paperwork of RECs, which normally feature physical rather than personal invasiveness, may not lend themselves to considering these issues. Qualitative researchers often complain about the lack of space on REC forms for them to highlight, and justify, the aspects of their research which they regard as ethically relevant. A research proposal which involves substantial personal invasiveness should include a systematic consideration of the threat to well-being and how the research team plans to manage these threats. There is no simple formula available here because social relations and contexts vary indefinitely but assessors can consider the following:

(i) Do the research team have the experience (or are they drawing on credible sources of experience) to understand and manage the sensitivities at issue?

(ii) Is the research project likely to generate expectations (e.g. personal support) on the part of the (possibly vulnerable) participants that the research team is not going to meet? What arrangements have the researchers put in place to deal with these expectations? Here it is obviously most important that researchers do not confuse the fact that participants value the experience of research with its beneficence. They must, for example, also consider the impact of the research process being 'withdrawn'.

(iii) Where it seems appropriate, have the researchers given an account of how they are going to handle interpersonal and social relationships during the research? For example, is there a potential role-conflict or confusion (e.g. in the case of nurse-researchers)? How will the boundaries of the research be defined for researchers and participants?

In sensitive areas assessors should expect to see an acknowledgement of the importance of potential risks to subjects, along with a thoughtful and practical account of how they will be handled.

Assessing respect for participants

It should go without saying that researchers must respect the autonomy of research participants. Involvement in research must be voluntary and the participant's wish for privacy honoured. These are fixed points. But, again,

qualitative research raises its own challenges in this area. There is no reason to assume that qualitative research is at a disadvantage when it comes to respecting participants – in some ways it is better placed – as all that is needed is a recognition of its distinctiveness. We will discuss questions of consent and confidentiality in turn:

Consent

(a) The unfolding nature of the qualitative research process means that researchers are sometimes not in a position to provide 'full information' about the process at the start and therefore cannot obtain a 'global' informed consent at that stage. Rather, the negotiating of consent has to be seen as a longitudinal process. Formal consent to participate should still be obtained from the outset but that consent should be re-visited informally from time to time (and even sometimes formally if the direction of the research changes substantially), and research participants should clearly understand that they can withdraw from involvement at any point. (In principle this is no different from any other type of research, but the style of qualitative research brings this issue to a head in practice.)

(b) Researching settings and groups in-depth also creates challenges for consent. Suppose you are studying the cultures and practices on a hospital ward. How do you obtain consent? If, say, a small minority of staff (even ignoring patients in this instance) object to your presence on the ward, is that enough to rule out that ward? This is obviously a tricky area. How often do you need to confirm consent and with whom? How much should having the agreement of the relevant people in the hierarchy weigh? What if everyone agrees for the first three months of the project and then a newly appointed staff member objects? Like all ethical issues there are no easy answers here; it is ultimately a matter of careful practical judgement based upon explicit argument and principles.

Confidentiality

(a) It is important that researchers only 'offer' the level of confidentiality and protection of anonymity that they can deliver. In case-study work, for example, where the researchers concentrate their attention in one setting, there are particular difficulties in protecting confidentiality. Unless agreement has been obtained to the contrary, data should not be published which identify the institution or individuals within it. This sometimes means being prepared to carefully 'disguise' the setting in question (and this would typically be made explicit). Even so, where there are a comparatively small number of possible settings hiding identities is by no means easy. (Imagine a London based academic who has found time to research the hospital management practices at a 'large' metropolitan teaching hospital – many people could make good informed guesses about where the research has been done, and who, for instance, the 'Head of Personnel' referred to is). This is a very real problem for qualitative research and researchers should (i) be realistic about what they can 'offer', (ii) be scrupulous about protecting those who want confidentiality, (iii) set higher thresholds for what goes into publications compared with 'internal' reports for the research team or institution in question.

(b) Qualitative researchers will normally collect large quantities of data that might, in other circumstances, be regarded as 'gossip'. That is to say they will not only be asking research participants to talk about themselves but inviting them to talk quite freely about what is of interest to them. Naturally, this may include perceptions and stories which relate to many others (their colleagues, their bosses, their patients etc.). It is clearly essential that researchers take care to protect the interest in privacy of these other people. The fact that they may not themselves be research participants should make no difference.

Assessors should expect researchers to set out their practical approach to these issues of consent and confidentiality in 'social spaces', and the rationale for their approach.

Implications for Research Ethics Committees

RECs must ensure that they either have members who have a feel for qualitative research, or they have easy access to a group of qualitative assessors or advisers.

In many cases there may be a need to review the paperwork and procedures of RECs to ensure that they are suitable for qualitative research appraisal.

In particular there is a need:

(a) To make sure that certain aspects of qualitative research proposals are not assessed using the wrong criteria.

For example: (i) It is usually inappropriate to consider statistical representativeness or statistical generalisability. (ii) Generally qualitative research studies pose little risk of harm to health or physical well-being. They will, by contrast, typically depend upon a degree of personal and social invasiveness – although in some cases it will not take long to establish that the invasiveness, and the associated risks of harm, are minimal.

(b) To make sure that certain aspects of qualitative research proposal are not under-scrutinised.

For example: (i) It is essential that researchers are familiar with the appropriate techniques of rigour for

their work, and specifically that they have a critically reflective approach to it. (ii) Some qualitative research studies are potentially highly invasive socially and emotionally. In these cases the justification for the research, and the safeguards proposed need very careful consideration indeed.

REFERENCES

Atkinson, P. (1992). *Understanding Ethnographic Texts*. London: Sage.

Black, N. (1994). Why we need qualitative research. *Journal of Epidemiology and Community Health*, **48**, 425–6.

Bryman, A. (1988). *Quantity and Quality in Social Research*. London: Unwin.

Glaser, B. & Strauss, A. (1967). *The Discovery of Grounded Theory*. Chicago: Aldine Publishing.

De Laine, M. (2000). *Fieldwork, Participation and Practice: Ethics and Dilemmas in Qualitative Research*. London: Sage.

Denzin, N.K. (1970). *The Research Act*. New Jersey: Prentice Hall.

Greenhalgh, T. & Taylor, R. (1997). Papers that go beyond numbers. *British Medical Journal*, **315**, 740–3.

Hammersley, M. (1990). *Reading Ethnographic Research*. London: Longman.

Hammersley, M. & Atkinson, P. (1995). *Ethnography. Principles in Practice*. London: Routledge.

Lincoln, Y. & Guba, E. (1985). *Naturalistic Inquiry*. London: Sage Publications.

Mays, N. & Pope, C. (1995). Rigour and qualitative research. *British Medical Journal*, **311**, 109–12.

McNiff, J. (1988). *Human Inquiry in Action: Developments in New Paradigm Research* London: Sage Publications.

Miles, M. & Huberman, A. (1994). *Qualitative Data Analysis*. London: Sage Publications.

Pope, C. & Mays, N. (1995). Reaching the parts other methods cannot reach: an introduction to qualitative methods in health and health service research. *British Medical Journal*, **311**, 42–5.

Strauss, A. (1987). *Qualitative Analysis for Social Scientists*. Cambridge: Cambridge University Press.

Strauss, A. & Corbin, J. (1990). *Basics of Qualitative Research: Grounded Theory Procedures and Techniques*. London: Sage.

ADDITIONAL QUALITATIVE RESEARCH REFERENCES

Following is an annotated bibliography which was created by Dr Tom Farsides, Lecturer in Social Psychology at the University of Sussex for participants on the King's College Centre for Medical Law and Ethics' Short Course on The Ethics for Research on Humans.

Highly recommended

Bryman, A. (1988). *Quantity and Quality in Social Research*. London: Routledge.

A very sensitive and sensible evaluation of the strengths and weaknesses of qualitative and quantitative research methods.

Creswell, J.W. (1998). *Qualitative Inquiry and Research Design: Choosing Among Five Traditions*. London: Sage.

The first book to turn to when attempting to answer specific questions about methodological and conceptual similarities and differences between any of the five traditions considered; life history, phenomenology, grounded theory, ethnography, and case study. A glaring omission, however, is a comparative treatment of ethical concerns.

Greenhalgh, T. & Hurwitz, B. (eds.) (1998). *Narrative Based Medicine: Dialogue and Discourse in Clinical Practice*. London: BMJ Books.

In particular, Chapters 3 ('The median isn't the message,' by Stephen Jay Gould, pp. 29–33) and 24 ('Narrative in an evidence based world,' by Trisha Greenhalgh, pp. 247–265) illustrate why a sparse knowledge of quantitative sample norms sometimes needs to be supplemented or replaced by a detailed knowledge of particulars that may (or may not) deviate from those norms.

LeCompte, M.D. & Goetz, J.P. (1982). Problems of reliability and validity in ethnographic research. *Review of Educational Research*, **51**, 31–60.

Attempt to establish parallels for reliability and validity criteria within qualitative research in pursuit of objectivity. They discuss such concepts as history and maturation, observer effects, selection and regression, mortality, spurious conclusions, and external validity.

Murphy, E., Dingwall, R., Greatbatch, D., Parker S. & Watson, P. (1998). Qualitative research methods in health technology assessment: A review of the literature. *Health Technology Assessment, 2 (16)*. Available on-line from links found at:
http://www.soton.ac.uk/~hta. Currently located at:
http://www.hta.nhsweb.nhs.uk/fullmono/mon216.pdf

A long but plain speaking and thorough overview of qualitative methods as they apply to 'real world' research. Particularly recommended are the 'Executive summary' and Chapters 1, 4, and 5. For those concerned solely with ethical issues, Chapter 5 ('Criteria for assessing qualitative research') alone might suffice.

Robson, C. (1993). *Real World Research: A Resource for Social Scientists and Practitioner Researchers*. Oxford: Blackwell.

A fantastic resource book. Beyond compare as a first-resort when conducting 'real-world' research using more or less any methodology. Has one chapter on 'the analysis of qualitative data.' An appendix contains a (now slightly out of date) statement of the British Psychological Society's views of 'ethical principles for conducting research with human participants.' Another appendix provides guidelines on writing and recognising good (and not so good) research proposals.

Miles, M.B. & Huberman, A.M. (1994). *Qualitative Data Analysis: An Expanded Source Book*, 2nd edn. London: Sage.

A very practical 'realist' overview and attempted synthesis of qualitative methods. Chapters 2, 6 and 10 are 'essential' chapters for learning about how 'realist' qualitative research may be fruitfully pursued. Chapter 11, 'Ethical issues in analysis,' adopts the simple

straightforward and practical approach as the rest of the book and is highly recommended for interested LREC members.

For more specific interests

Case study

Stake, R. (1994). Case studies. In *Handbook of Qualitative Research* ed. N.K. Denzin & Y.S. Lincoln pp. 236–247. London: Sage.

A chapter-length overview of case study research in a qualitative collection of much broader interest. Contains references to the earlier classics of Lincoln & Guba (1985) and Yin (1989).

Conversation analysis

Silverman, D. (2001). *Interpreting Qualitative Data : Methods for Analyzing Talk, Text and Interaction*, 2nd edn. London: Sage.

Champions reliability by using high specification and low inference of category generation.

Discourse analysis

Potter, J. & Wetherell, M. (1987). *Discourse and Social Psychology: Beyond Attitudes and Behaviour*. London: Sage.

The most important exposition of discourse analysis. Makes explicit that discourse analysts 'do not intend to use the discourse as a pathway to entities or phenomena lying "beyond" the text . . . Rather, the focus is on the discourse *itself* : how it is organized and what it is doing' (p. 49). Discourse analysts are 'interested in language use rather than the [attitudes and behaviour of] people generating the language' (p. 161). Thus, discourse analysts attempt to identify the 'functions' discourses serve and how those functions may be served by the discourse. They attempt to do this without reference to anything beyond (interpretations of) the text at their disposal.

Grounded theory

Strauss, A.L. (1987). *Qualitative Analysis for Social Scientists*. Cambridge: Cambridge University Press.

Part 2 of the introductory chapter, entitled 'grounded theory analysis: main elements' (pp. 22–39) is an excellent overview of grounded theory. This details the main methodological rules of thumb by which grounded theorists attempt to generate theory from data, as opposed to using data to test theories.

Strauss, A.L. & Corbin, J.M. (1998). *Basics of Qualitative Research: Techniques and Procedures for Developing Grounded Theory*. London: Sage.

For those who prefer more up to date references. Develops the classic Strauss & Corbin (1990) text which is both highly cited and eminently readable.

Interviewing

Kvale, S. (1996). *Interviews: An introduction to qualitative research interviewing*. London: Sage.

Much cited, but of interest to LREC members primarily for its Chapter 6, 'Ethical issues in interview inquiries.' This usefully considers ethical issues that may be particularly relevant at different stages of the research processes, from identifying the scientific value of the knowledge sought to considering the consequences of publishing findings.

Other recent and/or important texts

Bryman, A. (2001). *Social Research Methods.* Oxford University Press. ISBN: 0198742045. Paperback.

Bryman, A. & Burgess, R.G. (eds.) (1994). *Analyzing Qualitative Data.* Routledge. ISBN: 041506063X Paperback – 232 pages.

Bryman, A. & Cramer, D. (2001). *Quantitative data analysis with SPSS Release 10 for Windows*, revised edn. Routledge. ISBN: 0415244005 Paperback – 336 pages.

Creswell, J.W. (1994). *Research Design: Qualitative and Quantitative Approaches.* Sage Publications. ISBN: 0803952554 Paperback.

Fielding, N.G. & Lee, R.M. (1998). *Computer analysis and qualitative research* (New techniques for social research). Sage Publications. ISBN: 0803974833 Paperback.

Henwood, K.L. & Pidgeon, N.F. (1992). Qualitative research and psychological theorising. *British Journal of Psychology*, **83 (1)**, 97–112.

Elliot, R., Fischer, C.T. & Rennie, D.L. (1999). Evolving guidelines for publication of qualitative research studies in psychology and related fields. *British Journal of Clinical Psychology*, **38**, 215–29.

Elliot, R., Fischer, C.T. & Rennie, D.L. (2000). Also against methodolatry: a reply to Reicher. *British Journal of Clinical Psychology*, **39**, 7–10.

Madill, A., Jordan A. & Shirley, C. (2000). Objectivity and reliability in qualitative analysis: realist, contextualist and radical constructionist epistemologies. *British Journal of Psychology*, **91**, 1–20.

Punch, K.F. (1998). *Introduction to Social Research: Quantitative and Qualitative Approaches.* Sage Publications. ISBN: 0761958134 Paperback.

Reicher, S. (2000). Against methodolatry: Some comments on Elliot, Fischer & Rennie. *British Journal of Clinical Psychology*, **39**, 1–6.

Tacq, J. (1996). *Multivariate Analysis Techniques in Social Science Research: From Problem to Analysis.* Sage Publications. ISBN: 076195273X Paperback.

Weiss, R.S. (1995). *Learning from Strangers: The Art and Method of Qualitative Interview Studies.* Free Press. ISBN: 0684823128 Paperback – 246 pages.

Wilkinson, S. (1998). Focus groups in health research: Exploring the meanings of health and illness: *Journal of Health Psychology*, **3 (3)**, 329–348.

USEFUL WEBSITES

'On doing qualitative research linked to ethical healthcare: An introduction to methodologies of qualitative research'
'Qualitative research: A vital resource for ethical healthcare'
both available on:

http://www.wellcome.ac.uk/en/1/mismisethres.html

Complementary and alternative medicine: challenges for research ethics committees

Julie Stone

Department of Human Science and Medical Ethics, Barts and The London,
Queen Mary's School of Medicine and Dentistry, London, UK

Introduction

Within the last 30 years, there has been a huge growth in usage of complementary and alternative therapies (CAM) both in the UK and world wide (Eisenberg et al., 1998). A report to the Department of Health estimated that up to 5 million patients in the UK may have consulted a CAM practitioner in the preceding year (Mills and Budd, 2000) and a recent Report by the House of Lords Select Committee on science and technology recognised that use of CAM in the UK is widespread and growing (House of Lords, 2000).

Whereas in the past, orthodox medicine was hostile towards CAM approaches, doctors are increasingly interested in the potential benefits CAM may offer their patients, particular those patients suffering from chronic, undifferentiated diseases for which conventional medicine has little to offer. A 1995 study estimated that 39.5% of GP practices in England were providing access to CAM therapists for their NHS patients (Thomas et al., 1995). A recent survey of UK GPs carried out by the BMA (BMA, 2000) found that 79% of those responding felt that acupuncture should be made available to patients on the NHS. The most popular therapies currently are the so-called 'big five', namely: acupuncture, homoeopathy, herbalism, osteopathy and chiropractic (the last two of which are subject to statutory regulation). Other popular therapies include aromatherapy, reflexology and healing. Most consultations with CAM practitioners occur in the private sector, with patients paying for sessions out of their own pockets. Most CAM practitioners are not medically qualified, although growing numbers of doctors, nurses, midwives and physiotherapists also utilise CAM techniques.

The current policy trend, both in the UK and the US, is towards the integration of conventional and CAM approaches (Rees and Weil, 2001). In the UK, this is likely to be evidenced by greater access to CAM treatments available through the NHS. For integration to occur, a sound evidence base must be established (BMA, 2000). Many CAM practitioners are committed to evidence-based CAM. The Research Council for Complementary Medicine's CISCOM database contains nearly 70 000 CAM references, including over 5000 randomised control trials (RCTs). Certainly, there have been concerns about the methodological rigour of much CAM research which has been conducted in the past. Systematic reviews have concluded that larger, well-designed studies are necessary before making authoritative guidance (Nahin and Straus, 2001). Centres of research excellence now exist and research methodology has a much higher profile in the education and training of CAM practitioners than in the past. Both the UK and US governments are currently funding research into the use of CAM.

Most of the concerns in this area turn on whether the research into CAM treatments is sufficiently scientific. If CAM is to be provided on the NHS, this will need to be on the basis of evidence. Such evidence may include qualitative as well as quantative aspects. However, many CAM therapists are not interested in exploring explanatory models for their therapy. Some CAM practitioners, coming to healing from a non-scientific background, are concerned that the entire framework underpinning medical research is based on the predominating biomedical paradigm which is starkly at odds with their beliefs about disease causation and appropriate treatment. Conventional research uses concepts of health and disease, cause and effect and massifying (extracting findings from the general population to the individual) which do not capture the holistic experience which aims to take account of the uniqueness of the individual patient (Stone, 2002).

Other therapists feel that the efficacy of their therapy does not need to be proven in scientific terms because the therapy has had a long history of safe and effective use. Acupuncture and herbal medicine are examples of healing traditions which go back thousands of years and for which much empirical data exists, but not necessarily in the form that modern-day researchers would find acceptable. However, the argument that a long history of safe usage obviates the need for further research is unsustainable as a basis for integration, since providers need evidence not only as to the efficacy of the therapy in question, but also as to the comparative efficacy between CAM approaches and conventional approaches to the extent that this can be ascertained.

Implications of integration on CAM research

The implications of integration are important in a research context for three reasons:
(i) Integration will be into an increasingly evidence-based culture and this will require a stronger research base for CAM than currently exists.
(ii) Integration into a dominant biomedical paradigm presupposes that the research will be comparable in standard and design to scientific research of allopathic treatments.
(iii) Integration of CAM will be into an already cash-starved NHS and so will require evidence as to cost effectiveness as well as efficacy.

Why scientific research into CAM may be difficult or inappropriate

CAM relationships differ from conventional treatment in a number of critical ways which may make research difficult:
• Holistic relationships rely on highly individualised methods of treatment and prescribing, which vary according to the individual, rather than being based on the presenting symptom. The effect of this is that product-based therapies (such as homoeopathy and herbalism) are extremely difficult to fit within a 'regular' RCT framework. For example, in a clinical setting, 100 patients with seemingly identical hayfever symptoms might each be prescribed a different remedy by a homoeopath or herbal medical practitioner, based on the individual's unique constitution and a broader diagnostic base than that used in conventional medicine.
• Many therapists routinely combine a range of therapeutic modalities in a single treatment session. Most conventional researchers attempt to evaluate the effect of a specific intervention and would consider that allowing practitioners to utilise different approaches with different patients would introduce too many variables into a study.
• RCTs may be able to evaluate CAM treatments with specific effects but are not the best tool for measuring non-specific effects, including the healing effect of the therapeutic encounter itself. Since many practitioners believe that there is a synergistic relationship between specific and non-specific effects, a clinical trial which only evaluated specific effects would be of limited value.
• In many therapies, the precise mechanism for how the therapy may work is, as yet, unknown.
• Many practitioners lack the training or experience to conduct high quality research, although several centres of excellence exist.
• Most practitioners work in single-handed, private practice and cannot afford to take time out to conduct research, or to participate in the numerous activities required to underwrite research, e.g. time to peer review research proposals, or to serve as advisors or trustees to research charities.
• Since most CAM patients pay privately for their treatment, there is not an obvious source of CAM patients upon whom CAM research can be conducted. Consideration needs to be given as to whether waiving/reducing fees in return for participation in a trial would count as unacceptable coercion which would invalidate the participant's consent.
• There has been a reluctance to fund CAM therapies by the major sources of research funding, although the main medical research charities are demonstrating increasing interest in this area.
• There has been publication and reviewer bias against CAM research in the past, with many mainstream medical journals being unwilling to publish what they perceive as 'soft evidence', and NHS funders unwilling to accept evidence published in CAM journals or non-peer-reviewed journals (Resch *et al.*, 2000).

What research questions need to be answered?

Vincent and Furnham (1997) identify five key areas for CAM research. These will be of varying importance depending on the developmental stage of a therapy and what research has already been carried out. The questions they identify are:
(i) Does the therapy have a beneficial effect on any individual disease or disorder?
(ii) Does the treatment have any advantage over existing treatments in terms of efficacy, safety, patient preference, cost and availability?

(iii) Is this effect primarily, or even partly, due to the specific and intended action of the treatment as opposed to placebo?

(iv) What mechanism might underlie the therapy's actions?

(v) The reliability and validity of diagnosis, the value of individual techniques, the role of the practitioner and perhaps the attitude of the patient.

Need to develop appropriate research methodologies for evaluating CAM

As discussed, the RCT, whilst considered the gold standard for evaluating drug treatments, may not be the most appropriate mechanism for evaluating CAM. Accordingly, the onus lies on CAM therapists to devise appropriate research methodology. Since CAM lacks the research infrastructure, established research groups are encouraged to consider collaborating with CAM practitioners (BMA, 2000). Other points to bear in mind are:

• Subjective outcome measures will form an important element of much CAM research, since CAM draws heavily on the patient's subjective experience of illness.

• Objective outcome measures may nonetheless be possible and desirable in much CAM research – this may require someone other than the treating practitioner to collect data to eliminate bias.

• The use of a placebo may not be possible, appropriate or desirable. Much debate exists, for example, over the use of 'sham' acupuncture as a placebo, since even superficial needling may exert a beneficial effect.

• Patient preference needs to be built into the trial design (particularly if the patients are fee-paying) (Fitter & Thomas, 1997), since this is likely to optimise outcomes and give a more realistic picture of the interaction than randomisation, possibly against the patient's preferences.

• Double blinding is unlikely to be feasible, e.g. in manipulative therapies/acupuncture.

• Pragmatic trials (which measure the outcomes of therapies as they are practised in real life situations) may provide more helpful data than exploratory RCTs (in which the practitioner's interventions are circumscribed and bear no resemblance to the reality of the CAM therapeutic encounter). Rather than attempting to eliminate it, the pragmatic trial seeks to maximise any placebo effect along with specific treatment effects.

• CAM therapies may not show benefits as quickly as conventional treatment and this needs to be factored into research design.

• The definition of what counts as an acceptable end point may vary from patient to patient. Since most CAM practitioners reject Cartesian assumptions about the mind/body split, a successful CAM outcome may not necessarily manifest in a physical 'cure' but in improvements in the patient's emotional and spiritual outlook.

Implications for Research Ethics Committees

Although there is limited NHS provision, at the present time most CAM encounters take place in the private sector. Although RECs are only mandated to vet research related to NHS patients, they are able, *and arguably obliged*, to consider any application affecting the well-being of human subjects. As moves towards integration increase, LRECs/MRECs are likely to see a significant increase in CAM applications in the coming months and years, so need to be aware of the particular issues that CAM research raises. The main problem which is likely to beset CAM research is that LREC/MREC members may know very little about CAM therapeutics. This, together with the medically dominated constitution of most ethics committees may lead to scepticism about CAM applications. Ethics committees should not dismiss or trivialise applications merely because they have little belief in, or experience of, non-conventional approaches to health and healing, or because they remain unconvinced as to the value of qualitative research. The duty of RECs is to protect research participants from harm and to promote ethically sound research. Whilst CAM therapies are, for the main part, considerably safer than conventional medical treatments, the parameters of what constitutes acceptable risk/benefit may be rather different in CAM than in conventional medicine and is far more likely to be subjectively determined by the patient.

Given the need for sound research in this area, LRECs/MRECs should facilitate research wherever possible, providing assistance with trial design if necessary, and making constructive comments if it is felt that a protocol is unacceptable in its present form. RECs should consider CAM applications with an open mind. Unless LRECs/MRECs have particular expertise in deciding these issues, they should co-opt onto the committee someone with the appropriate expertise to advise on a CAM application. The Research Council for Complementary Medicine (information@rccm.org.uk) and the Foundation for Integrated Medicine (enquiries@fimed.org) may be useful resources in this regard.

REFERENCES

British Medical Association. (2000). *Acupuncture: Efficacy, Safety and Practice*. Harwood Academic Publishers.

Eisenberg, D.M., Davis, R.B. and Ettner, S.I. (1998). Trends in alternative medicine use in the United States, 1990–1997: results of a follow-up national survey. *Journal of the American Medical Association*, **280**, 1569–1575.

Fitter, M.J. and Thomas, K.J. (1997). Evaluating complementary therapies for use in the National Health Service: 'horses for courses'. Part 1: the design challenge. *Complementary Therapies in Medicine*, **5**, 90–93.

House of Lords. (2000). *Complementary and Alternative Medicine*. London: Stationery Office.

Mills, S.Y. and Budd, S. (2000). *Professional Organisation of Complementary and Alternative Medicine in the United Kingdom*. Exeter University: The Centre for Complementary Health Studies.

Nahin, R. and Straus, S. (2001). Research into complementary and alternative medicine: problems and potential. *British Medical Journal*, **322**, 161–164.

Rees, L. and Weil, A. (2001). Integrated Medicine. *British Medical Journal*, **322**, 119–120.

Resch, K.I., Ernst, E. and Garrow, J. (2000). A randomized controlled study of reviewer bias against an unconventional therapy. *Journal of the Royal Society of Medicine*, **93**, 164–167.

Stone, J. (2002). *An Ethical Framework for Complementary and Alternative Therapists*. London: Routledge.

Thomas K.J., Fall, M., Parry, G. and Nicholl, J. (1995). National Survey of Access to Complementary Health Care via General Practice. DoH Report. Sheffield: Medical Care Research Unit.

Vincent, C. and Furnham, A. (1997). *Complementary Medicine. A Research Perspective*. Chichester: John Wiley.

USEFUL WEBSITES

House of Lords Science and Technology Sixth Report –
Complementary and Alternative Medicine
[http://www.parliament.the-stationery-office.co.uk/pa/ld199900/
ldselect/ldsctech/123/12301.htm

National Center for Complementary and Alternative
Medicine
http://nccam.nih.gov/

The Research Council for Complementary Medicine
http://www.rccm.org.uk/

The White House Commission on Complementary and Alternative
Medicine Policy
http://www.whccamp.hhs.gov/

The ethical review of student research in the context of the governance arrangements for research ethics committees

Richard Ashcroft[1] and Michael Parker[2]

[1]Department of Primary Health Care and General Practice, Imperial College of Science, Technology and Medicine, London, UK
[2]Oxford Centre for Ethics and Communication Skills in Health Care (Ethox), Oxford University, UK

Introduction

Students of health care and the biomedical and social sciences generally require some training in the methods of research in their disciplines. At upper undergraduate and postgraduate levels, such training is often deepened by requiring students to carry out research projects themselves. The situation regarding the ethical review of such projects has been unclear in the UK and elsewhere for some time. Recent guidance from the UK Department of Health has created some clarity in this area, but there is still much room for interpretation and debate. In this brief chapter, we discuss this guidance and set out some general principles for the review of student projects.

Student research and research governance

Current thinking on the ethics of research lays great stress on the implementation of effective structures and processes for quality management of research and ensuring that research protects the interests of participants while facilitating wider health services, social and scientific goals. This approach is known as 'research governance'. In 2000, the UK Government's Department of Health issued guidance on a general approach to research governance throughout the UK National Health Service (NHS), the *Research Governance Framework for Health and Social Care*.[1] As part of the implementation programme for this framework, in 2001 the Department of Health's Central Office for Research Ethics Committees (COREC) issued *Governance Arrangements for Research Ethics Committees* (GAFREC).[2]

---

[1] Available at http://www.doh.gov.uk/research/rd3/nhsrandd/researchgovernance/govhome.htm

[2] Available at http://www.doh.gov.uk/research/documents/gafrec.doc
All references in the text are to paragraph numbers in this document.

This replaced previously existing guidance specifying the role and responsibilities of Research Ethics Committees (RECs) in the NHS, and sets out the responsibilities of RECs, researchers and sponsors *vis-à-vis* the ethics and governance of research projects in the NHS.

GAFREC recommends that research conducted outside the NHS or in a social care context be reviewed, either by an NHS REC, or by an independent REC complying with the general principles of GAFREC.

The only statement in GAFREC relating to student research is as follows:

10.4 Research to be undertaken by students primarily for educational purposes (e.g. as a requirement for a University degree course) shall be considered according to the same ethical and operational standards as are applied to other research. In such cases the supervisor takes on the role and responsibilities of the sponsor. In reaching its decision, the REC will wish to consider the broader overall benefits gained by such research.

In the context of the GAFREC document as a whole, this could be read, narrowly, to imply that certain types of research, because they fall outside the express remit of NHS RECs, are more loosely regulated than others. For instance, students conducting physiological experiments on each other in a university laboratory, or students interviewing members of the public about their health beliefs (provided they did not identify participants through NHS lists), might be thought the kind of research outside the scope of GAFREC. Conversely, any research by students which does fall within GAFREC's scope now appears to be much more tightly regulated than it has been in the past. We would argue that this is mistaken, because GAFREC, rather than being a set of rules, is a recommendation of quality and ethical standards, which, while binding (as management decisions) on the NHS and its staff, represent current best practice for human participants' research in all contexts. In the remainder of this chapter we will set out some processes and standards, consistent with GAFREC, which make sensible review of student research clear and practicable.

Governance of student projects

Paragraph 10.4 makes certain key points clear:
- The same ethical standards apply to student projects as to any other research.
- The same operational standards apply to student projects as to any other research.
- The supervisor of the student's work has the role of sponsor.
- Review should take into account the broad social goals served by allowing students to do 'training' projects, but these goals remain secondary to the dignity, safety, rights and well-being of the participants in research.

This paragraph is supplemented by an earlier paragraph, 10.2, which reads as follows:

10.2 Where a potential applicant is inexperienced, there should be an identified supervisor of adequate quality and experience who will counter-sign the application form, and then share the responsibility for the ethical and scientific conduct of the research. A current signed CV of the supervisor should be submitted with the application.

10.2 and 10.4 together address the requirements of a previous paragraph, which reads as follows:

10.1 The application shall be submitted by the "principal investigator" who is the person designated as taking overall responsibility within the team of researchers for the design, conduct and reporting of the study. It follows that the applicant should be of adequate qualification and expertise to fulfil this important role.

The Research Governance Framework requires every project to have an identified principal investigator, funder, sponsor, employing organisation (for the investigators), care organisation (host of the research), and responsible care professional (where patient care is involved or may be necessary to support the research investigation) (Research Governance Framework 3.3.1 Box C). In much student research, the costs are minimal or zero, so that the roles of the funder and sponsor coincide; most students are not carrying out research as employees, although their supervisor normally will be an employee of a healthcare organisation, research organisation, university or college.

According to paragraphs 10.1,2,4 of GAFREC, and paragraph 3.3.1 of the Research Governance Framework, student research is always to be governed by a set of mechanisms and identified responsibilities which support students in their research and protect participants. The degree of responsibility falling on the student varies according to their experience and qualifications to carry out the research; the more inexperienced the student, the greater the responsibility falling on the supervisor and host institution to ensure that the research is carried out effectively and ethically. In practice, this will mean tailoring research projects to the student's ability and experience, both to achieve satisfactory educational goals and to minimise the risk of harm to participants. But it will also require certain duties from supervisors and educational institutions.

At section 9.8, GAFREC makes it clear that research which merely duplicates existing knowledge or is methodologically inadequate is unethical. This implies that students should demonstrate that the project they wish to undertake is innovative. At 9.13a, it states that the proposal for review must establish that the proposed methods and resources requested are appropriate to the question at hand, the ethical standards required, and the completion of the project in reasonable time. At 9.13g it requires the applicant to show that the site and supervision arrangements for research are adequate. Further, at 10.5–10.6 it is clear that the application requirements to RECs are the same, whatever the nature of the application – whether or not this is a student project.

This is a tall order for most students. Some suggestions following from this are as follows:
- Students should concentrate their efforts on producing literature-based research reports, until such time as they acquire sufficient knowledge and experience to identify a genuine research question (however modest).
- Students wishing to practise research techniques should begin by working under a supervisor's direction with the supervisor as principal investigator, and with appropriate employment or equivalent contracts, and liability arrangements as necessary. Working as an experienced researcher's assistant will not normally necessitate an application in the student's own right.
- Where a student has identified an innovative research question, he or she should work with a supervisor who will work to an agreed code of practice, consistent with the Research Governance Framework, to guarantee the quality of the research method and the ethical safeguards required.
- The responsibility taken by the student for the research project will grow according to the student's experience, training and qualifications, and mastery of the methods and management skills required. At a certain point, the sponsor, supervisor and student will agree that the student is the appropriate principal applicant, and will take

over all the responsibilities implied in GAFREC and the Research Governance document.

- Where the student is a health care professional, the professional standards which apply to them apply equally to the research. This may transfer some of the legal liability and moral responsibility to their shoulders, but in practice where the professional is a trainee learning a new technique (here, research methods), the responsibility remains shared with the supervisor, sponsor and host institution.
- All students carrying out research are obliged to maintain the same high ethical standards as their seniors. This applies to consent, information, risk control and proper technique. In particular, where the student is carrying out research on other students, care must be taken not to exploit the 'peer relationship'; where research is carried out with patients or members of the public, they must be informed that the research is being carried out by a student and that it is primarily for educational reasons, unless the research objective is very clearly primary (as in a PhD, for instance).

Paragraph 10.4 seems to open the door to a relaxation of scientific standards, or replacing those standards by 'educational standards'. Thus, it would be reasonable to say that the aim of most student projects is not to add to the stock of human knowledge, but rather to contribute to their training, and the stock of social good is advanced by adding another trained professional to the cadre. Under this theory, student projects should state that they are educational projects, that the researcher is a student and that he or she aims to learn how to do something, rather than to contribute to science. These aims should certainly be made clear to participants. In practice, however, it is very hard to distinguish, as a general rule, where the line between educational and scientific aims is to be drawn. In addition, patients in health care settings may find it highly confusing to learn that their doctor may be highly qualified in one way, as their doctor, but a novice in another way, as a researcher. We recommend that RECs bear in mind that some projects are far more 'educational' than 'scientific' in nature, and look on educational projects sympathetically; but GAFREC makes it clear that formally no special case is to be made, and indeed higher governance standards are required.

In most educational institutions, students working under a particular supervisor, or undertaking a particular course or module will present their work for review in batches at certain times of year, predictable in advance. GAFREC implies that the principal investigator is responsible for ensuring the scientific and ethical standards are met in a project, and that application for review is made in proper form at the appropriate time. This entails – for most student research at undergraduate or Masters' level – the supervisor acting as principal applicant, or in some cases as co-principal. For more advanced students the supervisor acts as sponsor (who is responsible for ensuring that REC review is sought, that the scientific quality of the work is up to the mark – usually by independent review – and that appropriate management and monitoring is in place).

This responsibility necessitates a kind of contract between student, supervisor and institution to the effect that:

- the student will have met the supervisor and discussed the project in detail
- the supervisor will make a project timetable with the student
- the student will prepare protocol and application material in good time for the supervisor
- the supervisor will review the project in detail before signing it off as principal or co-principal investigator, where necessary submitting the project to independent scientific review (possibly by a Faculty or Departmental committee)
- the supervisor will take overall responsibility for ensuring that the student has the support and oversight necessary to conduct the project safely and efficiently, in time for writing up and submission for examination
- the supervisor will be responsible for sending a copy of the final report to the REC. Here 'responsible' means either doing it or seeing that it is done, as appropriate. Failure to carry out these responsibilities should be a disciplinary matter (for supervisor and student alike).

All of these requirements on the student and supervisor should be set out in the institution's code of practice, which should also cover the working conditions and expectations for student research assistantships, work experience, part time work, and 'elective' projects (particularly for medical students).

REC review of student projects

GAFREC does not make reviewing student projects easier or more lenient. However it does structure the process, in such a way as to make it clearer what kinds of project are acceptable from students. By casting matters in terms of quality and ethical standards, it becomes clearer what work we can expect from students at differing levels of experience, what projects are or are not appropriate, and what level of responsibility is to be attributed to students and supervisors alike. This will mean that certain kinds of project become less likely to be submitted, while others become more likely. It may mean a rise in workload for many committees, but a fall in workload for others. Two proposals may simplify matters.

First, it is clear that RECs should work with educational institutions to establish very clear understandings about what kinds of project, and what application process, are acceptable in the light of GAFREC and the Research Governance Framework. This kind of partnership and communication, while maintaining independence, is mandated by paragraph 1.10 of GAFREC, which begins 'the protection of research participants is best served by close co-operation and efficient communication amongst all those who share the responsibility for it.'

Second, on consideration of the strict time standards now imposed on REC review (on receipt of a valid application, the REC must report within 60 days), it is clear that RECs will be strict about what amounts to a valid application and efficient in reporting to applicants.(7.10–7.16) Inadequately presented applications will not be reviewed; valid applications will be reported on within 60 days. This is a long time in student time, but a short period in the real world! Given that most RECs review many proposals in addition to student proposals, GAFREC authorises Health Authorities to establish as many RECs in their area as necessary in order to ensure that all protocols in an area are reviewed within 60 days.(4.8, 7.16) It also authorises Health Authorities to establish a single administrative office to service all RECs in their area (4.8), and to recover the costs of review from funders or sites outside the NHS. (7.22) On this basis, it is possible for a Health Authority, in consultation with educational institutions, to establish a REC on lines consistent with GAFREC which reviews only – or mainly – student research projects, and sits to a timetable determined by the points on the student calendar when bulk applications are to be expected. An alternative would be to establish a subcommittee of an existing REC, although GAFREC appears to require the same standards to be used as in the full REC. (Standards for 'expedited review' are to be published shortly, in part B of GAFREC, which sets out model standing orders and similar details.)

Conclusion

Much ambiguity remains regarding the review of student projects. Are such projects properly understood as 're-search'? If not, do they fall into GAFREC's remit? How are projects outside the broad reach of the NHS to be reviewed, and how is this requirement to be enforced? Are standards for research methodology in student projects being set too high? But we believe that the GAFREC standards do at least provide a clearer and more straightforward approach to student projects than hitherto. We strongly believe in the importance of helping students to learn research methods in a safe and constructive environment. What appears clear from GAFREC is that the responsibilities of supervisors and educational institutions to provide students with appropriate training, support and oversight are much greater than before. Given that protection of the interests of patients, the public and student volunteers themselves is so important, this raising of standards is only appropriate.

Acknowledgement

This paper was prepared by the authors following a presentation on the ethical review of student research at an Association of Research Ethics Committees conference on 'Qualitative Research Review and Student Research', held in Bristol in July 2000. Following this meeting, AREC set up a working party to develop a set of guidelines for the review of student research. Whilst an earlier and very different version of this paper was used as the starting point for discussions at the working party, it should not be taken as representative of the views of AREC, its members, or the members of the working party.

The ethics of genetic research

Ruth Chadwick

Institute for Environment, Philosophy and Public Policy, Lancaster University, UK

Introduction: what is genetic research?

New scientific work in human genetics and the increasing use of large-scale genetic databases may require new thinking about the ethics of genetic research. Genetic research covers both research on single gene disorders such as cystic fibrosis, and research into any genetic contribution to common multifactorial diseases such as heart disease, diabetes and the cancers. It also covers research into mental disorders such as schizophrenia, into behavioural differences such as learning disabilities, personality or behavioural traits and the genetic variations responsible for differential response to drugs (the basis for pharmacogenetics). Genetic research also includes gene therapy trials. For the purpose of this chapter, non-human genetic research such as research on plants or animals will not be covered.

There has been a debate about the extent to which genetics and genetic research raise distinctive ethical issues. Some writers argue for forms of genetic exceptionalism. They have pointed out that genetic information about an individual has implications for their blood relatives, that it is predictive and that it may be obtained before any symptoms of a disorder are apparent. Others think that genetics does not raise ethical issues that are wholly distinctive, although it raises issues that may be different in degree.

The ethical issues most often discussed in relation to genetic research are that:

- genetic research could lead to discrimination against and stigmatisation of individuals and populations, and be misused to promote racism or for eugenic purposes
- patenting and commercialisation may hamper access to genetic discoveries for research and medical purposes
- the importance of genetic causes of social and other human problems may be exaggerated

- genetic research, or some of its applications, might be used in ways that fail to respect the values, traditions and integrity of populations, families and individuals
- the scientific community may not engage adequately with the public in planning and conducting genetic research (HUGO, 1996).

During the years 1990–2000, a great deal of genetic research was aimed at the decoding of the human genome. The HUGO (Human Genome Organisation) Ethics Committee made a number of recommendations in 1996 that responded to these concerns, as did many other international, national and professional ethics committees. Recommendations typically covered requirements for competence on the part of the researcher and for the researcher to consult with participants; to seek informed consent; to respect the choices of research subjects; to maintain confidentiality; to achieve collaboration between individuals, populations and researchers; to identify any conflicts of interest and to provide appropriate compensation without undue inducements.

Distinctive ethical issues may be raised by genetic research on specific sorts of research populations (Clarke et al., 2001). There are populations such as that of the UK which are ethnically and genetically very varied. The UK has been regarded as a good site for a national collection that would associate genetic differences with disease risk. Then there are populations, such as that of Iceland, which have remained geographically isolated and which contain much less genetic variation. This is one reason why it has been claimed that Iceland is such a good population on which to study the minute differences between otherwise more genetically similar individuals that might make them differ in their susceptibility to common diseases (Gulcher and Stefansson, 2000).

Research on groups affected by particular disorders also raises specific issues. Such research may identify genetic factors responsible for individual differences in responses to particular pharmaceutical products used in treatment, so providing the basis for pharmacogenetics. While it has always been evident that individuals respond differently to drugs, standard clinical trials do not provide information about the genetic factors responsible for differential drug response. Pharmacogenetics seeks and uses genetic information about differential individual responses to drugs so must obtain information on genetic variation. Requirements for informed consent, confidentiality and privacy are all more demanding where participants in drug trials are given genetic tests.

Informed consent

The doctrine of informed consent claims that research participants should be informed of the aims, methods, risks and benefits of research in which they are asked to participate, and that their consent be voluntary and free from coercion. In genetic research it is hard to obtain genuinely informed consent.

Individuals' understanding of genetic research and information may be limited. Media representations of genetic discoveries may foster misconceptions. Understanding of the risks and benefits of uses of genetic information may be sketchy. The risks created by use of genetic information by third parties, such as insurers, or by possible stigmatisation or discrimination may be hard to comprehend. Research participants may misunderstand the implications of the genetic information that they receive.

Storage of samples

These risks have to be assessed in a context in which the ethical and regulatory framework is still developing, so it is not clear what protections for individuals will be in place in the future. This is a particular issue in the long-term storage of DNA samples and/or the setting up of genetic information databases (cf. House of Lords, 2001).

A research protocol may allow for samples to be taken to investigate the genetic factors involved in a particular condition, or in drug response to treatment for that condition. To track drug response, however, may require long term storage of samples, and over time it may become clear that there are other aspects of genetic research that could usefully be done on those samples. It is questionable whether research participants can properly consent to 'genetic research' being done on their samples at some future date without being clear about the detailed nature of that

research. This has led to a discussion on the relative merits of 'broad' and 'narrow' consent. Broad consent allows that participants might be able to consent to certain types of genetic research being done on their samples. Narrow consent would require explicit detail of exactly what conditions would be investigated (cf MRC, 2001; Chadwick and Berg, 2001).

Confidentiality and access

Genetic information may be stored in a variety of ways. Samples may be fully anonymised, personally identified through labelling, or coded in such a way as to maintain a (restricted) link between the genetic information and the research participant. There are advantages and disadvantages of each of these methods, both to researchers and to research participants. The greater the possibility of linking genetic information with personally identifying information, the greater the risk of a breach of confidentiality. However, the greater the security of the information, the less the possibility of feeding back information to participants. Information provided to research participants must make it clear what the procedures are for controlling access and safeguarding security. It also needs to address the issue of whether, and to what extent, feedback will be available.

Right to know and not to know

The idea of a right not to know appears incongruous, given that a major thrust of medical ethics in recent years has been towards giving patients more information to facilitate their autonomous choice. The idea of a right not to know has developed along with the knowledge that genetic information may not only be distressing but also imprecise. The offer of predictive genetic information is not often accompanied by any possibility of preventive action and, in these circumstances, the burden of increasing amounts of genetic information may be too great. Conversely, there is a view that if there is genetic information available that may be relevant to the health or health care of an individual, then the individual has a right to that information.

Some researchers choose to make the results of the research as a whole available, but not to provide feedback to individuals, even if in principle it would be possible. Making the research results available may or may not include an offer of post-research testing and counselling to research participants (cf. Clarke et al., 2001).

Classification according to types of genetic information

Although all genetic information is sensitive, both because of worries about possible misuse by third parties and because of the way in which we may believe it to be one of the most deeply personal aspects of ourselves, some genetic information is particularly sensitive.

Research into the genetic basis of mental disorders has given rise to particular concerns about the possible implications for individuals who may be identified as having a genetic predisposition to mental disorder. Other areas where genetic research is particularly sensitive include research on the genetic factors involved in 'intelligence', behaviour and lifestyle. For example, the very fact that the genetic basis of homosexuality might be chosen as a research topic could be interpreted as evidence of a discriminatory attitude towards homosexuality, independently of what use might be made of the results. There are also worries about the implications of research into behavioural differences between ethnic groups (Nuffield Council on Bioethics, 2001).

Gene therapy

Gene therapy trials are likely to become more common as the functions of an increasing number of genes are identified. While a distinction has commonly been drawn between somatic gene therapy and germline therapy, this distinction has been challenged on both practical and moral grounds. Somatic gene therapy affects only the body cells of an individual and thus can be covered by the same rules as other clinical trials, the only caveat being concerns about the extent to which consent can be genuinely informed in the context of genetics. Germline gene therapy, however, affects future generations and there are worries not only about the irreversibility of effects on future generations but also about the fact that they cannot give informed consent.

Changing paradigms in ethics and science

Although it is now frequently argued that it is a mistake to speak in terms of a gene 'for' a given condition, when a gene is identified that is implicated in a condition it gives rise to expectations that this will lead to a therapy. There are research ethics issues associated both with piloting testing for the genetic factor in question and with trials of any gene therapy that might be developed.

It is worth noting that there is a shifting paradigm in science from the testing of hypotheses in the laboratory to the use of large genetic databases to generate and test hypotheses. Although this kind of research may not involve human research participants directly, the results may still have relevance or ethical implications for them.

REFERENCES

Chadwick, R. and Berg, K. (2001). Solidarity and equity: new ethical frameworks for genetic databases. *Nature Reviews Genetics*, **2**, 318–321.

Clarke A., English, V., Harris, H. and Wells, F. (2001). Ethical considerations [on pharmacogenetics]. *International Journal of Pharmaceutical Medicine*, **15**, 89–94.

Gulcher, J.R. and Stefansson, K. (2000). The Icelandic healthcare database and informed consent. *New England Journal of Medicine*, **342**, 1827–1830.

House of Lords, Select Committee on Science and Technology (2001). *Human Genetic Databases: Challenges and Opportunities*. London: House of Lords.

HUGO ELSI Committee (1996). Statement on the Principled Conduct of Genetic Research. *Genome Digest*, **3**, p. 3.

Medical Research Council (2001). Human tissue and biological samples for use in research: operational and ethical guidelines, London: MRC.

Murray, T. (1997). Genetic exceptionalism and future diaries: is genetic information different from other medical information? In *Genetic Secrets: Protecting Privacy and Confidentiality*, ed. M.A. Rothstein. Yale: Yale University Press.

Nuffield Council on Bioethics (2001). *Genetics and Human Behaviour: the ethical context*. Public Consultation Document, London, Nuffield Council on Bioethics.

O'Neill, Onora (2001). Informed Consent and Genetic Information. *Studies in History and Philosophy of Biological and Biomedical Sciences*, **32**, 689–704.

USEFUL WEBSITES

Advisory Committee on Genetic Testing, 1998, *Genetic Testing for Late Onset Disorders*
http://www.doh.gov.uk/pub/docs/doh/lodrep.pdf

deCODE Genetics. The Icelandic Health Sector Database
http://www.decode.com/resources/ihd/

British Society for Human Genetics
http://www.bshg.org.uk/

Gene Therapy Advisory Committee
http://www.doh.gov.uk/genetics/gtac/index.htm

Genetic Interest Group
http://www.gig.org.uk

The Nuffield Council on Bioethics – Genetics and Human Behaviour: the ethical context
http://www.nuffieldbioethics.org/behaviouralgenetics/index.asp

Public Health Genetics
http://www.medinfo.cam.ac.uk/phgu/

Research or audit?

Anthony Madden

Department of Anaesthesia, Southmead Hospital, Bristol, UK

It is sometimes hard to find the dividing line between research and audit. The following is designed to make the distinction clearer.

Medical research

- May involve experiments on human subjects, whether patients, patients as volunteers, or healthy volunteers.
- Is a systematic investigation which aims to increase the sum of knowledge.
- May involve allocating patients randomly to different treatment groups.
- May involve a completely new treatment.
- May involve extra disturbance or work beyond that required for normal clinical management.
- Usually involves an attempt to test a hypothesis.
- May involve the application of strict selection criteria to patients with the same problem before they are entered into the research study.

Medical audit

- Never involves experiments, whether on healthy volunteers, or patients as volunteers.
- Is a systematic approach to the peer review of medical care in order to identify opportunities for improvement and to provide a mechanism for bringing them about.
- Never involves allocating patients randomly to different treatment groups.
- Never involves a completely new treatment.
- Never involves disturbance to the patients beyond that required for normal clinical management.
- May involve patients with the same problem being given different treatments, but only after full discussion of the known advantages and disadvantages of each treatment. The patients are allowed to choose freely which treatment they get.

USEFUL WEBSITES

The Audit Commission
http://www.audit-commission.gov.uk/home/

Clinical Research and Audit Group
http://www.show.scot.nhs.uk/crag/

The Commission for Health Improvement
http://www.chi.gov.uk/

The National Audit Office
http://www.nao.gov.uk/

Randomised controlled trials

Hazel Inskip[1] and Richard W. Morris[2]

[1]MRC Environmental Epidemiology Unit, University of Southampton, UK
[2]Royal Free and University College Medical School, London, UK

A randomised controlled trial is the standard method for assessing a new treatment or procedure. Such trials provide a more definitive answer than observational studies about differences between groups. To assess whether a treatment is effective or not, a group of patients allocated to a new treatment is compared with a group that receives an existing treatment or placebo.

In observational studies we can only observe what happens to individuals without intervening in any way. We can never rule out confounding as an explanation for any differences found. In an RCT, allocation of the treatment is done randomly to rule out the effects of confounding. RCTs are similar to cohort studies except that we have randomly allocated the 'exposure' (treatment) to the individuals in the study.

The design of an RCT is vital in ensuring that the observed results can be attributed to the treatment(s) under consideration. Poorly designed studies are often biased and are therefore uninterpretable.

Study designs

The simplest design is where two groups of patients are assessed. One is given the new treatment and the other is given an existing treatment or a placebo. Allocation of patients to the two groups is done randomly. However, there are many more complex designs. Some examples are given below.

1 **Multi-centre studies** are increasingly being conducted where large numbers of patients need to be recruited. It is important that the same procedures are used in each centre.

2 **Cross-over studies** are those in which the patients act as their own controls. Each patient receives both the new treatment and the old treatment or placebo sequentially. Each patient is allocated randomly to his/her first treatment. Usually a 'wash-out' period between the two treatments is required to ensure that the effects of the first treatment period do not carry over into the second. The effect of the new treatment is assessed by comparing the results from each of the two treatments within each patient. The advantage of this type of trial is that differences between patients do not have to be considered. This is particularly useful if the outcome measure is hard to ascertain, such as the patient's assessment of pain. A disadvantage is that it is hard to rule out carry-over effects.

3 **Sequential trials** are designed in rather a different way. They can only be used easily if there is a defined end-point for each person. This might be death or recurrence of disease. Every time such an event occurs, the results of the trial are assessed; if a predetermined difference between treatments has been reached then the trial is stopped. A modified version is a 'group sequential trial', where the data are inspected by an independent monitoring committee after recruitment of patients has reached given fractions of the total intended.

4 **Multiple treatments**. Some trials assess the effect of two or more new treatments and some consider combinations of treatments.

Randomisation

Patients must be recruited to the trial before they are allocated to a treatment group. If this is not done there is a risk of biases operating in the allocation. In any study the doctor must feel satisfied that on present knowledge the patient may do as well in either treatment group. However, allocation biases are very subtle, and to avoid them the recruitment must be done before allocation.

The general preferred method of randomisation is to prepare a set of sealed envelopes in advance. Each envelope contains an indicator describing the treatment group that the particular patient will receive. The envelopes are numbered on the outside, and issued sequentially. When the first patient has been recruited to the study the first envelope is opened to reveal the treatment arm to which the patient is allocated. Variations on this method exist – and in multi-centre trials there may be a central office that is telephoned whenever a patient is recruited.

Patients are usually the 'unit' of randomisation. However, for certain studies whole groups of patients may make up the unit. For example, if a new ward management policy is being assessed, the entire ward will have to be a unit of randomisation. In other circumstances there may be practical reasons for group randomisation. If there is concern about 'spill-over' or 'contamination' of the treatment from one group to another – such as if the treatment is mainly in the form of advice given – then randomisation may be by GP surgery for example. Such studies need to be very large as the analysis has to be by the unit of randomisation and not by the individual patients in each unit. The study size is the number of units – not the number of patients.

Eligibility of study participants

Strict rules need to be established about the type of patient who is to be considered for the trial. Examples of the restrictions that might be made are:

Age: It may not be appropriate to treat children.

Sex: For some disorders it may be appropriate to consider one sex only.

Severity of disease: The treatment may only be appropriate for patients whose disease is at a certain stage.

Residence: If a specialist hospital treats patients referred from a long distance there may be a bias towards patients with more complex presentations of the disease (patients with simpler conditions may be treated locally) so a restriction to the normal catchment area of the hospital may be appropriate.

However, as soon as a trial starts there often seem to be fewer eligible patients than anticipated. It is important not to make the eligibility criteria too tight, as recruitment may then be very difficult. Importantly too, the tighter the eligibility criteria, the less generalisable are the results. A treatment that is only shown to be successful in, say, women aged 60–64 with systolic blood pressures between 120 and 130 mmHg and a body mass index between 20 and 24 kg/m^2 is unlikely to be very helpful in routine medical practice.

A related problem is whether the patients will find it hard to comply with the trial protocol. Will many patients withdraw from the trial? If, say, the trial is in the very elderly, will many of them die from other conditions before the trial ends? A trial that is unable to assess a high percentage of its participants at the end of the trial will be hard to interpret. The preferred analysis is called 'intention to treat' in which all the patients are included in the analysis even if they have stopped taking the treatment. If it is impossible to assess many of the patients, the trial will inevitably be weakened; the results may be hard to interpret and it may not be possible to generalise them to other patients in the population.

Assessment of the effect of treatment (blinding)

Ideally neither the patient nor the person assessing the outcome of the treatment knows which treatment the patient has received. This is known as a double-blind study. A single blind study is where either the patient or the person assessing the outcome knows the treatment. For drug treatments, ideally the various treatments are made to look and taste identical and a double-blind trial is possible. To compare exercise with traction for the treatment of back pain, it is impossible to blind the patient; but it should be possible for someone who was not involved in treating the patient to assess how well he/she has done on the treatment – though of course the patient may mention which treatment he/she has received. As far as possible the study should incorporate as much blinding as possible. This avoids subjective preferences for particular treatments affecting the assessment in each patient.

Points to be considered by an Ethics Committee

Many medical journals now require a CONSORT (CONsolidated Standards Of Reporting Trials) statement to be provided when reporting an RCT. The reference is given below, with the web address that provides full details of each point of the statement. Those describing the methods are particularly relevant to an Ethics Committee and cover many of the issues described above. However, many trials never reach the publication stage because problems have arisen along the way, and there are some additional points that a committee might wish to consider, such as:

(i) Are the eligibility criteria well described and is there likely to be a large enough pool of patients to recruit the number required for the study in the specified time?

(ii) Are the eligibility criteria such that the study can be generalised to a reasonable section of the general population?

(iii) Are drop-outs likely to be a major problem? If so, what steps have been taken to minimise this?

Publication bias

As the synthesis of research evidence on particular medical topics has become more popular, the dangers of publication bias have become more apparent. Negative studies (those with statistically non-significant differences) have a lower chance of being published than positive (statistically significant) studies. This phenomenon is especially marked for small studies, where spurious large effects will sometimes appear by chance. Small negative studies are unlikely to be published. Thus small studies have special potential to mislead the research community. It is particularly important that ethics committees ensure that proper study size calculations have been carried out. Partly to address the problem of publication bias, the Cochrane collaboration tries to maintain a prospective register of trials as they are begun. Those conducting trials should be encouraged to obtain an International Standard Randomised Controlled Trial Number through the trial sponsors.

Cautionary note

RCTs are a gold standard and should be conducted wherever possible to test out a new procedure or treatment. There may, however, be situations in which an RCT is impossible. This may occur when, for example, the unit of randomisation would have to be extremely large and it would be impossible to recruit enough units for a meaningful analysis. Examples would include the assessment of a change in hospital-wide policy. To recruit sufficient hospitals and assess the effect on all the patients within them would mean that a study of this type might never be conducted. Sometimes compromises need to be made and a weaker form of assessment may be better than none – but the case for not doing an RCT needs to be justified.

REFERENCES

Matthews, J.N.S. *An Introduction to Randomised Controlled Clinical Trials*, Arnold Texts in Statistics, 2000. *A general textbook on RCTs, though written by a statistician so somewhat technical in places – but a good description of the issues.*

Moher, D., Schulz, K.F., Altman, D.G. for the CONSORT group. (2001). The CONSORT statement: revised recommendations for improving the quality of parallel-group randomised trials. *Lancet*, **357**, 1191–1194 *or* http://www.consort-statement.org *The CONSORT statement mentioned above. The website contains much more information than the Lancet paper.*

Gardner, M.J., Machin, D. & Campbell, M.J. (1986). Use of checklists for the assessment of the statistical content of medical studies. *Br Med J*, **292**, 810–812. *Describes the lists that are used to assess papers submitted to the British Medical Journal. A general list and a list for clinical trials are described and each has a section on design issues.*

http://www.sghms.ac.uk/depts/phs/staff/jmb/pbstnote.htm. *This website contains the Statistical Notes that have been published in the BMJ. This is a series of over 40 articles that have been published intermittently since 1994 giving basic introductions (about a page long) to a variety of statistical topics. Quite a few of them are about randomised controlled trials.*

Determining the study size

Hazel Inskip[1] and Richard W. Morris[2]

[1] MRC Environmental Epidemiology Unit, University of Southampton, UK
[2] Royal Free and University College Medical School, London, UK

On most Ethics Committee application forms there is a question asking how the size of the study was determined. This is an important question as study size has ethical implications. Studies that are too small tend to give inconclusive results; they waste money and time, and study participants are inconvenienced. They can give inaccurate answers, which jeopardise future research. An apparently large effect found in a small trial may make a further trial unethical. Conversely, important true effects may be missed.

Usually a formal study size calculation has to be made and the answers to this question on the form are amongst the most complicated to understand. Sometimes confidence intervals are used to explain the study size (usually for descriptive rather than comparative studies) and these are discussed at the end of this chapter. Formal study size calculations are used when the purpose of the study is to compare two or more groups of subjects. There are five areas that must be considered:

- Difference of interest
- Variability of measurements
- Significance level (p-value)
- Power of the study to detect a difference
- The proportion of the study population that is 'exposed' or taking the treatment

People without a statistical training may find it difficult to assess the study size statements and will have to rely on a statistician. However, they can assess whether the difference of interest seems reasonable.

The five points will be considered in turn.

Difference of interest

For quantitative variables (e.g. height, weight, blood pressure), the difference of interest is usually expressed as a difference between means (averages), for example:

5 mmHg difference in blood pressure between two treatment groups

100 g difference in birthweight between two groups

For categorical variables, especially for those with only two categories (e.g. dead/alive, disease occurs/does not occur), the difference may be expressed in terms of relative risks, odds ratios, hazard ratios, risk ratios, standardised mortality ratios, rate ratios (or any statistic with the term 'relative' or 'ratio' in the name). All these ratios can be interpreted in much the same way, for example:

a ratio of   1.2 indicates a 20% increase in risk

0.8 indicates a 20% reduction in risk

5 indicates a fivefold increase in risk

1 indicates no difference in risk

e.g. (i) the odds ratio for hip osteoarthritis associated with being overweight vs. normal weight is 1.7 (i.e. the risk of hip osteoarthritis in those who are overweight is 1.7 times the risk in those of normal weight, or in other words, the risk of hip osteoarthritis is increased by 70% if the person is overweight); (ii) the hazard ratio for breast cancer recurrence with adjuvant tamoxifen therapy is 0.6 (i.e. the risk for those on tamoxifen is reduced to 60% of the risk in those not on the therapy or, in other words, tamoxifen reduces the risk of recurrence by 40%).

Studies that are only large enough to detect huge effects are not worth doing. For example: (a) a study that is only capable of detecting an average reduction in blood pressure of 40 mmHg or more is a waste of time as no new drug would be able to make such a huge difference, (b) a study of lung cancer claiming to be able to detect an odds ratio of 5 for high v. low exposure to diesel exhaust fumes is too small, as such a large odds ratio is very unlikely truly to exist.

Variability of measurements

Variability of quantitative variables

This is particularly relevant for differences in means. Variables whose values vary widely between people in the population will require larger sample sizes than those that do not. Variability is summarised by 'variance', or 'standard deviation'. Variance and standard deviation describe the variability of individual measurements in the population being studied.

The statistical explanations for these terms are as follows:
- Variance is approximately the average of the squares of the difference of each observation from the mean.
- Standard deviation $= \sqrt{\text{variance}}$

Four standard deviations is approximately the range of the measurements in the population. The range is the difference between the largest and the smallest measurement.

'Variability' of categorical variables

This is more complex. Essentially we consider proportions (e.g. the proportion of people getting the disease or the proportion dying). If the proportion is close to zero or close to one then larger numbers are needed, but as the proportions get nearer to a half we need smaller numbers, e.g. in a cohort study looking at the risk of leukaemia in workers exposed to radiation, a very small proportion of workers will get leukaemia (approximately 0.01% per year) so very large numbers are required. However, if we were looking at back pain in nurses, approximately 20% per year will get the 'disease' so this is easier to estimate and smaller numbers are required.

Significance level (*P*-value)

A *P*-value is a probability. It is the probability that the study will seem to find an effect when one does not really exist (sometimes called a Type I error). For example, suppose a drug being tested is actually useless, the study might – by chance – seem to find that those on the drug did better than those on placebo. The probability of this happening is the *P*-value. Commonly the *P*-value chosen is 0.05, which means that there is a 1 in 20 chance of observing a difference that is not really there. Results in papers often quote $P < 0.05$. Smaller *P*-values mean that the findings are even less likely to be due to chance, e.g. $P < 0.001$ (less than 1 in 1000).

Power of the study to detect a difference

Power is also a probability. It is the probability that we will be able to detect an important difference if it is really there. When a study misses a difference, or effect, which is actually present, this is a Type II error. The more powerful the study, the lower the probability of making a Type II error. This depends on the difference of interest. Large differences will be easier to detect so the power will be higher. The following table shows how we might be in error. Of course we do not know the 'truth' but we hope that our study will get close to it.

		Study findings	
		Difference found	*Difference not found*
'Truth'	Real difference	Correct	Type II error
	No difference	Type I error	Correct

Commonly 80% power is chosen. This means that we have an 80% chance of detecting the difference of interest if it really exists. It also means that there is a 20% chance of missing it. Sometimes higher power is used. Rarely should powers less than 80% be considered.

The proportion of the population exposed

Often in randomised controlled trials half the study participants are given the new treatment and half are given the standard treatment. In this case the proportion 'exposed' is 50%. In epidemiological studies, however, there may only be a small proportion of the population that is exposed. If an exposure of interest is rare (or extremely common) then many more people will need to be studied than if about half the population is exposed. For example, if only about 0.1% of the population smoked then it would have taken a much larger study to show that smoking caused lung cancer than when the proportion smoking was about 50%.

Examples of the answers given to the question 'How was the size of the study determined?'
- Assuming 95% power, a 5% significance level and a standard deviation of 20 mmHg in systolic blood pressure, we expect that with 420 patients in each arm of the trial we could detect a reduction of 5 mmHg in systolic blood pressure in those on the intervention drug compared to the placebo.
- With 80% power and $P < 0.05$ and 1100 patients in each arm of the trial we should be able to detect an increase in the 5-year survival rate from 75% to 80% by treating

breast cancer patients with a new drug as opposed to the standard drug.

- We are studying a group of asthmatic children who experience an average of five episodes of asthma per year with a standard deviation of 2. In 340 children, comparing the top quarter of the distribution of NO_2 exposure to the lowest quarter we expect to be able to detect a difference of 1 episode per year, with 80% power and $P < 0.05$.
- In a 15-year follow-up of middle aged men we expect 10% of them to die from ischaemic heart disease. We aim to test whether the death rate is as high as 15% in men who are positive for antibodies to *Chlamydia pneumoniae* (a relative risk of 1.5). We estimate that 20% of men will be positive for antibodies and with 80% power and a 5% level of significance, we need to study 2500 men.

Notes

1 For a statistician to replicate the study size calculations, he/she needs all the information that is given in each of the scenarios above.

2 There are problems with study size calculations as they are crude. Allowance must be made for drop-outs; the study size obtained from the calculations is the number who do not drop out. Therefore the number recruited will need to be inflated appropriately according to the expected drop-out rate.

3 In epidemiology, much larger numbers are needed to take account of other factors such as age and sex. Adjustments have to be made in the analysis for these factors, as we have not done a randomised study such that there is a balance of these factors across the different groups.

4 Sometimes very large studies are set up to address many questions and formal study size calculations may not really be appropriate.

5 Also, be aware that sometimes people derive a study size to suit the numbers available. Check that the difference of interest is realistic.

Confidence intervals

Confidence intervals may be quoted in the scientific background on the ethics form. They may also be given as a justification of the study size as the researchers may say that their study size allows them to estimate the parameter of interest with a confidence interval of a specific width.

Examples:

- a mean difference of 5 mmHg (95%CI: 2.4–7.6) in systolic blood pressure
- a difference of 225 g in birthweight (95%CI: 216–234 g)
- an odds ratio of 2.7 (95%CI: 1.5–4.9)
- a hazard ratio of 0.4 (95%CI: 0.2–0.9).

Usually 95% confidence intervals are quoted as above, though other percentages are possible, if unusual. The formal definition of a 95% confidence interval is not straightforward: if we did 100 studies we would expect the 95% confidence intervals of 95 of the studies to include the true difference/odds ratio etc. More simply (and not formally correct), it gives us an estimate of the range within which the true value of the difference/odds ratio etc. is likely to lie. We 'think' that the true value is likely to lie within our confidence interval. We cannot be absolutely certain, as we have quoted a 95% confidence interval, rather than a 100% confidence interval (which would be infinitely wide).

Also, it is worth noting that the confidence interval only takes account of the variability due to chance. If the study were poorly designed and it was biased, then the confidence interval could easily fail to include the true value of the difference or ratio under consideration.

SUGGESTED READING

Lemeshow, S., Hosmer, D.W., Klar, J. and Lwanga, S.K. (1990). *Adequacy of Sample Size in Health Studies*. Chichester: John Wiley. (ISBN 0 471 92517 9). *Provides methods for assessing sample size of a variety of different study types, including many pages of tables giving the required sample size in a variety of situations.*

Machin, D., Campbell, M., Fayers, P. and Pinol, A. (1997). *Sample Size Tables for Clinical Studies*. 2nd edn. Blackwell Science. (ISBN 0 86542 870 0). *Similar type of book to Lemeshow et al. Contains program on floppy disk tucked inside back cover.*

Altman, D. and Machin, D. (2001). Statistics with confidence – Confidence intervals and statistical guidelines. *BMJ*, London, 2nd edn. (ISBN 0727913751). *Gives the methods for calculating confidence intervals for a variety of statistics and also provides sets of guidelines and checklists for authors of papers.*

http://ebook.stat.ucla.edu/calculators/powercalc/. *A website that allows study sizes to be calculated for difference types of assessment.*

Risk assessment for research participants

Kenneth Calman

University of Durham, UK

This chapter tries to provide a way by which research participants can assess the risks of being involved in a particular research project. At the heart of the process will be the balance and a judgement made by the individual between the perceived benefits of the research and the possible risks.

Uncertainty is a key word in the assessment of risk. It should also be noted that any potential benefits may not be for the person taking part in the research, but for subsequent patients and/or populations. By definition, carrying out research means that the outcome is not known and thus potential benefits and risks not known. If they were clear, the procedure, treatment, intervention, would be classified as good practice, not research, as the risks would have been already assessed. It is thus difficult to assess the risks of taking part in a research project as much is unknown. This section can only give an indication of the terms and language used and the kinds of issues which might be considered by people before taking part in a research project.

Some definitions

Before considering some of the possible categories of risk, it is worth being clear about what certain terms mean.
(a) A hazard is any set of circumstances that may have harmful consequences.
(b) The risk is the probability of the hazard causing an adverse effect.
Thus a hazard, such as a drug, is not a risk until it is administered. The risk, the probability of an adverse effect occurring, will depend on various factors including the nature of the drug itself, the dose, the condition of the patient, and many others. Probability is at the heart of this and while it is possible to give a figure such as a 25% chance of a risk, or one in a million risk of an adverse event occurring, it is

not possible to predict for the individual whether or not they will be affected. This is the problem of uncertainty.

Risk as a universal feature of all procedures

It is not possible to conceive of a procedure, investigation, or process which would be without any risk, no matter how small or insignificant. It would be wrong to consider that there are procedures which are not potentially hazardous and for which there will be no risk.

The perception of risk

One of the most important factors in the assessment of risk is the perception by the person of the importance of risk. Thus, the patient's illness may substantially affect the way in which a risk is perceived. For example, people with a life threatening disease may (but not always) be prepared to accept a higher risk from a procedure in the hope that it might improve their condition. This is in contrast with people who are 'well' in whom any risk (the probability of an adverse effect occurring) may be less acceptable.

The person's choice and consent

The end point of the process is the consent given by the person to be part of the research project having considered all aspects of the process and asked all relevant questions. Implicit in this is that the person is given, in one form or another, all relevant information. Individual people have rights and responsibilities. The outcome of the project may not benefit them, but other patients, and, over the years generations of people have given their consent for research projects which have seen significant benefits for the next group of patients. This has been with considerable courage and with the benefits to others in mind. Uncertainty will always be there and assessing the balance is very difficult. It will always be a matter of judgement.

The process and the questions to ask

Assessing the risk requires that the project be carefully explained and that the choice is made and consent given without coercion or undue pressure being applied. There should be an opportunity to ask questions as appropriate. Information can be presented in different ways, and this can influence choice. Ability to withdraw from the project should be part of the process.

The categories of risk

While many of the risks relate to the physical consequences, there are other possible risks and they are discussed here.

Risk of physical damage

This is the commonest group of risks to be discussed. These will depend on the procedure or intervention (surgery, drug treatment, X-ray investigation, etc.) and may be very specific for the procedure. In some cases because of previous research or results from similar procedures, some of the side effects will already be predictable. In other instances this will not be the case and the possible side effects will be quite uncertain. This should be borne in mind during the discussion. Remember, research is not risk free.

Psychological consequences of research

While the physical aspects are rightly highlighted, it should not be forgotten that there are also potential psychological consequences. Research may require the person to attend a clinic more frequently and to have more tests and investigations. This on the one hand may be reassuring and positive and on the other be negative and upsetting. For some people with particular illnesses (e.g. HIV infection) being part of a research project may be associated with a stigma. If the person refuses to take part then there may be a feeling of guilt.

Social consequences of research

Being part of a research project may also have social consequences. Families may be involved and may have additional stress. There may be financial costs in transport or special diets, and the problems of side effects (physical or psychological) may impact on those nearest and dearest.

Conclusions

For each of these headings the person will have to make a choice and to weigh up the benefits and the risks. A judgement will have to be made based on the evidence available before consent is given. Uncertainty will still be present and there may be unknown risks to be faced. Taking part in a research project requires both courage and a wish to do something from which others might benefit. All of us should be grateful for such motives and feelings.

15

Absorbed radiation in patient and volunteer studies submitted to the ethical committee: a memorandum

Keith Britton and Rosemary Foley

Department of Nuclear Medicine, St Bartholomew's Hospital London, UK

Introduction

Radiation is a natural phenomenon.

The current method of measuring absorbed radiation is the effective dose equivalent in units called millisieverts, mSv. This allows different types of radiation from different sources, X-rays, gamma rays, cosmic rays, etc. to be compared. Normal exposure in London is about 0.18 mSv per month including that from cosmic rays and natural radioactive potassium and radon in our bodies. The computed risk of death from 0.1 mSv is one in a million, which is the same risk as smoking one and a half cigarettes in a lifetime or drinking half a litre of wine in a lifetime or, indeed, the risk of death for a man aged 42 living for a day or a man aged 60 living 20 minutes.[1a]

Perception of risk

The popular perception of radiation risk is much greater than in fact it is. Studies in the USA of League of Women Voters and college students put the risk of nuclear power first and business and professional club members put the risk at eighth of a list of 30 agents, whereas in fact it was 20th (the risk was 1500 times less than average cigarette smoking, 1000 times less than average alcohol consumption, 500 times less than motor vehicle driving, 30 times less than swimming and 10 times less than bicycling).[1b] The lifespan shortening on a population basis associated with medical X-ray is 6 days, of which the nuclear medicine contribution is 4 hours as compared with natural background radiation 8 days; accidents in the home 95 days; accidents at work 74 days; and heart disease 2100 days as examples.[1c]

The Ionising Radiation Regulations 1999 and the approved code of practice

The Ionising Radiation Regulations 1999 (IRR99)[2,3] has defined the effective dose limit to any member of the public, including persons under the age of 16, to be no more than 1 mSv in one calendar year, and the dose limit for occupationally exposed workers 20 mSv. Should circumstances dictate, it is acceptable for an occupationally exposed person to receive a maximum of 100 mSv effective absorbed dose, in a period of 5 consecutive years with the proviso that a maximum dose of 50 mSv can be received in one calendar year. In order for occupationally exposed workers to avoid 'classification', the annual limit should be kept below 6 mSv. The level of exposure for pregnant women should be less than 1 mSv. (The natural radiation background in London is 2.2 mSv per year.) Typical diagnostic studies and their effective dose equivalents are given for Nuclear Medicine Notes for Guidance on the Clinical Administration of Radiopharmaceuticals [4] and for X-rays.[5] The training and requirements for carrying out a procedure involving ionising radiation are set out in the Ionising Radiation (Medical Exposure) Regulations 2000.[6]

It is normal nuclear medicine practice to relate the absorbed radiation dose from the nuclear medicine procedures to that of the same organ undergoing an X-ray procedure. This is partly because many patients are familiar with X-ray studies of the organ about which they are concerned and partly because it serves as a familiar frame of reference to the referring clinician. It is usually not appropriate to relate absorbed radiation dose to that of a chest X-ray since the dose for a chest X-ray, depending upon the machinery used, varies from 0.01–0.1 mSv. It is not generally realised that the risks from the injected chemical exceed those from radiation.

Table 1. Risks of contrast material and radiopharmaceuticals

Cause	Risk	Ref
Death from routinely used water soluble intravenous X-ray contrast material:	1 in 40 000	7
Reaction to routinely used water soluble intravenous contrast materials:	1 in 15	7
	1 in 6	8
Reaction to radiopharmaceutical injections:	1 in 2500	9
Reaction to penicillin	1 in 10	10

The risks from the injection of contrast media and radiopharmaceuticals are shown in Table 1.

Thus it can be seen that the risks from the radiation involved for diagnostic X-ray and nuclear medicine studies are much less than those from the pharmaceutical preparation itself.

Given this information, the question is how to convey the very low risk associated with diagnostic X-ray and nuclear medicine procedures to a public that has an exaggerated perception of risk from radiation.

Pregnancy and radiation

The radiation sensitivity of the fertilised ovum is of the same order as that of the unfertilised ovum so that the so-called 10-day rule (that studies of the lower abdomen involving the use of X-rays should be limited to the first 10 days after the start of the last menstrual period) was never radiobiologically sound[11] and not directly applicable to nuclear medicine procedures.[12]

Women who are pregnant are most sensitive to radiation to the foetus during the period of organogenesis, which occurs between weeks 7 and 17 of the pregnancy. No pregnant patient, or any patient who is uncertain as to whether or not she is pregnant, should normally be considered for a research study that involves the use of ionising radiation. In practice, the risk to a patient found to be pregnant following the study, where the effective absorbed dose to the abdomen was 0.5 mSv, would only give a one in 100 000 chance of damage to the foetus. If the effective dose was 5 mSv, the risk would be increased to one in 10 000. This compares with the 'natural' risk of a congenital abnormality occurring in a delivered baby of 1 in 40. The abdomen of a pregnant person should not receive an effective dose of more than 1 mSv during the declared term of pregnancy. The dose limit to the abdomen of an occupationally exposed woman of reproductive capacity should be restricted to a maximum

of 13 mSv in any period of 3 consecutive months, or to avoid classification, 4 mSv during the 3-month period.[2,3,4,6]

Consent forms

We propose that, for investigations involving an absorbed radiation dose of less than 1 mSv, the phrase on the Consent Form is:

the study involves administration of (X-rays)/(a tiny amount of radioactivity) at a level considered to be of negligible risk for members of the public by the International Commission on Radiation Protection.

And for 1–5 mSv:

the study involves administration of (X-rays)/(a small amount of radioactivity) at a level considered to be of very low risk for members of the public by the International Commission on Radiation Protection.

In the text of the submission to the Ethical Committee, we propose that the Effective Dose in mSv should be stated for each study that involves the diagnostic use of X-rays or of a nuclear medicine procedure.

Postscript

Current absorbed radiation dose assessment is based on the assumption that all radiation, however low, represents a risk and that no radiation represents no risk. Such an argument would not apply to any other physical environment affecting human beings. It is based on a 'linear hypothesis' with data from higher levels of radiation extrapolated back to zero over the range of very low level radiation in the absence of data in that range. Increasing experimental data suggest that this hypothesis is not tenable at very low level radiation[13] and that there may be a threshold somewhere between 20 and 200 mSv. The 1994 report from the United Nations' UNSCEAR committee stated that with 'the statistical limitations of the current evidence, no conclusions could be drawn about the dose–response relationship below 200 mGy.[14]

Indeed, there is experimental evidence of the beneficial effects of low-level radiation in animals and plants, even ignoring the supposed benefits of radon-containing hot spring spa water. This beneficial effect is called Radiation Hormesis and the prestigious radiation protection journal *Health Physics* devoted a special issue to this subject.[15]

Published originally as: Britton K E. Absorbed Radiation in Patients: a memorandum for the ethical committee in *Clinical Nuclear Medicine* 2nd edn. pp. 620–623, ed. M.N.

Maisey, K.K.E. Britton, D.L. Gilday, London, Chapman & Hall 1991. Modified for this publication in 2001.

REFERENCES

1a Brill, A.R. (1985). *Low Level Radiation Effects: A Fact Book*. New York: The Society of Nuclear Medicine. Table 6.1.

1b Brill, A.R. (1985). *Low Level Radiation Effects: A Fact Book*. New York: The Society of Nuclear Medicine. Table 6.4.

1c Brill, A.R. (1985). *Low Level Radiation Effects: A Fact Book*. New York: The Society of Nuclear Medicine. Table 6.3.

2 *Ionising Radiation Regulations 1999*, No.3232 (IRR99). The Stationery Office.

3 *The Approved Code of Practice and Guidance, Working with Ionising Radiation*. HSE Books, L121.2000.

4 Notes for guidance on the clinical administration of Radiopharmaceuticals and use of sealed radioactive sources. Administration of radioactive substances Advisory Committee. *Nuclear Medicine Communications* 2000; 21 Suppl: S1-S95.

5 Shrimpton, P.C. & Wall, B.F. (1986). Doses to patients from medical radiological examinations in Great Britain. *Radiation Protection Bulletin*, **7**, 10–14.

6 *The Ionising Radiation (Medical Exposure) Regulations 2000*, No 1059. The Stationery Office.

7 Ansell, G. (1996). *Complications in Diagnostic Imaging and Interventional Radiology*, 3rd edn, ed. G. Ansell, M.A. Bettmann, J.A. Kaufman & R.A. Wilkins, Chap. 13 Complications of intravascular iodinated contrast media, pp. 245–300. Table 13.5. p. 264. Cambridge: Blackwell Science.

8 Panto, P.N. & Davies, P. (1986). *British Journal of Radiology*, **59**, 41–44.

9 Keeling, D.H. and Sampson, C.B. (1984). *British Journal of Radiology*, **57**, 1091–6.

10 *Drug and Therapeutic Bulletin* 1975, **13**, 9.

11 Mole, R.H. (1987). The so-called 10-day rule. *Lancet*, **ii**, 1138–40.

12 Longmead, W.A., Crown, V.P.D., Jewkes, R.J. et al. (1983). *Radiation Protection of the Patient in Nuclear Medicine, A Manual of Good Practice*. OUP: Oxford Medical Publications. pp. 79–83.

13 Feinendegen, L.E., Bond, V.P., Sondhaus, C.A. & Altman, K.P. (1999). Cellular signal adaptation with damage control at low doses versus the predominance of DNA damage at high doses. *Academie Science, Paris*, **322**, 245–51.

14 *Sources and Effects of Ionising Radiation*, UNSCEAR 1994 (Annex B: adaptive responses to radiation in cells and organisms). New York, 1994.

15 (1987), Radiation hormesis. *Health Physics*, **52**, 517–680.

16

A guide to the use of radioactive materials and radiological procedures for research purposes

Niall Moore

Department of Radiology, University of Oxford and Oxford Radcliffe Hospital, UK

Anyone wishing to administer radioactive substances to patients or volunteers must do so in accordance with regulations from the Administration of Radioactive Substances Advisory Committee (ARSAC). Notes from ARSAC guiding practitioners are formulated in accordance with the Medicines (Administration of Radioactive Substances) Regulations 1978, and the Medicines (Radioactive Substances) Order 1978.

The Medicines (Administration of Radioactive Substances) Regulations 1978 relate to the protection of the patient or volunteer during the clinical or research use of radioactive substances. According to these Regulations, it is an offence for anyone to administer a radioactive medicinal product to a human being unless he or she is a doctor or dentist holding a certificate issued by the Health Ministers in respect of that product, or a person acting in accordance with the directions of such a doctor or dentist. The Health Ministers receive advice from ARSAC relevant to the granting of certificates. The Health Ministers define the duration, and conditions for renewal, of a certificate and may suspend, revoke or vary a certificate.

The Medicines (Radioactive Substances) Order 1978 regulates specifically the administration of Radioactive Medicinal Products (RMPs), which are defined as medicinal products that contain or generate a radioactive substance and that contain or generate that substance, in order, when administered to a human being, to utilise the radiation admitted therefrom.

ARSAC requires that a Certificate is needed by any doctor or dentist wishing to administer RMPs to people on a regular basis for one or more of the three following reasons:
(a) All clinical trials as defined in section 31 (a) of the Medicines Act (1968) where a CTC or CTX has been granted, or a DDX has been agreed.
(b) The administration of RMPs where the subject is not expected to benefit from the tests.

(c) Additional radiation exposure above that incurred in the routine management of patients.

Practitioners should normally be of Consultant status, and should be those who have responsibility for carrying out procedures. Applications for certification must include information about the equipment, facilities and scientific support available. Applications are made by sending the fully completed standard application form to the Department of Health; applications usually take 8 or more weeks to process. Applicants are expected to: know and understand the RMP to be used; judge the suitability of the products for the tests requested and the effects they may have; be familiar with the measures necessary to ensure a proper standard of radiation protection; understand how the test is carried out; be able to judge whether the test has been effectively performed and interpret the results accordingly.

Where a research investigation differs significantly from that outlined in the original application, the practitioner should inform the secretariat of the ARSAC.

Any person who contravenes the regulations shall be guilty of an offence and shall be liable on conviction to the penalties prescribed in Section 67(4) of the Medicines Act (1968).

Guidance on administration

Detailed guidelines on recommended activities are given in Appendix 1 of ARSAC 1993. It should be noted that the activity administered should be the minimum consistent with adequate information from the investigation. Alternative non-ionising techniques should always be considered in women of child-bearing potential. Only such investigations as are imperative should be conducted during pregnancy.

Table 1. Common radiological tests. Doses and risks for a UK population

Examination	Effective dose (mSv)	CXRs	NBR [a]	Lifetime risk of cancer Fatal [1]	Non-fatal [1]	Hereditary effects [1]	Total detriment [b]	Fatal cancer [1]	Total Detriment [b]
				Risk per 10 000. All ages – both sexes				*Risk per 10 000. 18–64 – both sexes*	
CXR	0.02	1	3 d	**0.012**	0.008	0.001	**0.021**	*0.01*	*0.02*
SXR	0.1	5	2 w	**0.06**	0.04	0.01	**0.11**	*0.05*	*0.09*
Pelvis	1.0	50	6 m	**0.6**	0.4	0.1	**1.1**	*0.5*	*0.9*
Abdomen	1.5	75	9 m	**0.9**	0.6	0.1	**1.6**	*0.75*	*1.3*
L Spine	2.4	120	14 m	**1.4**	0.9	0.2	**2.5**	*1.02*	*2.1*
IVU	4.6	230	2.5 y	**2.7**	1.8	0.4	**4.9**	*2.3*	*4.1*
Ba meal	5.0	250	2.5 y	**3.0**	2.0	0.5	**5.5**	*2.5*	*4.5*
Ba enema	9.0	450	4.5 y	**4.5**	3.0	0.9	**8.4**	*4.5*	*8.0*
CT head	2.0	100	1 y	**1.2**	0.8	0.2	**2.2**	*1.0*	*1.8*
CT chest	9.0	450	4.5 y	**5.3**	3.6	0.9	**9.8**	*4.5*	*8.0*
CT abdomen	12.0	600	6 y	**7.1**	4.8	1.2	**13.1**	*6.0*	*10.7*
CT pelvis	10.0	500	5 y	**5.9**	4.0	1.0	**10.9**	*5.0*	*8.9*
CT chest/abdo	20.0	1000	10 y	**11.8**	7.9	2.0	**21.7**	*10.0*	*17.8*
CT abdo/pelvis	17.0	850	8.5 y	**10.0**	6.7	1.7	**18.4**	*8.5*	*15.1*
CT chest/abdo/ pelvis	26.0	1300	13 y	**15.3**	10.3	2.6	**28.2**	*13.0*	*23.1*
Kidney scan	0.7	35	4 m	**0.4**	0.3	0.07	**0.77**	*0.4*	*0.6*
Lung perfusion scan	1.2	60	7 m	**0.7**	0.5	0.1	**1.3**	*0.6*	*1.1*
Bone scan	3.8	190	1.8 y	**2.2**	1.5	0.3	**4.0**	*1.8*	*3.1*
Brain perfusion scan	6.9	350	3.5 y	**4.1**	2.7	0.7	**7.5**	*3.5*	*6.1*
Heart perfusion scan	18.0	900	9 y	**10.6**	7.1	1.8	**19.5**	*9.0*	*16.0*

Notes.

1. Risks are estimates for lifetime probability of detriment. 40-year observations are 50% of lifetime detriment.

2. Risks are 200% in paediatric group.

3. Risks are 20% in geriatric (> 70 year) group.

[a] Natural background radiation.

[b] Includes fatal cancer, non-fatal cancer and severe hereditary risks.

Sources:

[1] National Radiological Protection Board. *Estimates of Late Radiation Risks to the UK Population.* Vol 4. No. 4. 1993

General considerations when using RMP for research purposes

Age Wherever possible, healthy volunteers should be aged over 50 years. Persons under 18 years of age should be excluded, unless problems specific to their age group are under investigation.

Numbers Should be restricted to the minimum necessary to obtain the information required.

Multiple studies It is unacceptable that an individual be exposed to a substantial cumulated radiation dosage.

Women The possibility of early pregnancy in those of child-bearing age should always be considered. Pregnant and breast-feeding women should not, normally, be involved in any project.

Classified radiation workers Should not normally be accepted as volunteers in a research project.

Approval of Research Ethics Committees

Every clinical research investigation using RMPs should be checked and approved by an REC. The ARSAC application should be made at the same time and should include a one-page summary of the submission to the REC. The ultimate approval for the project as a whole will be with the REC, which should ensure that the applicant holds all the necessary authorisations.

The Ionising Radiation (Medical Exposure) Regulations 2000

The IR(ME)R incorporate the core concept of justification when a medical exposure is made. The need for justification of an exposure 'shall show a sufficient net benefit when the total potential diagnostic or therapeutic benefits it produces, including the direct health benefits to an individual and the benefits to society, against the individual detriment that the exposure might cause, taking into account the efficacy, benefits and risks of available alternative techniques having the same objective but involving less or no exposure to ionising radiation'.

The new regulations also address the use of medical exposures in research ionising radiation-based techniques used in medical research programmes. Research projects involving ionising radiation should be submitted to a local research ethics committee for approval before commencement (Regulation 7(4)). The justification described above must be applied equally to subjects taking part in medical research as to patients involved in medical diagnosis or treatment. IR(ME)R provides for the optimisation process, which involves ensuring that doses arising from exposures are kept as low as reasonably practicable. Departments should keep a record of acceptable exposure values for radiographic techniques and nuclear medicine procedures. Regulation 7(4)(c) requires dose constraints to be applied where no direct medical benefit for the individual is expected from the exposure. The constraints must be set by the employer (usually the hospital trust) and must not be exceeded. The constraints should be set at a level to facilitate the research, and be deemed appropriate by the radiology department and agreed by the LREC. This concept is reiterated in Regulation (1)(c) where the LREC can recommend that a research project is undertaken with a proviso that a certain dose is not exceeded.

17

Indemnity in medical research

Janet Jeffs[1] and Richard Mayon-White[2]

[1]Legal Services, Oxford Radcliffe Hospitals, UK
[2]Public Health and Health Policy, Oxfordshire Health Authority, UK

Medical research carries risks for the subjects who take part. The subjects accept these risks, because they are interested in the area of the research and in the general good achieved by better medical knowledge. If the research is a clinical trial, there is also the chance, however random, of obtaining an effective new treatment. From time to time, things go wrong – a trial drug causes harm, an accident occurs, or a subject feels aggrieved – and the investigators may need to find money to redress the wrong. Indemnity involves both protection for the investigator (by various forms of insurance) and the payment to injured parties (if appropriate). This chapter examines these two aspects of indemnity, the first by notes for investigators on the insurance schemes and the second by showing the pathways by which a subject might claim financial compensation.

Forms of indemnity

Indemnity by the employing organisation

National Health Service (NHS) Staff and people who have **paid or honorary contracts with NHS hospitals** are covered by the NHS indemnity for clinical trials involving NHS patients. This scheme compensates for injury arising from negligence, for example, a failure to follow a research protocol, an accident caused by poor maintenance of a building or harm resulting from personal medical information falling into the wrong hands. In the re-organised NHS, the costs of a successful claim fall primarily on the employing NHS trust, which may have to borrow from the Department of Health to settle very large clinical negligence claims, unless it is a member of the Clinical Negligence Scheme for Trusts (CNST) run by the NHS Litigation

Authority (NHSLA). Non-clinical accidents will be partly covered by commercial insurance taken out by Trusts or under the Liabilities to Third Parties Scheme (LTPS) also run by the NHSLA. Claims arising from incidents occurring before a hospital became a trust are the responsibility of the health authority which managed the hospital at the time of the incident. Money used for compensation is money lost to treat patients. Therefore, NHS managers will look critically at research projects that run the risk of large claims and at investigators who stray from their protocols. Investigators may expect that the NHS employers will require that:

(a) the research has passed an ethical review,

(b) any drugs used have product licences or exemption certificates, and

(c) any sponsoring drug company provides standard indemnity, described below.

The NHS can make *ex gratia* payments of up to £50,000 to subjects injured as a result of medical research, without the injured person having to allege or prove negligence by the NHS hospital or its staff. The hospital has to obtain the agreement of the Department of Health and has to bear the costs itself.

Employees of other organisations

Employees of other organisations such as universities or drug companies, engaged in medical research outside the NHS, should obtain insurance from their parent organisation. Usually the organisation will have a policy with a commercial insurance company, with premiums affected by the type of medical research conducted by their employees. The insurers will often ask for details of proposed research so that they can get an opinion on the risks involved, particularly when the research is not the usual type for that organisation. Therefore, investigators should

Possible routes for compensation for patient or volunteer injured either on NHS premises, in the community or elsewhere.

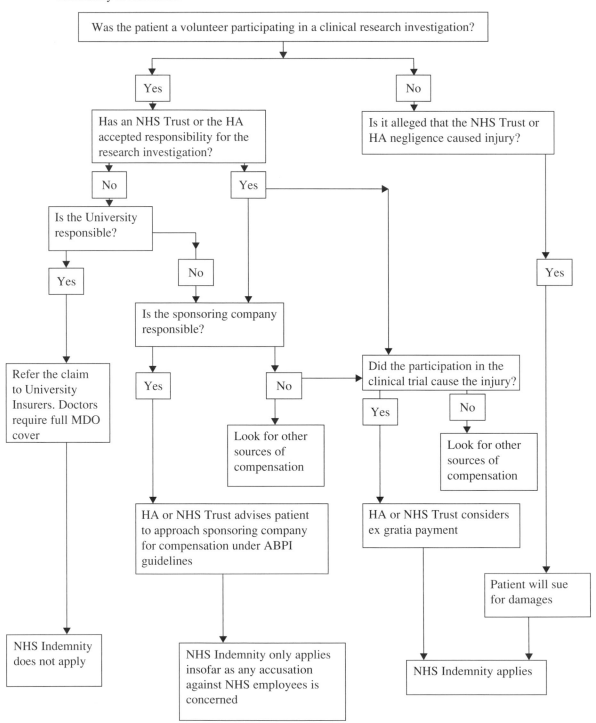

Figure 1 NHS indemnity for clinical research investigations flow chart.

register proposed research with their employers to ensure that cover is arranged.

Indemnity by drug companies

In the majority of drug trials, a company that supplies the drug(s) and sponsors the trial will give indemnity to the NHS body and the investigators, *provided* that the protocol is followed. The Association of the British Pharmaceutical Industry (ABPI) has a code of practice, which gives standard terms for this indemnity.

Investigators should be careful about three points.

(a) The drug company indemnity form is correctly worded, signed and dated. Otherwise the medical investigators may find that their subjects, who are their patients, have a legal tangle in getting compensation which they would get easily if the contract had been correct in every detail.

(b) The drug company's liability does not cover adverse effects of treatments given outside the strict terms of the protocol, despite good medical reasons for a deviation from the protocol in some circumstances. It is becoming common practice for the patient information sheets prepared by drug companies for trials to tell the subjects about the compensation under the ABPI terms. Whilst this practice may reassure some subjects and their investigators, the restrictions set by the protocol should be clearly understood.

(c) The investigators should check that the drug company is not protected from proper claims by being beyond the jurisdiction of a British court. This might happen with a foreign company without a British base, or with a company that went bankrupt or had insufficient funds. If an injured subject cannot get compensation from the drug company, he or she will reasonably claim against the investigator.

Indemnity by companies providing medical devices for investigation

For any research involving medical devices that is sponsored by the company providing the device, there are similar considerations. The Association of British Health-Care Industries (ABHI) has devised guidelines similar to those of the ABPI. These cover the clinical investigation of a medical device, either involving healthy volunteers or patient volunteers.

If the research into a medical device is initiated by a doctor or other clinician, rather than by the company, then the ABHI would not provide indemnity. Investigators should approach either their employers or their medical defence organisation (see below)

Medical defence organisations

General practitioners engaged in research outside hospitals do not have cover from the NHS scheme, because they are independent contractors not employees. They, and doctors in private hospital practice, use medical defence organisations, with annual subscriptions that are related to the income from their practice. Some universities employing medical doctors for non-clinical teaching and research require (and help with the fees) that these doctors subscribe to medical defence organisations, as was once the case in the NHS. For hospital doctors doing research in the NHS, there are advantages in subscribing to a defence organisation. These hospital doctors may need independent support if they find themselves at odds with their employers. This might happen if they faced an accusation that they had wrongly deviated from a protocol, or had conducted research without the proper authorisation. It might happen when the employer was inclined to settle a claim, but on terms that left a doctor's reputation damaged. There are 'grey areas' where work is done outside the doctor's terms of employment – an example not from medical research is the 'Good Samaritan' help at a road accident. For these problems that might arise in ordinary practice, it is advisable for all doctors to belong to a medical defence organisation. The basic subscription would cover NHS employees, including their research work, provided that the main indemnity comes from the employing organisation and the drug companies above. Doctors who are paid by drug companies for their work in clinical trials should check that their subscriptions are appropriate for the extra income received.

Indemnity for Research Ethics Committees (RECs)

It may be alleged that an injury resulting from a study was foreseeable, and that the ethics committee concerned should not have approved of the research. RECs are NHS bodies, but as they are not legal entities members are individually liable. Members must therefore ensure that they are explicitly covered by NHS indemnity as recommended in NHSE Circular HSG (91)5 paragraph 2.11 and Governance Arrangements for NHS Research Ethics Committees 4.14.

Pathways for compensation for subjects injured in medical research

Investigators are expected to take great care that their patients or healthy volunteers will not be injured by medical research. But, if harm does occur, the last thing that anyone wants is a confused and protracted battle over compensation. Figure 1 summarises the routes to compensation, depending on whether the injury was caused by the research. If the injury was caused by medical research, and all the main routes to compensation have failed, there is one source left to try: the Samuel Hanson Rowbotham Fund, administered by the Registrar to the University of Birmingham, Edgbaston, Birmingham B15 2TT.

18

The prevention and management of fraud and misconduct: the role of the LREC

Jennifer Blunt[1] and Frank Wells[2]

[1] North West MREC, UK
[2] Medicolegal Investigations Ltd, UK

Introduction

In an ideal world, fraud or even misconduct in clinical research would not exist; but we do not live in such a world. Accepting, therefore, that they can happen, research ethics committees – particularly local committees – have important roles to play in trying to prevent their occurrence and, if either does occur, to assist in their investigation.

Fraud is much less common than carelessness, though its incidence is difficult to quantify. Nevertheless some element of fraud in clinical trials has been variously estimated (Horton, 1996; Wells, 2001) at between 0.1 and 1% of research projects. As justification for this estimate, there are about 3000 sponsored clinical trials taking place at any one time in the United Kingdom. If the higher figure is assumed, this means that 30 studies may be currently being conducted that could include fraudulent or inaccurately compiled data. Even one case of fraud or other misconduct is one too many. Fraud is likely to exploit patients, deceive the sponsor and may skew the scientific database. Reports of proven cases of fraud in biomedical research are usually greeted with dismay and an element of surprise. Society expects doctors conducting research to be honest and honourable as well as competent – as, indeed, the vast majority of them are.

Definition of research misconduct

At a consensus conference held under the auspices of the Royal College of Physicians in Edinburgh in 1999, a number of definitions of misconduct were discussed. Research misconduct was viewed as including fabrication, falsification and/or suppression of data and plagiarism, as well as unintentional action that undermines the scientific value of the work. The conference concluded with an agreed broad definition of misconduct as 'behaviour by a researcher, intentional or not, that falls short of good ethical and scientific standards' (RCPE, 2000, p. 2).

Occasionally, suspect data are submitted to a sponsoring company or funding charity, or to a contract research organization. Such submissions are more likely to be sloppy than fraudulent, but extreme sloppiness is itself a form of research misconduct. However, outright fraud, which is the most serious type of misconduct, includes an element of intent: it is the generation of false data with the intent to deceive.

Examples of research misconduct and fraud

Research misconduct may comprise a range of inadequacies, including failure to obtain ethics committee approval, failure to obtain (clear) consent from research subjects, changing data, adding missing data and publishing false reports. There are also various examples of publication irregularity, including unacknowledged duplicate publication and publication of a single report in several parts spread over different journals (so-called 'salami slicing') in order to exaggerate the importance of the work. Another publication irregularity is 'gift authorship'. Here, the name of a distinguished colleague not involved in the work is added to the list of authors in an attempt to enhance the status of the report, or the name of a less distinguished colleague similarly not involved is added so as to provide another reference for inclusion in a curriculum vitae or a list of publications.

Overt fraud in clinical research includes forging ethics committee approval, forging patient signatures, fabricating clinical results, inventing pathology laboratory data, completing diary cards as if by a patient, dividing blood samples from one patient into several aliquots purportedly from different patients and taking lengthy electrocardiogram tracings, which are then divided into convenient strips purportedly recorded at different times or on different patients. Clearly, this list of examples, all of which have been seen recently, is not comprehensive, but it demonstrates that patients are exploited, sponsors are defrauded and fraudulent science is published. It is one of the tasks of a research ethics committee to minimize such fraud and other misconduct as far as possible.

Causes of fraud and misconduct

There are several reasons why research misconduct may occur. They include carelessness, over-commitment and over-ambition. Fraud occurs when the doctor or researcher involved actively decides to make up data or to forge documents or signatures. A likely reason for generating false data – at least in the early stages – is a combination of laziness and greed. As time goes on, however, fraudsters find that they cannot afford to be lazy, and may have to spend an increasing amount of time covering their tracks. The Royal College of Physicians has suggested that doctors who are too lazy, too busy, too bored, too frustrated by the bureaucracy surrounding them or too greedy should not be recruited as investigators for research projects (RCP London, 1991, p. 4). This list of risk factors is a useful *aide memoire* for Research Ethics Committees, as well as for clinical trial sponsors and their contract organisation associates.

Research ethics committee review

Research Ethics Committees are expected to review two major elements of a research project: the protocol and the environment in which the project is to be carried out. A multi-centre research ethics committee has a particular responsibility to review the environment associated with the lead investigator, but a local committee has that responsibility for every project to be conducted in its own area. Local research ethics committees therefore have a very important role to play in preventing possible research misconduct, which it is their duty not to shirk. It is particularly important that these committees consider all the local circumstances that apply, including the suitability of the project for local participants bearing in mind current disease patterns and workload, the facilities available at the site and the experience of the investigator.

The **suitability of a local site** is judged by a site visit to determine whether the facilities contain the necessary equipment and whether staff have the necessary experience to conduct the research.

The **suitability of a local investigator** is assessed, bearing in mind published guidelines on good clinical practice (CPMP, 1991; European Commission, 1996), the volume of research being conducted by the investigator, and the track record of the researcher or doctor whose proposal is under review. The assessment of the researcher or doctor should not be based merely on scrutiny of the individual's cv. Where research is initiated by a pharmaceutical company or contract research organisation, it is their responsibility to ensure that only reliable investigators are recruited: companies should reject any potential investigator whose past research projects raise doubts. In general, the LREC is in a position to know relevant factors about a local investigator better than a remote company.

It is theoretically possible that local investigators could be registered as 'approved' on the basis of an initial screening test, so that determining their suitability could thereafter be a matter of an administrative checklist. This, however, may not be the most appropriate way to assess ethical suitability (Blunt, 2001); both Research Ethics Committees and investigators may, in time, become complacent about the research capabilities of an approved investigator.

Consent

The process by which subjects consent to participate in research is central to LREC approval and must include both a written statement of that to which consent is given and a signature from the person consenting. As part of the consent process, potential subjects must be given full information which is clearly expressed and does not contain details that could mislead. Model patient information sheets (PIS) are now available. There must be protection of patient data in line with the Data Protection Act 1998, with particular attention to systems for ensuring confidentiality of personal information and the security of these systems (Medical Research Council, 2000). Subjects must also be given time to decide whether or not to take part, and it must be made clear that the clinical care of any patient who does not give consent to take part in a research project or decides for whatever reason to withdraw from such a project will not in any way be jeopardized.

There are many guidelines on the conduct of research some of which an investigator ought to be familiar with (ABPI, 1996; Medical Research Council, 1997, 1998, 1999; Royal College of Pathologists, 1999; ICH GCP, 1996; Declaration of Helsinki, 2000).

Route(s) to take in cases of suspicion

Research ethics committees should maintain records that can provide information to any legitimate body that is investigating a case of suspected fraud. Time and again, those who have committed fraud and are discovered for the first time, are also found to have committed it before. Multiple episodes of fraud, within repeating patterns of misconduct, are not uncommon. RECs are, however, advisory bodies and have no executive functions; they are not themselves detective agencies, nor are they legal entities, and they have no authority to investigate suspected or admitted misconduct. Their current duty when they suspect misconduct is to bring the matter to the attention of their establishing body – usually the Health Authority/Board/Commission or Trust.

Although it is probable that the research governance procedures currently being introduced in the NHS will define responsibility for assessing the research competence and suitability of investigators, it will still be necessary for LRECs to ensure that this assessment has taken place. The following clause appears in Governance Arrangements for Research Ethics Committees (2001): 'A member of an REC who becomes aware of a possible breach of good practice in research should report this initially to the Chair and Administrator of the REC, who shall inform the appointing Authority. The Authority's officers shall be accountable for taking appropriate action.'

The duty of a research ethics committee is therefore to co-operate in the investigations led by others with competence to investigate. An LREC is in a prime position to assist, and may be the only source of comprehensive information about an individual investigator's research activity. A committee can usually provide a list of those projects that the committee has considered and approved for that particular investigator during the past 5 years. This information can be used by the forensic team to pursue matters further (Wells & Blunt, 1997). As a result of this process, it is probable that a committee will have been given information about a doctor who has, beyond doubt, committed research misconduct; in those circumstances it is necessary for the committee to bear this information in mind when it comes to assess any future project submitted by that particular doctor.

Conclusions

Research ethics committees have an essential function to ensure that only research that is scientifically sound and ethically viable is approved. Additionally, however, they have important roles to play in tackling research misconduct and fraud, bearing in mind that such behaviour exploits patients and undermines scientific integrity. They can therefore constitute a powerful preventative measure, and can co-operate in providing information when a case of misconduct is being investigated by a legitimate organisation outside the ethics committee. If research ethics committees carry out these roles comprehensively, they will provide an environment in which it is more difficult for research misconduct to occur, and will clearly be demonstrating their commitment to protect patients and the public against harm.

REFERENCES

Association of the British Pharmaceutical Industry (ABPI)(1996). *Good Clinical Research Practice Guidelines.*

Blunt, J. (2001). The Role of Research Ethics Committees. In *Fraud and Misconduct in Medical Research.* 3rd edn. London: BMJ Books.

Commission of the European Communities (1991). CPMP Working Party on Efficacy of Medicinal Products. Notes for guidance on good clinical practice for trials on medicinal products in the European Community.

Farthing, M., Leck, S. & Wells, F. (2001). *Fraud and Misconduct in Medical Research.* 3rd edn. London: BMJ Books.

Governance Arrangements for NHS Research Ethics Committees (2001). London: Central Office for Research Ethics Committees.

Horton, R. (Editorial) (1996). Dealing with deception. *Lancet,* 347, 843.

International Conference on Harmonisation of Technical Requirements for Regulation of Pharmaceuticals for Human Use (ICH)(1996). *Tripartite Guideline for Good Clinical Practice.* Geneva: IFPMA.

Medical Research Council (1997). MRC policy and procedure for inquiring into allegations of scientific misconduct. MRC, December 1997 MRC ethics series.

Medical Research Council (1998). Guidelines for good clinical practice in clinical trials. MRC, March 1998.

Medical Research Council (1999). Human Tissue and Biological Samples for use in Research: MRC interim operational and ethical guidelines. MRC Consultation, November 1999.

Medical Research Council (2000). Personal Information in Medical Research. MRC guidelines MRC/55/00 October 2000 MRC ethics series.

Royal College of Pathologists (1999). Consensus Statement of Recommended Policies for Uses of Human Tissue in Research, Education and Quality Control. RCPath.

Royal College of Physicians (1991). Fraud and Misconduct in Medical Research. London.

Royal College of Physicians of Edinburgh (2000). Proceedings: Supplement No 7.

Wells, F. & Blunt, J. (1997). *Bulletin of Medical Ethics,* September 1997, 1.

World Medical Association (2000). Geneva: Declaration of Helsinki (Edinburgh revision).

Protecting the interests of research participants
(A) General principles

19

Understanding clinical trials: a model for providing information to potential participants

Philippa Easterbrook[1] and Joan Houghton[2] (and edited and reproduced with their kind permission)

[1]Division of Medicine, Guy's, King's and St Thomas' School of Medicine, London, UK
[2]Formerly at CRC Clinical Trials Centre, Rayne Institute, London, UK

How to use this booklet

For many people the idea of being involved in research raises fears of 'experimentation' or of being a 'guinea-pig'. Understanding what is involved in taking part in a research study can ease many of these anxieties. This booklet answers the questions patients ask most often about clinical trials, and can help you decide about taking part in a trial. It is meant to add to the information your doctor has already given you.

The 'Glossary' defines some of the common technical words used in clinical trials.

What is a clinical trial?

Almost every week we hear of a new drug for the treatment of a disease, or of a new diagnostic test or surgical procedure. These new treatments, tests and procedures must be shown to be effective and safe before they can be marketed or used more widely. A clinical trial is a research study in patients to test the usefulness and safety of a promising new treatment or procedure.

Clinical trials are used to study new ways to prevent, diagnose or treat diseases. Most trials evaluate new drugs or drug combinations, for example, antibiotic treatments for an infectious disease, or chemotherapy for a specific cancer. Other trials might test new radiation treatments or surgical procedures, such as a comparison of radical mastectomy vs. lumpectomy for the treatment of breast cancer. The example of a drug trial will be used throughout the rest of the booklet.

Clinical trials begin only after preliminary studies in the laboratory and with animals have shown promising

results. Clinical trials are usually conducted in three steps or phases:

Phase I trials

These test the treatment in a few healthy people to learn whether it is safe to take and what happens when it enters the human body.

Phase II trials

These test the treatment in a few patients to see if it is active against the disease in the short term. If the treatment is not effective, no more trials will take place.

Phase III trials

These test the treatment on several hundred to several thousand patients, often at many different clinics or hospitals. These trials usually compare the new treatment either with a treatment already in use or, occasionally, with no treatment.

The results of the trials are sent to the national Licensing Authority, called the Medicines Control Agency. If the Licensing Authority agrees that the new treatment is effective and safe, it is licensed for marketing.

Why are clinical trials needed?

Clinical trials are the link between basic laboratory research and everyday medical practice. Through clinical trials, researchers learn which treatments are most likely to be effective for future patients. A few treatments are so powerful that their value is obvious without a clinical trial. For instance, we do not have doubts about the value of penicillin for pneumonia, or surgery for appendicitis. However, the effects of most treatments are much less dramatic and need to be tested in a clinical trial. Not every trial will find a drug that works, but trials can also improve care by finding a drug that clearly does not work.

Many medical advances have been possible only because of clinical trials. Clinical trials have shown researchers which new drugs or combinations of drugs are most effective for the treatment of cancer and heart disease, and which surgical techniques and diagnostic tests work best. Clinical trials are also being used to find better treatment for life-threatening diseases such as TB and AIDS.

Who can join a clinical trial?

To be eligible to take part in a particular clinical trial, a patient must meet the eligibility requirements of that trial. These vary for each trial, and may include a person's age or stage of disease. Not everyone will be allowed to enter a trial. For instance, patients with conditions such as high blood pressure may not be eligible to join some trials.

How are clinical trials organised?

Planning

A great deal of thought and planning goes on before any clinical trial is set up. The plan for a trial (the 'protocol') gives the background to exactly how the trial will be run, which types of patients will be studied, the treatments involved, the timetable of tests and visits for patients, the length of the study, etc.

Ethical approval

Before a study can begin, the local research ethics committee must approve the protocol as safe and ethical. The membership of this committee varies from hospital to hospital, but usually includes doctors, nurses, a lay person from the community and sometimes a lawyer or a chaplain. The ethics committee works independently of the researchers setting up the clinical trial.

Patient consent

Before you can join a trial, the researchers must first explain the study to you, answer any questions you may have and obtain your agreement to take part. This is the same as when you give your consent for a surgical operation; the nature of the operation, its benefits and its side effects should be explained to you before you agree to go ahead. The same applies to joining a clinical trial. The doctors or nurses should tell you why the trial is being run, the risks you may face, and how you may be helped. Usually you will be asked to sign a consent form, to show that you understand what has been explained to you. Signing this form does not commit you to the study.

Study design

The most common type of clinical trial is a 'comparison trial' in which one group of patients receiving a new treatment is compared to another group of patients receiving an existing, often a standard treatment. The patients who receive the new experimental treatment are called the 'test group' and those who receive the standard treatment, the 'control group'. In some diseases, no standard treatment exists. In these cases, the new treatment will often be compared to no treatment or to a 'placebo'. A placebo is an inactive substance or 'dummy drug' that looks like the drug being tested. Patients will not be given a placebo if there is any treatment available that might benefit them.

The glossary gives a description of other types of clinical trials.

How treatment is chosen

In many studies, the decision about whether a patient receives the test or the control treatment is made using a predetermined code or in a random fashion. 'Randomisation' is the best way to avoid bias. This means that the test and the control treatments can be compared more accurately. Also, since the researchers do not know which treatment will turn out to be better or safer, randomisation gives all patients an equal chance of receiving the more effective or safer treatment, whichever it turns out to be.

Patient follow-up

The researchers carefully follow the progress of patients in both the control and test groups. They look for whether patients who received the new therapy had a different response from patients in the control group. Did the new treatment prevent the disease or slow its progress? Did the symptoms go away? Did patients have fewer side effects with the experimental drug?

What is it like to be in a clinical trial?

Once you agree to take part in a clinical trial, the doctor in charge of the trial will find out which treatment you are to receive. He will probably also contact your general practitioner (GP) and provide him with details of the trial. Usually you can take the treatment at home, but some trials require treatment in hospital.

During the trial, you will have to follow a schedule of treatment, check-ups and blood tests, to see if the treatment is working. The researchers will keep a careful record of your progress. You may have to visit the doctor as rarely as once every 6 months, or as often as five times a week. You may also be asked to keep a list of any side effects you notice from the treatment, or a record of your daily activities, or what you eat. It is important that you tell the researchers if you make any changes from the treatment protocol, for example, if you do not take your treatment as prescribed, or if you stop taking it altogether.

What about stopping the trial?

In the protocol, the researchers usually give an estimate of how long the trial will last. While some trials last only a few weeks, others can go on for years. Sometimes a trial will be stopped earlier than planned. In many large trials, a special group of independent researchers, called a data monitoring and safety committee, check regularly on the results of the trial during its progress. If they find that one group of patients is doing much better than the other, they can stop the trial and offer all the patients the better treatment. They can also stop the trial if one group of patients develops serious new side effects.

Your doctor can decide to take you out of a trial if he feels your condition is getting worse and the therapy is not helping you. You can also decide to leave a trial at any time, without it interfering with the regular medical care you receive.

What are the benefits of joining a clinical trial?

Helping future patients

Patients can contribute to medical knowledge by helping researchers learn whether a treatment or new test will be able to help more patients in the future. This in itself can give patients a sense of accomplishment.

Early access to a new treatment

Patients in clinical trials are among the first to receive new treatments before they become widely available. Sometimes experimental drugs are the only treatment available for a disease. In other cases patients may be unable to take the usual treatment because of side effects or allergies. While it is possible that the new treatment may turn out to be disappointing, the researchers hope that it will be more effective or have fewer side effects than the current treatment.

Specialist care

Whether or not patients receive the new treatment, they will get the benefit of excellent medical care, with frequent check-ups by specialists in the field.

What are the risks of joining a clinical trial?

'Unproven' treatment

Until clinical trials are held, no one knows whether the new treatment being tested will prove to be better than treatment already available. There is always the chance that the new treatment will turn out to be ineffective or do more harm than good.

Side effects

Like any medical therapy, the treatments tested in clinical trials carry some risks. Before a clinical trial begins, the new treatment has already been through much testing in the laboratory to make sure it is safe. The researchers may know about some of the side effects already, but more side effects may show up during the trial. Most of these, such as tiredness or nausea, are mild, and usually go away on their own, or after treatment is stopped. Other side effects can be more serious, like kidney or liver damage.

Inconvenience

Patients may sometimes have to make frequent visits to the hospital or GP surgery for check-ups on their progress, and for laboratory tests. Most tests just require drawing of blood, but some may be more complicated and time consuming.

Other questions to ask your doctor

Every clinical trial is different. It is important to find out what the demands of a particular trial will be before you agree to take part. Here is a list of questions you may want to ask, to help you decide if the trial is right for you. Most of these questions should be answered when the researcher first tells you about the study.

- What is the purpose of the study?
- What kinds of treatment does the study involve?
- What additional tests will be required because of the trial?
- How will the study affect my daily life? Will I require additional visits to the doctor? Will my diet be limited? Will I have to spend time in hospital?
- What are the standard treatments available for my disease? From what is already known, how does the new treatment compare with them?
- What is likely to happen to my condition with or without this new treatment?
- How long is the study expected to last?

Thinking it over

Taking part in a clinical trial involves making a commitment. Only you can decide whether or not to join. You must consider all the benefits and risks, and keep your personal interests in mind. There is nothing wrong in saying 'no' or asking for more time to think about it. If possible, talk the decision over with a doctor or a trusted relative or friend. Ask your GP or hospital doctor if you have any other questions or would like something explained in more detail.

GLOSSARY

Clinical trial A research study in patients to find out whether a new way of treating a disease is better, worse or the same as the therapy used at present.

Control group A group of patients in a study who receive the standard treatment (the other group is called the 'test group'). The standard treatment is the best medical treatment that would normally be given to a patient. When there is no standard treatment, the control group may receive either no treatment or a placebo.

Controlled trial A clinical trial in which an experimental treatment is compared with either another experimental treatment, or against a standard treatment or placebo.

Crossover trial A clinical trial in which all patients receive both treatments at different times. Halfway through the study, one group is switched from the control treatment to the experimental treatment, and the other is switched from the experimental treatment to the control.

Dose comparison trial A clinical trial that compares different amounts of the same drug.

'Double-blind or 'single-blind' trial A 'double-blind' trial is a trial in which neither the patient nor the researcher knows who is receiving the control treatment. This is done to prevent the results of the trial being biased. In a 'single-blind' trial, patients do not know what treatments they are getting, but their doctors do.

Eligibility criteria 'Inclusion criteria' are conditions you must meet to join a trial. Some are obvious, like age, or what symptoms you have. Others, like blood test results require laboratory tests. 'Exclusion criteria' are conditions that would disqualify you from the trial. These may include taking drugs other than the drug being studied, or certain diseases. Often patients are excluded for safety reasons, because doctors know that the new drug may cause people with a certain illness or blood test result to get sicker.

Informed consent Consent following a full written or verbal explanation of a trial, including the risks and benefits of taking part.

Placebo A pill or liquid that may look and taste exactly like a real drug, but contains no active substance (a 'dummy drug'). A placebo is sometimes given to the control group in a trial, so that neither the patients nor their doctors know who is taking the test drug and who is taking the placebo.

Protocol A research plan that gives the background to the trial and the way patients should be treated.

Randomisation The process of selecting by chance the treatment a patient will receive in a trial.

Side effect Unintended adverse effect from a drug or other treatment.

Test group A group of patients in a study who receive the new treatment (the other group is called the 'control group').

CERES – Consumers for Ethical Research – also produces useful information sheets for research participants, including Medical Research and You, Genetic Research and You and Spreading the World on Research (On writing patient information leaflets)
Ceres – PO Box 1365, London N16 OBW; www.ceres.org.uk

20

The law relating to consent

Andrew Grubb[1], Rosamund Scott[2], Penney Lewis[2] and Phil Bates[2]

[1]Law School, Cardiff University, Wales, UK
[2]Centre of Medical Law and Ethics, School of Law, King's College, London, UK

General principles: treatment

Consent and battery

In general, medical treatment may only be given lawfully to a patient with that patient's consent. A doctor who acts without a patient's consent risks criminal prosecution for assault or, more likely, being sued for damages in the tort of battery. A signed consent form is only evidence (not conclusive) that a patient has given consent to a treatment. It is the reality of the patient's consent which is the concern of the law (*Chatterton v. Gerson* [1981]).

Exceptionally, medical treatment may be given without consent where the patient is unable to consent, for example, where the patient is unconscious in an emergency or where the patient is permanently unable to consent through mental disability and the treatment is reasonably necessary in that patient's best medical interests (*Re F (A Mental Patient: Sterilisation)* [1990]).

A valid consent in law requires three elements:
(i) the patient must be competent to consent;
(ii) the consent must be based upon adequate information;
(iii) the consent must be voluntarily given.

Competence to consent

A patient will be competent to give consent if he or she is capable of understanding what is involved in the medical treatment, including the procedure itself, its consequences and the consequences of non-treatment.

An adult patient (i.e. has attained the age of 18) will usually be presumed to be competent to understand a medical

The original version of this article was written by Andrew Grubb in 1994. The article was revised and updated by Rosamund Scott, Penney Lewis and Phil Bates of The School of Law, King's College, London in 2001, who take responsibility for its current accuracy.

procedure unless there is good reason to doubt it, for example, if he or she is mentally ill, mentally disabled or affected by external factors such as drugs, alcohol, extreme pain, panic or shock. In such cases the patient will only be competent to consent if he or she is capable of 'comprehending and retaining treatment information', 'believing it' and 'weighing it in the balance to arrive at a choice' (*Re C* [1994]). This test was approved in *Re MB (An Adult: Medical Treatment)* [1997], in which Lady Justice Butler-Sloss emphasised the importance of 'some impairment or disturbance of mental functioning render[ing] the person unable to make a decision'. This inability would occur when the patient could not fulfil the tasks required in the first and third limbs of the *Re C* test. (In *Re MB* the requirement of ability to believe seems to have become part of the ability to weigh the information.)

The position of a child is somewhat different. For legal purposes, childhood begins at birth, and ends when the child reaches 18. However, if a child is aged between 16 and 18, he or she will be presumed to have the capacity to consent to medical treatment to the same extent as an adult (Family Law Reform Act 1969, s.8(1)). A child under the age of 16 will be able to consent to medical treatment providing he or she is sufficiently mature and intelligent to be able to understand what is involved in the treatment (*Gillick v. West Norfolk and Wisbech A.H.A.* [1986]). In *Re C (Detention: Medical Treatment)* [1997], the judge adopted the three-stage test which had been developed in earlier cases involving adults: that is, asking whether the child is capable of (i) comprehending and retaining treatment information, (ii) believing it, and (iii) weighing it in the balance to arrive at choice. Applying this approach, a child's capacity to understand will depend upon the individual child and the nature of the medical treatment, in particular its complexity and seriousness. A child may be capable of understanding what is involved in some procedures, for example setting a broken arm, but insufficiently mature to understand others, for example a heart bypass operation. In relation to medical research, it is likely that a child would have to demonstrate a high level of understanding before being regarded as 'Gillick competent' for this purpose (see below).

The power to make decisions about a child's medical treatment is an aspect of 'parental responsibility' under the Children Act 1989. Therefore, consent to a child's medical treatment may be obtained from a person with parental responsibility (usually one of the parents), as well as from a competent child, or from a court. The parents' consent to treatment is then valid in law, providing that it is exercised in the 'best interests' of the child. The ability of parents to consent to a child's involvement in non-therapeutic research is considered below. For recent case-law on parental consent to medical treatment see especially *Re T (A Minor) (Wardship: Medical Treatment) [1996]* and *Re A (Conjoined Twins: Medical Treatment) (No. 2) [2001]*. As a matter of good professional practice, even where a child is unable to provide a legally valid consent, it is usually appropriate to involve the child as fully as possible in decision-making (see British Medical Association, 2001). Unfortunately, the allocation of parental responsibility is legally complex, and not all parents have parental responsibility, and not everyone with parental responsibility is a parent. In particular, mothers have parental responsibility automatically, but a father who is not married to the mother will only have parental responsibility for a child if he has made a parental responsibility agreement with the mother, or obtained a court order granting him responsibility. Local authorities obtain parental responsibility for a child who is subject to a Care Order, but not if the child is merely accommodated by the Local Authority. Adoption of a child ends the parental responsibility of the parents, and gives parental responsibility to the adoptive parents. In cases where the allocation of parental responsibility is uncertain, it may be necessary to seek specific legal advice. In Scotland, these issues are governed by the Children (Scotland) Act 1995.

A controversial development in the law has established that, while a competent child may consent to medical treatment, the child's refusal will not necessarily be valid. A parent (or other with parental responsibility) may give a valid consent to medical treatment notwithstanding the child's refusal. It may be that the parents may only do so if the child's life is threatened or the treatment is necessary to avoid serious permanent harm to the child (*Re W* [1992]). Despite this development in relation to medical treatment, it is very doubtful that it would ever be appropriate to override a child's refusal to participate in research in this way (see below).

Information

For a consent to be valid, a patient must understand in broad terms the basic nature and purpose of the medical procedure (*Chatterton v. Gerson* [1981]). A doctor has a legal obligation to volunteer this information to the patient. Also, a patient's apparent consent will be invalid if it is induced through fraud or misrepresentation as to the nature of the medical procedure (*Sidaway v. Bethlem Royal Hospital* [1985]).

Voluntariness

A patient's consent must be freely given without coercion or pressure. Whether a patient's consent is voluntary is a question of degree and will depend upon the individual circumstances of each case. However, where there is a danger of pressure or coercion, the court will be alive to that risk in determining whether the patient's consent is in fact freely given (*Freeman v. Home Office (No. 2)* [1984], *Re T* [1992]).

Consent and negligence

Alternatively, a doctor may be sued for damages in the tort of negligence if he or she fails to comply with his legal duty when obtaining a patient's consent and harm results to the patient. This legal duty may go beyond that seen above in the context of a battery action. It consists of the duty to provide information not only relating to the nature and purpose of the procedure, but also other information such as risks inherent in the procedure and available alternatives.

Traditionally understood, what this amounts to is that the doctor must volunteer to his patient all information which a reasonable doctor would provide having regard to the particular circumstances of the patient. In general, a doctor will satisfy this requirement if he or she responsibly exercises his or her clinical judgement in determining what information should be provided and his or her view is supported by a competent and responsible body of medical opinion. Exceptionally, however, the court may determine that the information is so necessary for the patient to make an informed decision whether to consent to the treatment or not that a doctor who fails to provide it would be in breach of his legal duty to the patient (*Sidaway v. Bethlem Royal Hospital* [1985]). More recently, in *Pearce v. United Bristol Healthcare N.H.S. Trust* [1998], the Court of Appeal defined the standard of disclosure by drawing together the decisions in *Sidaway* and *Bolitho v. City and Hackney H.A.* [1998]. (The latter is the most recent House of Lords' decision on clinical negligence, in which Lord Browne-Wilkinson held that a respectable or responsible body of medical opinion is one having a logical basis in which medical professionals have directed their minds to comparative risks and benefits to reach a 'defensible' conclusion on the matter.) In *Pearce* Lord Woolf M.R. held that 'if there is a significant risk which would affect the judgement of a reasonable patient, then in the normal course it is the responsibility of a doctor to inform the patient of that significant risk, if the information is needed so that the patient can determine for him or herself as to what course he or she should adopt'.

Additionally, a doctor will be in breach of his duty if he does not truthfully answer any questions his patient may put to him unless the doctor forms the view reasonably that to provide the information requested would be demonstrably harmful to the patient's physical or mental health (*Sidaway* [1985]). Recent Court of Appeal case-law has re-emphasised that 'if a patient asks a doctor about the risk, then the doctor is required to give an honest answer' (per Lord Woolf M.R. in *Pearce*).

Consent and research

These principles should be borne in mind when determining the application of the law of consent to research on patients or healthy volunteers. The law may not always, however, reach identical conclusions. It is important to distinguish between therapeutic research (where there is a dual intention, i.e. to treat the patient and obtain data of a generalisable nature) and non-therapeutic research (where there is only the latter intention). The crucial factor which distinguishes clinical research from treatment is the intention always to use the individual as a means of generating scientific data. The law in this area is untested because there is no governing legislation and, as yet, the courts have not been called upon to express a view.

When applying the general principles outlined above, all of which equally apply to research, those which call for special comment are:

(a) the individual's capacity to consent – competence;
(b) the information which must be given to a research subject;
(c) the position of the incompetent research subject.

Capacity to consent: competence

Therapeutic research

In general, an *adult patient* may validly consent to therapeutic research if he or she is competent to understand what is to be undertaken.

Whether *a child* (a minor) may validly consent to therapeutic research is more problematic. A child aged between 16 and 18 *may* be competent to give a valid consent to the same extent as an adult if section 8(1) of the Family Law Reform Act 1969 (which refers to 'treatment') applies to therapeutic research. If the Act does not apply (because the research is not 'treatment', or because the child is under the age of 16), it is necessary to ask whether a child can consent to research under the *Gillick* principle considered above. The law relating to treatment would suggest that a valid consent may be given to therapeutic research if the child is capable of understanding what is involved in what is proposed by the doctor. However, given the fact that the child would be consenting, in part, to research and what that entails, the court is likely to require a high standard of comprehension and, therefore, a child is less likely to have sufficient maturity and intelligence to consent to therapeutic research.

Furthermore, even if a child is competent to consent, it will usually be appropriate to seek the consent of the child's parents even if this is not required as a matter of strict law. The Department of Health's 1991 guidance for Research Ethics Committees took an even more cautious approach: 'Children who are under 16 years of age may ... be able to give full consent – providing they have sufficient understanding of what is proposed, as judged by the doctor attending them. Even for therapeutic purposes it would, however, be unacceptable not to have the consent of the parent or guardian where the child is under 16. Where the child is over 16 and under 18 generally parental consent should also be required – unless it is clearly in the child's best interests that the parents should not be informed.' (Department of Health, 1991). The latest version of this guidance (Department of Health, *Governance Arrangements for NHS Research Ethics Committees*, 2001), does not contain this statement, so the current view of the Department of Health on this issue is unclear.

Non-therapeutic research

Again, an adult healthy volunteer or patient would be presumed by the law to be competent to consent to non-therapeutic research. However, given the lack of benefit to the individual, the law is likely to set limits on the risk of harm that an individual may agree to be exposed to. It is likely that the court would only permit an adult to expose himself to what is frequently called 'minimal risk' or 'minimal burden'.

In the case of children aged between 16 and 18, section 8(1) of the Family Law Reform Act 1969 does not apply to non-therapeutic research, and so it is unclear whether a child of any age can consent to such research. Even if a competent child could legally consent to non-therapeutic research, a court would require a very high standard of competence before accepting that a particular child was competent to consent to non-therapeutic research. It may therefore be difficult for a child to give a valid consent to non-therapeutic research and, in any event, there are strict limits upon the level of risk for which a child should be able to volunteer. However, in relation to procedures involving 'minimal burden', the Royal College of Paediatrics and Child Health guidance suggests that young children may be able to understand what is involved in relatively simple non-therapeutic procedures:

'Where children are unable to give consent, by reason of insufficient maturity or understanding, their parents or guardians may consent to the taking of blood for non-therapeutic purposes, provided that they have been given and understand a full explanation of the reasons for blood sampling and have balanced its risk to their child. Many children fear needles, but with careful explanation of the reason for venepuncture and an understanding of the effectiveness of local anaesthetic cream, they often show altruism and allow a blood sample to be taken. We believe that this has to be the child's decision. We believe that it is completely inappropriate to insist on the taking of blood for non-therapeutic reasons if a child indicates either significant unwillingness before the start or significant stress during the procedure.' (Royal College of Paediatrics and Child Health, 2000).

Information

It was seen above that the law of consent to treatment requires that a doctor should adequately inform a patient about what is involved. When the procedure proposed is therapeutic or non-therapeutic research, the law requires a greater degree of disclosure.

Battery

A doctor's obligation to inform an individual in broad terms of the nature and purpose of the procedure would go further in cases of therapeutic or non-therapeutic research. In addition to the matters referred to above in the case of medical treatment, it would be essential for the patient or healthy volunteer to be told that they are to be a research subject. Further, a court may insist that the patient or healthy volunteer be informed that, for example, they may withdraw at any time from the research without adverse consequence to them, that they may be part of a controlled group in a clinical trial and (if relevant) that the trial is a randomised controlled trial.

Negligence

A researcher's duty of care would require disclosure to an individual not only of the fact that the individual is involved in research but also any information relevant to the patient or healthy volunteer's participation in the research. In addition to the risks inherent in the procedure, by way of example such information would include any future tests the individual might have to undergo, that he might have to stay in hospital longer or visit hospital more often in the future.

In the case of therapeutic research a doctor's duty would not be governed by the standards current in the medical profession. While a court might be guided by medical practice, the law will impose its own standards of disclosure to protect the interests of the research subject and to allow them to make a *fully* informed decision of whether to participate in the research. Obviously, in the case of non-therapeutic research, the standards current in the medical profession are irrelevant. The researcher might make reference to common practice among researchers but a court would adopt the same approach as mentioned above.

One particular point worth noting is that, in the case of therapeutic research, the law is unlikely to accept that information may be withheld from a patient out of a concern for the patient's health (the so-called 'therapeutic privilege'). This is undoubtedly true in the case of a healthy volunteer or patient agreeing to participate in non-therapeutic research.

Incompetent patients and healthy volunteers

The extent to which the law permits a child or an incompetent adult to be the subject of research is very problematic. This is acknowledged in recent GMC guidance:

'You should seek further advice where your research will involve adults who are not able to make decisions for themselves, or children. You should be aware that in these cases the legal position is complex or unclear, and there is currently no general consensus on how to balance the possible risks and benefits to such vulnerable individuals against the public interest in conducting research. You should consult the guidance issued by bodies such as the Medical Research Council and the medical royal colleges to keep up to date. You should also seek advice from the relevant research ethics committee where appropriate.' (General Medical Council, 1999, para 37)

It is helpful to consider adults and children separately.

Adults

It is clear that no one has legal power to consent to medical treatment on behalf of an adult who is incompetent. Instead, the law permits a doctor to *treat* an incompetent adult when the doctor reasonably believes that the treatment is in the 'best interests' of the individual in order to preserve his health, life or well-being (*Re F* [1990]). It is the application of this principle which would most probably also govern the lawfulness of research upon an incompetent adult.

While a court would, if called upon to do so, carefully scrutinise any decision to carry out *therapeutic research* upon an incompetent adult, the law would accept that such research could be carried out where it would have been justified in the case of a competent adult provided the researcher has satisfied a research ethics committee of this, i.e. of its scientific validity and of the need for, and ethical propriety of, such research.

A potential difficulty arises if the individual is to be placed in a randomised trial. In such a case, a doctor's duty to the patient may be compromised if he thinks (or, in a 'double-blind trial', is unable to tell whether) the patient is not receiving what, in his view, is the best treatment. In the case of a competent patient, this problem is overcome by the patient waiving his doctor's duty to act in what the doctor thinks is in his 'best interests' once the patient has full knowledge of the nature of the trial and agrees to participate. If this is correct, an incompetent patient is unable to waive the doctor's duty and hence randomisation would not be possible. The law is untested on this matter.

As regards *non-therapeutic research*, one view of the law is that it cannot lawfully be carried out on an incompetent adult since such research can never, as the law requires, be in the individual's 'best interests' (*Re F* [1990]). In one case, the court allowed an incompetent adult to donate bone marrow to her sister who was seriously ill because the emotional benefits to the donor doing so outweighed the small physical risks to her (*Re Y* [1996]). While this allows an individual to be considered, it probably has no application to cases of non-therapeutic research. While the law remains uncertain, an alternative view may be that non-therapeutic research on incompetent adults is lawful if it cannot be done on competent persons, it poses only 'minimal' or 'negligible risk', and it is 'not against the interests' of the incompetent person (MRC, *The Ethical Conduct of Research on the Mentally Incapacitated* (1991); Law Commission, *Mental Incapacity* (1995)).

Whereas the law in England and Wales is uncertain, Scottish Law is much clearer, because of the Adults with Incapacity (Scotland) Act 2000. Section 51 states that no surgical, medical, nursing, dental or psychological research shall be carried out on any adult who is incapable in relation to a decision about participation in the research unless research of a similar nature cannot be carried out on an adult who is capable in relation to such a decision. In addition, it is necessary to show that the purpose of the research is to obtain knowledge of the causes, diagnosis, treatment or care of the adult's incapacity; or the effect of any treatment or care given during his incapacity to the adult which relates to that incapacity. Finally, it is necessary to demonstrate that:

(a) the research is likely to produce real and direct benefit to the adult;
(b) the adult does not indicate unwillingness to participate in the research;
(c) the research has been approved by the Ethics Committee;
(d) the research entails no foreseeable risk, or only a minimal foreseeable risk, to the adult;
(e) the research imposes no discomfort, or only minimal discomfort, on the adult; and
(f) consent has been obtained from any guardian or welfare attorney who has power to consent to the adult's participation in research or, where there is no such guardian or welfare attorney, from the adult's nearest relative.

However, in cases where the research is not likely to produce real and direct benefit to the adult, it may nevertheless be carried out if it will contribute, through significant improvement in the scientific understanding of the adult's incapacity, to the attainment of real and direct benefit to the adult or to other persons having the same incapacity, provided the other circumstances or conditions mentioned above are fulfilled. In England, the Law Commission have made similar recommendations, but the Government has not yet introduced legislation on this issue.

Children

It is unclear to what extent a person with parental responsibility ('the proxy') can legally consent to the involvement of a child in medical research (especially non-therapeutic research). In *Re A (Conjoined Twins: Medical Treatment) (No. 2)* [2001], Ward L.J. confirmed that parental rights and powers exist for the performance of the parents' duties and responsibilities to the child, and must be exercised in the best interests of the child. Applying this principle to research, it seems that the proxy may consent to *therapeutic research* providing it is in the 'best interests' of the child having regard to the risk–benefit ratio of the procedure proposed, given the child's illness. Although it is more problematic, it seems likely that a proxy may consent to the child being placed in a randomised trial even though the doctor's duty to the child may thereby be compromised if he thinks (or, in the case of a 'double-blind trial', is unable to tell whether) his child patient is receiving what he considers the best treatment.

It is essential that the proxy should be fully informed of all relevant information pertaining to the therapeutic research including, if it is the case, the fact of randomisation. There is no legal basis for deliberately withholding information from a proxy based on the notion of 'therapeutic privilege'. However, a court would take into account the practical difficulties involved in communicating detailed information in certain contexts, for example when dealing with the parents of a seriously ill child (see BMA, 2001, Chapter 9). As a minimum, however, a person giving consent to research (including a proxy) should understand that it is research to which they are consenting, and that the results are not predictable (see General Medical Council, 1999, para 35).

If a child's involvement in research must always be in the child's best interests, then the legality of non-therapeutic research on children is very doubtful. However, this issue has never been considered directly by the courts. In *S v S* [1970], the House of Lords stated that a child could undergo a blood test to ascertain paternity, provided that this was *not against* the child's best interests. However, it could be argued that this is appropriate because establishing the identity of the child's father is a procedure which is intended to benefit the child. No such justification would be available in relation to the child's non-therapeutic research. On the other hand, parents routinely expose their children to all manner of small 'day-to-day' risks in the course of everyday life, and the law usually interferes only where the child is likely to be harmed by the parents' behaviour. Therefore, it could be argued that parents may consent to medical research provided that it is not against their child's interest. (See, for example, RCPCH (2000), British Medical Association (2001), and Montgomery (2001).) Although this view is now widely accepted, there should be strict limits on proxy consent, so a proxy would not be able to consent to non-therapeutic research which involves more than 'minimal risk' to the child (see Nicholson, 1986) or 'minimal burden' (see Department of Health, *Reference Guide to Consent for Examination or Treatment*, 2001).

REFERENCES AND FURTHER READING

Re A (Conjoined Twins: Medical Treatment) (No. 2) [2001] 1 F.L.R. 267.
Bolitho v. City and Hackney H.A. [1998] A.C. 232.
Re C (Detention: Medical Treatment) [1997] 2 F.L.R. 180.
Re C [1994] 1 All E.R. 819.
Chatterton v. Gerson [1981] 1 Q.B. 432.
Re F (A Mental Patient: Sterilisation) [1990] 2 A.C. 1.
Freeman v. Home Office (No. 2) [1984] Q.B. 524.
Gillick v. West Norfolk and Wisbech A.H.A. [1986] A.C. 112.
Re MB (An Adult: Medical Treatment) [1997] 38 B.M.L.R. 175.
Pearce v. United Bristol Healthcare N.H.S. Trust [1998] 48 B.M.L.R. 118.
S v S [1970] 3 All ER 107; [1972] AC 24; [1970] 3 WLR 366, House of Lords.
Sidaway v. Bethlem Royal Hospital [1985] 1 All E.R. 643.
Re T (A Minor) (Wardship: Medical Treatment) [1996] 35 B.M.L.R. 63.
Re T (Adult: Refusal of Treatment) [1992] 4 All E.R. 649.
Re W [1992] 4 All E.R. 627.
Re Y (Mental incapacity: bone marrow transplant) [1996] 2 FLR 787; [1997] 2 WLR 556.

Adults with Incapacity (Scotland) Act 2000.
Children Act 1989.
Children (Scotland) Act 1995.
British Medical Association (2001). *Consent, Rights and Choices in Health Care for Children and Young People.* BMJ Books.
Department of Health (1991). *Guideline on Local Research Ethics Committees,* HSG 91(5).
Department of Health (2001). *Governance Arrangements for NHS Research Ethics Committees* (Department of Health).
Department of Health (2001). *Reference Guide to Consent for Examination or Treatment.* Department of Health.
General Medical Council (1999). *Seeking Patients' Consent: The Ethical Considerations.* GMC.
Kennedy (1998). Research and experimentation. In Kennedy & Grubb, *Principles of Medical Law.* OUP, p. 730.
Law Commission (1995) *Mental Incapacity.* HMSO.
Montgomery, J. (2001). Informed consent and clinical research with children. In Doyal and Tobias (eds), *Informed Consent in Medical Research.* BMJ Books.
MRC (1991). *The Ethical Conduct of Research on the Mentally Incapacitated.* MRC.
Nicholson, R. (ed). (1986). *Medical Research with Children.* OUP.
Royal College of Paediatrics and Child Health: Ethics Advisory Committee (2000). 'Guidelines for the ethical conduct of medical research involving children' *Arch Dis Child,* 82, 177–182.

USEFUL WEBSITES

Data Protection Act 1998
http://www.hmso.gov.uk/acts/acts1998/19980029.htm

Human Fertilisation and Embryology Act 1990
http://www.hmso.gov.uk/acts/acts1990/
Ukpga_19900037_en_1.htm

Human Rights Act 1998
http://www.hmso.gov.uk/acts/acts1998/19980042.htm

Health and Social Care Act
http://www.hmso.gov.uk/acts/acts2001/20010015.htm

Scotland

Adults with Incapacity (Scotland) Act 2000
http://www.hmso.gov.uk/legislation/scotland/acts2000/
20000004.htm

Family Law Reform Act 1969 (not available on the web)

8 Consent by persons over 16 to surgical, medical and dental treatment

(1) The consent of a minor who has attained the age of sixteen years to any surgical, medical or dental treatment which, in the absence of consent, would constitute a trespass to his person, shall be as effective as it would be if he were of full age; and where a minor has by virtue of this section given an effective consent to any treatment

it shall not be necessary to obtain any consent for it from his parent or guardian.

(2) In this section 'surgical, medical or dental treatment' includes any procedure undertaken for the purposes of diagnosis, and this section applies to any procedure (including, in particular, the administration of an anaesthetic) which is ancillary to any treatment as it applies to that treatment.

(3) Nothing in this section shall be construed as making ineffective any consent which would have been effective if this section had not been enacted.

21

Writing information for potential research participants

Elizabeth Mellor[1], David K. Raynor[2] and Jonathan Silcock[2]

[1]Pharmacy Services, The Leeds Teaching Hospitals NHS Trust, UK
[2]Pharmacy Practice and Medicines Management, School of Healthcare Studies, University of Leeds, UK

Introduction

Good researchers show respect for participants' needs, rights, well-being and safety. In part, they do this by giving (potential) research participants clear and accurate written information. In this chapter we provide guidance on producing consent forms and information leaflets that are easy to read and understand. This will help researchers who prepare written information and research ethics committee (REC) members who review it. Researchers will need other sources of practical advice and we provide some references. For information on broader issues, you could contact Consumers for Ethics in Research (http://www.ceres.org.uk) or Consumers in NHS Research (http://www.hfht.org/ConsumersinNHSResearch/).

Information for potential participants should inform, educate and explain (Scotland, 1985). It must not coerce or unreasonably induce participation in research. Potential participants (patients, carers, users or volunteers) will usually have little medical knowledge and will possess a range of reading ages, education and intelligence. Participants with good reading and comprehension skills will not be insulted by simple and direct language.

Concern for participant welfare will guide study design and should be apparent in your writing. This chapter contains specific guidance on:
- content that is accurate, unambiguous and comprehensible
- style that is clear and direct (Anon, 2000)
- layout and presentation that indicates competence (Secker & Pollard, 1995).

Content of written information

Detailed guidance on what to write in consent forms and information leaflets can be obtained elsewhere, for example:

- your local REC
- the Central Office for Research Ethics Committees (COREC) (http://www.corec.org.uk)
- the US National Library of Medicine (http://www.clinicaltrials.gov)
- the International Conference on Harmonisation (http://www.ich.org)

Written information will contain all the details necessary to ensure that consent is informed and describe mechanisms for ensuring participant confidentiality. In this brief guidance we suggest wording that is based on the principles of plain English. Other examples can be found that are often based on previous custom and practice. It is vital for researchers to consider the suitability of wording for their own participants.

An invitation to participate voluntarily

The invitation to participate should be clear and direct. For example: 'We invite you to take part in a research project. You do not have to accept our invitation. If you decide to refuse, then you don't need to give us a reason.' A less appropriate alternative is: 'You are being invited to participate in a research project. Participation in this trial is entirely voluntary and you are free to decline entry into this study.' Passive verbs are used in this last sentence (see below) and the synonyms 'trial', 'project' and 'study' may cause confusion.

Be open to questions from potential participants who seek clarification or more information. You could state 'Please ask us if there is anything you don't understand. Please read this information carefully before you decide what to do. We will give you time to think and ask other people for advice.'

Project details

Give project details under appropriate sub-headings, which may be short, user-friendly questions such as 'What if something goes wrong?' A logical order might be:

- *Purpose*: give a brief rationale for the project and state what it hopes to achieve.
- *Selection*: state reasons why the potential participant was approached.
- *Process*: give full details of any procedures, testing and questionnaires.
- *Benefits*: assess potential impact on participants' health, including zero benefit for healthy volunteers or in non-therapeutic research.
- *Risks*: clearly identify and explain the risks of therapeutic research.
- *Special considerations*: highlight and discuss any unusual or novel interventions.
- *Protection*: describe the procedure for complaints and possible compensation for harm caused.

Rights to confidentiality and withdrawal

The Data Protection Act 1998 requires respect for confidentiality, so explain what you will do to achieve this (Anon, 2001). Clearly state that participants can withdraw at any time and that withdrawal will not affect normal medical care. If relevant, explain the normal treatment for the participants' clinical condition.

Simple rules for plain English

Talk directly to the reader

Descriptions of procedures will be much more meaningful if the potential participant is addressed as 'you' and the researchers are addressed as 'we'. For example, 'If you agree to take part, then we will put you into one of two groups.' Most people would be disturbed and confused by: 'random allocation into control and treatment groups will be performed by a computer.'

Use simple words and do not use jargon

Your writing should be formal and polite, but the vocabulary should be as simple as possible. Choosing words in English is often difficult because we have many everyday and sophisticated options, for example, 'give – administer' and 'test – analyse'. Medical science also has a wealth of jargon, for example, 'knee cap – patella' and 'pill – oral contraceptive'. Simple, short options should be chosen whenever they are accurate and precise.

If technical or medical words must be used, then a simple definition will be needed. For example, 'Leukaemia is a disease that makes white blood cells faulty. White blood cells are needed to help the body fight infection', or 'Left ventricular failure is a type of heart failure. In heart failure the heart does not pump enough blood round the body'.

Be positive and direct

Try to write in a positive and direct style. Make sentences short and without too much punctuation. If more than one comma or connecting word seem necessary, then consider more than one sentence or a bulleted list. Make sure that your main point is in the first part of a sentence and/or paragraph.

There is no need to use conditional language throughout your document to demonstrate the absence of coercion, e.g. 'you would be' (cf. Hughes & Foster, 1997, p. II.23). The simple present (we are) or future tense (you will) is easier to understand. For example: 'We will split you into two groups. In the first group you take a new medicine that we are testing. In the second group you take the most commonly used medicine. We need to compare the new and old medicines fairly. We do this by randomly choosing the group you go into. We could toss a coin to do this, but use a computer because it's quicker. The same number of people will take each medicine.'

Active is better than passive

Clear writing describes people doing things, not people having things done to them. So use active verbs not passive ones. For example, 'a blood sample will be taken' is passive, but 'we will take a blood sample' is active. Most people find the passive more difficult to understand. Subject, verb and object should usually remain in order, for example 'you – will take – the medicine' or 'we – will measure – your blood pressure'. Some passive construction is necessary, but it should not be used to make procedures sound less dangerous or to avoid clear responsibility.

Don't turn verbs into nouns

In formal documents, verbs are often turned into nouns (nominalisation). 'Allocation' is an abstract noun formed from the verb 'allocate'; 'decision' is formed from 'decide'. Like the passive, nominalisation obscures meaning and generates meaningless filler words (Russell, 1993, p. 95). For example, 'When your blood has been tested, a decision will be taken with respect to your continued participation in the trial.' This could read 'We will test your blood and decide if you should stay in the trial.'

Testing readability

Testing on real people is the only foolproof way to find out if your written information can be read and understood. A valid test of readability is a small pilot with participants similar to those in your main study. Readability statistics or formulae are for guidance only. The most commonly used formula is Flesch reading ease. This is based on 'words per sentence' and 'syllables per 100 words'. Higher scores (100) indicate easier reading than lower scores (0).

You may come across Flesch–Kincard grade level. US school students enter Grade 1 at age 6, so grade level 10 indicates a reading age of about 15. Any piece of text should have as few passive sentences as possible. We tested a randomly selected article from the *Sun* newspaper that had reading ease of 84.6, grade level of 2.6 and 3% passive sentences. The corresponding figures for a draft of this chapter were 54.2, 9.5 and 15%.

When you are preparing information for children (or people with learning difficulties), readability statistics may help you to modify your normal style. Readers should understand your writing after it has been read once. For more advice on plain English try the web pages of the:
• Plain English Campaign (www.plainenglish.co.uk).
• Plain Language Network
  (www.plainlanguagenetwork.org).
• US Government (www.plainenglish.gov).

Layout and presentation

Guide the reader

The layout and presentation of information is a matter of individual choice, but may significantly affect comprehension. Detailed written information may benefit from a short covering letter that incorporates an invitation to participate. A short introduction can be used to highlight important points and guide the reader through detailed text. Make an effort to select and use clear sub-headings. Group related points together under an appropriate heading.

Be open and accessible

A face-to-face meeting with a researcher (or associate) will give potential participants more chances to ask questions. You should usually allow at least 24 hours for decision making and consultation with friends, family, other healthcare professionals or carers. The actual time allowed may reflect: the complexity of the research, potential risks to the participants, normal practice; and the clinical condition of patients. Further questions or problems may arise after consent is given. Give details in any written information that let participants contact a researcher quickly and conveniently.

Look good

Written information should be printed in a professional font, and laser-printed originals make the clearest copies. A4 is the standard paper size, but it can be made into an A5 booklet or split into columns. Line spacing of 1.5 is comfortable for most people and text should usually be aligned left. Justified text, with unequal space between words, is harder to read and centred text is often confusing.

Densely packed text with many highlighted words is very hard for the reader to scan. Sparing use of *italic*, **bold** and <u>underlined</u> styles is advised. Bold is preferred when emphasis is necessary. Headings can be highlighted with additional space rather than underlining. Leaving plenty of clear space is especially important around bullet points and lists. For some groups, well-designed cartoons or pictograms may be a useful aid to understanding.

Consider your reader when choosing font size and style. Capitalised text is VERY HARD TO READ quickly; do not use it in the body of your document. For general use a 12-point serif font is easy to read, for example, Times New Roman. Older readers might find a larger sans serif font easier to read, for example, 14-point Ariel. The Royal National Institute for the Blind sometimes use 16-point text for partially sighted readers (Secker & Pollard, 1995, p. 19).

Conclusion

We have provided brief but clear guidance on providing written information for research participants. The quality of written information must be excellent in order to obtain informed consent. Excellence, in this context, means that participants readily understand what you have written and are able to accurately describe their role in your project. Good use of plain English reflects the importance of participant welfare in clinical research.

REFERENCES

Anon (2000). *How to Write Reports in Plain English*. New Mills: Plain English Campaign. Online at http://www.plainenglish.co.uk/reportguide.html

Anon (2001). *Research Governance Framework for Health and Social Care*. London: Department of Health. Online at http://www.doh.gov.uk/research

Hughes, T. & Foster, C. (1997). Communicating with the potential research subject. *Manual for Research Ethics Committees*, 5th edn.

Russell, R. (1993). *Grammar, Structure and Style: A Practical Guide to A-level English*. Oxford: Oxford University Press.

Scotland, A. (1985). Towards readability and style. *Community Medicine*, 7, 126–132.

Secker, J. & Pollard, R. (1995). *Writing Leaflets for Patients: Guidelines for Producing Written Information*. Edinburgh: Health Education Board for Scotland.

22

The law relating to confidentiality

Andrew Grubb[1], Ian Kennedy[2] and Sabine Michalowski[3]

[1]Law School Cardiff University, Wales, UK
[2]School of Public Policy, University College London, UK
[3]Department of Law, University of Essex, UK

Obligation to protect confidentiality

Those involved in clinical research owe an ethical and legal obligation to respect the confidences of research subjects. The obligation extends to all personal information, medical and other, given to or observed by the researcher in circumstances where the research subject expects it not to be disclosed. This expectation need not be explicitly stated but may be assumed from the context, e.g. it is always assumed in a physician–patient relationship, regardless of the existence of a contract between the physician and the patient. Health care professionals who disclose confidential information may be subject to disciplinary action by their professional body (e.g. the GMC or UKCC) and all researchers, whether health care professionals or not, may also be subject to legal action. Medical confidentiality is protected as part of the right to private life under Article 8(1) of the European Convention on Human Rights (*Z* v *Finland* [1997]), and consequently also under the Human Rights Act 1998.

Disclosure of information which does not reveal the identity of a research subject, e.g. epidemiological or aggregated data, is not a breach of the obligation of confidence. This is even true where anonymised patient information is sold for research purposes without the patient's consent (*R* v *Department of Health, ex parte Source Informatics Ltd* [1999]).

Exemptions from the duty of confidentiality

There are a number of exceptions to the obligation of confidentiality which may justify disclosure.

The original version of this article was written by Andrew Grubb and Ian Kennedy in 1994. The article was revised and updated by Sabine Michalowski of the Department of Law, University of Essex in 2001, who takes responsibility for its current accuracy.

Consent

Disclosure of confidential information is lawful if the patient consents to it. This consent may be expressed, whether verbal or in writing, or implied from the circumstances. Consent may be implied where a reasonable patient would expect disclosure to take place, for example, sharing of information between health care professionals involved in the patient's treatment. Ordinarily in a clinical trial the research protocol should refer to the need to obtain express permission if confidential information is to be used in a manner which will identify the research subject. The GMC guidelines (GMC, 2000) specify in paragraph 16 that a patient's consent to the disclosure of identifiable patient information can exceptionally be implied where the disclosure is needed for research purposes and is unlikely to have personal consequences for the patient; the anonymisation of the data and the obtaining of express consent is not practicable; and the patient has been told, or had access to written material informing him/her of the possibility of disclosure for that purpose.

Public interest justification

Disclosure may be justified if it is in the public interest. While both ethics and the law will jealously guard the right of a patient or healthy volunteer to confidentiality, there may be circumstances in which this right must be weighed against the public interest in disclosure where there is a real or serious risk that another, or the public at large, may be put in danger by the patient or the healthy volunteer (e.g. *W* v. *Egdell* [1990]). The doctor or researcher must conscientiously weigh the interests of others and reasonably conclude that the risks to them outweigh the patient's or healthy volunteer's right before disclosure will be ethical or lawful. Importantly, neither public curiosity nor the general benefit to society of research will suffice (*X* v. *Y* [1988]). Disclosure in criminal proceedings would not violate Article 8 of the ECHR or, correspondingly, the Human Rights Act 1998 (*Z* v *Finland* [1998]).

Statutes requiring disclosure

Disclosure of confidential information will be justified if required by statute, e.g. Abortion Act 1967 (notify Chief Medical Officer); or Public Health (Control of Diseases) Act 1984 (notifiable diseases). Under s.60 of the Health and Social Care Act 2001, the Secretary of State may make regulations requiring or authorising the disclosure of patient information for medical purposes, including medical research, if this is necessary in the interests of improving patient care or in the public interest.

Access to medical records

Under s.7 of the Data Protection Act 1998, a patient (or healthy volunteer) is entitled to obtain access to his or her medical records whether stored electronically or manually. Disclosure of part or all of the record to the patient may be withheld where that would be 'likely to cause serious harm to the physical or mental health of the data subject' (Article 5(1) of the Data Protection (Subject Access Modification) (Health) Order 2000), or where disclosure would identify information relating to another person. The patient's right of access to personal data pursuant to s.7 of the Data Protection Act 1998 does not extend to data which are processed (the term 'process' includes the mere fact that data are being held) only for research purposes, provided the data are not processed to support measures or decisions with respect to particular individuals, the processing is not done in such a way as to cause, or be likely to cause, substantial damage or distress to the data subject, and the results of the research are not made available in a form which identifies the data subject (s.33 of the Data Protection Act 1998).

This legislation does not raise any problems of confidentiality when disclosure is made to the patient (or healthy volunteer). However, the situation is more complex if the data subject is incompetent: under Article 5(3) and (4) of the Data Protection (Subject Access Modification) (Health) Order 2000, persons with parental responsibility (in the case of children), or persons who have been appointed by a court order to manage the research subject's affairs (in the case of incompetent adults), can, in principle, obtain access to medical records, unless one of the exceptions set out in Article 5(3) and (4) applies.

Confidentiality and its limits under the Data Protection Act 1998

The confidentiality of personal information contained in medical records, whether stored electronically or manually, is guaranteed by the provisions of the Data Protection Act 1998. However, the Act only protects individualised personal information and therefore does not apply to anonymised data.

According to the Data Protection Principles set out in Schedule 1 to the 1998 Act, personal data shall be processed fairly and lawfully. Data originally obtained for a specific purpose may be further processed for other research purposes if the data are not processed to support measures or decisions with respect to particular individuals and the processing is not done in such a way as to cause, or be likely to cause, substantial damage or distress to the data subject (s.33 Data Protection Act 1998). Data related to a person's health are regarded as sensitive personal data and receive particular protection under Schedule 3 of the Act. However, such data may be disclosed, for example, in order to protect vital interests of another person; if it is necessary in connection with legal proceedings; or if it is necessary for the administration of justice. (For a detailed analysis of the Data Protection Act 1998, see I. Kennedy and A. Grubb, *Medical Law*, Butterworths: London, 2000, 3rd edn, Chapter 7.)

Incompetent patients

Special problems arise concerning confidentiality in the case of children and the mentally disabled adult.

Children

As regards a child (i.e. a person under the age of 18), the ethical and legal obligation to respect confidence is related to the child's capacity to consent to treatment and research. If a child is **competent** to consent to *treatment*, then a doctor must not disclose the child's confidences. A child who has reached the age of 16 is presumed to be competent to consent to medical treatment (Family Law Reform Act 1969, s.8). A child under 16 may be competent to consent if of such maturity as to be able to understand what is involved (*Gillick* [1986]) (see above paper on The Law relating to Consent). While this analysis is true of treatment, the question is whether it applies either to therapeutic or non-therapeutic research.

As regards *therapeutic research*, the law is probably that a high level of maturity will be required of a child before a child under the age of 18 will be regarded as able to understand what is involved (subject, of course, to the circumstances of the child's illness and the nature of the proposed research). If the child is capable of understanding and thus of giving consent, confidential information obtained as a consequence of the research may not be disclosed.

As regards *non-therapeutic research*, the law undoubtedly would demand an even higher level of maturity of a child before regarding the child as competent to consent. This reflects an ethical concern to protect the child from possible exploitation or from decisions which the child might later regret. Obviously, much depends on the context of the proposed research, but the general principle of law is that a child may be presumed to lack competence to consent to non-therapeutic research. Given this conclusion, questions of confidentiality will rarely arise.

If a child is **incompetent** to consent to treatment, the power to consent rests with the child's parents (or others with 'parental responsibility' under the Children Act 1989). The parent must always act in the child's 'best interests'. The obligation to respect confidences is not breached in such circumstances by disclosing personal information about the child to the parent, provided it is in the child's best interests to do so. This is a matter of judgment for the doctor, but his/her decision can be reviewed by the courts if it is thought that he/she is acting unreasonably.

As regards *therapeutic research* on an incompetent child, a parent may give consent providing that the research is in the child's 'best interests' on the basis of a risk–benefit analysis. In such a case the disclosure of confidential information about the child gained in the research will not be a breach of confidence provided it is in the child's 'best interests' to do so. The same analysis as regards confidentiality applies to those (arguably rare) cases in which parents may consent to *non-therapeutic research* on an incompetent child.

Adults

No one is authorised in law to consent to *treatment* of an incompetent adult. The treatment is legally (and ethically) justified if it is shown to be in the 'best interests' of the adult incompetent (*re F* [1990]). Confidential information concerning the patient may not be disclosed to anyone other than those who, by virtue of their responsibility to care for the patient, must be involved in determining the patient's 'best interests' (ordinarily the medical team).

If *therapeutic research* can be shown on a risk–benefit analysis to be in the 'best interests' of an incompetent adult, those charged with the care of the adult would be entitled give consent. In such a case, the law relating to confidentiality is as set out above in the case of treatment.

As regards *non-therapeutic research* the legal position, whatever the ethical view, is problematic. If it is forbidden in law, no questions of confidentiality arise. If it is allowed under certain conditions, what has been said above about confidentiality applies.

REFERENCES

Gillick v. *West Norfolk and Wisbech A. H. A.* [1986] AC 112.

R v. *Department of Health, ex parte Source Informatics Ltd* [1999] 52 BMLR 65.

W v. *Egdell* [1990] 1 All ER 835.

X v. *Y* [1988] 2 All ER 648.

Z v. *Finland* (1998) 25 E.H.R.R. 371.

General Medical Council *Confidentiality: Protecting and Providing Information* (2000).

(B) Vulnerable participants

23

Research involving vulnerable participants: some ethical issues

Sue Eckstein

Centre of Medical Law and Ethics, King's College London, UK

One of the issues that causes concern and divergence of opinion for members of Research Ethics Committees is that of research involving vulnerable participants. Members of vulnerable groups are usually taken to include children, the mentally ill, people with cognitive impairment, elderly people and dying patients.

Common questions asked by REC members at the Centre of Medical Law and Ethics' Introductory Courses on the Ethics of Research on Humans have included whether research involving the terminally ill can ever be ethical, what constitutes minimal risk in the context of research involving children, how freely informed consent can be obtained in psychiatric studies and how effective research in dementia can be carried out.

Recognising the importance and complexity of these issues, the Centre of Medical Law and Ethics convened a series of Advanced Study Days bringing together practitioners and REC members to discuss the ethical issues raised in relation to paediatric research, psychiatric research, research into diseases of age and research into palliative care.

Whilst in no way exhaustive, the following pages outline some of the interesting issues covered during these meetings.

This chapter has drawn on the presentations and discussions of all the plenary speakers, panel members and participants at the Centre of Medical Law and Ethics' Advanced Study Days on Paediatric Research, Psychiatric Research, Research into Diseases of Age, and Research into Palliative Care during 2000 and 2001.

The author would like to thank the following, in particular, for their presentations which have been adapted for this chapter: Dr Julia Addington-Hall, Mr Phil Bates, Dr Antony Bayer, Dr Calliope (Bobbie) Farsides, Professor Jonathan Glover, Professor Michael Gunn, Dr Vic Larcher, Dr Karen Le Ball, Dr Steven Luttrell, Dr Donald Portsmouth, Dr Diana Rose, Professor Sir Michael Rutter, Dr Nigel Sykes, Dr Teresa Tate.

Ethical considerations in paediatric research

The Royal College of Paediatrics and Child Health (RCPCH) regards research into children's diseases as crucial in securing better evidence-based care for future children but stresses in its Guidelines on the Ethical Conduct on Medical Research Involving Children (2000) that such research should conform to the highest ethical standards.

Further to this, the Ethics Advisory Committee of the Royal College of Paediatrics and Child Health (RCPCH) holds the position that MRECs should have paediatric representation or consultation on paediatric topics. The argument for specific paediatric representation is that children are a unique, vulnerable client group whose interests are best served or protected by the advice of those who have developed considerable experience and expertise in the area. While LRECs may not have specific paediatric representation, it is important that committee members have a good understanding of the particular ethical issues involved in research with children.

Children are acknowledged as having a unique physiological and psychosocial status, thus making them different to adults in some important respects. However, they are equally deserving of evidence-based treatment and yet the fact that many medicines are not licensed for children renders them therapeutic orphans (Sutcliffe, 1999). A child's vulnerability (if real as opposed to assumed) and need for protection should not be used to prevent them from benefiting from research which is therapeutically useful. It is particularly important to establish that the lack of research is not purely driven by commercial or indemnity-related concerns.

Some of the problems raised by paediatric research arise out of the parents being responsible for giving or withholding consent. Some parents might feel morally obliged to contribute to therapeutic research which will benefit their children, but this obligation should not be motivated by a disproportionate sense of gratitude. Practitioners involved in the long-term care of children with a chronic or life-threatening disease should be particularly aware of the impact of the relationship between the team and the family, and the ways in which this might influence parents' attitudes.

Putting aside the legal issues relating to consent, there is a moral requirement to involve a child as much as is possible and/or appropriate in the consent process. This entails a number of specific duties when there is the possibility that the child could participate in a meaningful way. These duties include:

- testing the individual child's ability to participate in the consent process and proceeding accordingly;
- establishing what the child already knows about their condition, treatment and prognosis;
- ascertaining the extent to which the child wishes to be involved in the decision making process;
- discussing with the parents or guardians the extent to which they are prepared to involve the child in the process and final decision;
- providing information which will help the child to get a realistic sense of what will be involved in participating without causing undue harm.

The key to success in gaining informed consent lies in effective communication between researchers, families, associated professionals, professional bodies, LRECs and MRECs, research councils, charities, drug companies and educational institutions, and possibly parental or patient involvement in the design of the project.

Some areas of paediatric research are now recognised as raising particularly complex issues. In December 1999, the RCPCH issued a position statement on neonatal research – *Safe-guarding informed parental involvement in clinical research involving newborn babies and infants*. The need for ethical neonatal research is acknowledged, as is the difficulty of obtaining informed consent for clinical trials involving neonates. It is suggested that the concept of agreement in principle may be an appropriate step. It is also proposed that there be an obligation to provide a continuous consenting process. While good practice involves early and continuing education of the mother-to-be about the research, in reality this may be very difficult to implement. It may not be appropriate to give pregnant women information that could unnecessarily alarm them or alert them to unlikely eventualities. Some valuable neonatal research will need to be carried out in an unanticipated emergency situation, where the mother may not be receptive to information or in a position to give fully informed consent.

The complex ethical issues raised by neonatal research can only be touched on here, but given the interest shown by REC members and neonatologists, paediatric nurses and others involved in the care of newborn babies, it is likely that this topic will be the subject of future advanced study days.

Ethical considerations in psychiatric research

The Declaration of Helsinki (2000) states that 'considerations related to the well-being of the human subject should take precedence over the interests of science and society'. This is particularly important in psychiatric research where psychiatric patients may be more vulnerable than many others. People with psychiatric illnesses may suffer from impaired judgement, they may have difficulties in communicating, and their condition may vary dramatically over time. To add to this, they may be stigmatised as a group and sympathy for, and empathy with, people with psychiatric disorders may be weakened.

In almost every section of this *Manual* 'freely given informed consent' is a key issue. Definitions of consent require both voluntariness and non-coercion as well as sufficient competence. This raises difficult questions in terms of psychiatric patients' ability to give or withhold consent. Psychiatric patients are often hospitalised. There may be a correlation between being an in-patient in a psychiatric unit and a diminution of status, which could in turn lead to a lack of voluntariness. Psychiatrists and psychiatric nurses acknowledge that, even in the best treatment centres, the regime could be seen as potentially coercive because of the patients' dependence and (if they are compulsorily detained) their inability to leave.

The issue of competence is complex. Competence or incompetence cannot be assumed from the mere reading of a patient's diagnosis, yet in this area more than others it is felt that both researchers and research ethics committee members might be too ready to make uninformed assumptions and employ inaccurate stereotypes.

Thomas Grisso and Paul S. Appelbaum (1998) list four factors relevant to assessing competence. These are the ability to communicate a choice, the ability to understand relevant information, the ability to appreciate alternatives/ consequences and the ability to think rationally about the issue.

The last two factors raise particular difficulties in psychiatric research. 'The ability to appreciate alternatives and consequences' may be present in a purely cognitive sense in people with psychiatric illness, but at the same time there may be a lack of what might be called 'emotional appreciation'. As Jonathan Glover has noted, in such a case the person can spell out exactly what the implications are of the different courses of action, but yet convey a lightness or detachment that raises doubts about whether a purely intellectual grasp is really enough.

Jonathan Glover has noted that something similar can be said about 'the ability to think rationally about the issue'. Is someone who has the ability to make logical inferences and to assess evidence, but who has utterly bizarre priorities, thinking rationally? An illness like manic depression can result in oscillating priorities according to which end of the continuum the person is at the time. Thus one should not assume that consent at one time reflects a competent decision by the whole person.

While psychiatric conditions that characteristically impair competence present special ethical difficulties for research, it is important that these conditions are not excluded from sustained research that could result in significant improvements in the treatment of the illness. It is therefore desirable to identify strategies that allow some research and yet do not involve abandoning of ethical constraints.

A crucially important element of the consent process is the imparting of information to the potential participant. Researchers may need to be more imaginative in the way they devise patient information sheets. Information must be given in small chunks, and pictures or photographs may be appropriate. A separate and 'more sophisticated' carer information sheet can be provided. In paediatric psychiatric research, it is important to provide information to parents to make it easier for them to talk to their child, to enable the child to share the responsibility of the consenting process.

An interesting discussion arose during the Advanced Study Day on Psychiatric Research in relation to the use of advance directives. Although advance directives are more usually made about treatment than participation in research, it was thought that advance directives could have a useful role in research if they are made when the patient is still competent to consent, for instance in the early stages of Alzheimer's disease.

In the absence of competence on the part of the research participant, one might logically think of using proxies to give or refuse consent on the patient's behalf. However, aside from the lack of legal clarity around this issue, there are significant problems with this strategy. It is important to ensure the proxy's independence from the research team. Family members may be suitable proxies, but it is essential for researchers to be alert to possible conflicts of interest. A key problem is how to ensure dispassionate proxy consent.

Control groups raise particular problems within psychiatric medicine due to the potential costs to the patient associated with discontinuing or delaying treatment. Merely giving patients a placebo will normally deny them the best therapeutic methods, so new treatments should normally be tested against current best treatments rather than placebo. The requirement of best therapeutic methods makes it virtually impossible to justify 'challenge' studies that see what triggers an episode of illness. The same requirement raises difficulties for 'washout' studies, which involve taking the patient off medication, unless there is no reason to think the medication has been beneficial.

It is increasingly acknowledged that, until recently, the voice of mental health service users has been absent from research. User-led research has been seen as problematic by people who have limited understanding or experience of it. Users are mistakenly seen as unable to keep confidence and much user-led research has been turned down by RECs.

User-Focused Monitoring (UFM) was first pioneered and developed by The Sainsbury Centre for Mental Health in 1997. The Sainsbury Centre's report, *Users' Voices* (Rose, 2001) is probably the first time mental health service users with severe and enduring mental health problems have created, developed, carried out and analysed a major piece of research. Some 61 user interviewers were trained and carried out the eight projects which make up the report. They interviewed 500 service users living both in the community and in hospital in seven sites throughout England. Some key recommendations emerged from the report that are likely to have a significant effect on the care of mental health service users throughout the UK.

It is hoped that, as user-led research becomes more common, and the research findings are recognised as valuable, resistance to this form of research will decrease.

Psychiatry is a field in which ethical research is often extremely difficult, but in which it is also of vital importance. Improved treatment is an ethical priority, and so is respect for patients' rights. There are real intellectual challenges in trying to meet either ethical imperative without betraying the other.

Ethical considerations in research into diseases of age

Elderly participants in clinical research may be vulnerable for a variety of reasons. These reasons might include a characteristic deference to authority, dependence on others, which may lead to coercion, and a different concept of their own lives and interests to that of a researcher who is likely to be considerably younger than the research participant.

As with all research, it is essential to assess capacity before asking for consent. The elderly are often treated as incapacitated when they are not. The elderly may suffer from loss of short-term memory or dementia but it is important to remember that there are degrees of dementia; elderly patients with mild dementia generally have the capacity to consent. Different methods, in terms of time and skills, will need to be employed when assessing capacity to consent in people with dementia. Comments from Study Day participants suggested that various bodies are piloting new forms of information sheets and consent forms, for example, incorporating the consent form questions into the information sheet so that questions follow the relevant paragraphs. Information sheets that have a lower reading level and larger typeface are increasingly being produced. The family will need to be involved in the consent process. However, geriatricians and gerontologists are quick to point out that an adult is an adult and should have the right to express his or her point of view even if it is different from that of their relatives.

Elderly people living in nursing homes have been thought of as particularly vulnerable. While it is essential that they should have an independent protector of their interests, research carried out in nursing homes can be beneficial. Geriatricians report that many elderly residents of nursing homes value the contact they have with researchers and the opportunity to continue to contribute to society. Additionally, standards in nursing homes may be more likely to be maintained if researchers are known to visit periodically.

While there are problems associated with inclusion of the elderly in trials, their exclusion from research trials poses greater problems. There is no doubt that the elderly are excluded from research. For example, Antony Bayer noted that of nearly 500 papers relevant to the elderly published in leading medical journals in 1996–1997, 42% excluded the elderly, 35% without any apparent justification (Bugeja et al, BMJ, 1997). Of 225 consecutive studies submitted to a particular Local Research Ethics Committee, 5 (2%) were specifically about the elderly, 70 (31%) justifiably excluded the elderly and 85 (38%) had an unjustified, inappropriate and unnecessary upper age limit. Of 46 studies with MREC approval, 20 (43%) had an upper age limit that seemed inappropriate. In no case had the LREC or MREC requested justification for age restrictions. (Bayer & Tadd, BMJ, 2000).

Ageism is often implied. For example, comments such as 'need for patients to be reliable/fully competent/able to follow instructions' are made in protocols to justify the exclusion of research participants over 69. There is an assumption – not borne out in reality – that there will be poor compliance and a high dropout rate.

Elderly women may be doubly discriminated against in research. Elderly immigrants, and particularly female immigrants, may also be doubly discriminated against in research where there may be practical difficulties in obtaining informed consent. The grant-giving bodies that fund much research may have deadlines and financial constraints, which preclude the translations of materials.

Ethical considerations in research into palliative care

The goals of palliative care have been defined by WHO as 'the active, total care of patients whose disease is not responsive to curative treatment. Control of pain, other symptoms and psychological, social and spiritual problems is paramount. The goal of palliative care is the achievement of the best quality of life for patients and families.'

Many experts in palliative care believe that dying patients get a raw deal. Palliative care is not offered to a large enough proportion of patients, and palliative care services still tend to concentrate on particular groups. For instance, cancer patients are likely to have more access to palliative care services than people suffering from diseases such as motor neurone disease or heart failure. The Cochrane Initiative has revealed a paucity of trials in palliative care, thus making the dying another group of 'therapeutic orphans'.

This has happened for a variety of reasons including the ethical challenges posed by researching in a palliative care setting, society's sensitivities around death and dying, the reluctance of LRECs and MRECs to approve research with dying patients and the reluctance on the part of palliateurs to conduct certain forms of research. Care is the founding principle of hospices. Interests of care and research do not necessarily conflict, but research is usually not the motivation for staff entering hospice work. Few hospice staff have research training and consequently, research in hospices can suffer from 'gate-keeping' whereby hospice staff may feel it is in the best interests of their patients not to participate in research and may be reluctant to co-operate in the research process. However, discussions between palliative care practitioners at the Study Day suggested that they are increasingly confronting the issues raised by research with dying patients.

It could be argued that palliative care patients should only be excluded from research for the same sorts of reasons as any other type of patient. Stereotypical assumptions should not be made about what patients do and do not want, or how they will be affected by their participation in research, or indeed by the fact that they are dying.

There are direct therapeutic benefits of research for palliative care patients including better pain and symptom control, fine tuning of sedation, and better understanding of nutrition and hydration at the end of life. There are benefits to be gained from being a participant, which may include attention, understanding, worth, hope, being altruistic and being valued. Research into palliative care might also contribute to the appropriate expansion of services.

There are, of course, costs to be borne by palliative care patients involved in research. These could include the tying up of precious time, distress and the over-medicalisation of the dying process. Patients involved in palliative care trials may also be excluded from other potentially beneficial forms of treatment and may have their place of care determined by their involvement in a trial.

There are also practical problems inherent in conducting trials with patients close to death. The limited life-span of research participants means that they may not live long enough to see the trial through. Additionally, most palliative care facilities are small, which could have an effect on the numbers it is possible to recruit into trials. This could mean that, in some cases, qualitative research may be a more appropriate tool in the palliative care setting, but it is important to remember that this is by no means an easy option.

The issues of competency and consent, as well of randomisation, may be particularly problematical. Consent to participation in a trial should preferably be sought by a staff member not primarily involved in the patient's care. There is a high level of gratitude from patients towards hospice staff. Because of this, patients may feel that they should not refuse to take part in research and consent may therefore not be 'freely given'. Those involved in the care of the dying will need to have consideration for the family as well as for the patient.

It is important to engage the whole multi-professional team in defining hospice research priorities. Hospice staff should be involved in early discussions and planning of research studies, and in the progress of studies through ethical approval. They should be encouraged to attend research ethics committee meetings where possible, and be aware of the commencement of studies and how they are being asked to become involved.

During the course of all these Advanced Study Days, some interesting themes emerged that pointed both to the similarities between vulnerable groups and also helped to highlight the relevant differences.

Amongst them were the following.

- Researchers and members of research ethics committees should not be over-zealous in the protection of apparently vulnerable research participants.
- There is a duty to assess how far any one individual shares the vulnerability of the group with which they have been identified.
- It is important to appreciate that vulnerability can arise through the under-researching of a group's particular condition or from not exposing them to the research process.
- This might be one area where we should question the prominence given to informed consent and ask whether, in exceptional circumstances, ethical research can proceed with other forms of protection.

The more knowledge and understanding that both researchers and members of research ethics committees have of the difficult issues surrounding research involving people in vulnerable groups, the more a healthy balance will be established between protecting the interests of vulnerable participants and valuably expanding the research base in the areas of health care which serve them.

REFERENCES

Bayer, A. & Tadd, W. (2000). Unjustified exclusion of elderly people from studies submitted to research ethics committee for approval: descriptive study, *BMJ*, **321**, 992–993.

Bugeja, G. Kumar, A. & Banerjee, A. K. (1997). Exclusion of elderly people from clinical research: a descriptive study of published reports, *BMJ*, **315**, 1059.

Grisso, T. & Appelbaum, P. S. (1998). *Assessing Competence to Consent, A Guide for Physicians and Other Health Care Professionals*, New York: Oxford University Press.

RCPCH (1999). Safe-guarding informed parental involvement in clinical research involving newborn babies and infants. A position statement.

RCPCH Ethics Advisory Committee (2000). Guidelines on the Ethical Conduct of Medical Research Involving Children.

Rose, D. (2001). *Users' Voices – The Perspectives of Mental Health Service Users on Community and Hospital Care.* The Sainsbury Centre for Mental Health.

Sutcliffe, A. G. (1999). Editorial, *BMJ*, 19:70–71. (10 July).

International research

24

The ethics of research related to healthcare in developing countries

Nuffield Council on Bioethics

Introduction

There are many ethical and social issues raised by developed countries undertaking or sponsoring clinical research in developing countries. These include:

- the extent to which individuals in developing countries should be invited to take part in research which may expose them, and the populations from which they are drawn, to a possible risk of harm, yet offer them little or no direct benefit;
- the responsibilities of investigators to research participants and the wider population after research has shown that an intervention is successful;
- the applicability and relevance of existing guidelines;
- the appropriate standard of care for control and intervention groups in research;
- the appropriate provision of information, and the capacity for voluntary consent;
- effective review, and ongoing monitoring, by research ethics committees;
- the ability of developing countries to set their own research agendas.

Many people in developing countries suffer from poor health and reduced life expectancy. Poverty, coupled with limited scientific, administrative and political development often makes it very difficult for developing countries to improve healthcare. Those who seek to improve the health status of developing countries do so against this background, in which poor health is a reflection of the larger

Adapted, with permission, by Sue Eckstein from the Nuffield Council's Report on The Ethics of Research Related to Healthcare in Developing Countries.

The full report is available on: www.nuffieldbioethics.org/developingcountries

inequality in resources between developed and developing countries. Developing countries urgently need research related to healthcare that addresses their burden of disease. It follows, therefore, that externally sponsored research that seeks to bring health benefits, should, with appropriate safeguards, be encouraged in developing countries. Moreover, there is virtue in research that provides not only direct benefits to participants such as treatments for specific health needs but also indirect benefits arising from the influx of resources into a local community and the enhancement of expertise in research.

Social and cultural issues

The inequalities in resources between external sponsors of research into healthcare, and communities and governmental authorities in the developing countries, will often be so great that there is a real risk of exploitation in the context of externally sponsored research. It is crucial, therefore, that the duty to alleviate suffering, the duty to show respect for persons, the duty to be sensitive to cultural differences, and the duty not to exploit the vulnerable, are respected when research is planned and that appropriate safeguards are put in place.

When planning and conducting research, researchers and their sponsors have a duty to recognise the importance of national and local cultures and social systems, values and beliefs. In addition, external sponsors have an obligation to educate and train members of the local and national communities in the methods and skills of conducting research. The need for research projects to be subjected to review as to their ethical propriety is paramount.

Systems of biomedical care in developed countries are generally based on common scientific assumptions. There are, however, a variety of other systems of diagnosis and healing, which may vary a great deal across cultures and countries. This is particularly true of developing countries. Research into healthcare conducted along scientific lines in a particular society, or culture, will be affected by existing assumptions and practices. In any research in developing countries, therefore, these need to be addressed. Particular attention will need to be given to the means of informing potential participants about the proposed study and the process of seeking their consent. The differing conceptions of what respect for persons entails in many societies in the developing world and, in some circumstances, the need for the community to discuss issues and reach agreement as a first step in the approval of a research project, must be taken into account by researchers.

Research that pays no regard to the development of local infrastructures, or that fails to make appropriate use of local systems, skills and practitioners, may fail to maximise the benefit of the research to the community. The possibility and desirability of co-operation between practitioners of traditional medicines and scientific researchers on a particular research project should be considered on a case-by-case basis.

The framework of guidance

Researchers and sponsors who undertake research related to healthcare in developing countries are faced with difficult choices. On the one hand, they need to be sensitive to the local social and cultural context, while on the other they need to ensure that their clinical methods reflect the obligations imposed by the relevant national and international guidance.

Training in interpreting and applying the guidance is an important accompaniment to the guidance itself. Unless guidance is clearly understood by researchers, sponsors and the members of the research ethics committees, it will be of little real value. National and international sponsors of research, including government agencies and departments, charitable foundations and pharmaceutical companies should ensure that provision is made for education and training in the ethics of research of all of those professionals involved in research related to healthcare so that the requirements of relevant guidance on ethics are met. In addition, developing countries should be encouraged to take account of existing international and national guidance and to create national guidance for its clear and unambiguous application.

Consent

For consent to be genuine, health professionals must do their best to communicate information accurately and in an understandable and appropriate way. The information provided to participants must be relevant, accurate and sufficient to enable a genuine choice to be made. It must include such matters as the nature and purpose of the research, the procedures involved and the potential risks and benefits.

An awareness of the social and cultural context in which research is to be conducted is required, so that communities and individuals can be informed of any aspect of the research that may cause them particular concern. The process of obtaining consent also needs to be designed to provide opportunities for participants to ask questions of personal interest about the proposed research.

For consent to be genuine, it must be freely given. In some societies it would be considered culturally inappropriate for researchers to ask individuals to participate in research without consulting the community or receiving permission from community leaders. Three such situations can be distinguished: consultation is required with the community before individuals are approached about research; permission from a leader(s) of the community is required before any research is discussed with the community or individuals; the leader of the community is considered to have the authority to enrol participants in research. In each of these circumstances, to seek consent from an individual without seeking assent from leader(s) of the community, or creating public acceptance of research, may be considered disrespectful and may harm relationships within that community and between a community and researchers.

Although assent from others may be necessary before research is conducted, it is not sufficient: individual participants must receive appropriate information about the research and be asked to give consent. To ensure that individual participants can make up their own minds without undue communal pressure, anonymity for those who wish to decline to participate in research should be assured. It is therefore recommended that, in circumstances where consent to research is required, genuine consent to participate in research must be obtained from each participant. In some cultural contexts it may be appropriate to obtain agreement from the community or assent from a senior family member before a prospective participant is approached. If a prospective participant does not wish to take part in research, this must be respected. Researchers must not enrol such individuals and have a duty to facilitate their non-participation.

Participants in research may have a variety of motivations for taking part in research. The healthcare that a participant would receive as part of a research programme may amount to a significant inducement to take part. Researchers will need to be aware that, when research is conducted in developing counties, prospective participants may have little or no alternative means of receiving healthcare for a condition, other than through the facilities supported by the research, and thus the healthcare provided as part of the research will amount to a significant inducement to participate. In addition, benefits unrelated to the research protocol, such as financial payments, may be offered to compensate for travel costs or time devoted to the research.

The dividing line between acceptable and inappropriate inducements is a fine one. The larger an inducement, the more likely it is to be inappropriate, because it causes an individual to expose himself or herself to risks or potential harms that he or she would otherwise consider to be unacceptable. In addition, payments and other benefits unrelated to the research protocol will act as significantly greater inducements in developing countries than would similar amounts in more developed contexts. Dialogue is needed with sponsors, external and local researchers and communities to ensure that any inducements to take part in research are appropriate to the local context, especially in circumstances where the research exposes participants to a risk of harm. Decisions about appropriate levels of inducement will need to be justified to local research ethics committees.

There are circumstances in which, while genuine consent to research can be obtained, it may be inappropriate to ask participants in research to sign consent forms, no matter how well designed. One obvious example is when research is being conducted in an illiterate population. It is not consistent with the duty of respect for persons to require a prospective participant to 'sign' a written consent form that they are unable to read. In such circumstances other means of recording genuine consent to participate is required, to protect participants from being enrolled in research that they have not consented to. Information sheets and consent forms must be designed to assist participants to make informed choices. The information provided should be accurate, concise, clear, simple, specific to the proposed research and appropriate for the social and cultural context in which it is being given. Where it is inappropriate for consent to be recorded in writing, genuine consent must be obtained verbally. The process of obtaining consent and the accompanying documentation must be approved by a research ethics committee and, where only verbal consent

to research is contemplated, include consideration of an appropriate process for witnessing the consent.

Standards of care

There has been significant international debate about the standards of care that should be provided to participants during externally sponsored research in developing countries. Much debate has been focused on whether participants in the control group of a research trial should be provided with a universal standard of care, regardless of where the research is conducted. The different approaches that have been proposed when deciding the level of care that should be provided for those in the control group of a clinical trial can be divided into two broad categories:

- universal: the best treatment available anywhere in the world, wherever the research is conducted
- non-universal: the treatment available in a defined region.

Equal respect for participants in research does not necessarily entail that they should receive equal treatment, regardless of where the research may be conducted. Instead, the circumstances in which the research will be conducted must be critically assessed to establish whether or not the variations in circumstances provide a morally relevant reason for offering a different standard of care.

In determining the appropriate standard of care to be provided to participants in the control group of a research trial, a number of factors should be considered by sponsors, researchers, and research ethics committees. These include:

- the appropriate research design(s) to answer the research question (in some situations only one research design may be appropriate to answer the research question, in others a number of research designs, in which different standards of care are offered to the control group, may be possible);
- the seriousness of the disease and the effect of proven treatments;
- the existence of a universal standard of care for the disease or condition in question and the quality of the supporting evidence;
- the standard(s) of care in the host and sponsoring country(ies) for the disease being studied;
- the standard(s) of care which can be afforded by the host and sponsoring country(ies) for the disease being studied;
- the standard(s) of care which can effectively be delivered in the host country(ies) during research;

- the standard(s) of care which can be provided in the host country(ies) on a sustainable basis.

Taking the above considerations into account, in some circumstances, it will be clear that a control group in a clinical trial should receive a universal standard of care, wherever they live. In contrast, there are situations in which it is clear that, even if there were an agreed universal standard of care for a disease, it may not be possible for this standard to be provided to the control group in a research project. This may be because of practical considerations, for example because the country in which the research is to be conducted may not have the infrastructure to provide such treatment, or because research using such a standard of care would have little relevance to the country in which it is conducted. A suitable standard of care can only be defined in consultation with those who work within the country and must be justified to the relevant research ethics committees. Wherever appropriate, participants in the control group should be offered a universal standard of care for the disease being studied. Where it is not appropriate to offer a universal standard of care, the minimum standard of care that should be offered to the control group is the best intervention available for that disease as part of the national public health system.

Ethical review of research

The requirement that the ethics of research related to healthcare is subject to review is designed to protect participants in research. Each proposal for externally sponsored research in developing countries should receive three levels of assessment: relevance to priorities in healthcare within the country(ies); scientific validity; and ethical acceptability. While research ethics committees are not constituted to make decisions about whether or not the findings of research can be implemented within a country, they should, however, determine if the implications of possible research results have been discussed, including the possibility of ongoing provision of treatments shown to be successful. Research ethics committees must also be satisfied that appropriate scientific review of research has taken place.

There are a number of issues which research ethics committees need to consider when reviewing externally sponsored research. These include the appropriateness of procedures for giving information about the research to prospective participants and communities and recording consent; the standards of care that should be provided to participants in research and arrangements that have been made for post-trial access to interventions.

The mere presence of a research ethics committee in a country is not enough to ensure that research will be adequately reviewed. Committees may be ineffective for a variety of reasons, including a lack of financial and human resources, and a lack of training in, and experience of, ethical review. An effective system for ethical review is a crucial safeguard for participants in research. Developing countries may determine that the most appropriate means of reviewing externally sponsored research is via an independent national research ethics committee. In such circumstances the establishment, funding and proper operation of independent national research ethics committees should be the responsibility of national governments. No research should be conducted without review at the national or local level.

Regardless of whether the financial support for research ethics committees comes from government, research institutions or as a result of levying fees for review, it is crucial that the independence of research ethics committees be maintained. There is a need for creative approaches to providing support, especially financial support, for research ethics committees, without compromising their independence. Sponsors should determine how they can meet the costs of ethical review without compromising the independence of the research ethics committee and should be responsible for meeting the costs of reviewing externally sponsored research.

In order to ensure that acceptable ethical standards are observed in externally sponsored research, research should be approved through a system of ethical review of research in both the host and the sponsoring country. As regards the latter, if a sponsor provides funding, it must have the means of ensuring that the funds are being used in a manner that is ethically acceptable. However, the country in which the research is to be conducted must also be satisfied about the ethical acceptability of the research. It is recommended that externally sponsored research projects should be subject to independent ethical review in the sponsor's country(ies) in addition to the country(ies) in which the research is to be conducted.

What happens once research is over?

Once an externally sponsored research study is completed in a developing country, the researchers and their sponsors are confronted with a number of issues relating to the future provision of healthcare benefits to the participants in the research and to the wider community. Many have taken the view that to fail to provide treatment which has been shown to be successful to the participants in research is ethically unacceptable. In general, it is the responsibility of governments and not researchers or sponsors to determine the level of healthcare and the range of treatments and medicines that are provided to populations. It is recognised that sponsors are rarely in a position to agree to open-ended commitments once the research is completed, whether for the maintenance of facilities for healthcare or for the provision of interventions, but these are issues that need to be discussed and agreed by the research ethics committee, to the extent possible, before the research is initiated.

With regard to the provision of an intervention shown to be successful once the research is completed, there are three groups of people to be considered: members of the control group in a trial, all of the participants in the research project, and the wider community in which the research took place.

It is recommended that the following issues are clearly considered by researchers, sponsors, national healthcare authorities, international agencies and research ethics committees as part of any research protocol before research relating to healthcare involving the testing of new interventions is undertaken:

- the need, where appropriate, to monitor possible long-term deleterious outcomes arising from the research, for an agreed period of time beyond the completion of the research
- the possibility of providing participants with the intervention shown to be best (if they are still able to benefit from it), for an agreed period of time
- the possibility of introducing and maintaining the availability to the wider community of treatment shown to be successful.

USEFUL WEBSITES

International guidelines

CIOMS (1993). **International Ethical Guidelines for Biomedical Research Involving Human Subjects**
http://www.cioms.ch/frame_1993_texts_of_guidelines.htm

CIOMS (1991). **International Guidelines for Ethical Review of Epidemiological Studies**
http://www.cioms.ch/frame_1991_texts_of_guidelines.htm

Council of Europe (1997). **Convention for the Protection of Human Rights and Dignity of the Human Being with regard to the Application of Biology and Medicine: Convention on Human Rights and Biomedicine**
http://conventions.coe.int/treaty/en/treaties/html/164.htm

CPMP/ICH (1996). **Note for Guidance on Good Clinical Practice**
http://www.emea.eu.int/pdfs/human/ich/013595en.pdf

UNAIDS (2000). Ethical considerations in HIV preventive vaccine research. UNAIDS guidance document
www.unaids.org/publications/documents/vaccines/vaccines/Ethicsresearch.pdf

WHO (1995). **Guidelines for good clinical practice (GCP) for trials on pharmaceutical products**
http://www.who.int/medicines/library/par/ggcp/GCPGuidePharmatrials.pdf

WHO (2000). **Operational Guidelines for Ethics Committees that Review Biomedical Research**
www.who.int/tdr/publications/publications/ethics.htm

WMA (2000). **Declaration of Helsinki – Ethical Principles for Medical Research Involving Human Subjects, Adopted by the 52nd WMA General Assembly, Edinburgh, Scotland, October 2000**
http://www.wma.net/e/policy/17-c_e.html

National guidance

Agency for International Development (US) **22 CFR 225: Protection of Human Subjects**
http://www.access.gpo.gov/nara/cfr/waisidx_99/22cfr225_99.html

Department of Health and Human Services, National Institutes of Health, Office for Protection from Research Risks **Code of Federal Regulations Title 45 Part 46: Protection of Human Subjects**
http://ohrp.osophs.dhhs.gov/humansubjects/guidance/45cfr46.htm

Food and Drug Administration (FDA) (US) **21 CFR 50: Protection of Human Subjects**
http://www.access.gpo.gov/nara/cfr/waisidx_00/21cfr50_00.html

Food and Drug Administration (FDA) (US) **21 CFR 56: Institutional Review Boards**
http://www.access.gpo.gov/nara/cfr/waisidx_00/21cfr56_00.html

Food and Drug Administration (FDA) (US) **21 CFR 312: Investigational New Drug Application**
http://www.access.gpo.gov/nara/cfr/waisidx_99/21cfr312_99.html

Indian Council of Medical Research (2000). **Ethical Guidelines for Biomedical Research on Human Subjects**
http://www.icmr.nic.in/ethical.pdf

Health Research Council of New Zealand (HRC) (1998). **Guidelines for Researchers on Health Research Involving Maori**
http://www.hrc.govt.nz/Maoguide.htm

Medical Research Council (South Africa) (1993). **Guidelines on Ethics for Medical Research, 3rd Edition**
http://www.mrc.ac.za/ethics/ethics.htm
(A 4th edition is being prepared and will be made available at:
http://www.sahealthinfo.org/ethics/index.htm)

National Bioethics Advisory Commission (US) (2001). **Ethical and Policy Issues in International Research: Clinical Trials in Developing Countries**

• Volume I: Report and Recommendations of the National Bioethics Advisory Commission
• Volume II: Commissioned Papers
http://bioethics.georgetown.edu/nbac/pubs.html

National Health and Medical Research Council of Australia (1991). **Guidelines on Ethical Matters in Aboriginal and Torres Strait Islander Health Research**
http://www.health.gov.au/nhmrc/issues/asti.pdf

National Health Council of Brazil (1996). **Resolution No. 196/96 on Research Involving Human Subjects**

http://www.aids.gov.br/resolution_196.htm

South African Department of Health (2000). **Guidelines for Good Practice in the Conduct of Clinical Trials in Human Participants in South Africa**
http://www.hst.org.za/doh/clinical.htm

The National Commission for the Protection of Human Subjects of Biomedical and Behavioral Research (US) (1979). **The Belmont Report. Ethical Principles and Guidelines for the Protection of Human Subjects of Research**
http://ohrp.osophs.dhhs.gov/humansubjects/guidance/belmont.htm

Fundamental legal and ethical considerations

25

Ethical principles for medical research involving human subjects

Declaration of Helsinki, World Medical Association

Adopted by the 18th WMA General Assembly Helsinki, Finland, June 1964 and amended by the 29th WMA General Assembly, Tokyo, Japan, October 1975; 35th WMA General Assembly, Venice, Italy, October 1983; 41st WMA General Assembly, Hong Kong, September 1989; 48th WMA General Assembly, Somerset West, Republic of South Africa, October 1996 and the 52nd WMA General Assembly, Edinburgh, Scotland, October 2000

A Introduction

1 The World Medical Association has developed the Declaration of Helsinki as a statement of ethical principles to provide guidance to physicians and other participants in medical research involving human subjects. Medical research involving human subjects includes research on identifiable human material or identifiable data.

2 It is the duty of the physician to promote and safeguard the health of the people. The physician's knowledge and conscience are dedicated to the fulfillment of this duty.

3 The Declaration of Geneva of the World Medical Association binds the physician with the words, "The health of my patient will be my first consideration," and the International Code of Medical Ethics declares that, "A physician shall act only in the patient's interest when providing medical care which might have the effect of weakening the physical and mental condition of the patient."

4 Medical progress is based on research which ultimately must rest in part on experimentation involving human subjects.

5 In medical research on human subjects, considerations related to the well-being of the human subject should take precedence over the interests of science and society.

6 The primary purpose of medical research involving human subjects is to improve prophylactic, diagnostic and therapeutic procedures and the understanding of the aetiology and pathogenesis of disease. Even the best proven prophylactic, diagnostic, and therapeutic methods must continuously be challenged through research for their effectiveness, efficiency, accessibility and quality.

7 In current medical practice and in medical research, most prophylactic, diagnostic and therapeutic procedures involve risks and burdens.

8 Medical research is subject to ethical standards that promote respect for all human beings and protect their health and rights. Some research populations are vulnerable and need special protection. The particular needs of the economically and medically disadvantaged must be recognized. Special attention is also required for those who cannot give or refuse consent for themselves, for those who may be subject to giving consent under duress, for those who will not benefit personally from the research and for those for whom the research is combined with care.

9 Research Investigators should be aware of the ethical, legal and regulatory requirements for research on human subjects in their own countries as well as applicable international requirements. No national ethical, legal or regulatory requirement should be allowed to reduce or eliminate any of the protections for human subjects set forth in this Declaration.

B Basic principles for all medical research

10 It is the duty of the physician in medical research to protect the life, health, privacy, and dignity of the human subject.

11 Medical research involving human subjects must conform to generally accepted scientific principles, be based on a thorough knowledge of the scientific literature, other relevant sources of information, and on adequate laboratory and, where appropriate, animal experimentation.

12 Appropriate caution must be exercised in the conduct of research which may affect the environment, and the welfare of animals used for research must be respected.

13 The design and performance of each experimental procedure involving human subjects should be clearly formulated in an experimental protocol. This protocol should be submitted for consideration, comment, guidance, and where appropriate, approval to a specially appointed ethical review committee, which must be independent of the investigator, the sponsor or any other kind of undue influence. This independent committee should be in conformity with the laws and regulations of the country in which the research experiment is performed. The committee has the right to monitor ongoing trials. The researcher has the obligation to provide monitoring information to the committee, especially any serious adverse events. The researcher should also submit to the committee, for review, information regarding funding, sponsors, institutional affiliations, other potential conflicts of interest and incentives for subjects.

14 The research protocol should always contain a statement of the ethical considerations involved and should indicate that there is compliance with the principles enunciated in this Declaration.

15 Medical research involving human subjects should be conducted only by scientifically qualified persons and under the supervision of a clinically competent medical person. The responsibility for the human subject must always rest with a medically qualified person and never rest on the subject of the research, even though the subject has given consent.

16 Every medical research project involving human subjects should be preceded by careful assessment of predictable risks and burdens in comparison with foreseeable benefits to the subject or to others. This does not preclude the participation of healthy volunteers in medical research. The design of all studies should be publicly available.

17 Physicians should abstain from engaging in research projects involving human subjects unless they are confident that the risks involved have been adequately assessed and can be satisfactorily managed. Physicians should cease any investigation if the risks are found to outweigh the potential benefits or if there is conclusive proof of positive and beneficial results.

18 Medical research involving human subjects should only be conducted if the importance of the objective outweighs the inherent risks and burdens to the subject. This is especially important when the human subjects are healthy volunteers.

19 Medical research is only justified if there is a reasonable likelihood that the populations in which the research is carried out stand to benefit from the results of the research.

20 The subjects must be volunteers and informed participants in the research project.

21 The right of research subjects to safeguard their integrity must always be respected. Every precaution should be taken to respect the privacy of the subject, the confidentiality of the patient's information and to minimize the impact of the study on the subject's physical and mental integrity and on the personality of the subject.

22 In any research on human beings, each potential subject must be adequately informed of the aims, methods, sources of funding, any possible conflicts of interest, institutional affiliations of the researcher, the anticipated benefits and potential risks of the study and the discomfort it may entail. The subject should be informed of the right to abstain from participation in the study or to withdraw consent to participate at any time without reprisal. After ensuring that the subject has understood the information, the physician should then obtain the subject's freely-given informed consent, preferably in writing. If the consent cannot be obtained in writing, the non-written consent must be formally documented and witnessed.

23 When obtaining informed consent for the research project the physician should be particularly cautious if the subject is in a dependent relationship with the physician or may consent under duress. In that case the informed consent should be obtained by a well-informed physician who is not engaged in the investigation and who is completely independent of this relationship.

24 For a research subject who is legally incompetent, physically or mentally incapable of giving consent or is a legally incompetent minor, the investigator must obtain informed consent from the legally authorized representative in accordance with applicable law. These groups should not be included in research unless the research is necessary to promote the health of the population represented and this research cannot instead be performed on legally competent persons.

25 When a subject deemed legally incompetent, such as a minor child, is able to give assent to decisions about participation in research, the investigator must obtain that assent in addition to the consent of the legally authorized representative.

26 Research on individuals from whom it is not possible to obtain consent, including proxy or advance consent, should be done only if the physical/mental condition that prevents obtaining informed consent is a necessary characteristic of the research population. The specific reasons for involving research subjects with a condition that renders them unable to give informed consent should be stated in the experimental protocol for consideration and approval of the review committee. The protocol should state that consent to remain in the research should be obtained as soon as possible from the individual or a legally authorized surrogate.

27 Both authors and publishers have ethical obligations. In publication of the results of research, the investigators are obliged to preserve the accuracy of the results. Negative as well as positive results should be published or otherwise publicly available. Sources of funding, institutional affiliations and any possible conflicts of interest should be declared in the publication. Reports of experimentation not in accordance with the principles laid down in this Declaration should not be accepted for publication.

C Additional principles for medical research combined with medical care

28 The physician may combine medical research with medical care, only to the extent that the research is justified by its potential prophylactic, diagnostic or therapeutic value. When medical research is combined with medical care, additional standards apply to protect the patients who are research subjects.

29 The benefits, risks, burdens and effectiveness of a new method should be tested against those of the best current prophylactic, diagnostic, and therapeutic methods. This does not exclude the use of placebo, or no treatment, in studies where no proven prophylactic, diagnostic or therapeutic method exists.

30 At the conclusion of the study, every patient entered into the study should be assured of access to the best proven prophylactic, diagnostic and therapeutic methods identified by the study.

31 The physician should fully inform the patient which aspects of the care are related to the research. The refusal of a patient to participate in a study must never interfere with the patient-physician relationship.

32 In the treatment of a patient, where proven prophylactic, diagnostic and therapeutic methods do not exist or have been ineffective, the physician, with informed consent from the patient, must be free to use unproven or new prophylactic, diagnostic and therapeutic measures, if in the physician's judgement it offers hope of saving life, re-establishing health or alleviating suffering. Where possible, these measures should be made the object of research, designed to evaluate their safety and efficacy. In all cases, new information should be recorded and, where appropriate, published. The other relevant guidelines of this Declaration should be followed.

The World Medical Association, Inc

Note of clarification on paragraph 29 of the WMA Declaration of Helsinki

The WMA is concerned that paragraph 29 of the revised Declaration of Helsinki (October 2000) has led to diverse interpretations and possible confusion. It hereby reaffirms its position that extreme care must be taken in making use of a placebo-controlled trial and that in general this methodology should only be used in the absence of existing proven therapy. However, a placebo-controlled trial may be ethically acceptable, even if proven therapy is available, under the following circumstances:

- Where for compelling and scientifically sound methodological reasons its use is necessary to determine the efficacy or safety of a prophylactic, diagnostic or therapeutic method; or
- Where a prophylactic, diagnostic or therapeutic method is being investigated for a minor condition and the patients who receive placebo will not be subject to any additional risk of serious or irreversible harm.

All other provisions of the Declaration of Helsinki must be adhered to, especially the need for appropriate ethical and scientific review.

As approved by the WMA Council on 7 October 2001 at its 160th Session in Ferney-Voltaire, France.

Reproduced by kind permission of the World Medical Association

26

The Belmont Report: ethical principles and guidelines for the protection of human subjects of research

National Commission for the Protection of Human
Subjects of Biomedical and Behavioral Research

Report of the National Commission for the Protection of Human Subjects of Biomedical and Behavioral Research

Table of contents

Summary

On July 12, 1974, the National Research Act (Public Law 93348) was signed into law, thereby creating the National Commission for the Protection of Human Subjects of Biomedical and Behavioral Research. One of the charges to the Commission was to identify the basic ethical principles that should underlie the conduct of biomedical and behavioral research involving human subjects, and to develop guidelines, which should be followed to assure that such research is conducted in accordance with those principles.

In carrying out the above, the Commission was directed to consider: (i) the boundaries between biomedical and behavioral research and the accepted and routine practice of medicine, (ii) the role of assessment of risk-benefit criteria in the determination of the appropriateness of research involving human subjects, (iii) appropriate guidelines for the selection of human subjects for participation in such research, and (iv) the nature and definition of informed consent in various research settings.

The *Belmont Report* attempts to summarize the basic ethical principles identified by the Commission in the course of its deliberations. It is the outgrowth of an intensive four-day period of discussions that were held in February 1976 at the Smithsonian Institution's Belmont Conference Center, supplemented by the monthly deliberations of the Commission that were held over a period of nearly four years. It is a statement of basic ethical principles and guidelines that should assist in resolving the ethical problems that surround the conduct of research with human subjects.

By publishing the Report in the **Federal Register,** and providing reprints upon request, the Secretary intends that it may be made readily available to scientists, members of institutional review boards, and Federal employees. The two-volume Appendix, containing the lengthy reports of experts and specialists, who assisted the Commission in fulfilling this part of its charge, is available as DHEW Publication No. (OS) 780013 and No. (OS) 78-0014, for sale by the Superintendent of Documents, U.S. Government Printing Office, Washington, D.C. 20402.

Unlike most other reports of the Commission, the *Belmont Report* does not make specific recommendations for administrative action by the Secretary of Health, Education, and Welfare. Rather, the Commission recommended that the *Belmont Report* be adopted in its entirety, as a statement of the Department's policy. The Department requests public comment on this recommendation.

Members of the commission

Kenneth John Ryan, M.D., Chairman, Chief of Staff, Boston Hospital for Women.

Joseph V. Brady, Ph.D., Professor of Behavioral Biology, Johns Hopkins University.

Robert E. Cooke, M.D., President, Medical College of Pennsylvania.

Dorothy I. Height, President, National Council of Negro Women, Inc.

Albert R. Jonsen, Ph.D., Associate Professor of Bioethics, University of California at San Francisco.

Patricia King, J.D., Associate Professor of Law, Georgetown University Law Center.

Karen Lebacqz, Ph.D., Associate Professor of Christian Ethics, Pacific School of Religion.

*David W. Louisell, J. D., Professor of Law, University of California at Berkeley.

Donald W. Seldin, M.D., Professor and Chairman, Department of Internal Medicine, University of Texas at Dallas.

Eliot Stellar, Ph.D., Provost of the University and Professor of Physiological Psychology, University of Pennsylvania.

*Robert H. Turtle, LL.B., Attorney, VomBaur, Coburn, Simmons & Turtle, Washington, D.C.

*Deceased.

The Belmont Report

Scientific research has produced substantial social benefits. It has also posed some troubling ethical questions. Public attention was drawn to these questions by reported abuses of human subjects in biomedical experiments, especially during the Second World War. During the Nuremberg War Crime Trials, the *Nuremberg Code* was drafted as a set of standards for judging physicians and scientists who had conducted biomedical experiments on concentration camp prisoners. This Code became the prototype of many later *codes* intended to assure that research involving human subjects would be carried out in an ethical manner.

The codes consist of rules, some general, others specific, that guide the investigators or the reviewers of research in their work. Such rules often are inadequate to cover complex situations; at times they come into conflict, and they are frequently difficult to interpret or apply. Broader ethical principles will provide a basis on which specific rules may be formulated, criticized and interpreted.

Three principles, or general prescriptive judgments, that are relevant to research involving human subjects are identified in this statement. Other principles may also be relevant. These three are comprehensive, however, and are stated at a level of generalization that should assist scientists, subjects, reviewers and interested citizens to understand the ethical issues inherent in research involving human subjects. These principles cannot always be applied, so as to resolve beyond dispute particular ethical problems. The objective is to provide an analytical framework that will guide the resolution of ethical problems arising from research involving human subjects.

This statement consists of a distinction between research and practice, a discussion of the three basic ethical principles, and remarks about the application of these principles.

A Boundaries between practice and research

It is important to distinguish between biomedical and behavioral research, on the one hand, and the practice of accepted therapy on the other, in order to know what activities ought to undergo review for the protection of human subjects of research. The distinction between research and practice is blurred, partly because both often occur together (as in research designed to evaluate a therapy), and partly because notable departures from standard practice are often called "experimental", when the terms "experimental" and "research" are not carefully defined.

For the most part, the term "practice" refers to interventions that are designed solely to enhance the well-being of an individual patient or client and that have a reasonable expectation of success. The purpose of medical or behavioral practice is to provide diagnosis, preventive treatment or therapy to particular *individuals*. By contrast, the term "research" designates an activity designed to test an hypothesis, permit conclusions to be drawn, and thereby to develop or contribute to generalizable knowledge (expressed, for example, in theories, principles, and statements of relationships). Research is usually described in a formal protocol that sets forth an objective and a set of procedures designed to reach that objective.

When a clinician departs in a significant way from standard or accepted practice, the innovation does not, in and of itself, constitute research. The fact that a procedure is "experimental" in the sense of new, untested or different, does not automatically place it in the category of research. Radically new procedures of this description should, however, be made the object of formal research at an early stage, in order to determine whether they are safe and effective. Thus, it is the responsibility of medical practice committees, for example, to insist that a major innovation be incorporated into a formal research *project*.

Research and practice may be carried on together, when research is designed to evaluate the safety and efficacy of a therapy. This need not cause any confusion regarding whether or not the activity requires review; the general rule is, that if there is any element of research in an activity, that activity should undergo review for the protection of human subjects.

B Basic ethical principles

The expression "basic ethical principles" refers to those general judgments that serve as a basic justification for the many particular ethical prescriptions and evaluations of human actions. Three basic principles, among those generally accepted in our cultural tradition, are particularly relevant to the ethics of research involving human subjects: the principles of respect for persons, beneficence and justice.

1 Respect for persons

Respect for persons incorporates at least two ethical convictions: first, that individuals should be treated as autonomous agents, and second, that persons with diminished autonomy are entitled to protection. The principle of respect for persons thus divides into two separate moral requirements: the requirement to acknowledge autonomy, and the requirement to protect those with diminished autonomy.

An autonomous person is an individual capable of deliberation about personal goals, and of acting under the direction of such deliberation. To respect autonomy is to give weight to autonomous persons' considered opinions and choices, while refraining from obstructing their actions, unless they are clearly detrimental to others. To show lack of respect for an autonomous agent is to repudiate that person's considered judgments, to deny an individual the freedom to act on those considered judgments, or to withhold information necessary to make a considered judgment, when there are no compelling reasons to do so.

However, not every human being is capable of self-determination. The capacity for self-determination matures during an individual's life, and some individuals lose this capacity wholly or in part, because of illness, mental disability, or circumstances that severely restrict liberty. Respect for the immature and the incapacitated may require protecting them as they mature or while they are incapacitated.

Some persons are in need of extensive protection, even to the point of excluding them from activities which may harm them; other persons require little protection beyond making sure they undertake activities freely and with awareness of possible adverse consequences. The extent of protection afforded should depend upon the risk of harm, and the likelihood of benefit. The judgment that any individual lacks autonomy should be periodically reevaluated, and will vary in different situations.

In most cases of research involving human subjects, respect for persons demands that subjects enter into the research voluntarily and with adequate information. In some situations, however, application of the principle is not obvious. The involvement of prisoners as subjects of research provides an instructive example. On the one hand, it would seem that the principle of respect for persons requires that prisoners not be deprived of the opportunity to volunteer for research. On the other hand, under prison conditions they may be subtly coerced or unduly influenced to engage in research activities, for which they would not otherwise volunteer. Respect for persons would then dictate that prisoners be protected. Whether to allow prisoners to "volunteer" or to "protect" them presents a dilemma. Respecting persons, in most hard cases, is often a matter of balancing competing claims urged by the principle of respect itself.

2 Beneficence

Persons are treated in an ethical manner, not only by respecting their decisions and protecting them from harm, but also by making efforts to secure their well-being. Such treatment falls under the principle of beneficence. The term "beneficence" is often understood to cover acts of kindness or charity that go beyond strict obligation. In this document, beneficence is understood in a stronger sense, as an obligation. Two general rules have been formulated as complementary expressions of beneficent actions in this sense: (1) do not harm; and (2) maximize possible benefits, and minimize possible harms.

The Hippocratic maxim "do no harm" has long been a fundamental principle of medical ethics. Claude Bernard extended it to the realm of research, saying that one should not injure one person, regardless of the benefits that might come to others. However, even avoiding harm requires learning what is harmful; and, in the process of obtaining this information, persons may be exposed to risk of harm. Further, the Hippocratic Oath requires physicians to benefit their patients "according to their best judgment". Learning what will in fact benefit may require exposing persons to risk. The problem posed by these imperatives is to decide when it is justifiable to seek certain benefits despite the risks involved, and when the benefits should be foregone because of the risks.

The obligations of beneficence affect both individual investigators and society at large, because they extend both to particular research projects and to the entire enterprise of research. In the case of particular projects, investigators and members of their institutions are obliged to give forethought to the maximization of benefits and the reduction of risk that might occur from the research investigation. In the case of scientific research in general, members of the larger society are obliged to recognize the longer term benefits and risks that may result from the improvement of knowledge, and from the development of novel medical, psychotherapeutic, and social procedures.

The principle of beneficence often occupies a well-defined, justifying role in many areas of research involving human subjects. An example is found in research involving children. Effective ways of treating childhood diseases and fostering healthy development are benefits that serve to justify research involving children – even when individual research subjects are not direct beneficiaries. Research also makes it possible to avoid the harm that may result from the application of previously accepted routine practices that, on closer investigation, turn out to be dangerous. But the role of the principle of beneficence is not always so unambiguous. A difficult ethical problem remains, for example, about research that presents more than minimal risk, without immediate prospect of direct benefit to the children involved. Some have argued that such research is inadmissible, while others have pointed out, that this limit would rule out much research promising great benefit to children in the future. Here again, as with all hard cases, the different claims covered by the principle of beneficence may come into conflict and force difficult choices.

3 Justice

Who ought to receive the benefits of research and bear its burdens? This is a question of justice, in the sense of "fairness in distribution" or "what is deserved". An injustice occurs, when some benefit to which a person is entitled is denied without good reason, or when some burden is imposed unduly. Another way of conceiving the principle of justice is that, equals ought to be treated equally. However, this statement requires explication. Who is equal and who is unequal? What considerations justify departure from equal distribution? Almost all commentators allow that distinctions based on experience, age, deprivation, competence, merit and position do sometimes constitute criteria justifying differential treatment for certain purposes. It is necessary, then, to explain in what respects people should be treated equally. There are several widely accepted formulations of just ways to distribute burdens and benefits. Each formulation mentions some relevant property, on the basis of which burdens and benefits should be distributed. These formulations are (1) to each person an equal share, (2) to each person according to individual need, (3) to each person according to individual effort, (4) to each person according to societal contribution, and (5) to each person according to merit.

Questions of justice have long been associated with social practices, such as punishment, taxation and political representation. Until recently, these questions have not generally been associated with scientific research. However, they are foreshadowed, even in the earliest reflections on the ethics of research involving human subjects. For example, during the 19th and early 20th centuries, the burdens of serving as research subjects fell largely upon poor ward patients, while the benefits of improved medical care flowed primarily to private patients. Subsequently, the exploitation of unwilling prisoners as research subjects in Nazi concentration camps was condemned as a particularly flagrant injustice. In this country, in the 1940's, the Tuskegee syphilis study used disadvantaged, rural black men to study the untreated course of a disease that is by no means confined to that population. These subjects were deprived of demonstrably effective treatment in order not to interrupt the project, long after such treatment became generally available.

Against this historical background, it can be seen how conceptions of justice are relevant to research involving human subjects. For example, the selection of research subjects needs to be scrutinized in order to determine whether some classes (*e.g.*, welfare patients, particular racial and ethnic minorities, or persons confined to institutions) are being systematically selected, simply because of their easy availability, their compromised position, or their manipulability, rather than for reasons directly related to the problem being studied. Finally, whenever research supported by public funds leads to the development of therapeutic devices and procedures, justice demands both that these do not provide advantages only to those who can afford them, and that such research should not unduly involve persons from groups unlikely to be among the beneficiaries of subsequent applications of the research.

C Applications

Applications of the general principles to the conduct of research leads to consideration of the following requirements: informed consent, risk/benefit assessment, and the selection of subjects of research.

1 Informed consent

Respect for persons requires that subjects, to the degree that they are capable, be given the opportunity to choose what shall or shall not happen to them. This opportunity is provided, when adequate standards for informed consent are satisfied.

While the importance of informed consent is unquestioned, controversy prevails over the nature and possibility of an informed consent. Nonetheless, there is widespread agreement that the consent process can be analyzed as containing three elements: information, comprehension and voluntariness.

Information

Most codes of research establish specific items for disclosure, intended to assure that subjects are given sufficient information. These items generally include: the research procedure, their purposes, risks and anticipated benefits, alternative procedures (where therapy is involved), and a statement offering the subject the opportunity to ask questions and to withdraw at any time from the research. Additional items have been proposed, including how subjects are selected, the person responsible for the research, *etc.*

However, a simple listing of items does not answer the question of what the standard should be for judging how much and what sort of information should be provided. One standard frequently invoked in medical practice, namely the information commonly provided by practitioners in the field or in the locale, is inadequate, since research takes place precisely when a common understanding does not exist. Another standard, currently popular in malpractice law, requires the practitioner to reveal the information that reasonable persons would wish to know in order to make a decision regarding their care. This, too, seems insufficient, since the research subject, being in essence a volunteer, may wish to know considerably more about risks gratuitously undertaken than do patients who deliver themselves into the hand of a clinician for needed care. It may be, that a standard of "the reasonable volunteer" should be proposed: the extent and nature of information should be such that persons, knowing that the procedure is neither necessary for their care nor perhaps fully understood, can decide whether they wish to participate in the furthering of knowledge. Even when some direct benefit to them is anticipated, the subjects should understand clearly the range of risk, and the voluntary nature of participation.

A special problem of consent arises, where informing subjects of some pertinent aspect of the research is likely to impair the validity of the research. In many cases, it is sufficient to indicate to subjects that they are being invited to participate in research, of which some features will not be revealed until the research is concluded. In all cases of research involving incomplete disclosure, such research is justified, only if it is clear that (1) incomplete disclosure is truly necessary to accomplish the goals of the research, (2) there are no undisclosed risks to subjects that are more than minimal, and (3) there is an adequate plan for debriefing subjects, when appropriate, and for dissemination of research results to them. Information about risks should never be withheld for the purpose of eliciting the cooperation of subjects, and truthful answers should always be given to direct questions about the research. Care should be taken to distinguish cases, in which disclosure would destroy or invalidate the research, from cases in which disclosure would simply inconvenience the investigator.

Comprehension

The manner and context, in which information is conveyed is as important as the information itself. For example, presenting information in a disorganized and rapid fashion, allowing too little time for consideration, or curtailing opportunities for questioning, all may adversely affect a subject's ability to make an informed choice.

Because the subject's ability to understand is a function of intelligence, rationality, maturity and language, it is necessary to adapt the presentation of the information to the subject's capacities. Investigators are responsible for ascertaining that the subject has comprehended the information. While there is always an obligation to ascertain that the information about risk to subjects is complete and adequately comprehended, when the risks are more serious, that obligation increases. On occasion, it may be suitable to give some oral or written tests of comprehension.

Special provision may need to be made, when comprehension is severely limited – for example, by conditions of immaturity or mental disability. Each class of subjects that one might consider as incompetent (*e.g.*, infants and young children, mentally disabled patients, the terminally ill, and the comatose) should be considered on its own terms. Even for these persons, however, respect requires giving them the opportunity to choose, to the extent they are able, whether or not to participate in research. The objections of these subjects to involvement should be honored, unless the research entails providing them a therapy unavailable elsewhere. Respect for persons also requires seeking the permission of other parties in order to protect the subjects from harm. Such persons are thus respected, both by acknowledging their own wishes, and by the use of third parties to protect them from harm.

The third parties chosen should be those, who are most likely to understand the incompetent subject's situation, and to act in that person's best interest. The person authorized to act on behalf of the subject should be given an opportunity to observe the research, as it proceeds, in order to be able to withdraw the subject from the research, if such action appears in the subject's best interest.

Voluntariness

An agreement to participate in research constitutes a valid consent, only if voluntarily given. This element of informed consent requires conditions free of coercion and undue influence. Coercion occurs when an overt threat of harm is intentionally presented by one person to another, in order to obtain compliance. Undue influence, by contrast, occurs through an offer of an excessive, unwarranted, inappropriate or improper reward or other overture, in order to obtain compliance. Also, inducements that would ordinarily be acceptable may become undue influences, if the subject is especially vulnerable.

Unjustifiable pressures usually occur, when persons in positions of authority or commanding influence – especially where possible sanctions are involved – urge a course of action for a subject. A continuum of such influencing factors exists, however, and it is impossible to state precisely, where justifiable persuasion ends and undue influence begins. But undue influence would include actions, such as manipulating a person's choice through the controlling influence of a close relative, and threatening to withdraw health services to which an individual would otherwise be entitled.

2 Assessment of risks and benefits

The assessment of risks and benefits requires a careful arrayal of relevant data, including, in some cases, alternative ways of obtaining the benefits sought in the research. Thus, the assessment presents both an opportunity and a responsibility to gather systematic and comprehensive information about proposed research. For the investigator, it is a means to examine whether the proposed research is properly designed. For a review committee, it is a method for determining whether the risks that will be presented to subjects are justified. For prospective subjects, the assessment will assist the determination whether or not to participate.

The nature and scope of risks and benefits

The requirement that research be justified on the basis of a favorable risk/benefit assessment, bears a close relation to the principle of beneficence, just as the moral requirement that informed consent be obtained is derived primarily from the principle of respect for persons.

The term "risk" refers to a possibility that harm may occur. However, when expressions such as "small risk" or "high risk" are used, they usually refer (often ambiguously) both to the chance (probability) of experiencing a harm, and the severity (magnitude) of the envisioned harm.

The term "benefit" is used in the research context to refer to something of positive value related to health or welfare. Unlike "risk", "benefit" is not a term that expresses probabilities. Risk is properly contrasted to probability of benefits, and benefits are properly contrasted with harms rather than risks of harm. Accordingly, so-called risk/benefit assessments are concerned with the probabilities and magnitudes of possible harms, and anticipated benefits. Many kinds of possible harms and benefits need to be taken into account. There are, for example, risks of psychological harm, physical harm, legal harm, social harm and economic harm, and the corresponding benefits. While the most likely types of harms to research subjects are those of psychological or physical pain or injury, other possible kinds should not be overlooked.

Risks and benefits of research may affect the individual subjects, the families of the individual subjects, and society at large (or special groups of subjects in society). Previous codes and Federal regulations have required that risks to subjects be outweighed by the sum of both the anticipated benefit to the subject, if any, and the anticipated benefit to society in the form of knowledge to be gained from the research. In balancing these different elements, the risks and benefits affecting the immediate research subject will normally carry special weight. On the other hand, interests, other than those of the subject, may on some occasions be sufficient by themselves to justify the risks involved in the research, so long as the subjects' rights have been protected. Beneficence thus requires that we protect against risk of harm to subjects, and also that we be concerned about the loss of the substantial benefits that might be gained from research.

The systematic assessment of risks and benefits

It is commonly said that benefits and risks must be "balanced", and shown to be "in a favorable ratio". The metaphorical character of these terms draws attention to the difficulty of making precise judgments. Only on rare occasions will quantitative techniques be available for the scrutiny of research protocols. However, the idea of systematic, nonarbitrary analysis of risks and benefits should be emulated insofar as possible. This ideal requires those making decisions about the justifiability of research to be thorough in the accumulation and assessment of information about all aspects of the research, and to consider alternatives systematically. This procedure renders the assessment of research more rigorous and precise, while making communication between review board members and investigators less subject to misinterpretation, misinformation and conflicting judgments. Thus, there should first be a determination of the validity of the presuppositions of the research; then the nature, probability and magnitude of risk should be distinguished, with as much clarity as possible. The method of ascertaining risks should be explicit, especially where there is no alternative to the use of such vague categories as small or slight risk. It should also be determined whether an investigator's estimates of the probability of harm or benefits are reasonable, as judged by known facts or other available studies.

Finally, assessment of the justifiability of research should reflect at least the following considerations: (i) Brutal or inhumane treatment of human subjects is never morally justified. (ii) Risks should be reduced to those necessary to achieve the research objective. It should be determined whether it is in fact necessary to use human subjects at all. Risk can perhaps never be entirely eliminated, but it can often be reduced by careful attention to alternative procedures. (iii) When research involves significant risk of serious impairment, review committees should be extraordinarily insistent on the justification of the risk (looking usually to the likelihood of benefit to the subject – or, in some rare cases, to the manifest voluntariness of the participation). (iv) When vulnerable populations are involved in research, the appropriateness of involving them should itself be demonstrated. A number of variables go into such judgments, including the nature and degree of risk, the condition of the particular population involved, and the nature and level of the anticipated benefits. (v) Relevant risks and benefits must be thoroughly arrayed in documents and procedures used in the informed consent process.

3 Selection of subjects

Just as the principle of respect for persons finds expression in the requirements for consent, and the principle of beneficence in risk/benefit assessment, the principle of justice gives rise to moral requirements that there be fair procedures and outcomes in the selection of research subjects.

Justice is relevant to the selection of subjects of research at two levels: the social and the individual. Individual justice in the selection of subjects would require that researchers exhibit fairness: thus, they should not offer potentially beneficial research only to some patients, who are in their favor, or select only "undesirable" persons for risky research.

Social justice requires that distinction be drawn between classes of subjects that ought, and ought not, to participate in any particular kind of research, based on the ability of members of that class to bear burdens, and on the appropriateness of placing further burdens on already burdened persons. Thus, it can be considered a matter of social justice, that there is an order of preference in the selection of classes of subjects (*e.g.*, adults before children), and that some classes of potential subjects (*e.g.*, the institutionalized mentally infirm or prisoners) may be involved as research subjects, if at all, only on certain conditions.

Injustice may appear in the selection of subjects, even if individual subjects are selected fairly by investigators, and treated fairly in the course of research. Thus, injustice arises from social, racial, sexual and cultural biases institutionalized in society. Thus, even if individual researchers are treating their research subjects fairly, and even if institutional review boards are taking care to assure that subjects are selected fairly within a particular institution, unjust social patterns may nevertheless appear in the overall distribution of the burdens and benefits of research. Although individual institutions or investigators may not be able to resolve a problem that is pervasive in their social setting, they can consider distributive justice in selecting research subjects.

Some populations, especially institutionalized ones, are already burdened in many ways by their infirmities and environments. When research is proposed that involves risks and does not include a therapeutic component, other less burdened classes of persons should be called upon first to accept these risks of research, except where the research is directly related to the specific conditions of the class involved. Also, even though public funds for research may often flow in the same directions as public funds for health care, it seems unfair that populations dependent on public health care constitute a pool of preferred research subjects, if more advantaged populations are likely to be the recipients of the benefits.

One special instance of injustice results from the involvement of vulnerable subjects. Certain groups, such as racial minorities, the economically disadvantaged, the very sick, and the institutionalized, may continually be sought as research subjects, owing to their ready availability in settings, where research is conducted. Given their dependent status and their frequently compromised capacity for free consent, they should be protected against the danger of being involved in research solely for administrative convenience, or because they are easy to manipulate as a result of their illness or socioeconomic condition.

27

ICH Good Clinical Practice Guideline

International Conference on Harmonisation of Technical Requirements
for Registration of Pharmaceuticals for Human Use

Recommended for Adoption at *Step 4* of the ICH Process
on 1 May 1996 by the ICH Steering Committee

This Guideline has been developed by the appropriate ICH
Expert Working Group and has been subject to consultation by the regulatory parties, in accordance with the ICH
Process. At Step 4 of the Process the final draft is recommended for adoption to the regulatory bodies of the European Union, Japan and USA.

IFPMA
30 rue de St.-Jean
P.O. Box 758
1211 Geneva 13
Switzerland
Telefax: +41 (22) 338 32 30

Guideline for good clinical practice

ICH harmonised tripartite guideline

Having reached *Step 4* of the ICH Process at the ICH Steering Committee meeting on 1 May 1996, this guideline is
recommended for adoption to the three regulatory parties
to ICH.

Table of contents

Not all sections of text have been reproduced. The full text
is accessible on http://www.ifpma.org/ ich5e.html#gcp

Guideline for good clinical practice

Introduction

Good Clinical Practice (GCP) is an international ethical and scientific quality standard for designing, conducting, recording and reporting trials that involve the participation of human subjects. Compliance with this standard provides public assurance that the rights, safety and well-being of trial subjects are protected, consistent with the principles that have their origin in the Declaration of Helsinki, and that the clinical trial data are credible.

The objective of this ICH GCP Guideline is to provide a unified standard for the European Union (EU), Japan and the United States to facilitate the mutual acceptance of clinical data by the regulatory authorities in these jurisdictions.

The guideline was developed with consideration of the current good clinical practices of the European Union, Japan, and the United States, as well as those of Australia, Canada, the Nordic countries and the World Health Organization (WHO).

This guideline should be followed when generating clinical trial data that are intended to be submitted to regulatory authorities.

The principles established in this guideline may also be applied to other clinical investigations that may have an impact on the safety and well-being of human subjects.

1 Glossary

1.1 Adverse Drug Reaction (ADR)

In the pre-approval clinical experience with a new medicinal product or its new usages, particularly as the therapeutic dose(s) may not be established: all noxious and unintended responses to a medicinal product related to any dose should be considered adverse drug reactions. The phrase responses to a medicinal product means that a causal relationship between a medicinal product and an adverse event is at least a reasonable possibility, i.e. the relationship cannot be ruled out.

Regarding marketed medicinal products: a response to a drug which is noxious and unintended and which occurs at doses normally used in man for prophylaxis, diagnosis, or therapy of diseases or for modification of physiological function (see the ICH Guideline for Clinical Safety Data Management: Definitions and Standards for Expedited Reporting).

1.2 Adverse event (AE)

Any untoward medical occurrence in a patient or clinical investigation subject administered a pharmaceutical product and which does not necessarily have a causal relationship with this treatment. An adverse event (AE) can therefore be any unfavourable and unintended sign (including an abnormal laboratory finding), symptom, or disease temporally associated with the use of a medicinal (investigational) product, whether or not related to the medicinal (investigational) product (see the ICH Guideline for Clinical Safety Data Management: Definitions and Standards for Expedited Reporting).

1.3 Amendment (to the protocol)

See Protocol Amendment.

1.4 Applicable regulatory requirement(s)

Any law(s) and regulation(s) addressing the conduct of clinical trials of investigational products.

1.5 Approval (in relation to institutional review boards)

The affirmative decision of the IRB that the clinical trial has been reviewed and may be conducted at the institution site within the constraints set forth by the IRB, the institution,

Good Clinical Practice (GCP), and the applicable regulatory requirements.

1.6 Audit

A systematic and independent examination of trial related activities and documents to determine whether the evaluated trial related activities were conducted, and the data were recorded, analyzed and accurately reported according to the protocol, sponsor's standard operating procedures (SOPs), Good Clinical Practice (GCP), and the applicable regulatory requirement(s).

1.7 Audit certificate

A declaration of confirmation by the auditor that an audit has taken place.

1.8 Audit report

A written evaluation by the sponsor's auditor of the results of the audit.

1.9 Audit trail

Documentation that allows reconstruction of the course of events.

1.10 Blinding/masking

A procedure in which one or more parties to the trial are kept unaware of the treatment assignment(s). Single-blinding usually refers to the subject(s) being unaware, and double-blinding usually refers to the subject(s), investigator(s), monitor, and, in some cases, data analyst(s) being unaware of the treatment assignment(s).

1.11 Case report form (CRF)

A printed, optical, or electronic document designed to record all of the protocol required information to be reported to the sponsor on each trial subject.

1.12 Clinical trial/study

Any investigation in human subjects intended to discover or verify the clinical, pharmacological and/or other pharmacodynamic effects of an investigational product(s), and/or to identify any adverse reactions to an investigational product(s), and/or to study absorption, distribution, metabolism, and excretion of an investigational product(s) with the object of ascertaining its safety and/or efficacy. The terms clinical trial and clinical study are synonymous.

1.13 Clinical trial/study report

A written description of a trial/study of any therapeutic, prophylactic, or diagnostic agent conducted in human subjects, in which the clinical and statistical description, presentations, and analyses are fully integrated into a single report (see the ICH Guideline for Structure and Content of Clinical Study Reports).

1.14 Comparator (product)

An investigational or marketed product (i.e., active control), or placebo, used as a reference in a clinical trial.

1.15 Compliance (in relation to trials)

Adherence to all the trial-related requirements, Good Clinical Practice (GCP) requirements, and the applicable regulatory requirements.

1.16 Confidentiality

Prevention of disclosure, to other than authorized individuals, of a sponsor's proprietary information or of a subject's identity.

1.17 Contract

A written, dated, and signed agreement between two or more involved parties that sets out any arrangements on delegation and distribution of tasks and obligations and, if appropriate, on financial matters. The protocol may serve as the basis of a contract.

1.18 Coordinating committee

A committee that a sponsor may organize to coordinate the conduct of a multicentre trial.

1.19 Coordinating investigator

An investigator assigned the responsibility for the coordination of investigators at different centres participating in a multicentre trial.

1.20 Contract research organization (CRO)

A person or an organization (commercial, academic, or other) contracted by the sponsor to perform one or more of a sponsor's trial-related duties and functions.

1.21 Direct access

Permission to examine, analyze, verify, and reproduce any records and reports that are important to evaluation of a clinical trial. Any party (e.g., domestic and foreign regulatory authorities, sponsor's monitors and auditors) with direct access should take all reasonable precautions within the constraints of the applicable regulatory requirement(s) to maintain the confidentiality of subjects' identities and sponsor's proprietary information.

1.22 Documentation

All records, in any form (including, but not limited to, written, electronic, magnetic, and optical records, and scans, x-rays, and electrocardiograms) that describe or record the methods, conduct, and/or results of a trial, the factors affecting a trial, and the actions taken.

1.23 Essential documents

Documents which individually and collectively permit evaluation of the conduct of a study and the quality of the data produced (see 8. Essential Documents for the Conduct of a Clinical Trial).

1.24 Good clinical practice (GCP)

A standard for the design, conduct, performance, monitoring, auditing, recording, analyses, and reporting of clinical trials that provides assurance that the data and reported results are credible and accurate, and that the rights, integrity, and confidentiality of trial subjects are protected.

1.25 Independent data-monitoring committee (IDMC) (data and safety monitoring board, monitoring committee, data monitoring committee)

An independent data-monitoring committee that may be established by the sponsor to assess at intervals the progress of a clinical trial, the safety data, and the critical efficacy endpoints, and to recommend to the sponsor whether to continue, modify, or stop a trial.

1.26 Impartial witness

A person, who is independent of the trial, who cannot be unfairly influenced by people involved with the trial, who attends the informed consent process if the subject or the subject's legally acceptable representative cannot read, and who reads the informed consent form and any other written information supplied to the subject.

1.27 Independent Ethics Committee (IEC)

An independent body (a review board or a committee, institutional, regional, national, or supranational), constituted of medical professionals and non-medical members, whose responsibility it is to ensure the protection of the rights, safety and well-being of human subjects involved in a trial and to provide public assurance of that protection, by, among other things, reviewing and approving / providing favourable opinion on, the trial protocol, the suitability of the investigator(s), facilities, and the methods and material to be used in obtaining and documenting informed consent of the trial subjects.

The legal status, composition, function, operations and regulatory requirements pertaining to Independent Ethics Committees may differ among countries, but should allow the Independent Ethics Committee to act in agreement with GCP as described in this guideline.

1.28 Informed consent

A process by which a subject voluntarily confirms his or her willingness to participate in a particular trial, after having been informed of all aspects of the trial that are relevant to the subject's decision to participate. Informed consent is documented by means of a written, signed and dated informed consent form.

1.29 Inspection

The act by a regulatory authority(ies) of conducting an official review of documents, facilities, records, and any other resources that are deemed by the authority(ies) to be related to the clinical trial and that may be located at the site of the trial, at the sponsor's and/or contract research organization's (CRO's) facilities, or at other establishments deemed appropriate by the regulatory authority(ies).

1.30 Institution (medical)

Any public or private entity or agency or medical or dental facility where clinical trials are conducted.

1.31 Institutional review board (IRB)

An independent body constituted of medical, scientific, and non-scientific members, whose responsibility is to ensure the protection of the rights, safety and well-being of human subjects involved in a trial by, among other things, reviewing, approving, and providing continuing review of trial protocol and amendments and of the methods and material to be used in obtaining and documenting informed consent of the trial subjects.

1.32 Interim clinical trial/study report

A report of intermediate results and their evaluation based on analyses performed during the course of a trial.

1.33 Investigational product

A pharmaceutical form of an active ingredient or placebo being tested or used as a reference in a clinical trial, including a product with a marketing authorization when used or assembled (formulated or packaged) in a way different from the approved form, or when used for an unapproved indication, or when used to gain further information about an approved use.

1.34 Investigator

A person responsible for the conduct of the clinical trial at a trial site. If a trial is conducted by a team of individuals at a trial site, the investigator is the responsible leader of the team and may be called the principal investigator. See also Subinvestigator.

1.35 Investigator/institution

An expression meaning "the investigator and/or institution, where required by the applicable regulatory requirements".

1.36 Investigator's brochure

A compilation of the clinical and nonclinical data on the investigational product(s) which is relevant to the study of the investigational product(s) in human subjects (see 7. Investigator's Brochure).

1.37 Legally acceptable representative

An individual or juridical or other body authorized under applicable law to consent, on behalf of a prospective subject, to the subject's participation in the clinical trial.

1.38 Monitoring

The act of overseeing the progress of a clinical trial, and of ensuring that it is conducted, recorded, and reported in accordance with the protocol, Standard Operating Procedures (SOPs), Good Clinical Practice (GCP), and the applicable regulatory requirement(s).

1.39 Monitoring report

A written report from the monitor to the sponsor after each site visit and/or other trial-related communication according to the sponsor's SOPs.

1.40 Multicentre trial

A clinical trial conducted according to a single protocol but at more than one site, and therefore, carried out by more than one investigator.

1.41 Nonclinical study

Biomedical studies not performed on human subjects.

1.42 Opinion (in relation to independent ethics committee)

The judgement and/or the advice provided by an Independent Ethics Committee (IEC).

1.43 Original medical record

See Source Documents.

1.44 Protocol

A document that describes the objective(s), design, methodology, statistical considerations, and organization of a trial. The protocol usually also gives the background and rationale for the trial, but these could be provided in other protocol referenced documents. Throughout the ICH GCP Guideline the term protocol refers to protocol and protocol amendments.

1.45 Protocol amendment

A written description of a change(s) to or formal clarification of a protocol.

1.46 Quality assurance (QA)

All those planned and systematic actions that are established to ensure that the trial is performed and the data are generated, documented (recorded), and reported in compliance with Good Clinical Practice (GCP) and the applicable regulatory requirement(s).

1.47 Quality control (QC)

The operational techniques and activities undertaken within the quality assurance system to verify that the requirements for quality of the trial-related activities have been fulfilled.

1.48 Randomization

The process of assigning trial subjects to treatment or control groups using an element of chance to determine the assignments in order to reduce bias.

1.49 Regulatory Authorities

Bodies having the power to regulate. In the ICH GCP guideline the expression Regulatory Authorities includes the authorities that review submitted clinical data and those that conduct inspections (see 1.29). These bodies are sometimes referred to as competent authorities.

1.50 Serious adverse event (SAE) or serious adverse drug reaction (Serious ADR)

Any untoward medical occurrence that at any dose:
• results in death,
• is life-threatening,
• requires inpatient hospitalization or prolongation of existing hospitalization,
• results in persistent or significant disability/incapacity, or
• is a congenital anomaly/birth defect
(see the ICH Guideline for Clinical Safety Data Management: Definitions and Standards for Expedited Reporting).

1.51 Source data

All information in original records and certified copies of original records of clinical findings, observations, or other activities in a clinical trial necessary for the reconstruction and evaluation of the trial. Source data are contained in source documents (original records or certified copies).

1.52 Source documents

Original documents, data, and records (e.g., hospital records, clinical and office charts, laboratory notes, mem-

oranda, subjects' diaries or evaluation checklists, pharmacy dispensing records, recorded data from automated instruments, copies or transcriptions certified after verification as being accurate copies, microfiches, photographic negatives, microfilm or magnetic media, x-rays, subject files, and records kept at the pharmacy, at the laboratories and at medico-technical departments involved in the clinical trial).

1.53 Sponsor

An individual, company, institution, or organization which takes responsibility for the initiation, management, and/or financing of a clinical trial.

1.54 Sponsor-investigator

An individual who both initiates and conducts, alone or with others, a clinical trial, and under whose immediate direction the investigational product is administered to, dispensed to, or used by a subject. The term does not include any person other than an individual (e.g., it does not include a corporation or an agency). The obligations of a sponsor-investigator include both those of a sponsor and those of an investigator.

1.55 Standard Operating Procedures (SOPs)

Detailed, written instructions to achieve uniformity of the performance of a specific function.

1.56 Subinvestigator

Any individual member of the clinical trial team designated and supervised by the investigator at a trial site to perform critical trial-related procedures and/or to make important trial-related decisions (e.g., associates, residents, research fellows). See also Investigator.

1.57 Subject/trial subject

An individual who participates in a clinical trial, either as a recipient of the investigational product(s) or as a control.

1.58 Subject identification code

A unique identifier assigned by the investigator to each trial subject to protect the subject's identity and used in lieu of the subject's name when the investigator reports adverse events and/or other trial related data.

1.59 Trial site

The location(s) where trial-related activities are actually conducted.

1.60 Unexpected adverse drug reaction

An adverse reaction, the nature or severity of which is not consistent with the applicable product information (e.g., Investigator's Brochure for an unapproved investigational product or package insert/summary of product characteristics for an approved product) (see the ICH Guideline for Clinical Safety Data Management: Definitions and Standards for Expedited Reporting).

1.61 Vulnerable subjects

Individuals whose willingness to volunteer in a clinical trial may be unduly influenced by the expectation, whether justified or not, of benefits associated with participation, or of a retaliatory response from senior members of a hierarchy in case of refusal to participate. Examples are members of a group with a hierarchical structure, such as medical, pharmacy, dental, and nursing students, subordinate hospital and laboratory personnel, employees of the pharmaceutical industry, members of the armed forces, and persons kept in detention. Other vulnerable subjects include patients with incurable diseases, persons in nursing homes, unemployed or impoverished persons, patients in emergency situations, ethnic minority groups, homeless persons, nomads, refugees, minors, and those incapable of giving consent.

1.62 Well-being (of the trial subjects)

The physical and mental integrity of the subjects participating in a clinical trial.

2 The principles of ICH GCP

2.1

Clinical trials should be conducted in accordance with the ethical principles that have their origin in the Declaration of Helsinki, and that are consistent with GCP and the applicable regulatory requirement(s).

2.2

Before a trial is initiated, foreseeable risks and inconveniences should be weighed against the anticipated benefit for the individual trial subject and society. A trial should be initiated and continued only if the anticipated benefits justify the risks

2.3

The rights, safety, and well-being of the trial subjects are the most important considerations and should prevail over interests of science and society.

2.4

The available nonclinical and clinical information on an investigational product should be adequate to support the proposed clinical trial.

2.5

Clinical trials should be scientifically sound, and described in a clear, detailed protocol.

2.6

A trial should be conducted in compliance with the protocol that has received prior institutional review board (IRB)/independent ethics committee (IEC) approval/favourable opinion.

2.7

The medical care given to, and medical decisions made on behalf of, subjects should always be the responsibility of a qualified physician or, when appropriate, of a qualified dentist.

2.8

Each individual involved in conducting a trial should be qualified by education, training, and experience to perform his or her respective task(s).

2.9

Freely given informed consent should be obtained from every subject prior to clinical trial participation.

2.10

All clinical trial information should be recorded, handled, and stored in a way that allows its accurate reporting, interpretation and verification.

2.11

The confidentiality of records that could identify subjects should be protected, respecting the privacy and confidentiality rules in accordance with the applicable regulatory requirement(s).

2.12

Investigational products should be manufactured, handled, and stored in accordance with applicable good manufacturing practice (GMP). They should be used in accordance with the approved protocol.

2.13

Systems with procedures that assure the quality of every aspect of the trial should be implemented.

3 Institutional review board/independent ethics committee (IRB/IEC)

3.1 Responsibilities

3.1.1

An IRB/IEC should safeguard the rights, safety, and well-being of all trial subjects. Special attention should be paid to trials that may include vulnerable subjects.

3.1.2

The IRB/IEC should obtain the following documents: trial protocol(s)/amendment(s), written informed consent form(s) and consent form updates that the investigator proposes for use in the trial, subject recruitment procedures (e.g. advertisements), written information to be provided to subjects, Investigator's Brochure (IB), available safety information, information about payments and compensation available to subjects, the investigator's current curriculum vitae and/or other documentation evidencing qualifications, and any other documents that the IRB/IEC may need to fulfil its responsibilities.

The IRB/IEC should review a proposed clinical trial within a reasonable time and document its views in writing, clearly identifying the trial, the documents reviewed and the dates for the following:
- approval/favourable opinion;
- modifications required prior to its approval/favourable opinion;
- disapproval/negative opinion; and
- termination/suspension of any prior approval/favourable opinion.

3.1.3

The IRB/IEC should consider the qualifications of the investigator for the proposed trial, as documented by a current curriculum vitae and/or by any other relevant documentation the IRB/IEC requests.

3.1.4

The IRB/IEC should conduct continuing review of each ongoing trial at intervals appropriate to the degree of risk to human subjects, but at least once per year.

3.1.5

The IRB/IEC may request more information than is outlined in paragraph 4.8.10 be given to subjects when, in the judgement of the IRB/IEC, the additional information would add meaningfully to the protection of the rights, safety and/or well-being of the subjects.

3.1.6

When a non-therapeutic trial is to be carried out with the consent of the subject's legally acceptable representative (see 4.8.12, 4.8.14), the IRB/IEC should determine that the proposed protocol and/or other document(s) adequately addresses relevant ethical concerns and meets applicable regulatory requirements for such trials.

3.1.7

Where the protocol indicates that prior consent of the trial subject or the subject's legally acceptable representative is not possible (see 4.8.15), the IRB/IEC should determine that the proposed protocol and/or other document(s) adequately addresses relevant ethical concerns and meets applicable regulatory requirements for such trials (i.e. in emergency situations).

3.1.8

The IRB/IEC should review both the amount and method of payment to subjects to assure that neither presents problems of coercion or undue influence on the trial subjects. Payments to a subject should be prorated and not wholly contingent on completion of the trial by the subject.

3.1.9

The IRB/IEC should ensure that information regarding payment to subjects, including the methods, amounts, and schedule of payment to trial subjects, is set forth in the written informed consent form and any other written information to be provided to subjects. The way payment will be prorated should be specified.

3.2 Composition, functions and operations

3.2.1

The IRB/IEC should consist of a reasonable number of members, who collectively have the qualifications and experience to review and evaluate the science, medical aspects, and ethics of the proposed trial. It is recommended that the IRB/IEC should include:
(a) At least five members.
(b) At least one member whose primary area of interest is in a nonscientific area.
(c) At least one member who is independent of the institution/trial site.
Only those IRB/IEC members who are independent of the investigator and the sponsor of the trial should vote/provide opinion on a trial-related matter.
A list of IRB/IEC members and their qualifications should be maintained.

3.2.2

The IRB/IEC should perform its functions according to written operating procedures, should maintain written records of its activities and minutes of its meetings, and should comply with GCP and with the applicable regulatory requirement(s).

3.2.3

An IRB/IEC should make its decisions at announced meetings at which at least a quorum, as stipulated in its written operating procedures, is present.

3.2.4

Only members who participate in the IRB/IEC review and discussion should vote/provide their opinion and/or advise.

3.2.5

The investigator may provide information on any aspect of the trial, but should not participate in the deliberations of the IRB/IEC or in the vote/opinion of the IRB/IEC.

3.2.6

An IRB/IEC may invite nonmembers with expertise in special areas for assistance.

3.3 Procedures

The IRB/IEC should establish, document in writing, and follow its procedures, which should include:

3.3.1

Determining its composition (names and qualifications of the members) and the authority under which it is established.

3.3.2

Scheduling, notifying its members of, and conducting its meetings.

3.3.3

Conducting initial and continuing review of trials.

3.3.4

Determining the frequency of continuing review, as appropriate.

3.3.5

Providing, according to the applicable regulatory requirements, expedited review and approval/favourable opinion of minor change(s) in ongoing trials that have the approval/favourable opinion of the IRB/IEC.

3.3.6

Specifying that no subject should be admitted to a trial before the IRB/IEC issues its written approval/favourable opinion of the trial.

3.3.7

Specifying that no deviations from, or changes of, the protocol should be initiated without prior written IRB/IEC approval/favourable opinion of an appropriate amendment, except when necessary to eliminate immediate hazards to the subjects or when the change(s) involves only logistical or administrative aspects of the trial (e.g., change of monitor(s), telephone number(s)) (see 4.5.2).

3.3.8

Specifying that the investigator should promptly report to the IRB/IEC:

(a) Deviations from, or changes of, the protocol to eliminate immediate hazards to the trial subjects (see 3.3.7, 4.5.2, 4.5.4).

(b) Changes increasing the risk to subjects and/or affecting significantly the conduct of the trial (see 4.10.2).

(c) All adverse drug reactions (ADRs) that are both serious and unexpected.

(d) New information that may affect adversely the safety of the subjects or the conduct of the trial.

3.3.9

Ensuring that the IRB/IEC promptly notify in writing the investigator/institution concerning:

(a) Its trial-related decisions/opinions.

(b) The reasons for its decisions/opinions.

(c) Procedures for appeal of its decisions/opinions.

3.4 Records

The IRB/IEC should retain all relevant records (e.g., written procedures, membership lists, lists of occupations/affiliations of members, submitted documents, minutes of meetings, and correspondence) for a period of at least 3 years after completion of the trial and make them available upon request from the regulatory authority(ies).

The IRB/IEC may be asked by investigators, sponsors or regulatory authorities to provide its written procedures and membership lists.

4 Investigator

4.1 Investigator's qualifications and agreements

4.1.1

The investigator(s) should be qualified by education, training, and experience to assume responsibility for the proper conduct of the trial, should meet all the qualifications specified by the applicable regulatory requirement(s), and should provide evidence of such qualifications through up-to-date curriculum vitae and/or other relevant documentation requested by the sponsor, the IRB/IEC, and/or the regulatory authority(ies).

4.1.2

The investigator should be thoroughly familiar with the appropriate use of the investigational product(s), as described in the protocol, in the current Investigator's Brochure, in the product information and in other information sources provided by the sponsor.

4.1.3

The investigator should be aware of, and should comply with, GCP and the applicable regulatory requirements.

4.1.4

The investigator/institution should permit monitoring and auditing by the sponsor, and inspection by the appropriate regulatory authority(ies).

4.1.5

The investigator should maintain a list of appropriately qualified persons to whom the investigator has delegated significant trial-related duties.

4.2 Adequate resources

4.2.1

The investigator should be able to demonstrate (e.g., based on retrospective data) a potential for recruiting the required number of suitable subjects within the agreed recruitment period.

4.2.2

The investigator should have sufficient time to properly conduct and complete the trial within the agreed trial period.

4.2.3

The investigator should have available an adequate number of qualified staff and adequate facilities for the foreseen duration of the trial to conduct the trial properly and safely.

4.2.4

The investigator should ensure that all persons assisting with the trial are adequately informed about the protocol, the investigational product(s), and their trial-related duties and functions.

4.3 Medical care of trial subjects

4.3.1

A qualified physician (or dentist, when appropriate), who is an investigator or a sub-investigator for the trial, should be responsible for all trial-related medical (or dental) decisions.

4.3.2

During and following a subject's participation in a trial, the investigator/institution should ensure that adequate medical care is provided to a subject for any adverse events, including clinically significant laboratory values, related to the trial. The investigator/institution should inform a subject when medical care is needed for intercurrent illness(es) of which the investigator becomes aware.

4.3.3

It is recommended that the investigator inform the subject's primary physician about the subject's participation in the trial if the subject has a primary physician and if the subject agrees to the primary physician being informed.

4.3.4

Although a subject is not obliged to give his/her reason(s) for withdrawing prematurely from a trial, the investigator should make a reasonable effort to ascertain the reason(s), while fully respecting the subject's rights.

4.4 Communication with IRB/IEC

4.4.1

Before initiating a trial, the investigator/institution should have written and dated approval/favourable opinion from the IRB/IEC for the trial protocol, written informed consent form, consent form updates, subject recruitment procedures (e.g., advertisements), and any other written information to be provided to subjects.

4.4.2

As part of the investigator's/institution's written application to the IRB/IEC, the investigator/institution should provide the IRB/IEC with a current copy of the Investigator's Brochure. If the Investigator's Brochure is updated during the trial, the investigator/institution should supply a copy of the updated Investigator's Brochure to the IRB/IEC.

4.4.3

During the trial the investigator/institution should provide to the IRB/IEC all documents subject to review.

4.5 Compliance with protocol

4.5.1

The investigator/institution should conduct the trial in compliance with the protocol agreed to by the sponsor and, if required, by the regulatory authority(ies) and which was given approval/favourable opinion by the IRB/IEC. The investigator/institution and the sponsor should sign the protocol, or an alternative contract, to confirm agreement.

4.5.2

The investigator should not implement any deviation from, or changes of the protocol without agreement by the sponsor and prior review and documented approval/favourable opinion from the IRB/IEC of an amendment, except where necessary to eliminate an immediate hazard(s) to trial subjects, or when the change(s) involves only logistical or administrative aspects of the trial (e.g., change in monitor(s), change of telephone number(s)).

4.5.3

The investigator, or person designated by the investigator, should document and explain any deviation from the approved protocol.

4.5.4

The investigator may implement a deviation from, or a change of, the protocol to eliminate an immediate hazard(s) to trial subjects without prior IRB/IEC approval/favourable opinion. As soon as possible, the implemented deviation or change, the reasons for it, and, if appropriate, the proposed protocol amendment(s) should be submitted:

(a) to the IRB/IEC for review and approval/favourable opinion,
(b) to the sponsor for agreement and, if required,
(c) to the regulatory authority(ies).

4.6 Investigational product(s)

4.6.1

Responsibility for investigational product(s) accountability at the trial site(s) rests with the investigator/institution.

4.6.2

Where allowed/required, the investigator/institution may/should assign some or all of the investigator's/institution's duties for investigational product(s) accountability at the trial site(s) to an appropriate pharmacist or another appropriate individual who is under the supervision of the investigator/institution.

4.6.3

The investigator/institution and/or a pharmacist or other appropriate individual, who is designated by the investigator/institution, should maintain records of the product's delivery to the trial site, the inventory at the site, the use by each subject, and the return to the sponsor or alternative disposition of unused product(s). These records should include dates, quantities, batch/serial numbers, expiration dates (if applicable), and the unique code numbers assigned to the investigational product(s) and trial subjects. Investigators should maintain records that document adequately that the subjects were provided the doses specified by the protocol and reconcile all investigational product(s) received from the sponsor.

4.6.4

The investigational product(s) should be stored as specified by the sponsor (see 5.13.2 and 5.14.3) and in accordance with applicable regulatory requirement(s).

4.6.5

The investigator should ensure that the investigational product(s) are used only in accordance with the approved protocol.

4.6.6

The investigator, or a person designated by the investigator/institution, should explain the correct use of the investigational product(s) to each subject and should check, at intervals appropriate for the trial, that each subject is following the instructions properly.

4.7 Randomization procedures and unblinding

The investigator should follow the trial's randomization procedures, if any, and should ensure that the code is broken only in accordance with the protocol. If the trial is blinded, the investigator should promptly document and explain to the sponsor any premature unblinding (e.g., accidental unblinding, unblinding due to a serious adverse event) of the investigational product(s).

4.8 Informed consent of trial subjects

4.8.1

In obtaining and documenting informed consent, the investigator should comply with the applicable regulatory requirement(s), and should adhere to GCP and to the ethical principles that have their origin in the Declaration of Helsinki. Prior to the beginning of the trial, the investigator should have the IRB/IEC's written approval/favourable opinion of the written informed consent form and any other written information to be provided to subjects.

4.8.2

The written informed consent form and any other written information to be provided to subjects should be revised whenever important new information becomes available that may be relevant to the subject's consent. Any revised written informed consent form, and written information

should receive the IRB/IEC's approval/favourable opinion in advance of use. The subject or the subject's legally acceptable representative should be informed in a timely manner if new information becomes available that may be relevant to the subject's willingness to continue participation in the trial. The communication of this information should be documented.

4.8.3

Neither the investigator, nor the trial staff, should coerce or unduly influence a subject to participate or to continue to participate in a trial.

4.8.4

None of the oral and written information concerning the trial, including the written informed consent form, should contain any language that causes the subject or the subject's legally acceptable representative to waive or to appear to waive any legal rights, or that releases or appears to release the investigator, the institution, the sponsor, or their agents from liability for negligence.

4.8.5

The investigator, or a person designated by the investigator, should fully inform the subject or, if the subject is unable to provide informed consent, the subject's legally acceptable representative, of all pertinent aspects of the trial including the written information and the approval/ favourable opinion by the IRB/IEC.

4.8.6

The language used in the oral and written information about the trial, including the written informed consent form, should be as non-technical as practical and should be understandable to the subject or the subject's legally acceptable representative and the impartial witness, where applicable.

4.8.7

Before informed consent may be obtained, the investigator, or a person designated by the investigator, should provide the subject or the subject's legally acceptable representative ample time and opportunity to inquire about details of the trial and to decide whether or not to participate in the trial. All questions about the trial should be answered to the satisfaction of the subject or the subject's legally acceptable representative.

4.8.8

Prior to a subject's participation in the trial, the written informed consent form should be signed and personally dated by the subject or by the subject's legally acceptable representative, and by the person who conducted the informed consent discussion.

4.8.9
If a subject is unable to read or if a legally acceptable representative is unable to read, an impartial witness should be present during the entire informed consent discussion. After the written informed consent form and any other written information to be provided to subjects, is read and explained to the subject or the subject's legally acceptable representative, and after the subject or the subject's legally acceptable representative has orally consented to the subject's participation in the trial and, if capable of doing so, has signed and personally dated the informed consent form, the witness should sign and personally date the consent form. By signing the consent form, the witness attests that the information in the consent form and any other written information was accurately explained to, and apparently understood by, the subject or the subject's legally acceptable representative, and that informed consent was freely given by the subject or the subject's legally acceptable representative.

4.8.10
Both the informed consent discussion and the written informed consent form and any other written information to be provided to subjects should include explanations of the following:
(a) That the trial involves research.
(b) The purpose of the trial.
(c) The trial treatment(s) and the probability for random assignment to each treatment.
(d) The trial procedures to be followed, including all invasive procedures.
(e) The subject's responsibilities.
(f) Those aspects of the trial that are experimental.
(g) The reasonably foreseeable risks or inconveniences to the subject and, when applicable, to an embryo, fetus, or nursing infant.
(h) The reasonably expected benefits. When there is no intended clinical benefit to the subject, the subject should be made aware of this.
(i) The alternative procedure(s) or course(s) of treatment that may be available to the subject, and their important potential benefits and risks.
(j) The compensation and/or treatment available to the subject in the event of trial-related injury.
(k) The anticipated prorated payment, if any, to the subject for participating in the trial.
(l) The anticipated expenses, if any, to the subject for participating in the trial.
(m) That the subject's participation in the trial is voluntary and that the subject may refuse to participate or withdraw from the trial, at any time, without penalty or loss of benefits to which the subject is otherwise entitled.
(n) That the monitor(s), the auditor(s), the IRB/IEC, and the regulatory authority(ies) will be granted direct access to the subject's original medical records for verification of clinical trial procedures and/or data, without violating the confidentiality of the subject, to the extent permitted by the applicable laws and regulations and that, by signing a written informed consent form, the subject or the subject's legally acceptable representative is authorizing such access.
(o) That records identifying the subject will be kept confidential and, to the extent permitted by the applicable laws and/or regulations, will not be made publicly available. If the results of the trial are published, the subject's identity will remain confidential.
(p) That the subject or the subject's legally acceptable representative will be informed in a timely manner if information becomes available that may be relevant to the subject's willingness to continue participation in the trial.
(q) The person(s) to contact for further information regarding the trial and the rights of trial subjects, and whom to contact in the event of trial-related injury.
(r) The foreseeable circumstances and/or reasons under which the subject's participation in the trial may be terminated.
(s) The expected duration of the subject's participation in the trial.
(t) The approximate number of subjects involved in the trial.

4.8.11
Prior to participation in the trial, the subject or the subject's legally acceptable representative should receive a copy of the signed and dated written informed consent form and any other written information provided to the subjects. During a subject's participation in the trial, the subject or the subject's legally acceptable representative should receive a copy of the signed and dated consent form updates and a copy of any amendments to the written information provided to subjects.

4.8.12
When a clinical trial (therapeutic or non-therapeutic) includes subjects who can only be enrolled in the trial with

the consent of the subject's legally acceptable representative (e.g., minors, or patients with severe dementia), the subject should be informed about the trial to the extent compatible with the subject's understanding and, if capable, the subject should sign and personally date the written informed consent.

4.8.13

Except as described in 4.8.14, a non-therapeutic trial (i.e. a trial in which there is no anticipated direct clinical benefit to the subject), should be conducted in subjects who personally give consent and who sign and date the written informed consent form.

4.8.14

Non-therapeutic trials may be conducted in subjects with consent of a legally acceptable representative provided the following conditions are fulfilled:
(a) The objectives of the trial can not be met by means of a trial in subjects who can give informed consent personally.
(b) The foreseeable risks to the subjects are low.
(c) The negative impact on the subject's well-being is minimized and low.
(d) The trial is not prohibited by law.
(e) The approval/favourable opinion of the IRB/IEC is expressly sought on the inclusion of such subjects, and the written approval/favourable opinion covers this aspect.

Such trials, unless an exception is justified, should be conducted in patients having a disease or condition for which the investigational product is intended. Subjects in these trials should be particularly closely monitored and should be withdrawn if they appear to be unduly distressed.

4.8.15

In emergency situations, when prior consent of the subject is not possible, the consent of the subject's legally acceptable representative, if present, should be requested. When prior consent of the subject is not possible, and the subject's legally acceptable representative is not available, enrolment of the subject should require measures described in the protocol and/or elsewhere, with documented approval/favourable opinion by the IRB/IEC, to protect the rights, safety and well-being of the subject and to ensure compliance with applicable regulatory requirements. The subject or the subject's legally acceptable representative should be informed about the trial as soon as possible and consent to continue and other consent as appropriate (see 4.8.10) should be requested.

4.9 Records and reports

4.9.1

The investigator should ensure the accuracy, completeness, legibility, and timeliness of the data reported to the sponsor in the CRFs and in all required reports.

4.9.2

Data reported on the CRF, that are derived from source documents, should be consistent with the source documents or the discrepancies should be explained.

4.9.3

Any change or correction to a CRF should be dated, initialed, and explained (if necessary) and should not obscure the original entry (i.e. an audit trail should be maintained); this applies to both written and electronic changes or corrections (see 5.18.4 (n)). Sponsors should provide guidance to investigators and/or the investigators' designated representatives on making such corrections. Sponsors should have written procedures to assure that changes or corrections in CRFs made by sponsor's designated representatives are documented, are necessary, and are endorsed by the investigator. The investigator should retain records of the changes and corrections.

4.9.4

The investigator/institution should maintain the trial documents as specified in Essential Documents for the Conduct of a Clinical Trial (see 8.) and as required by the applicable regulatory requirement(s). The investigator/institution should take measures to prevent accidental or premature destruction of these documents.

4.9.5

Essential documents should be retained until at least 2 years after the last approval of a marketing application in an ICH region and until there are no pending or contemplated marketing applications in an ICH region or at least 2 years have elapsed since the formal discontinuation of clinical development of the investigational product. These documents should be retained for a longer period however if required by the applicable regulatory requirements or by an agreement with the sponsor. It is the responsibility of the sponsor to inform the investigator/institution as to when these documents no longer need to be retained (see 5.5.12).

4.9.6

The financial aspects of the trial should be documented in an agreement between the sponsor and the investigator/institution.

4.9.7

Upon request of the monitor, auditor, IRB/IEC, or regulatory authority, the investigator/institution should make available for direct access all requested trial-related records.

4.10 Progress reports

4.10.1

The investigator should submit written summaries of the trial status to the IRB/IEC annually, or more frequently, if requested by the IRB/IEC.

4.10.2

The investigator should promptly provide written reports to the sponsor, the IRB/IEC (see 3.3.8) and, where applicable, the institution on any changes significantly affecting the conduct of the trial, and/or increasing the risk to subjects.

4.11 Safety reporting

4.11.1

All serious adverse events (SAEs) should be reported immediately to the sponsor except for those SAEs that the protocol or other document (e.g., Investigator's Brochure) identifies as not needing immediate reporting. The immediate reports should be followed promptly by detailed, written reports. The immediate and follow-up reports should identify subjects by unique code numbers assigned to the trial subjects rather than by the subjects' names, personal identification numbers, and/or addresses. The investigator should also comply with the applicable regulatory requirement(s) related to the reporting of unexpected serious adverse drug reactions to the regulatory authority(ies) and the IRB/IEC.

4.11.2

Adverse events and/or laboratory abnormalities identified in the protocol as critical to safety evaluations should be reported to the sponsor according to the reporting requirements and within the time periods specified by the sponsor in the protocol.

4.11.3

For reported deaths, the investigator should supply the sponsor and the IRB/IEC with any additional requested information (e.g., autopsy reports and terminal medical reports).

4.12 Premature termination or suspension of a trial

If the trial is prematurely terminated or suspended for any reason, the investigator/institution should promptly inform the trial subjects, should assure appropriate therapy and follow-up for the subjects, and, where required by the applicable regulatory requirement(s), should inform the regulatory authority(ies). In addition:

4.12.1

If the investigator terminates or suspends a trial without prior agreement of the sponsor, the investigator should inform the institution where applicable, and the investigator/institution should promptly inform the sponsor and the IRB/IEC, and should provide the sponsor and the IRB/IEC a detailed written explanation of the termination or suspension.

4.12.2

If the sponsor terminates or suspends a trial (see 5.21), the investigator should promptly inform the institution where applicable and the investigator/institution should promptly inform the IRB/IEC and provide the IRB/IEC a detailed written explanation of the termination or suspension.

4.12.3

If the IRB/IEC terminates or suspends its approval/favourable opinion of a trial (see 3.1.2 and 3.3.9), the investigator should inform the institution where applicable and the investigator/institution should promptly notify the sponsor and provide the sponsor with a detailed written explanation of the termination or suspension.

4.13 Final report(s) by investigator

Upon completion of the trial, the investigator, where applicable, should inform the institution; the investigator/institution should provide the IRB/IEC with a summary of the trial's outcome, and the regulatory authority(ies) with any reports required.

5 Sponsor

5.8 Compensation to subjects and investigators

5.8.1

If required by the applicable regulatory requirement(s), the sponsor should provide insurance or should indemnify (legal and financial coverage) the investigator/the institution against claims arising from the trial, except for claims that arise from malpractice and/or negligence.

5.8.2

The sponsor's policies and procedures should address the costs of treatment of trial subjects in the event of trial-related injuries in accordance with the applicable regulatory requirement(s).

5.8.3

When trial subjects receive compensation, the method and manner of compensation should comply with applicable regulatory requirement(s).

5.11 Confirmation of review by IRB/IEC

5.11.1

The sponsor should obtain from the investigator/institution:

(a) The name and address of the investigator's/institution's IRB/IEC.

(b) A statement obtained from the IRB/IEC that it is organized and operates according to GCP and the applicable laws and regulations.

(c) Documented IRB/IEC approval/favourable opinion and, if requested by the sponsor, a current copy of protocol, written informed consent form(s) and any other written information to be provided to subjects, subject recruiting procedures, and documents related to payments and compensation available to the subjects, and any other documents that the IRB/IEC may have requested.

5.11.2

If the IRB/IEC conditions its approval/favourable opinion upon change(s) in any aspect of the trial, such as modification(s) of the protocol, written informed consent form and any other written information to be provided to subjects, and/or other procedures, the sponsor should obtain from the investigator/institution a copy of the modification(s) made and the date approval/favourable opinion was given by the IRB/IEC.

5.11.3

The sponsor should obtain from the investigator/institution documentation and dates of any IRB/IEC reapprovals/re-evaluations with favourable opinion, and of any withdrawals or suspensions of approval/favourable opinion.

5.15 Record access

5.15.1

The sponsor should ensure that it is specified in the protocol or other written agreement that the investigator(s)/institution(s) provide direct access to source data/documents for trial-related monitoring, audits, IRB/IEC review, and regulatory inspection.

5.15.2

The sponsor should verify that each subject has consented, in writing, to direct access to his/her original medical records for trial-related monitoring, audit, IRB/IEC review, and regulatory inspection.

5.16 Safety information

5.16.1

The sponsor is responsible for the ongoing safety evaluation of the investigational product(s).

5.16.2

The sponsor should promptly notify all concerned investigator(s)/institution(s) and the regulatory authority(ies) of findings that could affect adversely the safety of subjects, impact the conduct of the trial, or alter the IRB/IEC's approval/favourable opinion to continue the trial.

5.17 Adverse drug reaction reporting

5.17.1

The sponsor should expedite the reporting to all concerned investigator(s)/institutions(s), to the IRB(s)/IEC(s), where required, and to the regulatory authority(ies) of all adverse drug reactions (ADRs) that are both serious and unexpected.

5.17.2

Such expedited reports should comply with the applicable regulatory requirement(s) and with the ICH Guideline for Clinical Safety Data Management: Definitions and Standards for Expedited Reporting.

5.17.3

The sponsor should submit to the regulatory authority(ies) all safety updates and periodic reports, as required by applicable regulatory requirement(s).

5.21 Premature termination or suspension of a trial

If a trial is prematurely terminated or suspended, the sponsor should promptly inform the investigators/institutions, and the regulatory authority(ies) of the termination or suspension and the reason(s) for the termination or suspension. The IRB/IEC should also be informed promptly and provided the reason(s) for the termination or suspension by the sponsor or by the investigator/institution, as specified by the applicable regulatory requirement(s).

5.22 Clinical trial/study reports

Whether the trial is completed or prematurely terminated, the sponsor should ensure that the clinical trial reports are prepared and provided to the regulatory agency(ies) as required by the applicable regulatory requirement(s). The sponsor should also ensure that the clinical trial reports in marketing applications meet the standards of the ICH Guideline for Structure and Content of Clinical Study Reports. (NOTE: The ICH Guideline for Structure and Content of Clinical Study Reports specifies that abbreviated study reports may be acceptable in certain cases.)

5.23 Multicentre trials

For multicentre trials, the sponsor should ensure that:

5.23.1

All investigators conduct the trial in strict compliance with the protocol agreed to by the sponsor and, if required, by the regulatory authority(ies), and given approval/favourable opinion by the IRB/IEC.

5.23.2

The CRFs are designed to capture the required data at all multicentre trial sites. For those investigators who are collecting additional data, supplemental CRFs should also be provided that are designed to capture the additional data.

5.23.3

The responsibilities of coordinating investigator(s) and the other participating investigators are documented prior to the start of the trial.

5.23.4

All investigators are given instructions on following the protocol, on complying with a uniform set of standards for the assessment of clinical and laboratory findings, and on completing the CRFs.

5.23.5

Communication between investigators is facilitated.

Reproduced by kind permission of ICH

Governance arrangements for NHS research ethics committees

Department of Health

Governance arrangements for NHS research ethics committees, July 2001

Preface

1 For many years the NHS has had the benefit of a generally high standard of advice from its Research Ethics Committees (RECs), which were formally established in England under cover of HSG(91)5 for Local Research Ethics Committees (LRECs) and HSG(97)23 for Multicentre Research Ethics Committees (MRECs).

2 The Department of Health (DH) has also established additional committees that offer an ethical opinion on research proposals within certain very specialist areas. These include the Gene Therapy Advisory Committee (GTAC), and the United Kingdom Xenotransplantation Interim Regulatory Authority (UKXIRA).

3 The recently published DH *Research Governance Framework for Health and Social Care*[1] (RGF) indicated a need for a review of LRECs and MRECs. There are also new developments in the national and international legal and regulatory framework in which research must in future be conducted. In particular, significant changes are required in order to respond to the rigorous standards set by European Directive 2001/20/EC.

4 The accountability for the various aspects of research was clarified in the RGF. The current document describes the role and remit of RECs as part of this overall governance framework.

[1] The *Research Governance Framework for Health and Social Care* also contains comprehensive references to other documents relevant to this guidance. It may be found on the Department of Health website: http://www.doh.gov.uk/research

© Department of Health.

5 Whilst the research environment itself is changing, the need for a prior favourable ethics opinion before the categories of research defined later in this document may be started is central to Research Governance. The provision of this opinion will remain the prerogative of Research Ethics Committees.

6 This document provides a standards framework for the process of review of the ethics of all proposals for research in the NHS and Social Care which is efficient, effective and timely, and which will command public confidence. It sets out general standards and principles for an accountable system of RECs, working collaboratively to common high standards of review and operating process throughout the NHS. It should be read in conjunction with the *Research Governance Framework for Health and Social Care*.

7 This guidance replaces the previous guidance issued under cover of HSG(91)5 and HSG(97)23. It is Section A of a suite of documents. The topics to be covered are as follows:

- Section A concentrates on general principles and standards, and is based on previous DH guidance, on guidance published by the World Health Organisation, and on the current regulatory standards pertaining to pharmaceutical and other research.

- Section B offers more detailed and timely guidance on operating procedures and the requirements for general support for RECs. It will be up-dated as new or modified operating procedures are required, particularly in order to implement new European legislation.

- Section C is a regularly up-dated resource for RECs and others, collating current advice on particular ethical issues, as issued by the Department of Health itself, or by august bodies such as Royal Colleges, Research Councils or appropriate professional organisations.

8 Plans for implementation of these Governance Arrangements for NHS Research Ethics Committees should start now, with a view to establishing the necessary REC structures and procedures from April 2002. As an interim measure, existing RECs – and their membership and administration – may continue after that date, but should operate according to this new guidance. All new appointments and new operational and management arrangements made after that date should conform to these new governance arrangements. Implementation of new structures and processes should be complete by April 2003.

Further information may be obtained from:

Central Office for Research Ethics Committees (COREC)
Room 76 Block B
40 Eastbourne Terrace
London W2 3QR

Email: tstacey@doh.gsi.gov.uk

Section A: Statement of general standards and principles

1 Introduction

1.1 Research is essential to the successful promotion and protection of health and well-being and to modern and effective health and social care. It also contributes to the efficiency and effectiveness of the content, planning, delivery and monitoring of health and social care. The National Health and Social Services have a key role in enabling relevant research of good quality, and as part of the NHS, Research Ethics Committees (RECs) share in this duty.

1.2 There is now a quality and accountability framework within which research is to be undertaken in the NHS.

This framework is described in the DH *Research Governance Framework for Health and Social Care.* In that guidance, particular reference is made to the duties and accountability of all NHS organisations that agree to host any research, whether undertaken by its own employees or by others. The *Guide to collaboration in Research between the NHS and other research funders* sets out additional factors relevant to collaboration on R&D in the NHS.

1.3 The Research Governance Framework states that the dignity, rights, safety and well-being of participants must be the primary consideration in any research study. The Department of Health requires that all research falling within certain categories *(set out in 3.1)* is reviewed independently to ensure it meets the required ethical standards.

1.4 For research in the NHS, this independent review must be obtained from a Research Ethics Committee recognised for that purpose by the Department of Health. For research in Health and Social Care occurring outside the NHS, it recommended that an opinion should be obtained from an NHS REC, or from an REC meeting the general standards for NHS RECs laid down in this document.

1.5 The decision that a research project may proceed is an important management responsibility involving the availability of resources, financial implications, and ethical issues. Before undertaking or hosting any research, an NHS organisation must ensure that a favourable opinion on the ethics of the proposed research has been obtained from an appropriate REC. Research may not be started until this has been obtained.

1.6 The research sponsor is also required to ensure that a favourable opinion on the ethics of the proposed research has been obtained from an appropriate REC.

1.7 Irrespective of the host or sponsor of the proposed research, it is the responsibility of the named principal investigator to apply for approval by the REC. This person retains responsibility for the scientific and ethical conduct of the research.

1.8 The requirements concerning application to RECs set out in this document apply to all research conducted within the NHS. This includes research conducted by those already having clinical responsibility for the research participants, by other NHS staff, and by those who have no other association with the NHS beyond the particular research project.

1.9 Should it wish to do so, an NHS organisation itself may corporately seek advice directly from an REC about ethical issues relating to research that it wishes to commission or host.

1.10 The protection of research participants is best served by close co-operation and efficient communication amongst all those who share the responsibility for it. Whilst not sacrificing the independence of their decision on the ethics of a proposal, RECs should, where appropriate, work closely with actual and potential participants, researchers, funders, sponsors, employers, care organisations and professionals – and each other – in order to achieve this goal.

2 The role of Research Ethics Committees

2.1 Research Ethics Committees are the committees convened to provide the independent advice to participants, researchers, funders, sponsors, employers, care organisations and professionals on the extent to which proposals for research studies comply with recognised ethical standards.

2.2 The purpose of a Research Ethics Committee in reviewing the proposed study is to protect the dignity, rights, safety and well-being of all actual or potential research participants. It shares this role and responsibility with others, as described in the *Research Governance Framework for Health and Social Care.*

2.3 RECs are responsible for acting primarily in the interest of potential research participants and concerned communities, but they should also take into account the interests, needs and safety of researchers who are trying to undertake research of good quality. However, the goals of research and researchers, while important, should always be secondary to the dignity, rights, safety, and well-being of the research participants.

2.4 RECs also need to take into consideration the principle of justice. This requires that the benefits and burdens of research be distributed fairly among all groups and classes in society, taking into account in particular age, gender, economic status, culture and ethnic considerations. In this context the contribution of previous research participants should also be recalled.

2.5 RECs should provide independent, competent and timely review of the ethics of proposed studies. Although operating within the Governance Framework determined by the Department of Health, in their decision-making RECs need to have independence from political, institutional, profession-related or market influences. They need similarly to demonstrate competence and efficiency in their work, and to avoid unnecessary delay.

2.6 In common with all those involved in research in the NHS and Social Care environments, RECs should have due regard for the requirements of relevant regulatory agencies and of applicable laws. It is not for the REC to provide specific interpretation of regulations or laws, but it may indicate in its advice to the researcher and host institution where it believes further consideration needs to be given to such matters.

3 The remit of an NHS REC

3.1 Ethical advice from the appropriate NHS REC is required for any research proposal involving:
   a. patients and users of the NHS. This includes all potential research participants recruited by virtue of the patient or user's past or present treatment by, or use of, the NHS. It includes NHS patients treated under contracts with private sector institutions
   b. individuals identified as potential research participants because of their status as relatives or carers of patients and users of the NHS, as defined above
   c. access to data, organs or other bodily material of past and present NHS patients
   d. fetal material and IVF involving NHS patients
   e. the recently dead in NHS premises
   f. the use of, or potential access to, NHS premises or facilities
   g. NHS staff – recruited as research participants by virtue of their professional role.

3.2 If requested to do so, an NHS REC may also provide an opinion on the ethics of similar research studies not involving the categories listed above in section 3.1, carried out for example by private sector companies, the Medical Research Council (or other public sector organisations), charities or universities.

3.3 The appropriate REC in each case is one recognised for this purpose by the Health Authority within the area of which the research is planned to take place.

3.4 This will normally be one established by the Health Authority itself within its geographical area – currently called a Local Research Ethics Committee (LREC).

3.5 For the purposes of ethical review of the research proposal, a research "site" is defined as the geographical area covered by one Health Authority, whether the research is based in institution(s) or in the community. Even when the research may physically take place at several locations within that geographical boundary, a favourable ethical opinion on the research protocol is required from only one NHS REC within that Health Authority boundary.

3.6 Where the research is planned to take place at more than one "site" as defined above, different arrangements apply. *(See Chapter 8).*

3.7 For research involving gene therapy, application should be made to the Gene Therapy Advisory Committee (GTAC). *(Further details are given in Section B).*

3.8 For clinical research that involves xenotransplantation, application should be made to the United Kingdom Xenotransplantation Interim Regulatory Authority (UKXIRA). *(Further details are given in Section B).*

3.9 Certain types of research specified under the Human Fertilisation and Embryology Act, 1990, may not proceed without a licence from the Human Fertilisation and Embryology Authority, from whom further information may be obtained. Research Ethics Committee approval is also required. *(See Section B).*

3.10 Specific arrangements are in place for ethical review of research on prisoners. *(See Section B).*

3.11 Research on clients of Social Services (i.e. participants recruited by virtue of their past or present status as clients of Social Services), including those cared for under contracts with private sector care providers, should have the favourable opinion of a Research Ethics Committee which meets the same general standards as NHS RECs in respect of composition, review process and general operating procedures. *(Details of the arrangements for ethical review of research in Social Care taking place outside the NHS are under review, and will be published at a later date).*

4 Establishment and support of NHS RECs

4.1 Research Ethics Committees with the authority to offer an opinion on research within the NHS may only be established and governed by Health Authorities or the Department of Health.

4.2 Health Authorities are accountable for the establishment, support, training and monitoring of all NHS Local Research Ethics Committees (LRECs) within their boundary. Each Health Authority should identify a named officer who is not otherwise directly involved in REC administration who will have lead responsibility for the governance of Research Ethics Committees on behalf of the Chief Executive (who has overall accountability).

4.3 It is the responsibility of the appointing Authority to set an annual budget for the adequate support of the REC(s) for which it is accountable, irrespective of any income received from charges made for review in cases where this is appropriate.

4.4 The Department of Health is responsible for these functions for Multi-centre Research Ethics Committees (MRECs), for the Gene Therapy Advisory Committee (GTAC), and for the United Kingdom Xenotransplantation Interim Regulatory Authority (UKXIRA).

4.5 RECs are not accountable in any way to NHS Trusts, and in particular are separate from Trust R&D Departments in respect of the accountability for their operational processes and decision-making.

4.6 RECs are not in any way management arms of any NHS organisation, and have no management role. They are advisory committees to, not sub-committees of, NHS organisations.

4.7 A Health Authority is responsible for identifying the REC (or RECs) that routinely provides ethical advice on research proposals arising within its own boundaries. This will usually be an LREC or LRECs that it has itself established.

4.8 A Health Authority shall establish sufficient LRECs within its boundary to cope with the workload, and must provide adequate administrative support for their business. The RECs within a Health Authority boundary should work collaboratively, and a common administrative structure or network should be established, so that applications can be directed to the most appropriate committee.

4.9 Similarly, for practical management purposes neighbouring Health Authorities may agree to collaborate on the establishment, maintenance and administration of one or more shared LRECs, but the accountability of each Health Authority remains.

Education and training of REC members and administrators

4.10 REC members have a need for initial and continuing education and training regarding research ethics, research methodology and research governance.

4.11 Appointing Authorities shall provide, within the annual budget for its REC(s), resources for such training, guidance on which will be issued by the Department of Health.

Office operation and support

4.12 The appointing Authority is responsible for providing suitable and discrete facilities in which the work of the REC officers and administrators can be undertaken in a confidential manner. These facilities should include adequate provision for handling and storing confidential documents.

4.13 Administrative staffing of the REC office should be sufficient to provide a comprehensive service to the REC, to researchers and, where appropriate, to the NHS. The administrator should have a sound knowledge of the Research Governance Framework, be trained in the work of RECs, and be of sufficient seniority to provide detailed operational advice to the REC officers and to researchers.

Legal liability

4.14 The appointing Authority will take full responsibility for all the actions of a member in the course of their performance of his or her duties as a member of the REC other than those involving bad faith, wilful default or gross negligence. A member should, however, notify the appointing Authority if any action or claim is threatened or made, and in such an event be ready to assist the Authority as required.

5 Membership requirements and process

5.1 RECs should be constituted to ensure the competent review and evaluation of all ethical aspects of the research projects they receive, and to ensure that their tasks can be executed free from bias and influence that could affect their independence in reaching their decision.

5.2 The Health Authority is responsible for appointment of LREC members. The Department of Health or its appointed agent is responsible for the appointment of members of MRECs, GTAC and UKXIRA.

5.3 Appointment of members shall be by an open process, compatible with the Nolan standards. Vacancies should be filled following public advertisement in the press, and/or by advertisement via local professional and other networks as most appropriate to the vacancy to be filled. Potential candidates shall be required to complete an application form. The process for selection of members shall be laid down in Standard Operating Procedures.

5.4 An appointed member must be prepared to have published his/her full name, profession and affiliation. When making appointments, conflicts of interest should be avoided if at all possible. Where unavoidable there should be transparency with regard to such interests, and they should be recorded and published with the above personal details.

5.5 Normally an appointed member shall be required to attend in full at least two thirds of all scheduled REC meetings in each year, barring exceptional circumstances. *(See 6.15 below).*

5.6 As a condition of appointment, a member must agree to take part in initial and continued education appropriate to his or her role as an REC member.

5.7 An appointed member shall be expected to maintain confidentiality regarding meeting deliberations, applications, information on research participants, and related matters.

5.8 The appointed member shall be informed in writing of the terms of the appointment, including its duration, the policy for renewal, the disqualification procedure and the resignation procedure, the policy concerning declaration of interests, and details of allowable expenses.

5.9 The appointing Authority shall provide each appointed member with a personal statement regarding the indemnity provided, and its conditions.

5.10 Members should be appointed for fixed terms, normally five years. Terms of appointment may be renewed, but not normally more than two consecutive terms should be served on the same REC. A member may however subsequently serve on another REC. Simultaneous service on both an MREC and LREC is permitted.

5.11 The appointing Authority shall ensure that a rotation system for membership is in place that allows for continuity, the development and maintenance of expertise within the REC, and the regular input of fresh ideas.

6 Composition of an REC

6.1 An REC should have sufficient members to guarantee the presence of a quorum (see 6.11) at each meeting. The maximum should be 18 members. This should allow for a sufficiently broad range of experience and expertise, so that the scientific, clinical and methodological aspects of a research proposal can be reconciled with the welfare of research participants, and with broader ethical implications.

6.2 Overall the REC should have a balanced age and gender distribution. Members should be drawn from both sexes and from a wide range of age groups. Every effort should also be made to recruit members from black and ethnic minority backgrounds, as well as people with disabilities. This should apply to both expert and lay members.

6.3 RECs should be constituted to contain a mixture of "expert" and "lay" members. At least three members must be independent of any organisation where research under ethical review is likely to take place.

Expert members

6.4 The "expert" members of the committee shall be chosen to ensure that the REC has the following expertise:
  • relevant methodological and ethical expertise in:
    - clinical research
    - non-clinical research
    - qualitative or other research methods applicable to health services, social science and social care research.
  • clinical practice including:
    - hospital and community staff (medical, nursing and other)
    - general practice
  • statistics relevant to research
  • pharmacy

Lay members

6.5 At least one third of the membership shall be "lay" members who are independent of the NHS, either as employees or in a non-executive role, and whose primary personal or professional interest is not in a research area.

6.6 The "lay" membership can include non-medical clinical staff who have not practised their profession for a period of at least five years.

6.7 At least half of the "lay" members must be persons who are not, and never have been, either health or social care professionals, and who have never been involved in carrying out research involving human participants, their tissue or data.

Non-representative role

6.8 Despite being drawn from groups identified with particular interests or responsibilities in connection with health and social care issues, REC members are not in any way the representatives of those groups. They are appointed in their own right, to participate in the work of the REC as equal individuals of sound judgement, relevant experience and adequate training in ethical review.

NHS staff as members

6.9 NHS organisations should provide encouragement to their staff who wish to serve as members of RECs. The time required for undertaking such service and the necessary training should be protected, and form a recognised part of the individual's job plan.

Specialist referees

6.10 The Chair and Administrator may seek the advice of specialist referees on any relevant aspects of a specific research proposal that lie beyond the expertise of the members. These referees may be specialists in ethical aspects, specific diseases or methodologies, or they may be representatives of communities, patients, or special interest groups. Such referees are not voting members of the committee, and should not be involved in the business of the committee other than that related to the specific research proposal in question. Terms of reference for independent referees should be established. Their advice should be recorded in the minutes.

Quorum requirements

6.11 For meetings at which research ethical review is undertaken, a quorum shall consist of seven members. It shall include the Chair and/or Vice-Chair, at least one "expert" member with the relevant clinical and/or methodological expertise, one "lay" member as defined in 6.7 above, and at least one *other* member who is independent of the institution or specific location where the research is to take place.

Committee officers

6.12 The Chair and Vice-Chair shall be appointed as such by the appointing Authority after consultation with the REC Administrator and committee members. The appointees should have had at least one year's experience of the work of RECs. Those appointed should have received personal training in research ethics reviewing, and possess the relevant chairing skills. Potential candidates should be offered any necessary supplementary training prior to appointment.

6.13 To facilitate communication, the REC may wish to designate a suitably qualified individual as Scientific Officer, who will be the principal point of liaison with applicants for more detailed discussion of issues related to the content of applications, and who can if necessary represent the committee at scientific management discussions. Depending on their background and personal expertise, this could be the Chair, Vice-Chair or Administrator, but need not necessarily be so. This work may be shared by other REC members.

6.14 The process for appointment of all officers shall be laid down in the standard operating procedures.

Deputies

6.15 Where a member provides unique expertise to the REC (e.g. pharmacy or statistical advice) the REC may, if necessary, make arrangements to appoint deputies for individual members of the committee. These deputies must have undergone the same recruitment, selection and appointment procedure as the named members, and must also have been trained in ethical review. When deputising, these members are considered full members of the committee. The names of deputies should be recorded in the Annual Report.

6.16 However, attendance of the member at the scheduled meetings must be of sufficient frequency to ensure their effective contribution to the work of the committee.

Observers

6.17 Observers, who shall play no part in the committee's deliberations, may be invited subject to the minuted agreement of the REC, and subject to written invitation giving the terms under which observer status is permitted. Such observers should have no vested interest in, or scientific or management responsibility for, any applications being considered. Observers should be allowed only if they accept in writing the same duty of confidentiality as REC members.

7 Working procedures

7.1 Good standard operating procedures and accurate record keeping are important. Standard operating procedures shall be drawn up in line with national guidance, and approved by the appointing Authority. These standard operating procedures should be publicly available.

7.2 RECs shall have standard operating procedures that state:
- the Authority under which the REC is established
- the functions and duties of the REC
- membership requirements
- the terms and conditions of appointment
- the officers and the structure of the secretariat
- internal procedures
- quorum requirements
- procedures for considering applications

7.3 Standard operating procedures shall be compatible with European and UK law, and, where appropriate, to the relevant provisions in Good Clinical Practice.

7.4 RECs shall act in accordance with their written standard operating procedures. The appointing Authority is responsible for the governance of the REC in this respect, and should ensure that account is taken of all guidance issued by the Department of Health.

7.5 An REC shall make its decisions at scheduled meetings at which a quorum is present.

7.6 All reimbursement for work or expenses, if any, within or related to an REC should be recorded and made available, by the Authority, to the public on request.

7.7 The REC should keep a register of all the proposals that come before it. This register will be available for public consultation. Appropriate sections shall be shared with the relevant NHS bodies hosting the research, for the purposes of governance and management. The register should form the basis of the REC's Annual Report to its appointing Authority.

7.8 An REC should retain all relevant records for a period of at least three years after completion of a research project, and should make them available upon request to any regulatory authorities.

7.9 The REC should always be able to demonstrate that it has acted reasonably in reaching a particular decision. When research proposals are rejected by the REC, the reasons for that decision should be made available to the applicant.

7.10 RECs should consider valid applications in a timely manner. A decision should be reached and communicated to the applicant within 60 calendar days of the submission of a valid application.

7.11 After an initial review, any further written information or clarification may be requested from the applicant on one occasion only. During this period, the timeframe is suspended and does not recommence until a response satisfactory to the REC is received. A final decision should then be made and communicated to the applicant within the total of 60 days. For multicentre research, this time frame includes consideration of the locality issues.

7.12 Amendments submitted once the research has started shall be considered at its next meeting by the REC that approved the original protocol, and an answer given to the applicant within a total of 35 days. However, where the amendment is substantial (for example requiring additional interventions to research participants), it may need to be treated by the REC as a new application requiring full ethical review within the standard 60-day time frame.

7.13 It follows that there should be a sufficient frequency of REC meetings within a Health Authority "site" to complete the business in a timely manner. It is recommended that individual RECs meet monthly, but that the timing of meeting of the individual RECs within one Health Authority "site" should be staggered.

7.14 Any local procedures for expedited review (where appropriate) outside the normal committee cycle shall be described in the standard operating procedures. *(See Section B).*

7.15 The ethical review by the REC should occur in parallel with the consideration of the proposed research by NHS host organisations (usually by its R&D Directorate) and any relevant regulatory authorities, e.g. the Medicines Control Agency.

7.16 An REC should not be expected to accept a workload that compromises the quality of ethical review. When this is likely, the Authority should establish additional RECs, or make formal arrangements for other RECs (e.g. from neighbouring Health Authorities) to provide an opinion.

Confidentiality of proceedings

7.17 REC members do not sit on the committee in any representative capacity and need to be able to discuss freely the proposals that come before them. For these reasons REC meetings will normally be held in private.

7.18 However, a summary of details of the application shall be made publicly available once the final decision on the application is ratified by the REC. These shall include:
- the names of the researcher and sponsor
- and of the research site
- a simple summary of the research proposal comprehensible to a lay person
- the issues discussed by the committee and the committee's conclusions
- and its overall opinion.

Producing an annual report

7.19 Within six months of the end of each financial year, an LREC should submit its Annual Report to the appointing Authority, which shall consider it at a scheduled open meeting of the Authority to which the REC members are invited. In the case of LRECs, copies should be sent to all the NHS bodies within the Authority's boundaries.

7.20 The report, which should be available for public inspection, should include:
- the names, affiliations and occupations of committee members and of deputies (if used)

- number and dates of meetings held
- attendance of members
- a list of proposals considered, and the decisions reached on each
- the time taken from acceptance of application to final decision on each proposal
- a list of projects completed or terminated during the year
- the training undertaken by the committee and by its members

7.21 Similarly, each MREC shall produce its Annual Report (to include the same category items) for presentation to the Department of Health, and for publication.

Advice to non-NHS bodies

7.22 Not all medical, other health-related or social care research takes place within the NHS or public sector Social Services. All those conducting such external research should be encouraged to submit their research proposals to an NHS REC for advice, and the REC should accept for consideration all such valid applications that meet the relevant standards. In such cases, the REC should report to the appointing Authority the cost of its work so that the cost can be recovered from the outside body conducting the research, if appropriate.

Following up and reports

7.23 Once the REC has given a favourable opinion, the researcher is required to notify the committee, in advance, of any proposed deviation from the original protocol. The committee may then wish to review its decision.

7.24 No deviation from, or changes to, the protocol shall be initiated by the researcher without the prior written approval of the REC, save where this is necessary to eliminate immediate hazards to research participants or when the change involves only logistical or administrative aspects of the research. In these cases, the changes may be implemented immediately, but the REC must be informed within seven days. The REC may then reconsider its opinion.

7.25 The research sponsor is responsible for ensuring that arrangements are in place to review significant developments as the research proceeds (particularly those which put the safety of individuals at risk) and to approve any modifications to the design of the research protocol. These modifications must be submitted to the REC and a favourable opinion obtained before implementation (except when there are immediate hazards to research participants, when the process laid out in 7.24 above shall apply).

7.26 The REC should indicate at the time of approval any progress reports it requires from time to time from the applicant. It shall request a final report to be delivered within three months of completion.

7.27 The REC shall require, as a minimum, an annual report from the researcher, and shall reconsider its opinion at that stage. Where the REC considers the degree of risk demands it, more frequent reports and subsequent interim review shall be required.

7.28 Where the research is terminated prematurely, a report shall be required within 15 days, indicating the reasons for early termination.

7.29 RECs may also ask to receive reports of inspections by other authorities.

7.30 Reports to the committee should also be required if there are any other unusual or unexpected results which raise questions about the safety of the research. *(See Section B for further details)*.

7.31 Reports on success (or difficulties) in recruiting participants provide the REC with useful feedback on perceptions of the acceptability of the project among potential research participants. RECs may wish to request such reports where they anticipate potential difficulties.

7.32 On the basis of any such reports, the REC may wish to review its decision. Failure to produce such required reports without a reason acceptable to the REC may result in suspension of the REC's favourable opinion, in which case the research must cease.

7.33 Other than by means of these required progress reports, the REC has no responsibility for pro-active monitoring of research, the accountability for which lies with the host NHS institution, but the REC may wish to be reassured of the process for such monitoring in certain specific cases.

7.34 A member of an REC who becomes aware of a possible breach of good practice in research should report this initially to the Chair and Administrator of the REC, who shall inform the appointing Authority. The Authority's officers shall be accountable for taking appropriate action.

Second ethical review when an REC declines to give a favourable opinion

7.35 Exceptionally, a further review of the protocol may be undertaken by a second REC. *(Details of the procedure for a second REC review are given in Section B)*.

8 Multi-centre research

8.1 For the purpose of ethical review of research, a research "site" is defined as the geographical area covered by a single Health Authority, and includes all the research institutions and localities within it. *(See also paragraph 3.5)*.

8.2 For the present, multi-centre research will continue to be defined as research carried out within five or more "sites", i.e. the area covered by five or more Health Authority boundaries, irrespective of the number of LRECs within each Authority.

8.3 For research taking place in from two to four sites, application should be made to one LREC within each of the Health Authority boundaries. However, when a favourable opinion has been obtained from the first Health Authority's LREC, the second, third and fourth Health Authorities may, on the advice of their own LRECs, accept that opinion with further review by their own LREC only of the "locality issues". *(Further details of this process, which is similar to that which currently operates with MRECs, are provided in Section B)*.

8.4 If recruitment is planned in five (or more) sites, irrespective of whether existing LREC approval in up to four sites has been already given, application is then required to a Multi-centre Research Ethics Committee (MREC). A favourable opinion of an MREC then covers the whole of the United Kingdom.

8.5 If the MREC declines to give a favourable opinion on the application, any existing approval by LRECs still stands, but those LRECs shall be informed of the MREC's decision (and its reasons).

8.6 Once an MREC has declined approval, no further application using the same proposal may be made to any LREC.

Consideration of "locality" issues

8.7 The MREC (or "lead" LREC – see 8.3 above) undertakes the review of the ethics of the research protocol, including the content of the patient information sheet and consent form. No further ethical review of these items shall be undertaken by other RECs (except in the process of a "second review" described in 7.35 above).

8.8 The "locality issues" are limited to:
- the suitability of the local researcher
- the appropriateness of the local research environment and facilities
- specific issues relating to the local community, including the need for provision of information in languages other than English

8.9 The LREC should satisfy itself that the "locality issues" have been adequately considered, and that it can approve them. In undertaking consideration of the "locality issues" the REC should work closely with the NHS host organisation, which also has a responsibility for research conduct and safety.

8.10 LRECs and local NHS trusts should set up administrative mechanisms to facilitate such joint working. The detailed assessment of the "locality issues" may be undertaken on behalf of the NHS either directly by an LREC itself (or its officers), or by the NHS host (if it is a Trust) with the prior agreement of the LREC. In the latter case the Trust shall inform the LREC of the outcome of the process. The LREC shall consider the advice of the Trust and, if accepted, shall record its approval in LREC minutes. For multi-centre research, the research may not proceed until the LREC has informed the approving MREC of its lack of objection with respect to the "locality issues". *(Further details of this process are described in Section B).*

8.11 The consideration of "locality issues" should occur in parallel with the consideration of ethical review of the research protocol by the MREC or "lead" LREC.

8.12 The decision on the "locality issues" should be made and communicated within 60 days of receipt of a valid application for this purpose.

Multi-centre research where there is no "local" researcher

8.13 For multi-centre research where there is no "local" researcher, and where this is confirmed by the MREC (or "lead" LREC – see 8.3 above) during its review of the research protocol, no specific consideration of "locality" issues by an LREC may be needed and the overall process of review may thus be expedited. Approval by the host NHS organisation is still required before the research may proceed. *(Details of the operational process are given in Section B).*

9 The process of ethical review of a research protocol

The review

9.1 All properly submitted and valid applications shall be reviewed in a timely fashion and according to an established review procedure described in the REC's standard operating procedures. A valid application is one which has been submitted by an appropriate investigator, is complete, with all the necessary documents attached, and is signed and dated.

9.2 RECs shall meet regularly on scheduled dates that are announced in advance. Meetings should be planned in accordance with the needs of the workload, but RECs must meet the time standards for review.

9.3 REC members should be given enough time in advance of the meeting to review the relevant documents.

9.4 Meetings shall be minuted. There should be an approval procedure for the minutes.

9.5 The applicant (and if appropriate, the sponsor and/or other investigators) shall be invited to be available to elaborate on or clarify specific issues as required by the REC at its meeting. An REC should not cause unnecessary delay by deferring consideration of an application when the necessary further information it requires could have been obtained from the applicant at the first review meeting.

9.6 Independent expert referees may be invited by the Chairman to attend the meeting or to provide written comments, subject to applicable confidentiality agreements.

Elements of the review

9.7 The primary task of an REC lies in the ethical review of research proposals and their supporting documents, with special attention given to the nature of any intervention and its safety for participants, to the informed consent process, documentation, and to the suitability and feasibility of the protocol.

9.8 The Research Governance Framework makes it clear that the sponsor is responsible for ensuring the quality of the science. Paragraphs 2.3.1 and 2.3.2 state that:
- "It is essential that existing sources of evidence, especially systematic reviews, are considered carefully prior to undertaking research. Research which duplicates other work unnecessarily or which is not of sufficient quality to contribute something useful to existing knowledge is in itself unethical.
- All proposals for health and social care research must be subjected to review by experts in the relevant fields able to offer independent advice on its quality. Arrangements for peer review must be commensurate with the scale of the research."

9.9 Thus, protocols submitted for ethical review should already have had prior critique by experts in the relevant research methodology, who should also comment on the originality of the research. It is not the task of an REC to undertake additional scientific review, nor is it constituted to do so, but it should satisfy itself that the review already undertaken is adequate for the nature of the proposal under consideration.

9.10 If the committee is of the opinion that the prior scientific review commensurate with the scale of the research is not adequate (including adequate statistical analysis), it should require the applicant to resubmit the application having obtained further expert review.

9.11 In addition to considering prior scientific review, RECs need to take into account the potential relevance of applicable laws and regulations. It is not the role of the REC to offer a legal opinion, but it may advise the applicant and the host NHS body whenever it is of the opinion that further expert legal advice might be helpful to them.

Requirements for a favourable opinion

9.12 Before giving a favourable opinion, the REC should be adequately reassured about the following issues, as applicable:

9.13 Scientific design and conduct of the study:

a. the appropriateness of the study design in relation to the objectives of the study, the statistical methodology (including sample size calculation where appropriate), and the potential for reaching sound conclusions with the smallest number of research participants

b. the justification of predictable risks and inconveniences weighed against the anticipated benefits for the research participants, other present and future patients, and the concerned communities

c. the justification for use of control arms in trials, (whether placebo or active comparator), and the randomisation process to be used

d. criteria for prematurely withdrawing research participants

e. criteria for suspending or terminating the research as a whole

f. the adequacy of provisions made for monitoring and auditing the conduct of the research, including the constitution of a data safety monitoring committee (DSMC)

g. the adequacy of the research site, including the supporting staff, available facilities, and emergency procedures. For multi-centre research, these locality issues will be considered separately from the ethical review of the research proposal itself

h. the manner in which the results of the research will be reported and published.

9.14 Recruitment of research participants

a. the characteristics of the population from which the research participants will be drawn (including gender, age, literacy, culture, economic status and ethnicity) and the justification for any decisions made in this respect

b. the means by which initial contact and recruitment is to be conducted

c. the means by which full information is to be conveyed to potential research participants or their representatives

d. inclusion criteria for research participants

e. exclusion criteria for research participants.

9.15 Care and protection of research participants

a. the safety of any intervention to be used in the proposed research

b. the suitability of the investigator(s)'s qualifications and experience for ensuring good conduct of the proposed study

c. any plans to withdraw or withhold standard therapies or clinical management protocols for the purpose of the research, and the justification for such action

d. the health and social care to be provided to research participants during and after the course of the research

e. the adequacy of health and social supervision and psychosocial support for the research participants

f. steps to be taken if research participants voluntarily withdraw during the course of the research

g. the criteria for extended access to, the emergency use of, and/or the compassionate use of study products

h. the arrangements, if appropriate, for informing the research participant's general practitioner, including procedures for seeking the participant's consent to do so

i. a description of any plans to make the study product available to the research participants following the research

j. a description of any financial costs to research participants

k. the rewards and compensations (if any) for research participants (including money, services and/or gifts)

l. whether there is provision in proportion to the risk for compensation/treatment in the case of injury/disability/death of a research participant attributable to participation in the research; the insurance and indemnity arrangements

m. the nature and size of any grants, payments or other reward to be made to any researchers or research hosts

n. circumstances that might be lead to conflicts of interest that may affect the independent judgement of the researcher(s).

9.16 Protection of research participants' confidentiality

a. a description of the persons who will have access to personal data of the research participants, including medical records and biological samples

b. the measures taken to ensure the confidentiality and security of personal information concerning research participants

c. the extent to which the information will be anonymised

d. how the data/samples will be obtained, and the purposes for which they will be used

e. how long the data/samples will be kept

f. to which countries, if any, the data/samples will be sent

g. the adequacy of the process for obtaining consent for the above.

9.17 Informed consent process

a. a full description of the process for obtaining informed consent, including the identification of those responsible for obtaining consent, the time-frame in which it will occur, and the process for ensuring consent has not been withdrawn

b. the adequacy, completeness and understandability of written and oral information to be given to the research participants, and, when appropriate, their legally acceptable representatives

c. clear justification for the intention to include in the research individuals who cannot consent, and a full account of the arrangements for obtaining consent or authorization for the participation of such individuals

d. assurances that research participants will receive information that becomes available during the course of the research relevant to their participation (including their rights, safety and wellbeing)

e. the provisions made for receiving and responding to queries and complaints from research participants or their representatives during the course of a research project.

9.18 Community considerations

a. the impact and relevance of the research on the local community and on the concerned communities from which the research participants are drawn

b. the steps which had been taken to consult with the concerned communities during the course of designing the research

c. the extent to which the research contributes to capacity building, such as the enhancement of local healthcare, research, and the ability to respond to public health needs

d. a description of the availability and affordability of any successful study product to the concerned communities following the research

e. the manner in which the results of the research will be made available to the research participants and the concerned communities.

Expedited review

9.19 RECs shall establish any procedures necessary for the expedited review of research proposals. (*See Section B*). These procedures, which should be described in full in the Standard Operating Procedures, should specify the following:

a. the nature of the applications, amendments, and other considerations that will be eligible for expedited review

b. the quorum requirements for expedited review

c. the status of decisions (e.g. whether requiring confirmation by the full REC or not)

Decision-making

9.20 In making decisions on applications for the ethical review of research, an REC should take the following into consideration:

a. a member should withdraw from the meeting for the discussion and decision procedure concerning an application where there arises a conflict of interest; the conflict of interest should be indicated to the Chair prior to the review of the application, and recorded in the minutes

b. an REC should not review an application in which one of its own members is a named researcher; such applications should be submitted to another REC

c. by invitation of the Chair, independent experts or others may take part in the discussion of the proposal at the REC meeting; however, a final decision may only be taken when sufficient time has been allowed for review and discussion of an application in the absence of non-members (e.g. the investigator, representatives of the sponsor, independent experts) from the meeting, with the exception of REC administrative staff and approved observers

d. decisions should only be made at meetings where a quorum is present

e. the documents required for a full review of the application shall be complete and the relevant elements mentioned above should be considered before a decision is made

f. written comments from absent members shall be allowed to inform the discussion, but only those members who actually participate in the review by the committee at its meeting shall participate in the decision

g. there should be a pre-determined method for arriving at a decision; it is recommended that decisions be arrived at through consensus where possible. Where a consensus is not achievable, the REC should vote.

9.21 Advice that is not binding may be appended to the decision.

9.22 In cases of conditional decisions, clear suggestions for revision and the procedure for having the application re-reviewed should be specified.

9.23 An unfavourable opinion on an application should be supported by clearly stated reasons.

10 Submitting an application

10.1 The application shall be submitted by the "principal investigator" who is the person designated as taking overall responsibility within the team of researchers for the design, conduct and reporting of the study. It follows that the applicant should be of adequate qualification and expertise to fulfil this important role.

10.2 Where a potential applicant is inexperienced, there should be an identified supervisor of adequate quality and experience who will counter-sign the application form, and then share the responsibility for the ethical and scientific conduct of the research. A current signed CV of the supervisor should be submitted with the application.

10.3 RECs should ensure that their requirements for submitting an application for review are described in an application procedure that is readily available to prospective applicants.

10.4 Research to be undertaken by students primarily for educational purposes (e.g. as a requirement for a University degree course) shall be considered according to the same ethical and operational standards as are applied to other research. In such cases the supervisor takes on the role and responsibilities of the sponsor. In reaching its decision, the REC will wish to consider the broader overall benefits gained by such research.

Application requirements

10.5 These shall be published by the REC and shall include the following:

a. the name(s) and address(es) of the REC secretariat to which the application is to be submitted

b. the application form

c. the format for submission

d. any additional documentation

e. the language(s) in which core document(s) are to be submitted

f. the number of copies to be submitted

g. the deadlines for submission of the application in relation to the review dates

h. the means by which the application will be acknowledged, including the communication of the incompleteness of the application

i. the expected time for notification of the decision following review

j. the time frame to be followed in cases where the REC requests supplementary information or changes to the documents from the applicant

k. the fee structure, if any, for reviewing an application

l. the application procedure for amendments to the protocol, the recruitment material, the potential research participant information, and the information or methods used to obtain consent

m. the process for addressing any disputed decisions.

The documentation

10.6 All documentation required for a thorough and complete review of the ethics of proposed research should be submitted by the applicant. This may include, but is not limited to:

a. signed and dated application form

b. the protocol of the proposed research (clearly identified and dated), together with supporting documents and references, and details of any previous scientific peer review

c. a summary, synopsis or diagram ("flow-chart") of the protocol in non-technical language

d. a description of the ethical considerations involved in the research

e. diary cards and other questionnaires intended for research participants

f. when the research involves a study product (such as a pharmaceutical or device under investigation), an adequate summary of all safety, pharmacological, pharmaceutical and toxicological data available on the study product, together with the summary of the clinical experience with the study product to date (e.g. recent investigators brochure, published data, a summary of the product's characteristics)

g. the applicant(s)'s current curriculum vitae (updated, signed and dated).

h. material to be used (including advertisements) for the recruitment of potential research participants

i. a full description of the process to obtain and document consent

j. written and other forms of information for potential research participants (clearly identified and dated) in the language(s) understood by the potential research participants and, when required, in other languages

k. informed consent form (clearly identified and dated) in the language(s) understood by the potential research participants and, when required, in other languages

l. a statement describing any compensation for study participation (including expenses, and access to medical care) to be given to research participants.

m. a description of the arrangements for indemnity, if applicable

n. a description of the arrangements for insurance coverage for research participants, if applicable

o. a statement of agreement to comply with ethical principles set out in relevant guidelines, and the identity of such guidelines

p. all significant previous decisions (e.g. those leading to a negative decision or a modified protocol) by other RECs or regulatory authorities for the proposed study (whether in the same location or elsewhere) and an indication of the modification(s) to the protocol made on that account. The reasons for previous negative decisions should be provided.

11 Glossary

11.1 Clarification is given here of the meaning of some of the terms as used in this document, and as used in the *Research Governance Framework for Health and Social Care*. These meanings are broadly compatible with their use in other regulatory documents. Sometimes such documents use alternative words.

11.2 For some definitions, a list of some *"Key responsibilities"* is also given where they are relevant to the role of Research Ethics Committees. It should be noted that the responsibilities as listed here are not comprehensive, and further reference should be made to the text of the *Research Governance Framework for Health and Social Care* where there is a complete description.

11.3 **Participants:** – patients, users, relatives of the deceased, professional carers or members of the public agreeing to take part in the study. In some legal and regulatory documents the term "subject" is used instead.

11.4 **Research Ethics Committee** – the committee convened to provide independent advice to participants, researchers, funders, sponsors, employers, care organisations and professionals on the extent to which proposals for the study comply with recognised ethical standards.

Key responsibilities:

• ensuring that the proposed research is ethical and by so doing, protects the dignity, rights, safety and well-being of participants

• providing public reassurance of that protection

11.5 **Principal Investigator** – the person designated as taking overall responsibility within the team of researchers for the design, conduct and reporting of the study.

Researchers – those conducting the study at individual sites.

Key responsibilities:

• developing proposals that are ethical and seeking research ethics committee approval

• conducting research to the agreed protocol and in accordance with legal requirements and guidance e.g. on consent

• ensuring participant welfare while in the study

• feeding back results of research to participants

11.6 **Funder(s)** – organisation(s) providing funding for the study through contracts, grants or donations to an authorised member of either the employing and/or care organisation.

Sponsor – the individual, company, institution or organisation which takes responsibility for the initiation, management and/or financing of a clinical trial. The sponsor takes primary responsibility for ensuring that the design of the study meets appropriate standards and that arrangements are in place to ensure appropriate conduct and reporting; the sponsor is usually, but does not have to be, the main funder.

Key responsibilities:

• assuring the scientific quality of proposed research

• ensuring research ethics committee approval obtained

• ensuring arrangements in place for the management and monitoring of research

11.7 **Employing Organisation(s)** – the organisation(s) employing the principal investigator and/or other researchers. The organisation employing the principal investigator will normally hold the contract(s) with the funder(s) of the study. Organisations holding contracts with funder(s) are responsible for the management of the funds provided.

Key responsibilities:

• promoting a quality research culture

• ensuring researchers understand and discharge their responsibilities

- taking responsibility for ensuring the research is properly managed and monitored where agreed with sponsor

11.8 **Care Organisation** – the organisation(s) responsible for providing care to patients and/or users and carers participating in the study.

Responsible Care Professional – the doctor, nurse or social worker formally responsible for the care of the participant while they are taking part in the study

Key responsibilities:

- ensuring that research using their patients, users, carers or staff meets the standard set out in the RGF (drawing on the work of the research ethics committee and sponsor)
- ensuring research ethics committee approval obtained for all research
- retaining responsibility for research participants' care

11.9 **Favourable opinion** – the term used to describe the decision reached by a Research Ethics Committee that the proposed research complies with recognised ethical standards.

11.10 **Approval** – a term in common usage which merely affirms that the REC has given a favourable opinion.

It should be noted that, by itself, such approval by an REC does not entitle a researcher to proceed with the research. All research taking place within the NHS additionally requires the "approval" of the host NHS organisation – this is an absolute requirement. To proceed without this would constitute research misconduct.

Certain types of research will also require the "approval" of other authorities (e.g. the Medicines Control Agency).

11.11 **Rejection** – the term used to describe the decision reached by a Research Ethics Committee that the proposed research does **NOT** comply with recognised ethical standards. Whatever other approval might have been gained, the research may **NOT** proceed within the NHS.

11.12 **Health Authority** – a body established by the NHS to oversee health matters for the population of a defined area. At present these are "District Health Authorities" but from April 2002, these will be replaced by " Strategic Health Authorities". The term "Health Authority" as used in this document refers to the current organisations until April 2002, and subsequently to the Strategic Health Authorities.

The research governance framework for health and social care

Department of Health
March 2001

Research governance framework

Research is essential to the successful promotion of health and well-being. Many of the key advances in the last century have depended on research, and health and social care professionals and the public they serve are increasingly looking to research for further improvements.

This country is fortunate to be able to draw upon a wide range of research within the health and social care systems. Most of this is conducted to high scientific and ethical standards. However, recent events have made us all painfully aware that research can cause real distress when things go wrong. The proper governance of research is essential to ensure that the public can have confidence in, and benefit from, health and social care research.

This Research Governance Framework reflects a wide range of discussions with the NHS and all the Department of Health's partners in health and social care research. We have considered carefully the responses to our earlier consultation and the issues raised in meetings with stakeholders.

I am grateful to all who have helped us with this important task. We now need to continue to work together to ensure that this Research Governance Framework for Health and Social Care is implemented successfully. In this way, we can provide the public with the reassurance it has the right to expect, and ensure that we can continue to reap the benefits of research.

Lord Hunt of Kings Heath

Table of contents

This document builds on a range of earlier published work and draws extensively on the following documents:

The NHS Plan	2000
Research and Development for a First Class Service – R&D Funding in the New NHS	2000
An Organisation with a Memory – Report of an expert group on learning from adverse events in the NHS	2000
A First Class Service: Quality in the New NHS	1998
Clinical Governance – Quality in the New NHS	1998
The New NHS: Modern and Dependable	1997
A Quality Strategy for Social Care	2000
Modernising Social Services	1998

All the above are available on www.doh.gov.uk

Valuing Diversity – Equality and Diversity in Policy Making	2000
Diversity in the Civil Service/Public Service www.cabinet-office.gov.uk	2000
OST Guideline on Use of Scientific Advice in Policy Making http://www.dti.gov.uk/ost/ostbusiness/index_policy_making_old.htm	2000
MRC Guidelines for Good Clinical Practice in Clinical Trials http://www.mrc.ac.uk	1998

Research Governance

- Sets standards
- Defines mechanisms to deliver standards
- Describes monitoring and assessment arrangement
- Improves research quality and safeguards the public by:
  - Enhancing ethical and scientific quality
  - Promoting good practice
  - Reducing adverse incidents and ensuring lessons are learned
  - Preventing poor performance and misconduct
- Is for all those who:
  - Participate in research
  - Host research in their organisation
  - Fund research proposals or infrastructure
  - Manage research
  - Undertake research
- Is for managers and staff, in all professional groups, no matter how senior or junior.

---

1 Purpose and scope

1.1 The Government is committed to enhancing the contribution of research to health and social care, and to the partnership between services and science. Research is essential to the successful promotion and protection of health and well-being and to modern and effective health and social care services. At the same time, research can involve an element of risk, both in terms of return on investment and sometimes for the safety and well-being of the research participants. Proper governance of research is therefore essential to ensure that the public can have confidence in, and benefit from, quality research in health and social care. The public has a right to expect high scientific, ethical and financial standards, transparent decision-making processes, clear allocation of responsibilities and robust monitoring arrangements.

1.2 This document sets out a framework for the governance of research in health and social care. The standards in this framework apply to all research which relates to the responsibilities of the Secretary of State for Health – that is research concerned with the protection and promotion of public health, research undertaken in or by the Department of Health, its non-Departmental Public Bodies and the NHS, and research undertaken by or within social care services that might have an impact on the quality of those services. This includes clinical and non-clinical research, research undertaken by NHS staff using NHS resources, and research undertaken by industry, the charities, the research councils and universities within the health and social care systems.

1.3 The framework is offered as a model for the governance of research in other areas where poor practice could have a direct impact on the health or well-being of the public.

1.4 The framework is of direct relevance to all those who host, conduct, participate in, fund and manage health and social care research. It is not restricted to principal investigators, managers or to any one professional group. All service and academic staff, no matter how senior or junior, have a role to play in the proper conduct of research. Participants in research and the public in general can also help to ensure that standards are understood and met.

1.5 This framework seeks to promote improvements in research quality across the board. As with clinical governance and best value in social care, research governance involves bringing general performance up to that of those at the leading edge. The framework provides a context for the encouragement of creative and innovative research and for the effective transfer of learning, technology and best practice to improve care.

1.6 The framework also aims to prevent poor performance, adverse incidents, research misconduct and fraud, and to ensure that lessons are learned and shared when poor practice is identified. Achievement of these aims, drawing on the work of the Chief Medical Officer's expert group on learning from adverse events[1], will promote good practice, enhance the ethical and scientific quality of research and safeguard the public.

1.7 Health and social care generate and draw upon a wide range of innovative work and ideas from professionals, organisations and the public. Services must promote innovation and its benefits whilst protecting participants from risk and waste. Innovation embraces a much wider range of activities than those managed formally as research. Research can be defined as the attempt to derive generalisable new knowledge by addressing clearly defined questions with systematic and rigorous methods.

1.8 This document sets out the responsibilities and standards that must be applied to work managed within the formal research context. Other documents on clinical governance and on quality in the NHS and social care set out standards and systems for assuring the quality of innovative work in non-research contexts.

1.9 In common with other quality assurance and governance systems, this research governance framework describes:

- arrangements to define and communicate clear quality standards;
- delivery mechanisms to ensure that these standards are met, and
- arrangements to monitor quality and assess adherence to standards nationally.

1.10 Recent enquiries into adverse incidents relating to research have criticised the lack of clarity in relation to responsibilities and accountabilities for research in health and social care. This is of particular importance, given the very wide range of individuals and organisations that can be involved. The framework pays particular attention to clarifying responsibilities and accountabilities.

1.11 Listed are some of the individuals and organisations involved in health and social care research:

- Patients/users, their relatives and organisations representing them.
- The public.
- Research workers.
- Universities.
- Research charities.
- Research councils.
- Health and social care professionals and professional organisations.
- Health and social care organisations.
- Local authorities.
- The pharmaceutical and other industries.
- Department of Health.

1.12 Achieving high quality in research depends on cooperation between all those involved. Figure 1 illustrates how the Department of Health will continue to work with patients, users and care professionals, the public and its research partners to develop and implement this research governance framework to assure quality in health and social care research.

1.13 Following the model in Fig. 29.1 the remainder of this document is structured as follows:

- Section 2 (with the Annex) sets out standards.
- Section 3 details responsibilities.
- Section 4 outlines delivery systems, and
- Section 5 describes local and national monitoring systems.

2 Standards

2.1 Introduction

2.1.1 Clinical governance aims to continually improve the overall standards of clinical care in the NHS and to reduce unacceptable variations in clinical practice. A comparable strategy is in place to improve the quality of social care services. Correspondingly, research governance is aimed at continuous improvement of standards and the reduction of unacceptable variations in research practice across health and social care.

2.1.2 Standards for research governance are set out in the Annex and include legislative requirements, Department of Health requirements and other helpful guidance produced from a variety of established sources. Professional judgement is necessarily involved in the interpretation of many aspects of the guidance. Quality in research therefore depends on those responsible being appropriately qualified with the relevant skills and experience to use their professional judgement effectively in the delivery of dependable research.

[1] An Organisation with a Memory – Report of an expert group on learning from adverse events in the NHS, 2000.

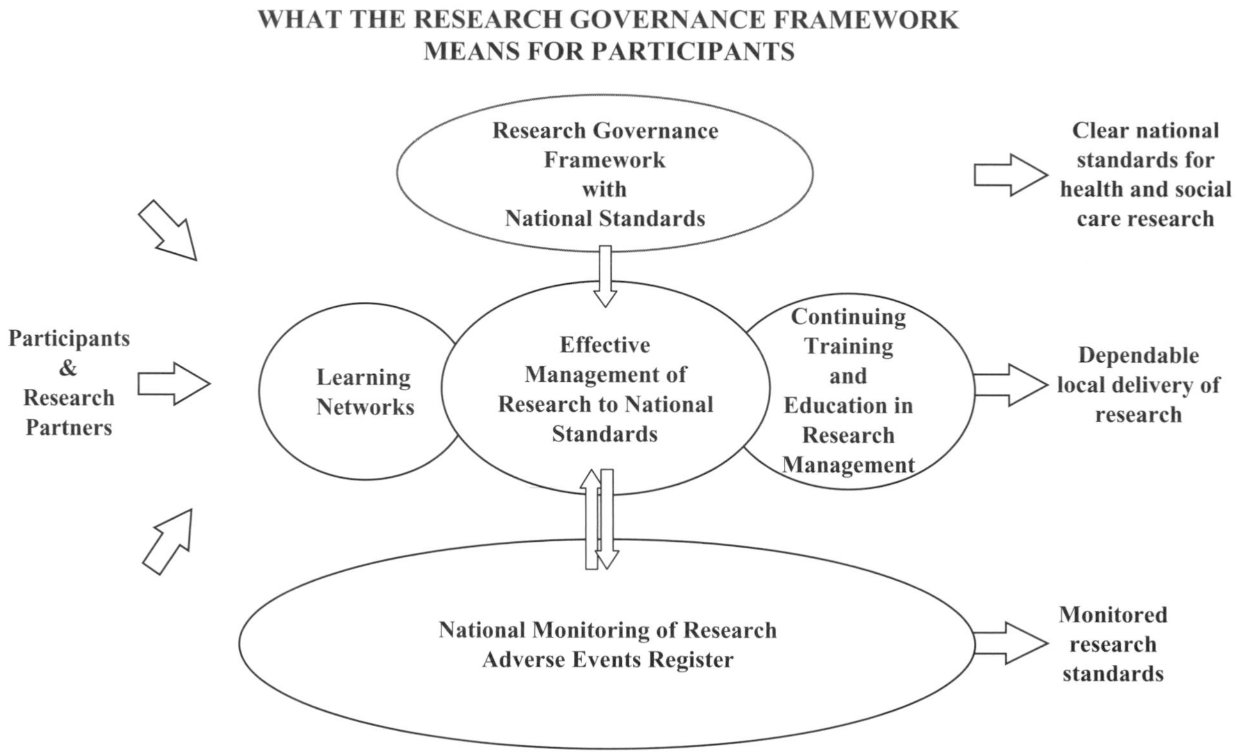

WHAT THE RESEARCH GOVERNANCE FRAMEWORK MEANS FOR PARTICIPANTS

Figure 1 Research governance framework for health and social care

2.1.3 Health and social care research is not the province of a single discipline, profession or organisation and no single document adequately captures the full range of legislation, standards and guidelines that need to be applied across this wide ranging body of work. They are presented here in five domains:
  • Ethics.
  • Science.
  • Information.
  • Health, Safety and Employment.
  • Finance and Intellectual Property.
  Where available, appropriate website addresses have been included to enable access to the current standards, legislation and guidance listed in the domains. Where these relate to more than one domain they have been cross-referenced.

2.1.4 Each domain has been grouped as follows:
  • standards set out in legislation and regulations;
  • other standards required by the Department of Health;
  • other established standards of good practice from recognised international and national authorities and professional organisations.

2.1.5 The contents of the Annex will be updated regularly. Key and enduring principles in each of the domains are set out in the following paragraphs.

2.2 Ethics

2.2.1 The dignity, rights, safety and well-being of participants must be the primary consideration in any research study. Box A describes a scenario to illustrate good practice in protecting research participants' rights.

2.2.2 The Department of Health requires that all research involving patients, service users, care professionals or volunteers, or their organs, tissue or data, is reviewed independently to ensure it meets ethical standards.

2.2.3 Informed consent is at the heart of ethical research. All studies must have appropriate arrangements for obtaining consent and the ethics review process must pay particular attention to those arrangements.

2.2.4 Particular care is needed when research involves tissue or organs of the deceased. The consent of their relatives must always be obtained, and it must be recognised that agreeing to such research involves relatives in difficult choices. Arrangements must be

Box A Protecting research participants' rights

What does it really feel like to be asked to participate?

The scenario: A Professor of Social Work was awarded a grant by the Department of Health to study support services for adoptive families. The research involved the study of adopted children and their parents. The study included children aged between 8 and 14.

The study also involved a survey of, and interviews with, a sample of adoptive parents. The research team sent the adoptive parents a letter and standard information sheet about the children's study. The information provided aimed to help them come to a decision about whether to support their child's participation in the research. It covered the project aims, interview arrangements, interview topics, and consent and confidentiality. It invited them to discuss over the' phone any aspect of the study with the research team.

Enclosed with the parents' letter and information sheet was an information pack for them to pass on to their child. The letter noted that the child might be puzzled by its arrival, and suggested that it might be helpful for them to explain that they have already taken part in the project. Before handing the pack to their adopted child, the parents had some questions about the study that the mother put to the lead researcher over the phone. The researcher clarified that the mother was speaking for herself and the child's adoptive father.

Parent – I've read the information, I think I understand it, but there are a few points I'm not sure about. I think my child may be keen to take part, but I'm worried she might find it upsetting.

Researcher – I can't really say that there's no possibility of something coming up that she may find upsetting. But if your daughter finds a question upsetting she won't have to answer it and she can stop the interview at any time. At the start of the interview we'll help her to rehearse telling us that she doesn't want to answer particular questions or that she doesn't want to go on. In the Information Sheet we noted down some of the topics we want to cover. Is there anything about your daughter's experience that it might be particularly helpful for the interviewer to be aware of?

Parent – No, I can't think of anything . . . , but will you tell me what she says?

Researcher – No, we'll reassure her that whatever she says won't be repeated to you, her teachers, or anyone else she knows. But we'll also let her know that *she* can tell other people about the interview if she wants to. If she talks about any problems which it seems you or other people aren't aware of, we'll explore whether she wants to talk about them with anybody else and, if appropriate, we'll gently encourage her to do so. In our other research with children we've found that once they've talked about a problem during an interview they're usually quite keen to talk about it with someone else.

Parent – How do I know it'll be worthwhile?

Researcher – At the moment we know very little about children's view of adoption. We particularly need to know if support services need to be improved for adopted children and their families. The study's been commissioned by the Department of Health and the findings will be fed directly into the Government's review of adoption. It has undergone ethical review.

Parent – If she says yes' can she pull out later?

Researcher – Yes. She can change her mind whenever she wants. We put that in writing for you and your daughter.

Parent – When the study's finished will you tell us what you've found out?

Researcher – Yes, we'll be writing a summary of our findings especially written for all the families who've taken part.

Parent – Do I have to make my mind up now?

Researcher – No, we don't need to know today, but it would be helpful if we knew by the 20th of next month – that's about four weeks away. Think about it for a while and call me again if you have any more questions.

Scenario: A week or so later the parent decided to pass on the information pack about the study to her eight-year-old daughter. This introduced the research team and explained that they were writing a book about adoption. It also explained the purpose and scope of the interview, and arrangements for gaining their consent and protecting their confidentiality. A few days later the child rang with her own questions:

Child – How long do you want to talk to me?

Researcher – For about an hour, but if you've only a few things to say it could be less than an hour. If you have a lot to say it could take longer.

Child – Will you tell anyone what I say?

Researcher – Only the people we work with at the university.

Child – Will you write down what I say?

Researcher – Maybe, but we'd really like to tape what you say if that's OK with you.

Child – Will anybody reading the book know me?

Researcher – No one will know your name except us.

Child – Will you all come to speak to me?

Researcher – No, just one of us.

Child – Can I change my mind?

Researcher – Yes, of course. You can change it at any time.

Child – What if I'm not sure?

Researcher – Take your time. We don't need to know straightaway. Talk to someone else about it if that helps, but it would be helpful if you could let me know in about three weeks time. If I have not heard from you by 20th, I will take it that you've decided that you don't want to take part.

This researcher is trying to do the right things in the right way. The principles of the research governance framework are reflected in her practice.

---

described for the respectful disposal of material once the research is completed, and for the reporting of the findings of the research to relatives.

2.2.5 The appropriate use and protection of patient data is also paramount. All those involved in research must be aware of their legal and ethical duties in this respect. Particular attention must be given to systems for ensuring confidentiality of personal information and to the security of these systems.

2.2.6 Participants or their representatives should be involved wherever possible in the design, conduct, analysis and reporting of research. Social care research has a long tradition of the involvement of participants in research. The Consumers in NHS Research Group has established the principle that major advisory bodies in NHS R&D programmes should normally have at least two consumer representatives.

2.2.7 Research and those pursuing it should respect the diversity of human culture and conditions and take full account of ethnicity, gender, disability, age and sexual orientation in its design, undertaking, and reporting. Researchers should take account of the multi-cultural nature of society. It is particularly important that the body of research evidence available to policy makers reflects the diversity of the population.

2.2.8 Some research may involve an element of risk to those participating in it. Risk must always be kept to a minimum and explained clearly to the relevant ethics committee and to participants. Arrangements for compensation in the unlikely event of non-negligent harm must always be explained.

2.2.9 Some essential research into important illnesses and treatments can only be conducted with animals.

When considering undertaking research which could involve the use of animals, wherever possible, alternatives such as cells, tissues, computers, bacteria, and plants must be used instead. Where animal use is unavoidable, there are strict controls, enforced by the Home Office. Before a researcher can use animals, a series of special licences must be obtained; primates are only to be used if less advanced animals could not provide the information; researchers must have the necessary skills, training and experience, and the research laboratory must have the facilities to care for the animals properly. In addition, there are three principles that should be followed: the replacement of animals by non-animal methods wherever possible; the reduction of numbers to the minimum necessary to obtain valid results where replacement is not possible; and refinement of all procedures to minimise adverse effects. The highest standards of animal husbandry and welfare under veterinary supervision must be maintained at all times and an ethical review process must operate in accordance with Home Office requirements listed in the Annex.

2.3 Science

2.3.1 It is essential that existing sources of evidence, especially systematic reviews, are considered carefully prior to undertaking research. Research which duplicates other work unnecessarily or which is not of sufficient quality to contribute something useful to existing knowledge is in itself unethical.

2.3.2 All proposals for health and social care research must be subjected to review by experts in the relevant fields able to offer independent advice on its quality. Arrangements for peer review must be commensurate with the scale of the research. For example, many organisations allow established research teams to determine details of the elements of an overall programme of research, which has been reviewed externally. For many student research projects the university supervisor may provide an adequate level of review.

2.3.3 Research involving medicines is regulated under the Medicines Act[2]. All trials of new medicinal products on people must be notified to the Medicines Control Agency who can offer advice and who undertake advisory inspections for such trials and the preparation of products used in them. Similarly, research involving new medical devices is regulated by the Medical Devices Agency.

2.3.4 Special regulations govern the use of human embryos, the release of genetically modified organisms and food or food processes. Further information is set out in the Annex.

2.3.5 Data collected in the course of research must be retained for an appropriate period to allow further analysis by the original or other research teams subject to consent, and to support monitoring of good research practice by regulatory and other authorities. Guidance on storage is set out in the Annex.

2.4 Information

2.4.1 Health and social care research is conducted for the benefit of patients, users, care professionals, and the public in general. There should be free access to information both on the research being conducted and on the findings of the research, once these have been subjected to appropriate scientific review. This information must be presented in a format understandable to the public. Reports need to be comprehensible and take language and other needs into account.

2.4.2 Some advances in health and social care need to be developed commercially if they are to be made widely available. Drugs, medical devices and aides for the disabled are examples. Successful commercial development often depends upon the protection of intellectual property or commercial confidentiality at critical points in the innovation process. The timing of the publication of research findings needs to take account of this.

2.4.3 All those pursuing health and social care research must open their work to critical review through the

[2] The Medicines Act, 1968.

accepted scientific and professional channels. Once established, findings must be made available to those participating in the research (including the relatives of deceased patients who have consented to the use of organs or tissue in the research) and to all those who could benefit from them, through publication and/or other appropriate means.

2.5 Health and safety

2.5.1 Research may involve the use of potentially dangerous or harmful equipment, substances or organisms. The safety of participants, and of research and other staff must be given priority at all times, and health and safety regulations must be strictly observed.

2.6 Finance

2.6.1 Financial probity and compliance with the law and with the rules laid down by H M. Treasury for the use of public funds are as important in research as in any other area.

2.6.2 Organisations employing researchers must be in a position to compensate anyone harmed as a result of their negligence. Any organisation offering participants compensation in the event of non-negligent harm must be in a position to do so.

2.6.3 Careful consideration must be given to the appropriate exploitation of intellectual property rights as set out in the Annex.

2.7 Quality research culture

2.7.1 Some standards set out in the Annex are clear-cut but many require judgement and interpretation. A quality research culture, where excellence is promoted and where there is visible and strong research leadership and expert management, is essential if researchers and managers are to understand and apply standards correctly. A quality research culture is thus essential for proper governance of health and social care research.

2.7.2 The key elements of a quality research culture are:
- Respect for participants' dignity, rights, safety and well-being.
- Valuing the diversity within society.
- Personal and scientific integrity.
- Leadership.
- Honesty.
- Accountability.
- Openness.
- Clear and supportive management.

Promotion of these principles and values is as important as the more detailed standards set out in the Annex.

2.7.3 Box B illustrates how research is managed in a health or social care organisation with a quality research culture.

3 Responsibilities and accountability

3.1 General

3.1.1 All those involved in research with human participants, their organs, tissue or data must be aware of and implement the law, and the basic principles relating to ethics, science, information, health and safety, and finance set out in this framework.

3.1.2 All those involved in research also have a duty to ensure that they and those they manage are appropriately qualified, both by education and experience, for the role they play in relation to any research. They must be aware of, and have ready access to, sources of information and support in undertaking that role.

3.2 Agreements

3.2.1 A complex array of organisations and individuals may be involved in a health or social care research study. It is essential that clear agreements describing allocation of responsibilities and rights are reached, documented and enacted.

3.2.2 Organisations that collaborate on a range of research work may find it helpful to develop and document framework agreements to facilitate the agreement of responsibilities for specific studies. Examples of collaborations where framework agreements will be necessary are:

- NHS trusts, primary care practices, groups or trusts and health authorities who work together regularly on research, whether or not in a formal network;
- universities and NHS trusts, primary care practices, groups or trusts, research networks and health authorities that work together regularly on research;
- local authorities and/or other social care providers, health authorities and primary care practices, groups or trusts that work together regularly on research whether or not in a formal research network;
- universities, local authorities and other social care providers who work together regularly on research.

3.2.3 It is particularly important that clear and documented agreements are in place for complex studies where there may be:

- work on more than one site; and/or
- researchers employed by more than one organisation; and/or
- patients, users and care professionals from more than one care organisation; and/or
- more than one funder.

3.3 Specific responsibilities

3.3.1 Box C describes the people and organisations involved in a health or social care research study. The key responsibilities of the people and organisations accountable for the proper conduct of a study are summarised in Box D.

3.3.2 The remainder of this section sets out these responsibilities in more detail. Box E illustrates these responsibilities with a scenario.

3.4 Responsibilities of participants

3.4.1 Effective and responsive services depend upon research. Through this framework and related provisions, the Government and its research partners strive to ensure that research conducted in health and social care in England offers the likelihood of real benefits either to those who participate, or those who use services subsequently, or both. All those using health and social care services should give serious consideration to invitations to become involved in the development or undertaking of research studies.

3.4.2 Researchers are responsible for selecting appropriate means of communication to ensure that potential participants are fully informed before deciding whether or not to join a study. Potential participants should not hesitate to ask if they do not understand the information and explanations given. Guidance on research with children and others who may have difficulty understanding the information given is listed in the Annex.

3.5 Responsibilities of researchers

3.5.1 Researchers bear the day-to-day responsibility for the conduct of research. They are responsible for ensuring that any research they undertake follows the agreed protocol, for helping care professionals to ensure that participants receive appropriate care while involved in research, for protecting the integrity and confidentiality of clinical and other records and data generated by the research, and for reporting

Box B Standards in a quality organisation undertaking research

Quality research culture

The organisation supports and promotes high quality research as part of a service culture receptive to the development and implementation of best practice in the delivery of care. There is strong leadership of research and a clear strategy linking research to national priorities and needs, the organisation's business, and to clinical governance (in NHS organisations) and delivery of best value (in social care). The organisation's research strategy values diversity in its patients or users and its staff and promotes their active participation in the development, undertaking and use of research.

Ethics

All research which involves patients, users or care professionals or their organs, tissue or data is referred to independent ethical review to safeguard the dignity, rights, safety and well-being of the participants.

Research is pursued with the active involvement of service users and carers including, where appropriate, those from hard to reach groups such as the homeless.

If organs or tissue are used following post mortems, informed consent is obtained from relatives, and there is a commitment to respectful disposal of material.

If animal use is unavoidable the highest standards of animal husbandry are maintained under veterinary supervision.

Science

There is commitment to the principle and practice of independent peer review, with scrutiny of the suitability of protocols and research teams for all work in the organisation.

There is close collaboration with partner organisations in higher education and care to ensure quality and relevance of joint work and avoidance of unnecessary duplication of functions.

The organisation's human resource strategy includes commitment to support research careers (full and part-time) by earmarking funds specifically for R&D training across the professions. The organisation plays its role in developing research capacity with appropriate

training and updating. This includes taking action to ensure that the diversity of the workforce reflects society and developing the capacity of consumers to participate.

The organisation promotes a high standard of health and safety in laboratory work.

Systems are in place to monitor compliance with standards and to investigate complaints and deal with irregular or inappropriate behaviour in the conduct of research.

The organisation assesses its research outputs and their impact and value for money.

Information

Information is available on all research being undertaken in the organisation. This is held on a database, which contains details of funding, intellectual property rights, recruitment, research outputs and impact.

The organisation ensures that patients, users and care professionals have easy access to information on research. Special arrangements are made to ensure access to information for those who are not literate in English or who may need information in different formats because of a disability eg braille.

Those agreeing to be involved in research (including the relatives of deceased patients who have consented to the use of organs or tissue in the research) are informed of the findings at the end of the study.

An information service provides access from a single point to all up-to-date regulatory and advisory documentation pertaining to research governance, together with procedural guidance, for example, for applications to research ethics committees.

There is a research dissemination strategy which addresses different media and writing styles for different audiences.

Finance

The organisation is aware of the activity involved in supporting research and of what it costs. Research expenditure is planned and accounted for.

The organisation demonstrates financial probity and compliance with the law and rules laid down by H M Treasury. It complies with all audit required by external funders or sponsors and has systems in place to deter, detect and deal with fraud.

When research findings have commercial potential the organisation takes action to protect and exploit them, in collaboration with its research partners and – when appropriate – commercial organisations.

Box C Description of the people and organisations involved in a health or social care research study

- **Participants** – patients, users, relatives of the deceased, professional carers or members of the public agreeing to take part in the study.
- **Researchers** – those conducting the study.
- **Principal Investigator** – the person designated as taking overall responsibility within the team of researchers for the design, conduct and reporting of the study.
- **Funder(s)** – organisation(s) providing funding for the study through contracts, grants or donations to an authorised member of either the employing and/or care organisation.
- **Sponsor** – the organisation taking primary responsibility for ensuring that the design of the study meets appropriate standards and that arrangements are in place to ensure appropriate conduct and reporting; the sponsor is usually, but does not have to be, the main funder.
- **Employing Organisation(s)** – the organisation(s) employing the principal investigator and/or other researchers. The organisation employing the principal investigator will normally hold the contract(s) with the funder(s) of the study. Organisations holding contracts with funders are responsible for the management of the funds provided.
- **Care Organisation** – the organisation(s) responsible for providing care to patients and/or users and carers participating in the study.
- **Responsible Care Professional** – the doctor, nurse or social worker formally responsible for the care of the participant while they are taking part in the study.

Research Ethics Committee – the committee convened to provide independent advice to participants, researchers, funders, sponsors, employers, care organisations and professionals on the extent to which proposals for the study comply with recognised ethical standards.

Box D Summary of key responsibilities of people and organisations accountable for the proper conduct of a study

Principal Investigator and other researchers	• Developing proposals that are ethical and seeking research ethics committee approval • Conducting research to the agreed protocol and in accordance with legal requirements and guidance e.g. on consent • Ensuring participant welfare while in the study • Feeding back results of research to participants
Research Ethics Committee	• Ensuring that the proposed research is ethical and respects the dignity, rights, safety and well-being of participants
Sponsor	• Assuring the scientific quality of proposed research • Ensuring research ethics committee approval obtained • Ensuring arrangements in place for the management and monitoring of research
Employing organisation	• Promoting a quality research culture • Ensuring researchers understand and discharge their responsibilities • Taking responsibility for ensuring the research is properly managed and monitored where agreed with sponsor

Care organisation/Responsible care professional	• Ensuring that research using their patients, users, carers or staff meets the standard set out in the research governance framework (drawing on the work of the research ethics committee and sponsor) • Ensuring research ethics committee approval obtained for all research • Retaining responsibility for research participants' care

Box E Specific responsibilities of key people involved in research

Who is responsible for what? – some questions and answers

The Scenario: A university Senior Lecturer in General Practice is awarded a grant by the Medical Research Council (MRC) to conduct a trial. The grant is paid to the university but the MRC is closely involved in the development of the trial design, and in the subsequent monitoring of the trial, and the study is based on MRC's General Practice Research Framework. It is agreed that MRC should take on the responsibilities of sponsor. The manufacturer of the drug being trialled has agreed to provide it free. The drug already has a licence. The research is taking place in a number of general practices which have agreed to participate.

Patient

Q: I did tell my GP that I might be interested in joining the study, but that does not commit me definitely, does it?

A: Your GP has agreed to join this study and invite her patients to participate. Whether or not you agree is entirely up to you.

Q: How can I know the study is worthwhile?

A: Well the study has been approved as scientifically sound and worthwhile by the ethical Medical Research Council and as by the Research Ethics Committee.

Q: How can I find out more about it?

A: You can take away this patient information leaflet to study, and you can ask your GP or anyone on the research team for further details.

Q: What if the drug involved does not agree with me?

A: Your GP is responsible for your care. She is satisfied with the arrangement to monitor participants in the trial. We will advise her immediately if we detect any problems, and you can approach her at any time.

G.P.

Q: How do I know that this study is well designed?

A: The study is sponsored by the Medical Research Council and has therefore been through their review system, but you must decide whether or not you want to collaborate with it.

Q: Who is responsible for the care of my patients if they agree to take part?

A: You are. The protocol explains the procedures the research team will follow and the circumstances in which they will alert you to anything they observe in your patients. You must ensure you are satisfied with these arrangements and discuss them with the principal investigator if you are not.

Q: Who is responsible for ensuring that the study is conducted according to the protocol and that data are monitored to detect any possible problems?

A: The principal investigator is responsible for ensuring that you and every other person involved in the study is well informed, and able to carry out their roles properly. If you have any concerns about this, you should contact the principal investigator and, if you are not satisfied with the response, you should raise the in this matter with the research sponsor, which case is the MRC.

Q: Who is responsible for the quality of the drugs?

A: The pharmaceutical company supplying the drugs is taking responsibility for their quality.

Q: One of my patients seems much worse since I entered him into the trial. He is keen to continue, but I am concerned. What should I do?

A: You have primary responsibility for the patient's care. If you are concerned that the research is bad for the patient you should advise him to withdraw. You can explain that you will be talking to the researcher and that if the treatment under the project is the cause of his problems this will be very valuable information in itself.

G.P. continued

It is very important that you notify the principal investigator of any concerns you have about treatment under the project.

Q: I have agreed to join the study, but a number of my patients are having trouble understanding what they are being asked to take part in and why. It's taking up an enormous amount of time. What should I do?

A: You should talk to the principal investigator about how communications can be improved. If there are still problems you are free to withdraw.

Principal investigator

Q: Who do I report an adverse event to?

A: Any worrying reaction must be reported immediately to the patient's GP. Any adverse drug reaction, as well as reporting it to the patient's GP, must be reported to the drug manufacturer, the Medicines Control Agency, the Trial Steering Committee, the Research Ethics Committee and the Data Monitoring Committee. The Steering Committee will decide whether or not to notify the sponsor.

Q: I am concerned that the staff in the university labs are not following appropriate health and safety rules. What do I do?

A: You should raise this concern through the university's local health and safety systems.

Q: I want to go on a training course, who should I talk to?

A: The university as your employer is responsible for your training.

Q: To whom do I talk about my suspicion that a university colleague is fabricating data?

A: The university as employer has primary responsibility. You should use the university's local system for dealing with suspected misconduct. The sponsor also has an interest. You should keep them informed, particularly if you have any concerns following your approach to the university. They have powers to withdraw funding. You could also consider consulting other organisations such as the General Medical Council with authority to regulate the conduct of the person concerned.

Q: I think we could improve the design of this study. What do I do?

A: You should discuss this with the Trial Steering Committee. If they agree, you will need to draw up a revised protocol and submit it through both ethical review and the MRC's scientific review system. You should not implement changes to a protocol without these formal agreements.

Q: I think I have generated some important intellectual property. What should I do?

A: Ownership of intellectual property will be addressed in your University's contract of employment with you and in their contract with the sponsor. There may also be an agreement between the university and the NHS locally. You need to report the findings to the University's responsible officer, who will advise you on the procedures to be followed.

any failures in these respects, adverse drug reactions and other events or suspected misconduct through the appropriate systems.

3.6 Responsibilities of the principal investigator

3.6.1 A senior individual must be designated as the principal investigator for any research undertaken in or through the NHS or social services or using participants' organs, tissue or data. This person will take responsibility for the conduct of the research and is accountable for this to their employer, and, through them, to the sponsor of the research and to the care organisation(s) within which the research takes place or through which participants, their organs, tissue or data are accessed.

3.6.2 Principal investigators must have suitable experience and expertise in the design and conduct of research

so that they are able either to undertake the design, conduct, analyses and reporting of the study to the standards set out in this framework or to lead and manage others with delegated responsibility for some of these aspects.

3.6.3 It is the principal investigator's responsibility to ensure that:
- The dignity, rights, safety and well-being of participants are given priority at all times by the research team.
- The research is carried out in accordance with this research governance framework.
- Controlled trials are registered.
- The Chief Executive of the care organisation(s) involved and/or any other individual(s) with responsibilities within this framework are informed that the study is planned, and that their approval is given before the research commences.

- When a study involves participants under the care of a doctor, nurse or social worker for the condition to which the study relates, those care professionals are informed that their patients or users are being invited to participate and agree to retain overall responsibility for their care.
- When the research involves a service user or carer or a child, looked after or receiving services under the auspices of the local authority, that the agency director or her deputy agrees to the person (and/or their carer) being invited to participate and is fully aware of the arrangements for dealing with any disclosures or other relevant information.
- Unless participants or the relevant research ethics committee request otherwise, participants' care professionals are given information specifically relevant to their care which arises in the research.
- The study complies with all legal and ethical requirements.
- Each member of the research team is qualified by education, training and experience to discharge his/her role in the study.
- Students and new researchers have adequate supervision, support and training.
- The research follows the protocol approved by the relevant ethics committee and the research sponsor.
- Any proposed changes or amendments to or deviations from the protocol are submitted for approval to the ethics committee, the research sponsor and any other appropriate body.
- Procedures are in place to ensure collection of high quality, accurate data and the integrity and confidentiality of data during processing and storage.
- Arrangements are made for the appropriate archiving of data when the research has finished.
- Reports on the progress and outcomes of the work required by the sponsor, funders, or others with a legitimate interest are produced on time and to an acceptable standard.
- The findings from the work are opened to critical review through the accepted scientific and professional channels.
- Once established, findings from the work are disseminated promptly and fed back as appropriate to participants.
- He or she accepts a key role in detecting and preventing scientific misconduct by adopting the role of guarantor on published outputs.
- Arrangements are in place for the management of financial and other resources provided for the study,

including for the management of any intellectual property arising.
- All data and documentation associated with the study are available for audit at the request of the appropriate auditing authority.

3.7 Responsibilities of research funders

3.7.1 Organisations that fund research, have a responsibility for ensuring that the work is a proper use of the funds they control and provides value for money.

3.7.2 Organisations wishing to fund research which requires the collaboration of the NHS or social care services in England must either be willing and able to discharge the responsibilities of research sponsor or collaborate with another organisation which is prepared and able to do so. Potential collaborators include the Department of Health itself and the NHS and/or university bodies to which the Department has delegated authority to act as research sponsor for work within programmes of social care or NHS research funded by the Department or the NHS.

3.8 Responsibilities of research sponsor

3.8.1 The research sponsor plays a critical role in assuring the quality of research. Any research requiring the collaboration of the NHS or social care services in England must have an organisation willing and able to take on the responsibilities of research sponsor. The responsibilities of sponsor of research undertaken for research training purposes are carried out by the research supervisor.

3.8.2 The research sponsor is responsible for assessment of the quality of the research as proposed, the quality of the research environment within which the research will be undertaken and the experience and expertise of the principal investigator and other key researchers involved. They are responsible for ensuring that arrangements are in place for the research team to access resources and support to deliver the research as proposed and that agreements are in place which specify responsibilities for the management and monitoring of research. They are also responsible for ensuring that arrangements are in place to review significant developments as the research proceeds, particularly those which put the safety of individuals at risk, and to approve modifications to the design.

3.8.3 The sponsor is responsible for ensuring that arrangements are in place for the management and monitoring of research. In cases where it is inappropriate for the organisation employing the principal investigator or initiating the research to take responsibility for the proper management and monitoring of research, the sponsor should either take that responsibility or agree with another organisation involved that it should take responsibility.

3.8.4 Where research sponsors provide substantial blocks of funding to teams with expertise and track record they may delegate responsibility for specific design and management of research to that team, provided the sponsor manages performance.

3.8.5 Where research has no external sponsor, care organisations must accept the responsibility of the sponsor. For example, an NHS trust must be willing and able to act as the sponsor for research which does not have an external sponsor (sometimes called "own account" research).

3.8.6 It is the research sponsor's responsibility to ensure that:

- The research proposal respects the dignity, rights, safety and well-being of participants and the relationship with care professionals.
- The research proposal is worthwhile, of high scientific quality and represents good value for money.
- The research proposal has been approved by an appropriate research ethics committee[3].
- Appropriate arrangements are in place for the registration of trials.
- The principal investigator, and other key researchers, have the necessary expertise and experience and have access to the resources needed to conduct the proposed research successfully.
- The arrangements and resources proposed will allow the collection of high quality, accurate data and the systems and resources being proposed are those required to allow appropriate data analysis and data protection.
- Intellectual property rights and their management are appropriately addressed in research contracts or terms of grant awards.
- Arrangements proposed for the work are consistent with the Department of Health research governance framework.

[3] See Section 3.12 for details of research ethics committees. The Department of Health is working to extend the present coverage of committees to review the ethics of social care research. If it is not possible to have a social care research proposal reviewed by an appropriate committee, the sponsor must satisfy itself that the research is ethical.

- Organisations and individuals involved in the research all agree the division of responsibilities between them.
- There is a clear written agreement identifying the organisation responsible for the ongoing management and monitoring of the study, whether this is the organisation employing the researchers, the sponsor, or another organisation.
- Arrangements are in place for the sponsor and other stakeholder organisations to be alerted if significant developments occur as the study progresses, whether in relation to the safety of individuals or to scientific direction.
- An agreement has been reached about the provision of compensation in the event of non-negligent harm and any organisation, including the sponsor itself, offering such compensation has made the necessary financial arrangements.
- Arrangements are proposed for disseminating the findings.
- All scientific judgements made by the sponsor in relation to responsibilities set out here are based on independent and expert advice.
- Assistance is provided to any enquiry, audit or investigation related to the funded work.

3.9 Responsibilities of universities and other organisations employing researchers

3.9.1 Employers of staff undertaking health and social care research have responsibility for developing and promoting a quality research culture in their organisation and for ensuring that their staff are supported in, and held to account for, the professional conduct of research. This will involve careful attention to training, career planning and development, and the use of clear codes of practice and systems for monitoring compliance, dealing with non-compliance or misconduct, and learning from complaints. These responsibilities apply to both private and public sector employers.

3.9.2 Organisations that employ principal investigators and other researchers have responsibility for ensuring that those researchers understand and discharge the responsibilities set out for them in this framework. They should also be prepared to take on some or all of the responsibility for ensuring that a study is properly managed and for monitoring its progress. The nature of the responsibilities taken on by the employing organisation should be agreed with the sponsor and care provider. The sponsor has ultimate responsibility for ensuring that appropriate arrangements are in place for the management and monitoring of any study they sponsor.

3.9.3 Employers should ensure that agreements are in place between them and their staff and between them and research funders and care organisations about ownership, exploitation and income from any intellectual property that may arise from research conducted by their employees. They have a responsibility for ensuring that employees identify and protect intellectual property.

3.9.4 Universities and other employers of staff engaged in research are responsible for:

- Compliance with all current employment and health and safety legislation.
- Demonstrating the existence of clear codes of practice in other areas for their staff and mechanisms to monitor and assess compliance.
- Ensuring that the principal investigator and/or other research staff are aware of, understand and comply with this framework.
- Discharging their agreed role in the management and monitoring of work undertaken by their organisation.
- Demonstrating systems for continuous professional development of staff at all levels.
- Having agreements and systems in place to identify, protect and exploit intellectual property.
- Ensuring that they are able to compensate anyone harmed as a result of negligence on the part of their staff and, if they have agreed to do so, for non-negligent harm arising from the research.
- Having in place systems to detect and address fraud, and other scientific or professional misconduct by their staff.
- Having in place systems to process, address and learn lessons from any complaints brought against their employees.
- Permitting and assisting in any investigation arising from complaints received in respect of actions taken by their employees.

3.10 Responsibilities of organisations providing care

3.10.1 All organisations providing health or social care in England must be aware of all research being undertaken in their organisation, or involving participants, organs, tissue or data obtained through the organisation. They should ensure that their patients, users and care professionals are provided with information about any research which may have a direct impact on their care, their experience of care, or their work in the organisation. They must ensure that only activity which is being managed formally as research within the provisions of this framework, is presented as research.

3.10.2 Organisations providing care are responsible for ensuring that any research involving their patients, users and carers or staff meet the standards set out in this framework, in particular that it has an identified research sponsor willing and able to discharge its responsibilities, and that clear and documented agreements are in place about the allocation of responsibilities between all parties involved. Accountability for this lies with the Chief Executive or Agency Director but he or she may delegate responsibility for ensuring compliance to an appropriately qualified and senior member of staff. The care provider remains responsible for the quality of all aspects of the care of their patients or users, whether or not they are involved in research and whoever that research may be conducted and funded by.

3.10.3 Chief Executives of NHS organisations are accountable for quality under the Duty of Care. Researchers not employed by the NHS organisation who interact with individuals in a way which has direct bearing on the quality of their care should hold an NHS honorary contract. Further guidance on issues of employment and accountability of university staff working in the NHS will be issued when a review of these areas led by the Department for Education and Employment reports.

3.10.4 A summary of the main responsibilities of organisations providing care are to:

- Retain responsibility for the quality of all aspects of participants' care whether or not some aspects of care are part of a research study.
- Be aware and maintain a record of all research work being undertaken through or within the organisation, including research undertaken by students as part of their training.
- Ensure patients or users and carers are provided with information on research that may affect their care.
- Be aware of any current legislation relating to research work and ensure that these are implemented effectively within the organisation.
- Ensure that all research has been approved by an appropriate research ethics committee.[4]

---

4 See footnote to paragraph 3.8.6

- Ensure that all research has an identified sponsor who understands, accepts and is able to discharge their duties as set out in this framework.
- Ensure that written agreements are in place regarding responsibilities for all research involving an external partner, funder and/or sponsor, including agreement with the University or other employer in relation to student supervision.
- Ensure that the necessary links with clinical governance and best value processes are made.
- Ensure that non-NHS employed researchers hold honorary NHS contracts where appropriate and that there is clear accountability and understanding of who is responsible for what.
- Put in place and maintain the necessary systems to identify and learn from errors and failures.
- Put in place and maintain the necessary systems to process, address and learn lessons from complaints arising from any research work being undertaken through or within the organisation.
- Ensure that significant lessons learnt from complaints and from internal enquiries are communicated to funders, sponsors and other partners.
- Permit and assist with any monitoring, auditing or inspection required by relevant authorities.

3.11 Responsibilities of care professionals

3.11.1 Health and social care staff retain responsibility for the care of their patients or users, when they are participating in research.

3.11.2 Before agreeing to their patients or users being approached, they must satisfy themselves that the research has been the subject of approval by appropriate scrutinising authorities within their organisation or agency, and that any research that relates directly to the care they provide complies with this framework.

3.12 Responsibilities relating to research ethics committees

3.12.1 Those establishing research ethics committees should ensure that the committees:
  - have clearly defined remits and terms of reference that are consistent with the system of ethics committees established through the powers of the Secretary of State for Health;
  - have clearly defined arrangements for appointing and replacing members;
  - have and meet clear performance targets;

- are adequately resourced, supported and trained;
- provide clear and independent advice, within their remit and terms of reference.

3.12.2 Research ethics committees and their members must act in good faith and provide impartial and independent advice within their remits and terms of reference. Their primary responsibility is to ensure that the research respects the dignity, rights, safety and well-being of individual research participants. They should also work efficiently to facilitate the good conduct of high quality research that offers benefits to participants, services and society at large. Unjustified delay to such research is itself unethical.

3.12.3 Research within the NHS, which involves individuals, their organs, tissue or data must have the prior approval of an NHS research ethics committee. The NHS is responsible for establishing, supporting and monitoring the performance of NHS research ethics committees (RECs). Those outside the NHS may also seek the advice of these committees.

3.12.4 Whilst operating within a Department of Health and NHS management framework, RECs must maintain independence when formulating their advice on the ethics of the proposed research if their advice is to be seen to be impartial. NHS research ethics committees are managerially independent of NHS Trust R&D structures.

3.12.5 Social care research involving work in NHS settings must be approved by the relevant NHS REC. For other social care research, the Association of Directors of Social Services (ADSS) Research Group advises the ADSS and individual directors and social services departments on the ethics, quality and relevance of proposals for multi-site studies. The Department of Health is discussing with ADSS how arrangements could best be developed to provide a more comprehensive system for the ethical review of social care research. Meanwhile, a number of universities run ethics committees which may be able to advise on social care research studies, and sponsors should take responsibility for ensuring that work is ethical when there is no appropriate committee to review it.

3.12.6 The decision on whether or not research in an NHS organisation should ultimately proceed rests with that organisation. No research should proceed without prior REC approval. However, even though REC approval may have been obtained, an NHS organisation may need to consider other factors before permitting the research to proceed. Similarly, Directors of Social Services are responsible for approving social care research conducted within their local authorities.

3.12.7 It is not the role or responsibility of the research ethics committees described above to give legal advice, nor are they liable for any of their decisions in this respect. Irrespective of the decision of a research ethics committee on a particular application, it is the researcher and the NHS or social care organisation who have the responsibility not to break the law. If a research ethics committee is of the opinion that implementation of a research proposal might contravene the law, it should advise both researcher and the appropriate authority of its concerns. The researcher and the organisation will need then to seek legal advice.

3.12.8 NHS research ethics committees require researchers working in the NHS to keep them informed of the progress of a study. Research ethics committees are responsible for reviewing their advice on the ethical acceptability of a study in the light of such information. However, the principal investigator and his or her employer, the research sponsor and the care organisation, and not the research ethics committee, are responsible for ensuring that a study follows the agreed protocol and for monitoring its progress.

4 Delivery systems

4.1 Organisations undertaking, sponsoring, funding or hosting health and social care research must have systems in place to ensure that they and their staff understand and follow the standards and good practice set out in this frame-work.

4.2 All research sponsors must have systems in place, or have access to systems to undertake expert independent review – appropriate to the scale and complexity of research proposals – to allow the organisation to satisfy itself on the scientific and ethical standing of the work, its strategic relevance and value for money. They must also ensure that systems are in place – managed either by themselves or by one of the organisations involved in the research, such as the host university, a funding body, or care provider – to ensure that all research they sponsor is conducted according to the agreed protocol, to monitor its general progress and to discuss and agree modifications to the protocol if the need arises.

4.3 All health and social care providers must have systems in place to ensure that they are aware of, and have given permission for, all research being conducted in or through their organisation, whether or not it is externally funded. Care providers should only give permission for research which has a sponsor. Care providers may only themselves take on the role of sponsor if they have systems in place to discharge those responsibilities. Whoever acts as sponsor, care providers must satisfy themselves that systems are in place, either in their own organisation or elsewhere, to ensure that all research conducted in or through their organisation conforms to appropriate scientific and ethical standards, and offers value for public money.

4.4 All those establishing research ethics committees must have systems in place to convene, support and monitor the performance of research ethics committees.

4.5 All research ethics committees should have systems in place to identify, and record and address conflicts of interest that may compromise, or be seen to compromise, the independence of their advice. They must also have systems in place to record their decisions and the reasons for them, and to record operational details of their meetings and handling of applications. References to formal guidance on this are in the Annex.

4.6 All delivery systems should be designed to detect failures to adhere to requirements, regardless of whether such failures arise by intent or oversight. Such systems should involve routine and random monitoring and audit as appropriate. Additionally, delivery systems should require, facilitate and support reporting of critical incidents, near misses, systems failures and misconduct either by self-reporting or whistle-blowing.

4.7 The Department of Health will work with key stakeholders to develop and issue guidance from time to time to help organisations discharge their responsibilities for research governance effectively and efficiently. This will cover both systems in individual organisations and systems for agreeing and discharging responsibilities between two or more organisations, e.g. a care provider and a university, or a number of care providers in a multi-centre study. Initial guidance will focus on the most important and challenging areas. Early attention will be given to guidelines on arrangements for studies involving the use of organs, in consultation with the Retained Organs Commission.

4.8 Regional Offices of the Department of Health will work with NHS providers to ensure that they understand their responsibilities, have systems in place to discharge them and take account of relevant guidance. Arrangements for social care will be developed as part of the implementation of the new quality framework outlined in *A Quality Framework for Social Care*.

4.9 Research governance depends critically on research workers and research managers understanding their responsibilities and having the skills needed to discharge them. The Department of Health will work with other research funders and the universities to promote the coverage of research governance in relevant degree courses and continuing education for these groups.

4.10 There is much good practice in research and many opportunities for individuals and organisations to learn from one another. The Department of Health will promote the development of learning networks to support this. The NHS R&D Management Forum is a good example of such a network.

5 Monitoring, inspection and sanctions

5.1 Organisations and individuals must be able to demonstrate adherence to this framework to reassure patients, service users and care professionals of the quality of their services and to assure their reputation in high quality research and care.

5.2 There are already powerful incentives to adhere to many of the principles and standards set out in the framework. These include the law, the duties of care in the NHS and social care and the high professional and ethical standards upheld by the majority of care professionals and researchers. Mechanisms, which monitor the quality of clinical work, such as audit, risk management and staff appraisal can assist in the monitoring of research governance. Nevertheless, a coherent system is needed to monitor performance against this framework, to identify best practice and shortfalls, to enhance public confidence and help to prevent adverse events. Where minimum acceptable standards are not met, sanctions are needed. The Department of Health will work with its partners to develop a coherent system for monitoring research governance and addressing shortcomings.

5.3 New arrangements will be established to work with and through structures, which already exist in health and social care systems, government departments, the universities and the charities to promote and monitor quality. These arrangements will be robust and will monitor the extent to which the standards set out in this framework are being followed by:
- sponsors of research (including the Department of Health);
- health and social care organisations participating in research;
- universities and other organisations employing researchers;

- other organisations on which this framework depends.

5.4 Reports of this monitoring will be presented to the Secretary of State for Health, to the organisations monitored and to those with responsibilities for these organisations. Organisations failing to meet expected standards will be required to produce recovery plans for agreement and implementation.

5.5 Under the new arrangements a list of recognised sponsors of health and social care research will be maintained. Health and social care organisations can consult this list to ascertain the standing of those wishing to fund research in their organisation. Research funders and research organisations may apply to be included in the list, subject to them providing a satisfactory account of the adequacy of their systems.

5.6 Clinical trials of medicinal products on patients must continue to be notified to the Medicines Control Agency (MCA). New regulations to be introduced in compliance with a proposed European Directive on the conduct of clinical trials will require all trials of medicines to be subject to inspection by the MCA. The Agency offers advisory inspections now against relevant good clinical practice and good manufacturing practice guidelines, in advance of the statutory requirement. Similar arrangements apply to medical devices and are the responsibility of the Medical Devices Agency (MDA). The arrangements described above for monitoring research governance will work closely with the MCA and the MDA to avoid duplication and to share best practice.

5.7 The Chief Medical Officer's expert group on learning from adverse events in the NHS reported on ways in which the NHS can learn more effectively from adverse health care events, so that recurrence can be prevented. It has made a number of recommendations, including the establishment of a new national system for reporting adverse health care events and "near misses". Monitoring of research governance will work alongside the new national system for adverse events in the NHS and existing systems for adverse events reporting in social care.

5.8 There is growing public and professional concern about research misconduct and fraud, though its extent is unknown. The Department of Health will continue to work with others on research misconduct, including consideration of the possibility of a co-ordinating group or body to take responsibility for investigation on behalf of all relevant stakeholders. The Director of Counter Fraud Services has overall responsibility for all work to counter fraud and corruption within the NHS.

Monitoring of research governance will check that appropriate systems are in place to detect and investigate possible fraud and to take appropriate action if fraud is found. In addition, health and social care organisations should themselves ensure that universities and any other organisations with whom they develop local partnerships have appropriate systems for detecting, investigating and addressing fraud by their employees.

5.9 Failures in NHS organisations to comply with this framework will be addressed through the normal lines of accountability and performance management. The Department of Health will look to those with responsibilities for other organisations to address any shortcomings in them. Department of Health and NHS funds for health and social care research will only be allocated to those competent to manage them and the work they support.

5.10 Failures on the part of staff in the Department of Health, the NHS or Social Services to meet responsibilities relating to this framework will be addressed through the normal management channels. Monitoring arrangements will check that other organisations have appropriate systems in place to address failures by their staff. University employees with NHS honorary contracts may have these removed, subject to a joint NHS/university investigation. The position of such staff is currently the subject of a review (see paragraph 3.10.3).

5.11 In the case of misconduct, some professional groups will be subject to disciplinary action by their professional bodies. Doctors are responsible to the General Medical Council for their professional conduct as researchers, as well as clinicians. Similarly, nurses, health visitors and midwives are responsible to the United Kingdom Central Council and state registered practitioners are responsible to the individual board of the Council for Professions Supplementary to Medicine for their professional conduct as researchers as well as clinicians. Misconduct by social care professionals will be one of the responsibilities of the General Social Care Council.

30

EU Clinical Directive 2001/20/EC of the European Parliament and of the Council of 4 April 2001 on the approximation of the laws, regulations, and administrative provisions of the Member States relating to the implementation of good clinical practice in the conduct of clinical trials on medicinal products for human use

The European Parliament and the Council of the European Union

Having regard to the Treaty establishing the European Community, and in particular Article 95 thereof,

Having regard to the proposal from the Commission[1],

Having regard to the opinion of the Economic and Social Committee[2],

Acting in accordance with the procedure laid down in Article 251 of the Treaty[3],

Whereas:

(1) Council Directive 65/65/EEC of 26 January 1965 on the approximation of provisions laid down by law, regulation or administrative action relating to medicinal products[4] requires that applications for authorisation to place a medicinal product on the market should be accompanied by a dossier containing particulars and documents relating to the results of tests and clinical trials carried out on the product. Council Directive 75/318/EEC of 20 May 1975 on the approximation of the laws of Member States relating to analytical, pharmacotoxicological and clinical standards and protocols in respect of the testing of medicinal products[5] lays down uniform rules on the compilation of dossiers including their presentation.

(2) The accepted basis for the conduct of clinical trials in humans is founded in the protection of human rights and the dignity of the human being with regard to the application of biology and medicine, as for instance reflected in the 1996 version of the Helsinki Declaration. The clinical trial subject's protection is safeguarded through risk assessment based on the results of toxicological experiments prior to any clinical trial, screening by ethics committees and Member States' competent authorities, and rules on the protection of personal data.

(3) Persons who are incapable of giving legal consent to clinical trials should be given special protection. It is incumbent on the Member States to lay down rules to this effect. Such persons may not be included in clinical trials if the same results can be obtained using persons capable of giving consent. Normally these persons should be included in clinical trials only when there are grounds for expecting that the administering of the medicinal product would be of direct benefit to the patient, thereby outweighing the risks. However, there is a need for clinical trials involving children to improve the treatment available to them. Children represent a vulnerable population with developmental, physiological and psychological differences from adults, which make age- and development-related research important for their benefit. Medicinal products, including vaccines, for children need to be tested scientifically before wide-spread use. This can only be achieved by ensuring that medicinal products which are likely to be of significant clinical value for children are fully studied. The clinical trials required for this purpose should be carried out under conditions affording the best possible protection for the subjects. Criteria for the protection

[1] OJ C 306, 8.10.1997, p. 9 and
OJ C 161, 8.6.1999, p. 5.

[2] OJ C 95, 30.3.1998, p. 1.

[3] Opinion of the European Parliament of 17 November 1998 (OJ C 379, 7.12.1998, p. 27). Council Common Position of 20 July 2000 (OJ C 300, 20.10.2000, p. 32) and Decision of the European Parliament of 12 December 2000. Council Decision of 26 February 2001.

[4] OJ 22, 9.2.1965, p. 1/65. Directive as last amended by Council Directive 93/39/EEC (OJ L 214, 24.8.1993, p. 22).

© Office for Official Publication of the European Communities.

[5] OJ L 147, 9.6.1975, p. 1. Direcctive as last amended by Commission Directive 1999/83/EC (OJ L 243, 15.9.1999, p. 9).

of children in clinical trials therefore need to be laid down.

(4) In the case of other persons incapable of giving their consent, such as persons with dementia, psychiatric patients, etc., inclusion in clinical trials in such cases should be on an even more restrictive basis. Medicinal products for trial may be administered to all such individuals only when there are grounds for assuming that the direct benefit to the patient outweighs the risks. Moreover, in such cases the written consent of the patient's legal representative, given in cooperation with the treating doctor, is necessary before participation in any such clinical trial.

(5) The notion of legal representative refers back to existing national law and consequently may include natural or legal persons, an authority and/or a body provided for by national law.

(6) In order to achieve optimum protection of health, obsolete or repetitive tests will not be carried out, whether within the Community or in third countries. The harmonisation of technical requirements for the development of medicinal products should therefore be pursued through the appropriate fora, in particular the International Conference on Harmonisation.

(7) For medicinal products falling within the scope of Part A of the Annex to Council Regulation (EEC) No 2309/93 of 22 July 1993 laying down Community procedures for the authorisation and supervision of medicinal products for human and veterinary use and establishing a European Agency for the Evaluation of Medicinal Products[1], which include products intended for gene therapy or cell therapy, prior scientific evaluation by the European Agency for the Evaluation of Medicinal Products (hereinafter referred to as the 'Agency'), assisted by the Committee for Proprietary Medicinal Products, is mandatory before the Commission grants marketing authorisation. In the course of this evaluation, the said Committee may request full details of the results of the clinical trials on which the application for marketing authorisation is based and, consequently, on the manner in which these trials were conducted and the same Committee may go so far as to require the applicant for such authorisation to conduct further clinical trials. Provision must therefore be made to allow the Agency to have full information on the conduct of any clinical trial for such medicinal products.

(8) A single opinion for each Member State concerned reduces delay in the commencement of a trial without

---

[1] OJ L 214, 24.8.1993, p. 1. Regulation as amended by Commission Regulation (EC) No 649/98 (OJ L 88, 24.3.1998, p. 7).

jeopardising the well-being of the people participating in the trial or excluding the possibility of rejecting it in specific sites.

(9) Information on the content, commencement and termination of a clinical trial should be available to the Member States where the trial takes place and all the other Member States should have access to the same information. A European database bringing together this information should therefore be set up, with due regard for the rules of confidentiality.

(10) Clinical trials are a complex operation, generally lasting one or more years, usually involving numerous participants and several trial sites, often in different Member States. Member States' current practices diverge considerably on the rules on commencement and conduct of the clinical trials and the requirements for carrying them out vary widely. This therefore results in delays and complications detrimental to effective conduct of such trials in the Community. It is therefore necessary to simplify and harmonise the administrative provisions governing such trials by establishing a clear, transparent procedure and creating conditions conducive to effective coordination of such clinical trials in the Community by the authorities concerned.

(11) As a rule, authorisation should be implicit, i.e. if there has been a vote in favour by the Ethics Committee and the competent authority has not objected within a given period, it should be possible to begin the clinical trials. In exceptional cases raising especially complex problems, explicit written authorisation should, however, be required.

(12) The principles of good manufacturing practice should be applied to investigational medicinal products.

(13) Special provisions should be laid down for the labelling of these products.

(14) Non-commercial clinical trials conducted by researchers without the participation of the pharmaceuticals industry may be of great benefit to the patients concerned. The Directive should therefore take account of the special position of trials whose planning does not require particular manufacturing or packaging processes, if these trials are carried out with medicinal products with a marketing authorisation within the meaning of Directive 65/65/EEC, manufactured or imported in accordance with the provisions of Directives 75/319/EEC and 91/356/EEC, and on patients with the same characteristics as those covered by the indication specified in this marketing authorisation. Labelling of the investigational medicinal products intended for trials of this nature should be subject to simplified

provisions laid down in the good manufacturing practice guidelines on investigational products and in Directive 91/356/EEC.

(15) The verification of compliance with the standards of good clinical practice and the need to subject data, information and documents to inspection in order to confirm that they have been properly generated, recorded and reported are essential in order to justify the involvement of human subjects in clinical trials.

(16) The person participating in a trial must consent to the scrutiny of personal information during inspection by competent authorities and properly authorised persons, provided that such personal information is treated as strictly confidential and is not made publicly available.

(17) This Directive is to apply without prejudice to Directive 95/46/EEC of the European Parliament and of the Council of 24 October 1995 on the protection of individuals with regard to the processing of personal data and on the free movement of such data[1].

(18) It is also necessary to make provision for the monitoring of adverse reactions occurring in clinical trials using Community surveillance (pharmacovigilance) procedures in order to ensure the immediate cessation of any clinical trial in which there is an unacceptable level of risk.

(19) The measures necessary for the implementation of this Directive should be adopted in accordance with Council Decision 1999/468/EC of 28 June 1999 laying down the procedures for the exercise of implementing powers conferred on the Commission[2];

Have adopted this directive:

ARTICLE 1

Scope

1 This Directive establishes specific provisions regarding the conduct of clinical trials, including multi-centre trials, on human subjects involving medicinal products as defined in Article 1 of Directive 65/65/EEC, in particular relating to the implementation of good clinical practice. This Directive does not apply to non-interventional trials.

2 Good clinical practice is a set of internationally recognised ethical and scientific quality requirements which must be observed for designing, conducting, recording and reporting clinical trials that involve the participation

of human subjects. Compliance with this good practice provides assurance that the rights, safety and well-being of trial subjects are protected, and that the results of the clinical trials are credible.

3 The principles of good clinical practice and detailed guidelines in line with those principles shall be adopted and, if necessary, revised to take account of technical and scientific progress in accordance with the procedure referred to in Article 21(2).

These detailed guidelines shall be published by the Commission.

4 All clinical trials, including bioavailability and bioequivalence studies, shall be designed, conducted and reported in accordance with the principles of good clinical practice.

ARTICLE 2

Definitions

For the purposes of this Directive the following definitions shall apply:

(a) 'clinical trial': any investigation in human subjects intended to discover or verify the clinical, pharmacological and/or other pharmacodynamic effects of one or more investigational medicinal product(s), and/or to identify any adverse reactions to one or more investigational medicinal product(s) and/or to study absorption, distribution, metabolism and excretion of one or more investigational medicinal product(s) with the object of ascertaining its (their) safety and/or efficacy;

This includes clinical trials carried out in either one site or multiple sites, whether in one or more than one Member State;

(b) 'multi-centre clinical trial': a clinical trial conducted according to a single protocol but at more than one site, and therefore by more than one investigator, in which the trial sites may be located in a single Member State, in a number of Member States and/or in Member States and third countries;

(c) 'non-interventional trial': a study where the medicinal product(s) is (are) prescribed in the usual manner in accordance with the terms of the marketing authorisation. The assignment of the patient to a particular therapeutic strategy is not decided in advance by a trial protocol but falls within current practice and the prescription of the medicine is clearly separated from the decision to include the patient in the study. No additional diagnostic or monitoring procedures shall be applied to the patients and epidemiological methods shall be used for the analysis of collected data;

---

[1] OJ L 281, 23.11.1995, p. 31.
[2] OJ L 184, 17.7.1999, p. 23.

(d) 'investigational medicinal product': a pharmaceutical form of an active substance or placebo being tested or used as a reference in a clinical trial, including products already with a marketing authorisation but used or assembled (formulated or packaged) in a way different from the authorised form, or when used for an unauthorised indication, or when used to gain further information about the authorised form;

(e) 'sponsor': an individual, company, institution or organisation which takes responsibility for the initiation, management and/or financing of a clinical trial;

(f) 'investigator': a doctor or a person following a profession agreed in the Member State for investigations because of the scientific background and the experience in patient care it requires. The investigator is responsible for the conduct of a clinical trial at a trial site. If a trial is conducted by a team of individuals at a trial site, the investigator is the leader responsible for the team and may be called the principal investigator;

(g) 'investigator's brochure': a compilation of the clinical and non-clinical data on the investigational medicinal product or products which are relevant to the study of the product or products in human subjects;

(h) 'protocol': a document that describes the objective(s), design, methodology, statistical considerations and organisation of a trial. The term protocol refers to the protocol, successive versions of the protocol and protocol amendments;

(i) 'subject': an individual who participates in a clinical trial as either a recipient of the investigational medicinal product or a control;

(j) 'informed consent': decision, which must be written, dated and signed, to take part in a clinical trial, taken freely after being duly informed of its nature, significance, implications and risks and appropriately documented, by any person capable of giving consent or, where the person is not capable of giving consent, by his or her legal representative; if the person concerned is unable to write, oral consent in the presence of at least one witness may be given in exceptional cases, as provided for in national legislation.

(k) 'ethics committee': an independent body in a Member State, consisting of healthcare professionals and non-medical members, whose responsibility it is to protect the rights, safety and wellbeing of human subjects involved in a trial and to provide public assurance of that protection, by, among other things, expressing an opinion on the trial protocol, the suitability of the investigators and the adequacy of facilities, and on the methods and documents to be used to inform trial subjects and obtain their informed consent;

(l) 'inspection': the act by a competent authority of conducting an official review of documents, facilities, records, quality assurance arrangements, and any other resources that are deemed by the competent authority to be related to the clinical trial and that may be located at the site of the trial, at the sponsor's and/or contract research organisations facilities, or at other establishments which the competent authority sees fit to inspect;

(m) 'adverse event': any untoward medical occurrence in a patient or clinical trial subject administered a medicinal product and which does not necessarily have a causal relationship with this treatment;

(n) 'adverse reaction': all untoward and unintended responses to an investigational medicinal product related to any dose administered;

(o) 'serious adverse event or serious adverse reaction': any untoward medical occurrence or effect that at any dose results in death, is life-threatening, requires hospitalisation or prolongation of existing hospitalisation, results in persistent or significant disability or incapacity, or is a congenital anomaly or birth defect;

(p) 'unexpected adverse reaction': an adverse reaction, the nature or severity of which is not consistent with the applicable product information (e.g. investigator's brochure for an unauthorised investigational product or summary of product characteristics for an authorised product).

ARTICLE 3

Protection of clinical trial subjects

1 This Directive shall apply without prejudice to the national provisions on the protection of clinical trial subjects if they are more comprehensive than the provisions of this Directive and consistent with the procedures and time-scales specified therein. Member States shall, insofar as they have not already done so, adopt detailed rules to protect from abuse individuals who are incapable of giving their informed consent.

2 A clinical trial may be undertaken only if, in particular:

(a) the foreseeable risks and inconveniences have been weighed against the anticipated benefit for the individual trial subject and other present and future patients. A clinical trial may be initiated only if the Ethics Committee and/or the competent authority comes to the conclusion that the anticipated therapeutic and public health benefits justify the risks and may be continued only if compliance with this requirement is permanently monitored;

(b) the trial subject or, when the person is not able to give informed consent, his legal representative has had the opportunity, in a prior interview with the investigator or a member of the investigating team, to understand the objectives, risks and inconveniences of the trial, and the conditions under which it is to be conducted and has also been informed of his right to withdraw from the trial at any time;

(c) the rights of the subject to physical and mental integrity, to privacy and to the protection of the data concerning him in accordance with Directive 95/46/EC are safeguarded;

(d) the trial subject or, when the person is not able to give informed consent, his legal representative has given his written consent after being informed of the nature, significance, implications and risks of the clinical trial; if the individual is unable to write, oral consent in the presence of at least one witness may be given in exceptional cases, as provided for in national legislation;

(e) the subject may without any resulting detriment withdraw from the clinical trial at any time by revoking his informed consent;

(f) provision has been made for insurance or indemnity to cover the liability of the investigator and sponsor.

3 The medical care given to, and medical decisions made on behalf of, subjects shall be the responsibility of an appropriately qualified doctor or, where appropriate, of a qualified dentist.

4 The subject shall be provided with a contact point where he may obtain further information.

ARTICLE 4

Clinical trials on minors

In addition to any other relevant restriction, a clinical trial on minors may be undertaken only if:

(a) the informed consent of the parents or legal representative has been obtained; consent must represent the minor's presumed will and may be revoked at any time, without detriment to the minor;

(b) the minor has received information according to its capacity of understanding, from staff with experience with minors, regarding the trial, the risks and the benefits;

(c) the explicit wish of a minor who is capable of forming an opinion and assessing this information to refuse participation or to be withdrawn from the clinical trial

at any time is considered by the investigator or where appropriate the principal investigator;

(d) no incentives or financial inducements are given except compensation;

(e) some direct benefit for the group of patients is obtained from the clinical trial and only where such research is essential to validate data obtained in clinical trials on persons able to give informed consent or by other research methods; additionally, such research should either relate directly to a clinical condition from which the minor concerned suffers or be of such a nature that it can only be carried out on minors;

(f) the corresponding scientific guidelines of the Agency have been followed;

(g) clinical trials have been designed to minimise pain, discomfort, fear and any other foreseeable risk in relation to the disease and developmental stage; both the risk threshold and the degree of distress have to be specially defined and constantly monitored;

(h) the Ethics Committee, with paediatric expertise or after taking advice in clinical, ethical and psychosocial problems in the field of paediatrics, has endorsed the protocol; and

(i) the interests of the patient always prevail over those of science and society.

ARTICLE 5

Clinical trials on incapacitated adults not able to give informed legal consent

In the case of other persons incapable of giving informed legal consent, all relevant requirements listed for persons capable of giving such consent shall apply. In addition to these requirements, inclusion in clinical trials of incapacitated adults who have not given or not refused informed consent before the onset of their incapacity shall be allowed only if:

(a) the informed consent of the legal representative has been obtained; consent must represent the subject's presumed will and may be revoked at any time, without detriment to the subject;

(b) the person not able to give informed legal consent has received information according to his/her capacity of understanding regarding the trial, the risks and the benefits;

(c) the explicit wish of a subject who is capable of forming an opinion and assessing this information to refuse participation in, or to be withdrawn from, the clinical trial at any time is considered by the investigator or where appropriate the principal investigator;

(d) no incentives or financial inducements are given except compensation;

(e) such research is essential to validate data obtained in clinical trials on persons able to give informed consent or by other research methods and relates directly to a life-threatening or debilitating clinical condition from which the incapacitated adult concerned suffers;

(f) clinical trials have been designed to minimise pain, discomfort, fear and any other foreseeable risk in relation to the disease and developmental stage; both the risk threshold and the degree of distress shall be specially defined and constantly monitored;

(g) the Ethics Committee, with expertise in the relevant disease and the patient population concerned or after taking advice in clinical, ethical and psychosocial questions in the field of the relevant disease and patient population concerned, has endorsed the protocol;

(h) the interests of the patient always prevail over those of science and society; and

(i) there are grounds for expecting that administering the medicinal product to be tested will produce a benefit to the patient outweighing the risks or produce no risk at all.

ARTICLE 6

Ethics Committee

1 For the purposes of implementation of the clinical trials, Member States shall take the measures necessary for establishment and operation of Ethics Committees.

2 The Ethics Committee shall give its opinion, before a clinical trial commences, on any issue requested.

3 In preparing its opinion, the Ethics Committee shall consider, in particular:

(a) the relevance of the clinical trial and the trial design;

(b) whether the evaluation of the anticipated benefits and risks as required under Article 3(2)(a) is satisfactory and whether the conclusions are justified;

(c) the protocol;

(d) the suitability of the investigator and supporting staff;

(e) the investigator's brochure;

(f) the quality of the facilities;

(g) the adequacy and completeness of the written information to be given and the procedure to be followed for the purpose of obtaining informed consent and the justification for the research on persons incapable of giving informed consent as regards the specific restrictions laid down in Article 3;

(h) provision for indemnity or compensation in the event of injury or death attributable to a clinical trial;

(i) any insurance or indemnity to cover the liability of the investigator and sponsor;

(j) the amounts and, where appropriate, the arrangements for rewarding or compensating investigators and trial subjects and the relevant aspects of any agreement between the sponsor and the site;

(k) the arrangements for the recruitment of subjects.

4 Notwithstanding the provisions of this Article, a Member State may decide that the competent authority it has designated for the purpose of Article 9 shall be responsible for the consideration of, and the giving of an opinion on, the matters referred to in paragraph 3(h), (i) and (j) of this Article.

When a Member State avails itself of this provision, it shall notify the Commission, the other Member States and the Agency.

5 The Ethics Committee shall have a maximum of 60 days from the date of receipt of a valid application to give its reasoned opinion to the applicant and the competent authority in the Member State concerned.

6 Within the period of examination of the application for an opinion, the Ethics Committee may send a single request for information supplementary to that already supplied by the applicant. The period laid down in paragraph 5 shall be suspended until receipt of the supplementary information.

7 No extension to the 60-day period referred to in paragraph 5 shall be permissible except in the case of trials involving medicinal products for gene therapy or somatic cell therapy or medicinal products containing genetically modified organisms. In this case, an extension of a maximum of 30 days shall be permitted. For these products, this 90-day period may be extended by a further 90 days in the event of consultation of a group or a committee in accordance with the regulations and procedures of the Member States concerned. In the case of xenogenic cell therapy, there shall be no time limit to the authorisation period.

ARTICLE 7

Single opinion

For multi-centre clinical trials limited to the territory of a single Member State, Member States shall establish a procedure providing, notwithstanding the number of Ethics Committees, for the adoption of a single opinion for that Member State.

In the case of multi-centre clinical trials carried out in more than one Member State simultaneously, a single opinion shall be given for each Member State concerned by the clinical trial.

ARTICLE 8

Detailed guidance

The Commission, in consultation with Member States and interested parties, shall draw up and publish detailed guidance on the application format and documentation to be submitted in an application for an ethics committee opinion, in particular regarding the information that is given to subjects, and on the appropriate safeguards for the protection of personal data.

ARTICLE 9

Commencement of a clinical trial

1 Member States shall take the measures necessary to ensure that the procedure described in this Article is followed for commencement of a clinical trial.

   The sponsor may not start a clinical trial until the Ethics Committee has issued a favourable opinion and inasmuch as the competent authority of the Member State concerned has not informed the sponsor of any grounds for non-acceptance. The procedures to reach these decisions can be run in parallel or not, depending on the sponsor.

2 Before commencing any clinical trial, the sponsor shall be required to submit a valid request for authorisation to the competent authority of the Member State in which the sponsor plans to conduct the clinical trial.

3 If the competent authority of the Member State notifies the sponsor of grounds for non-acceptance, the sponsor may, on one occasion only, amend the content of the request referred to in paragraph 2 in order to take due account of the grounds given. If the sponsor fails to amend the request accordingly, the request shall be considered rejected and the clinical trial may not commence.

4 Consideration of a valid request for authorisation by the competent authority as stated in paragraph 2 shall be carried out as rapidly as possible and may not exceed 60 days. The Member States may lay down a shorter period than 60 days within their area of responsibility if that is in compliance with current practice. The competent authority can nevertheless notify the sponsor before the end of this period that it has no grounds for non-acceptance.

   No further extensions to the period referred to in the first subparagraph shall be permissible except in the case of trials involving the medicinal products listed in paragraph 6, for which an extension of a maximum of 30 days shall be permitted. For these products, this 90-day period may be extended by a further 90 days in the event of consultation of a group or a committee in accordance with the regulations and procedures of the Member States concerned. In the case of xenogenic cell therapy there shall be no time limit to the authorisation period.

5 Without prejudice to paragraph 6, written authorisation may be required before the commencement of clinical trials for such trials on medicinal products which do not have a marketing authorisation within the meaning of Directive 65/65/EEC and are referred to in Part A of the Annex to Regulation (EEC) No 2309/93, and other medicinal products with special characteristics, such as medicinal products the active ingredient or active ingredients of which is or are a biological product or biological products of human or animal origin, or contains biological components of human or animal origin, or the manufacturing of which requires such components.

6 Written authorisation shall be required before commencing clinical trials involving medicinal products for gene therapy, somatic cell therapy including xenogenic cell therapy and all medicinal products containing genetically modified organisms. No gene therapy trials may be carried out which result in modifications to the subject's germ line genetic identity.

7 This authorisation shall be issued without prejudice to the application of Council Directives 90/219/EEC of 23 April 1990 on the contained use of genetically modified micro-organisms[1] and 90/220/EEC of 23 April 1990 on the deliberate release into the environment of genetically modified organisms[2].

8 In consultation with Member States, the Commission shall draw up and publish detailed guidance on:

   (a) the format and contents of the request referred to in paragraph 2 as well as the documentation to be submitted to support that request, on the quality and manufacture of the investigational medicinal product, any toxicological and pharmacological tests, the protocol and clinical information on the investigational medicinal product including the investigator's brochure;

   (b) the presentation and content of the proposed amendment referred to in point (a) of Article 10 on substantial amendments made to the protocol;

   (c) the declaration of the end of the clinical trial.

[1] OJ L 117, 8.5.1990, p. 1. Directive as last amended by Directive 98/81/EC (OJ L 330, 5.12.1998, p. 13).

[2] OJ L 117, 8.5.1990, p. 15. Directive as last amended by Commission Directive 97/35/EC (OJ L 169, 27.6.1997, p. 72).

ARTICLE 10

Conduct of a clinical trial

Amendments may be made to the conduct of a clinical trial following the procedure described hereinafter:

(a) after the commencement of the clinical trial, the sponsor may make amendments to the protocol. If those amendments are substantial and are likely to have an impact on the safety of the trial subjects or to change the interpretation of the scientific documents in support of the conduct of the trial, or if they are otherwise significant, the sponsor shall notify the competent authorities of the Member State or Member States concerned of the reasons for, and content of, these amendments and shall inform the ethics committee or committees concerned in accordance with Articles 6 and 9.

On the basis of the details referred to in Article 6(3) and in accordance with Article 7, the Ethics Committee shall give an opinion within a maximum of 35 days of the date of receipt of the proposed amendment in good and due form. If this opinion is unfavourable, the sponsor may not implement the amendment to the protocol.

If the opinion of the Ethics Committee is favourable and the competent authorities of the Member States have raised no grounds for non-acceptance of the above-mentioned substantial amendments, the sponsor shall proceed to conduct the clinical trial following the amended protocol. Should this not be the case, the sponsor shall either take account of the grounds for non-acceptance and adapt the proposed amendment to the protocol accordingly or withdraw the proposed amendment;

(b) without prejudice to point (a), in the light of the circumstances, notably the occurrence of any new event relating to the conduct of the trial or the development of the investigational medicinal product where that new event is likely to affect the safety of the subjects, the sponsor and the investigator shall take appropriate urgent safety measures to protect the subjects against any immediate hazard. The sponsor shall forthwith inform the competent authorities of those new events and the measures taken and shall ensure that the Ethics Committee is notified at the same time;

(c) within 90 days of the end of a clinical trial the sponsor shall notify the competent authorities of the Member State or Member States concerned and the Ethics Committee that the clinical trial has ended. If the trial has to be terminated early, this period shall be reduced to 15 days and the reasons clearly explained.

ARTICLE 11

Exchange of information

1 Member States in whose territory the clinical trial takes place shall enter in a European database, accessible only to the competent authorities of the Member States, the Agency and the Commission:

(a) extracts from the request for authorisation referred to in Article 9(2);

(b) any amendments made to the request, as provided for in Article 9(3);

(c) any amendments made to the protocol, as provided for in point (a) of Article 10;

(d) the favourable opinion of the Ethics Committee;

(e) the declaration of the end of the clinical trial; and

(f) a reference to the inspections carried out on conformity with good clinical practice.

2 At the substantiated request of any Member State, the Agency or the Commission, the competent authority to which the request for authorisation was submitted shall supply all further information concerning the clinical trial in question other than the data already in the European database.

3 In consultation with the Member States, the Commission shall draw up and publish detailed guidance on the relevant data to be included in this European database, which it operates with the assistance of the Agency, as well as the methods for electronic communication of the data. The detailed guidance thus drawn up shall ensure that the confidentiality of the data is strictly observed.

ARTICLE 12

Suspension of the trial or infringements

1 Where a Member State has objective grounds for considering that the conditions in the request for authorisation referred to in Article 9(2) are no longer met or has information raising doubts about the safety or scientific validity of the clinical trial, it may suspend or prohibit the clinical trial and shall notify the sponsor thereof.

Before the Member State reaches its decision it shall, except where there is imminent risk, ask the sponsor and/or the investigator for their opinion, to be delivered within one week.

In this case, the competent authority concerned shall forthwith inform the other competent authorities, the Ethics Committee concerned, the Agency and the Commission of its decision to suspend or prohibit the trial and of the reasons for the decision.

2 Where a competent authority has objective grounds for considering that the sponsor or the investigator or any other person involved in the conduct of the trial no longer meets the obligations laid down, it shall forthwith inform him thereof, indicating the course of action which he must take to remedy this state of affairs. The competent authority concerned shall forthwith inform the Ethics Committee, the other competent authorities and the Commission of this course of action.

ARTICLE 13

Manufacture and import of investigational medicinal products

1 Member States shall take all appropriate measures to ensure that the manufacture or importation of investigational medicinal products is subject to the holding of authorisation. In order to obtain the authorisation, the applicant and, subsequently, the holder of the authorisation, shall meet at least the requirements defined in accordance with the procedure referred to in Article 21(2).

2 Member States shall take all appropriate measures to ensure that the holder of the authorisation referred to in paragraph 1 has permanently and continuously at his disposal the services of at least one qualified person who, in accordance with the conditions laid down in Article 23 of the second Council Directive 75/319/EEC of 20 May 1975 on the approximation of provisions laid down by law, regulation or administrative action relating to proprietary medicinal products[1], is responsible in particular for carrying out the duties specified in paragraph 3 of this Article.

3 Member States shall take all appropriate measures to ensure that the qualified person referred to in Article 21 of Directive 75/319/EEC, without prejudice to his relationship with the manufacturer or importer, is responsible, in the context of the procedures referred to in Article 25 of the said Directive, for ensuring:

(a) in the case of investigational medicinal products manufactured in the Member State concerned, that each batch of medicinal products has been manufactured and checked in compliance with the requirements of Commission Directive 91/356/EEC of 13 June 1991 laying down the principles and guidelines of good manufacturing practice for medicinal products for human use[2], the product specification file and the information notified pursuant to Article 9(2) of this Directive;

(b) in the case of investigational medicinal products manufactured in a third country, that each production batch has been manufactured and checked in accordance with standards of good manufacturing practice at least equivalent to those laid down in Commission Directive 91/356/EEC, in accordance with the product specification file, and that each production batch has been checked in accordance with the information notified pursuant to Article 9(2) of this Directive;

(c) in the case of an investigational medicinal product which is a comparator product from a third country, and which has a marketing authorisation, where the documentation certifying that each production batch has been manufactured in conditions at least equivalent to the standards of good manufacturing practice referred to above cannot be obtained, that each production batch has undergone all relevant analyses, tests or checks necessary to confirm its quality in accordance with the information notified pursuant to Article 9(2) of this Directive.

Detailed guidance on the elements to be taken into account when evaluating products with the object of releasing batches within the Community shall be drawn up pursuant to the good manufacturing practice guidelines, and in particular Annex 13 to the said guidelines. Such guidelines will be adopted in accordance with the procedure referred to in Article 21(2) of this Directive and published in accordance with Article 19a of Directive 75/319/EEC.

Insofar as the provisions laid down in (a), (b) or (c) are complied with, investigational medicinal products shall not have to undergo any further checks if they are imported into another Member State together with batch release certification signed by the qualified person.

4 In all cases, the qualified person must certify in a register or equivalent document that each production batch satisfies the provisions of this Article. The said register or equivalent document shall be kept up to date as operations are carried out and shall remain at the disposal of the agents of the competent authority for the period specified in the provisions of the Member States concerned. This period shall in any event be not less than five years.

[1] OJ L 147, 9.6.1975, p. 13. Directive as last amended by Council Directive 93/39/EC (OJ L 214, 24.8.1993, p. 22).

[2] OJ L 193, 17.7.1991, p. 30.

5 Any person engaging in activities as the qualified person referred to in Article 21 of Directive 75/319/EEC as regards investigational medicinal products at the time when this Directive is applied in the Member State where that person is, but without complying with the conditions laid down in Articles 23 and 24 of that Directive, shall be authorised to continue those activities in the Member State concerned.

ARTICLE 14

Labelling

The particulars to appear in at least the official language(s) of the Member State on the outer packaging of investigational medicinal products or, where there is no outer packaging, on the immediate packaging, shall be published by the Commission in the good manufacturing practice guidelines on investigational medicinal products adopted in accordance with Article 19a of Directive 75/319/EEC.

In addition, these guidelines shall lay down adapted provisions relating to labelling for investigational medicinal products intended for clinical trials with the following characteristics:

- the planning of the trial does not require particular manufacturing or packaging processes;
- the trial is conducted with medicinal products with, in the Member States concerned by the study, a marketing authorisation within the meaning of Directive 65/65/EEC, manufactured or imported in accordance with the provisions of Directive 75/319/EEC;
- the patients participating in the trial have the same characteristics as those covered by the indication specified in the abovementioned authorisation.

ARTICLE 15

Verification of compliance of investigational medicinal products with good clinical and manufacturing practice

1 To verify compliance with the provisions on good clinical and manufacturing practice, Member States shall appoint inspectors to inspect the sites concerned by any clinical trial conducted, particularly the trial site or sites, the manufacturing site of the investigational medicinal product, any laboratory used for analyses in the clinical trial and/or the sponsor's premises.

The inspections shall be conducted by the competent authority of the Member State concerned, which shall inform the Agency; they shall be carried out on behalf of the Community and the results shall be recognised by all the other Member States. These inspections shall be coordinated by the Agency, within the framework of its powers as provided for in Regulation (EEC) No 2309/93. A Member State may request assistance from another Member State in this matter.

2 Following inspection, an inspection report shall be prepared. It must be made available to the sponsor while safeguarding confidential aspects. It may be made available to the other Member States, to the Ethics Committee and to the Agency, at their reasoned request.

3 At the request of the Agency, within the framework of its powers as provided for in Regulation (EEC) No 2309/93, or of one of the Member States concerned, and following consultation with the Member States concerned, the Commission may request a new inspection should verification of compliance with this Directive reveal differences between Member States.

4 Subject to any arrangements which may have been concluded between the Community and third countries, the Commission, upon receipt of a reasoned request from a Member State or on its own initiative, or a Member State may propose that the trial site and/or the sponsor's premises and/or the manufacturer established in a third country undergo an inspection. The inspection shall be carried out by duly qualified Community inspectors.

5 The detailed guidelines on the documentation relating to the clinical trial, which shall constitute the master file on the trial, archiving, qualifications of inspectors and inspection procedures to verify compliance of the clinical trial in question with this Directive shall be adopted and revised in accordance with the procedure referred to in Article 21(2).

ARTICLE 16

Notification of adverse events

1 The investigator shall report all serious adverse events immediately to the sponsor except for those that the protocol or investigator's brochure identifies as not requiring immediate reporting. The immediate report shall be followed by detailed, written reports. The immediate and follow-up reports shall identify subjects by unique code numbers assigned to the latter.

2 Adverse events and/or laboratory abnormalities identified in the protocol as critical to safety evaluations shall be reported to the sponsor according to the reporting requirements and within the time periods specified in the protocol.

3 For reported deaths of a subject, the investigator shall supply the sponsor and the Ethics Committee with any additional information requested.

4 The sponsor shall keep detailed records of all adverse events which are reported to him by the investigator or investigators. These records shall be submitted to the Member States in whose territory the clinical trial is being conducted, if they so request.

ARTICLE 17

Notification of serious adverse reactions

1(a) The sponsor shall ensure that all relevant information about suspected serious unexpected adverse reactions that are fatal or life-threatening is recorded and reported as soon as possible to the competent authorities in all the Member States concerned, and to the Ethics Committee, and in any case no later than seven days after knowledge by the sponsor of such a case, and that relevant follow-up information is subsequently communicated within an additional eight days.

(b) All other suspected serious unexpected adverse reactions shall be reported to the competent authorities concerned and to the Ethics Committee concerned as soon as possible but within a maximum of fifteen days of first knowledge by the sponsor.

(c) Each Member State shall ensure that all suspected unexpected serious adverse reactions to an investigational medicinal product which are brought to its attention are recorded.

(d) The sponsor shall also inform all investigators.

2 Once a year throughout the clinical trial, the sponsor shall provide the Member States in whose territory the clinical trial is being conducted and the Ethics Committee with a listing of all suspected serious adverse reactions which have occurred over this period and a report of the subjects' safety.

3(a) Each Member State shall see to it that all suspected unexpected serious adverse reactions to an investigational medicinal product which are brought to its attention are immediately entered in a European database to which, in accordance with Article 11(1), only the competent authorities of the Member States, the Agency and the Commission shall have access.

(b) The Agency shall make the information notified by the sponsor available to the competent authorities of the Member States.

ARTICLE 18

Guidance concerning reports

The Commission, in consultation with the Agency, Member States and interested parties, shall draw up and publish detailed guidance on the collection, verification and presentation of adverse event/reaction reports, together with decoding procedures for unexpected serious adverse reactions.

ARTICLE 19

General provisions

This Directive is without prejudice to the civil and criminal liability of the sponsor or the investigator. To this end, the sponsor or a legal representative of the sponsor must be established in the Community.

Unless Member States have established precise conditions for exceptional circumstances, investigational medicinal products and, as the case may be, the devices used for their administration shall be made available free of charge by the sponsor.

The Member States shall inform the Commission of such conditions.

ARTICLE 20

Adaptation to scientific and technical progress

This Directive shall be adapted to take account of scientific and technical progress in accordance with the procedure referred to in Article 21(2).

ARTICLE 21

Committee procedure

1 The Commission shall be assisted by the Standing Committee on Medicinal Products for Human Use, set up by Article 2b of Directive 75/318/EEC (hereinafter referred to as the Committee).

2 Where reference is made to this paragraph, Articles 5 and 7 of Decision 1999/468/EC shall apply, having regard to the provisions of Article 8 thereof.

The period referred to in Article 5(6) of Decision 1999/468/EC shall be set at three months.

3 The Committee shall adopt its rules of procedure.

ARTICLE 22

Application

1 Member States shall adopt and publish before 1 May 2003 the laws, regulations and administrative provisions necessary to comply with this Directive. They shall forthwith inform the Commission thereof.

   They shall apply these provisions at the latest with effect from 1 May 2004.

   When Member States adopt these provisions, they shall contain a reference to this Directive or shall be accompanied by such reference on the occasion of their official publication. The methods of making such reference shall be laid down by Member States.

2 Member States shall communicate to the Commission the text of the provisions of national law which they adopt in the field governed by this Directive.

ARTICLE 23

Entry into force

This Directive shall enter into force on the day of its publication in the Official Journal of the European Communities.

ARTICLE 24

Addressees

This Directive is addressed to the Member States.
Done at Luxembourg, 4 April 2001.

For the European Parliament	*For the Council*
The President	*The President*
N. Fontaine	**B. Rosengren**

31

European convention on human rights and biomedicine (ETS 164) and additional protocol on the prohibition of cloning human beings

Council of Europe

Oviedo, 4.IV.1997

Preamble

The member States of the Council of Europe, the other States and the European Community, signatories hereto,

Bearing in mind the Universal Declaration of Human Rights proclaimed by the General Assembly of the United Nations on 10 December 1948;

Bearing in mind the Convention for the Protection of Human Rights and Fundamental Freedoms of 4 November 1950;

Bearing in mind the European Social Charter of 18 October 1961;

Bearing in mind the International Covenant on Civil and Political Rights and the International Covenant on Economic, Social and Cultural Rights of 16 December 1966;

Bearing in mind the Convention for the Protection of Individuals with regard to Automatic Processing of Personal Data of 28 January 1981;

Bearing also in mind the Convention on the Rights of the Child of 20 November 1989;

Considering that the aim of the Council of Europe is the achievement of a greater unity between its members and that one of the methods by which that aim is to be pursued is the maintenance and further realisation of human rights and fundamental freedoms;

Conscious of the accelerating developments in biology and medicine;

Convinced of the need to respect the human being both as an individual and as a member of the human species and recognising the importance of ensuring the dignity of the human being;

Conscious that the misuse of biology and medicine may lead to acts endangering human dignity;

Affirming that progress in biology and medicine should be used for the benefit of present and future generations;

Stressing the need for international co-operation so that all humanity may enjoy the benefits of biology and medicine;

Recognising the importance of promoting a public debate on the questions posed by the application of biology and medicine and the responses to be given thereto;

Wishing to remind all members of society of their rights and responsibilities;

Taking account of the work of the Parliamentary Assembly in this field, including Recommendation 1160 (1991) on the preparation of a convention on bioethics;

Resolving to take such measures as are necessary to safeguard human dignity and the fundamental rights and freedoms of the individual with regard to the application of biology and medicine,

Have agreed as follows:

Chapter I General provisions

Article 1 Purpose and object

Parties to this Convention shall protect the dignity and identity of all human beings and guarantee everyone, without discrimination, respect for their integrity and other rights and fundamental freedoms with regard to the application of biology and medicine.

Chapter 5 on scientific research has been expanded. The final version may appear at the end of 2002. See the website for more information: www.coe.int

© Council of Europe.

Each Party shall take in its internal law the necessary measures to give effect to the provisions of this Convention.

Article 2 Primacy of the human being

The interests and welfare of the human being shall prevail over the sole interest of society or science.

Article 3 Equitable access to health care

Parties, taking into account health needs and available resources, shall take appropriate measures with a view to providing, within their jurisdiction, equitable access to health care of appropriate quality.

Article 4 Professional standards

Any intervention in the health field, including research, must be carried out in accordance with relevant professional obligations and standards.

Chapter II Consent

Article 5 General rule

An intervention in the health field may only be carried out after the person concerned has given free and informed consent to it.

This person shall beforehand be given appropriate information as to the purpose and nature of the intervention as well as on its consequences and risks.

The person concerned may freely withdraw consent at any time.

Article 6 Protection of persons not able to consent

1 Subject to Articles 17 and 20 below, an intervention may only be carried out on a person who does not have the capacity to consent, for his or her direct benefit.
2 Where, according to law, a minor does not have the capacity to consent to an intervention, the intervention may only be carried out with the authorisation of his or her representative or an authority or a person or body provided for by law.

   The opinion of the minor shall be taken into consideration as an increasingly determining factor in proportion to his or her age and degree of maturity.
3 Where, according to law, an adult does not have the capacity to consent to an intervention because of a mental disability, a disease or for similar reasons, the intervention may only be carried out with the authorisation of his or her representative or an authority or a person or body provided for by law.

   The individual concerned shall as far as possible take part in the authorisation procedure.
4 The representative, the authority, the person or the body mentioned in paragraphs 2 and 3 above shall be given, under the same conditions, the information referred to in Article 5.
5 The authorisation referred to in paragraphs 2 and 3 above may be withdrawn at any time in the best interests of the person concerned.

Article 7 Protection of persons who have a mental disorder

Subject to protective conditions prescribed by law, including supervisory, control and appeal procedures, a person who has a mental disorder of a serious nature may be subjected, without his or her consent, to an intervention aimed at treating his or her mental disorder only where, without such treatment, serious harm is likely to result to his or her health.

Article 8 Emergency situation

When because of an emergency situation the appropriate consent cannot be obtained, any medically necessary intervention may be carried out immediately for the benefit of the health of the individual concerned.

Article 9 Previously expressed wishes

The previously expressed wishes relating to a medical intervention by a patient who is not, at the time of the intervention, in a state to express his or her wishes shall be taken into account.

Chapter III Private life and right to information

Article 10 Private life and right to information

1 Everyone has the right to respect for private life in relation to information about his or her health.
2 Everyone is entitled to know any information collected about his or her health. However, the wishes of individuals not to be so informed shall be observed.
3 In exceptional cases, restrictions may be placed by law on the exercise of the rights contained in paragraph 2 in the interests of the patient.

Chapter IV Human genome

Article 11 Non-discrimination

Any form of discrimination against a person on grounds of his or her genetic heritage is prohibited.

Article 12 Predictive genetic tests

Tests which are predictive of genetic diseases or which serve either to identify the subject as a carrier of a gene responsible for a disease or to detect a genetic predisposition or susceptibility to a disease may be performed only for health purposes or for scientific research linked to health purposes, and subject to appropriate genetic counselling.

Article 13 Interventions on the human genome

An intervention seeking to modify the human genome may only be undertaken for preventive, diagnostic or therapeutic purposes and only if its aim is not to introduce any modification in the genome of any descendants.

Article 14 Non-selection of sex

The use of techniques of medically assisted procreation shall not be allowed for the purpose of choosing a future child's sex, except where serious hereditary sex-related disease is to be avoided.

Chapter V Scientific research

Article 15 General rule

Scientific research in the field of biology and medicine shall be carried out freely, subject to the provisions of this Convention and the other legal provisions ensuring the protection of the human being.

Article 16 Protection of persons undergoing research

Research on a person may only be undertaken if all the following conditions are met:
  i there is no alternative of comparable effectiveness to research on humans;
  ii the risks which may be incurred by that person are not disproportionate to the potential benefits of the research;
  iii the research project has been approved by the competent body after independent examination of its scientific merit, including assessment of the importance of the aim of the research, and multidisciplinary review of its ethical acceptability,
  iv the persons undergoing research have been informed of their rights and the safeguards prescribed by law for their protection;
  v the necessary consent as provided for under Article 5 has been given expressly, specifically and is documented. Such consent may be freely withdrawn at any time.

Article 17 Protection of persons not able to consent to research

1 Research on a person without the capacity to consent as stipulated in Article 5 may be undertaken only if all the following conditions are met:
  i the conditions laid down in Article 16, sub-paragraphs i to iv, are fulfilled;
  ii the results of the research have the potential to produce real and direct benefit to his or her health;
  iii research of comparable effectiveness cannot be carried out on individuals capable of giving consent;
  iv the necessary authorisation provided for under Article 6 has been given specifically and in writing; and
  v the person concerned does not object.
2 Exceptionally and under the protective conditions prescribed by law, where the research has not the potential to produce results of direct benefit to the health of the person concerned, such research may be authorised subject to the conditions laid down in paragraph 1, sub-paragraphs i, iii, iv and v above, and to the following additional conditions:
  i the research has the aim of contributing, through significant improvement in the scientific understanding of the individual's condition, disease or disorder, to the ultimate attainment of results capable of conferring benefit to the person concerned or to other persons in the same age category or afflicted with the same disease or disorder or having the same condition;
  ii the research entails only minimal risk and minimal burden for the individual concerned.

Article 18 Research on embryos *in vitro*

1 Where the law allows research on embryos *in vitro*, it shall ensure adequate protection of the embryo.
2 The creation of human embryos for research purposes is prohibited.

Chapter VI Organ and tissue removal from living donors for transplantation purposes

Article 19 General rule

1 Removal of organs or tissue from a living person for transplantation purposes may be carried out solely for the therapeutic benefit of the recipient and where there is no suitable organ or tissue available from a deceased person and no other alternative therapeutic method of comparable effectiveness.
2 The necessary consent as provided for under Article 5 must have been given expressly and specifically either in written form or before an official body.

Article 20 Protection of persons not able to consent to organ removal

1 No organ or tissue removal may be carried out on a person who does not have the capacity to consent under Article 5.
2 Exceptionally and under the protective conditions prescribed by law, the removal of regenerative tissue from a person who does not have the capacity to consent may be authorised provided the following conditions are met:

 i there is no compatible donor available who has the capacity to consent;
 ii the recipient is a brother or sister of the donor;
 iii the donation must have the potential to be life-saving for the recipient;
 iv the authorisation provided for under paragraphs 2 and 3 of Article 6 has been given specifically and in writing, in accordance with the law and with the approval of the competent body;
 v the potential donor concerned does not object.

Chapter VII Prohibition of financial gain and disposal of a part of the human body

Article 21 Prohibition of financial gain

The human body and its parts shall not, as such, give rise to financial gain.

Article 22 Disposal of a removed part of the human body

When in the course of an intervention any part of a human body is removed, it may be stored and used for a purpose other than that for which it was removed, only if this is done in conformity with appropriate information and consent procedures.

Chapter VIII Infringements of the provisions of the Convention

Article 23 Infringement of the rights or principles

The Parties shall provide appropriate judicial protection to prevent or to put a stop to an unlawful infringement of the rights and principles set forth in this Convention at short notice.

Article 24 Compensation for undue damage

The person who has suffered undue damage resulting from an intervention is entitled to fair compensation according to the conditions and procedures prescribed by law.

Article 25 Sanctions

Parties shall provide for appropriate sanctions to be applied in the event of infringement of the provisions contained in this Convention.

Chapter IX Relation between this Convention and other provisions

Article 26 Restrictions on the exercise of the rights

1 No restrictions shall be placed on the exercise of the rights and protective provisions contained in this Convention other than such as are prescribed by law and are necessary in a democratic society in the interest of public safety, for the prevention of crime, for the protection of public health or for the protection of the rights and freedoms of others.
2 The restrictions contemplated in the preceding paragraph may not be placed on Articles 11, 13, 14, 16, 17, 19, 20 and 21.

Article 27 Wider protection

None of the provisions of this Convention shall be interpreted as limiting or otherwise affecting the possibility for a Party to grant a wider measure of protection with regard to the application of biology and medicine than is stipulated in this Convention.

Chapter X Public debate

Article 28 Public debate

Parties to this Convention shall see to it that the fundamental questions raised by the developments of biology and medicine are the subject of appropriate public discussion in the light, in particular, of relevant medical, social, economic, ethical and legal implications, and that their possible application is made the subject of appropriate consultation.

Chapter XI Interpretation and follow-up of the Convention

Article 29 Interpretation of the Convention

The European Court of Human Rights may give, without direct reference to any specific proceedings pending in a court, advisory opinions on legal questions concerning the interpretation of the present Convention at the request of:
- the Government of a Party, after having informed the other Parties;
- the Committee set up by Article 32, with membership restricted to the Representatives of the Parties to this Convention, by a decision adopted by a two-thirds majority of votes cast.

Article 30 Reports on the application of the Convention

On receipt of a request from the Secretary General of the Council of Europe any Party shall furnish an explanation of the manner in which its internal law ensures the effective implementation of any of the provisions of the Convention.

Chapter XII Protocols

Article 31 Protocols

Protocols may be concluded in pursuance of Article 32, with a view to developing, in specific fields, the principles contained in this Convention.

The Protocols shall be open for signature by Signatories of the Convention. They shall be subject to ratification, acceptance or approval. A Signatory may not ratify, accept or approve Protocols without previously or simultaneously ratifying accepting or approving the Convention.

Chapter XIII Amendments to the Convention

Article 32 Amendments to the Convention

1 The tasks assigned to "the Committee" in the present article and in Article 29 shall be carried out by the Steering Committee on Bioethics (CDBI), or by any other committee designated to do so by the Committee of Ministers.
2 Without prejudice to the specific provisions of Article 29, each member State of the Council of Europe, as well as each Party to the present Convention which is not a member of the Council of Europe, may be represented and have one vote in the Committee when the Committee carries out the tasks assigned to it by the present Convention.
3 Any State referred to in Article 33 or invited to accede to the Convention in accordance with the provisions of Article 34 which is not Party to this Convention may be represented on the Committee by an observer. If the European Community is not a Party it may be represented on the Committee by an observer.
4 In order to monitor scientific developments, the present Convention shall be examined within the Committee no later than five years from its entry into force and thereafter at such intervals as the Committee may determine.
5 Any proposal for an amendment to this Convention, and any proposal for a Protocol or for an amendment to a Protocol, presented by a Party, the Committee or the Committee of Ministers shall be communicated to the Secretary General of the Council of Europe and forwarded by him to the member States of the Council of Europe, to the European Community, to any Signatory, to any Party, to any State invited to sign this Convention in accordance with the provisions of Article 33 and to any State invited to accede to it in accordance with the provisions of Article 34.
6 The Committee shall examine the proposal not earlier than two months after it has been forwarded by the Secretary General in accordance with paragraph 5. The Committee shall submit the text adopted by a two-thirds majority of the votes cast to the Committee of Ministers for approval. After its approval, this text shall be forwarded to the Parties for ratification, acceptance or approval.
7 Any amendment shall enter into force, in respect of those Parties which have accepted it, on the first day of the month following the expiration of a period of one month after the date on which five Parties, including at least four member States of the Council of Europe, have informed the Secretary General that they have accepted it.
In respect of any Party which subsequently accepts it, the amendment shall enter into force on the first day of the month following the expiration of a period of one month

after the date on which that Party has informed the Secretary General of its acceptance.

Chapter XIV Final clauses

Article 33 Signature, ratification and entry into force

1 This Convention shall be open for signature by the member States of the Council of Europe, the non-member States which have participated in its elaboration and by the European Community.
2 This Convention is subject to ratification, acceptance or approval. Instruments of ratification, acceptance or approval shall be deposited with the Secretary General of the Council of Europe.
3 This Convention shall enter into force on the first day of the month following the expiration of a period of three months after the date on which five States, including at least four member States of the Council of Europe, have expressed their consent to be bound by the Convention in accordance with the provisions of paragraph 2 of the present article.
4 In respect of any Signatory which subsequently expresses its consent to be bound by it, the Convention shall enter into force on the first day of the month following the expiration of a period of three months after the date of the deposit of its instrument of ratification, acceptance or approval.

Article 34 Non-member States

1 After the entry into force of this Convention, the Committee of Ministers of the Council of Europe may, after consultation of the Parties, invite any non-member State of the Council of Europe to accede to this Convention by a decision taken by the majority provided for in Article 20, paragraph d, of the Statute of the Council of Europe, and by the unanimous vote of the representatives of the Contracting States entitled to sit on the Committee of Ministers.
2 In respect of any acceding State, the Convention shall enter into force on the first day of the month following the expiration of a period of three months after the date of deposit of the instrument of accession with the Secretary General of the Council of Europe.

Article 35 Territories

1 Any Signatory may, at the time of signature or when depositing its instrument of ratification, acceptance or approval, specify the territory or territories to which this Convention shall apply. Any other State may formulate the same declaration when depositing its instrument of accession.
2 Any Party may, at any later date, by a declaration addressed to the Secretary General of the Council of Europe, extend the application of this Convention to any other territory specified in the declaration and for whose international relations it is responsible or on whose behalf it is authorised to give undertakings. In respect of such territory the Convention shall enter into force on the first day of the month following the expiration of a period of three months after the date of receipt of such declaration by the Secretary General.
3 Any declaration made under the two preceding paragraphs may, in respect of any territory specified in such declaration, be withdrawn by a notification addressed to the Secretary General. The withdrawal shall become effective on the first day of the month following the expiration of a period of three months after the date of receipt of such notification by the Secretary General.

Article 36 Reservations

1 Any State and the European Community may, when signing this Convention or when depositing the instrument of ratification, acceptance, approval or accession, make a reservation in respect of any particular provision of the Convention to the extent that any law then in force in its territory is not in conformity with the provision. Reservations of a general character shall not be permitted under this article.
2 Any reservation made under this article shall contain a brief statement of the relevant law.
3 Any Party which extends the application of this Convention to a territory mentioned in the declaration referred to in Article 35, paragraph 2, may, in respect of the territory concerned, make a reservation in accordance with the provisions of the preceding paragraphs.
4 Any Party which has made the reservation mentioned in this article may withdraw it by means of a declaration addressed to the Secretary General of the Council of Europe. The withdrawal shall become effective on the first day of the month following the expiration of a period of one month after the date of its receipt by the Secretary General.

Article 37 Denunciation

1 Any Party may at any time denounce this Convention by means of a notification addressed to the Secretary General of the Council of Europe.

2 Such denunciation shall become effective on the first day of the month following the expiration of a period of three months after the date of receipt of the notification by the Secretary General.

Article 38 Notifications

The Secretary General of the Council of Europe shall notify the member States of the Council, the European Community, any Signatory, any Party and any other State which has been invited to accede to this Convention of:

a any signature;

b the deposit of any instrument of ratification, acceptance, approval or accession;

c any date of entry into force of this Convention in accordance with Articles 33 or 34;

d any amendment or Protocol adopted in accordance with Article 32, and the date on which such an amendment or Protocol enters into force;

e any declaration made under the provisions of Article 35;

f any reservation and withdrawal of reservation made in pursuance of the provisions of Article 36;

g any other act, notification or communication relating to this Convention.

In witness whereof the undersigned, being duly authorised thereto, have signed this Convention.

Done at Oviedo (Asturias), this 4th day of April 1997, in English and French, both texts being equally authentic, in a single copy which shall be deposited in the archives of the Council of Europe. The Secretary General of the Council of Europe shall transmit certified copies to each member State of the Council of Europe, to the European Community, to the non-member States which have participated in the elaboration of this Convention, and to any State invited to accede to this Convention.

Additional Protocol to the Convention for the Protection of Human Rights and Dignity of the Human Being with regard to the Application of Biology and Medicine, on the prohibition of cloning human beings (ETS No. 168) and explanatory report to the Protocol

The member States of the Council of Europe, the other States and the European Community Signatories to this Additional Protocol to the Convention for the Protection of Human Rights and Dignity of the Human Being with regard to the Application of Biology and Medicine,

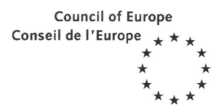

Council of Europe
Conseil de l'Europe

DIR/JUR (98) 7

Noting scientific developments in the field of mammal cloning, particularly through embryo splitting and nuclear transfer;

Mindful of the progress that some cloning techniques themselves may bring to scientific knowledge and its medical application;

Considering that the cloning of human beings may become a technical possibility;

Having noted that embryo splitting may occur naturally and sometimes result in the birth of genetically identical twins;

Considering however that the instrumentalisation of human beings through the deliberate creation of genetically identical human beings is contrary to human dignity and thus constitutes a misuse of biology and medicine;

Considering also the serious difficulties of a medical, psychological and social nature that such a deliberate biomedical practice might imply for all the individuals involved;

Considering the purpose of the Convention on Human Rights and Biomedicine, in particular the principle mentioned in Article 1 aiming to protect the dignity and identity of all human beings,

Have agreed as follows:

Article 1

1 Any intervention seeking to create a human being genetically identical to another human being, whether living or dead, is prohibited.

2 For the purpose of this article, the term human being "genetically identical" to another human being means a human being sharing with another the same nuclear gene set.

Article 2

No derogation from the provisions of this Protocol shall be made under Article 26, paragraph 1, of the Convention.

Article 3

As between the Parties, the provisions of Articles 1 and 2 of this Protocol shall be regarded as additional articles to the Convention and all the provisions of the Convention shall apply accordingly.

Article 4

This Protocol shall be open for signature by Signatories to the Convention. It is subject to ratification, acceptance or approval. A Signatory may not ratify, accept or approve this Protocol unless it has previously or simultaneously ratified, accepted or approved the Convention. Instruments of ratification, acceptance or approval shall be deposited with the Secretary General of the Council of Europe.

Article 5

1 This Protocol shall enter into force on the first day of the month following the expiration of a period of three months after the date on which five States, including at least four member States of the Council of Europe, have expressed their consent to be bound by the Protocol in accordance with the provisions of Article 4.

2 In respect of any Signatory which subsequently expresses its consent to be bound by it, the Protocol shall enter into force on the first day of the month following the expiration of a period of three months after the date of the deposit of the instrument of ratification, acceptance or approval.

Article 6

1 After the entry into force of this Protocol, any State which has acceded to the Convention may also accede to this Protocol.

2 Accession shall be effected by the deposit with the Secretary General of the Council of Europe of an instrument of accession which shall take effect on the first day of the month following the expiration of a period of three months after the date of its deposit.

Article 7

1 Any Party may at any time denounce this Protocol by means of a notification addressed to the Secretary General of the Council of Europe.

2 Such denunciation shall become effective on the first day of the month following the expiration of a period of three months after the date of receipt of such notification by the Secretary General.

Article 8

The Secretary General of the Council of Europe shall notify the member States of the Council of Europe, the European Community, any Signatory, any Party and any other State which has been invited to accede to the Convention of:

a any signature;

b the deposit of any instrument of ratification, acceptance, approval or accession;

c any date of entry into force of this Protocol in accordance with Articles 5 and 6;

d any other act, notification or communication relating to this Protocol.

In witness whereof the undersigned, being duly authorised thereto, have signed this Protocol.

Done at Paris, this twelfth day of January 1998, in English and in French, both texts being equally authentic, in a single copy which shall be deposited in the archives of the Council of Europe. The Secretary General of the Council of Europe shall transmit certified copies to each member State of the Council of Europe, to the non-member States which have participated in the elaboration of this Protocol, to any State invited to accede to the Convention and to the European Community.

Explanatory report to the additional protocol to the convention on human rights and biomedicine on the prohibition of cloning human beings

1 This Protocol builds on certain provisions of the Convention on Human Rights and Biomedicine, in particular the following: Article 1 provides that Parties to this Convention shall protect the dignity and identity of all human beings and guarantee everyone, without discrimination, respect for their integrity and other rights and fundamental freedoms with regard to the application of biology and medicine; Article 13, which provides that an intervention seeking to modify the human genome may only be undertaken for preventive, diagnostic or therapeutic purposes and only if its aim is not to introduce any modification in the genome of any descendants; Article 18.1, which ensures the protection of the embryo *in vitro* in the

framework of research and Article 18.2 which prohibits the creation of embryos for research purposes.

2 Cloning of cells and tissue is considered worldwide to be an ethically acceptable valuable biomedical technique. However, there are different views about the ethical acceptability of cloning undifferentiated cells of embryonic origin. Whatever attitudes towards such cloning techniques exist, the standards set forth in the Convention on Human Rights and Biomedicine as mentioned above form clear barriers against the misuse of human embryos, as their adequate protection is guaranteed and their creation for research purposes is prohibited by Article 18 of the Convention. Therefore, one has to distinguish between three situations: cloning of cells as a technique, use of embryonic cells in cloning techniques, and cloning of human beings, for example by utilising the techniques of embryo splitting or nuclear transfer. Whereas the first situation is fully acceptable ethically, the second should be examined in the protocol on embryo protection. The consequences of the third situation, that is the prohibition of cloning human beings, are within the scope of this Protocol.

3 Deliberately cloning humans is a threat to human identity, as it would give up the indispensable protection against the predetermination of the human genetic constitution by a third party. Further ethical reasoning for a prohibition to clone human beings is based first and foremost on human dignity which is endangered by instrumentalisation through artificial human cloning. Even if in the future, in theory, a situation could be conceived, which might seem to exclude the instrumentalisation of artificially cloned human offspring, this is not considered a sufficient ethical justification for the cloning of human beings. As naturally occurring genetic recombination is likely to create more freedom for the human being than a predetermined genetic make up, it is in the interest of all persons to keep the essentially random nature of the composition of their own genes.

4 This Protocol does not take a specific stand on the admissibility of cloning cells and tissue for research purposes resulting in medical applications. However, it can be said that cloning as a biomedical technique is an important tool for the development of medicine, especially for the development of new therapies. The provisions in this Protocol shall not be understood as prohibiting cloning techniques in cell biology.

5 However, the Protocol does enshrine clear barriers against any attempt artificially to produce genetically identical human beings. The Protocol is not concerned with hormone stimulation to treat infertility in women and which might result in the birth of twins. It explicitly restricts genetic identity to sharing the same nuclear gene set, meaning that any intervention by embryo splitting or nuclear transfer techniques seeking to create a human being genetically identical to another human being, whether living or dead, is prohibited.

6 In conformity with the approach followed in the preparation of the Convention on Human Rights and Biomedicine, it was decided to leave it to domestic law to define the scope of the expression "human being" for the purposes of the application of the present Protocol.

7 The term "nuclear" means that only genes of the nucleus – not the mitochondrial genes – are looked at with respect to identity, which is why the prohibition of cloning human beings also covers all nuclear transfer methods seeking to create identical human beings. The term "the same nuclear gene set" takes into account the fact that during development some genes may undergo somatic mutation. Thus monozygotic twins developed from a single fertilised egg will share the same nuclear gene set, but may not be 100% identical with respect to all their genes. It is important to note that the Protocol does not intend to discriminate in any fashion against natural monozygotic twins.

8 This Protocol is an important step in drawing up clear ethical and legal provisions in the area of reproductive medicine. Together with the provisions in Articles 1, 13, 14 and 18 of the Convention, it enshrines important ethical principles which should form the basis for further developments of biology and medicine in this field not only today but also in the future.

The research process
(A) General guidelines

32

Good research practice

Medical Research Council

Updates to this guidance are available on MRC's website: **www.mrc.ac.uk** Copies available from MRC External Communications **020 7636 5422** ©2000 Medical Research Council. December 2000.

Contents

1 Introduction and scope

The MRC expects **all** scientists, both clinical and non-clinical, funded by the Council (ie, MRC employees, visiting workers in MRC establishments, and recipients of MRC grants or training awards) to adopt the highest achievable standards in the conduct of their research. This means exhibiting impeccable scientific integrity and following the principles of good research practice.

The *MRC Policy and Procedure for Inquiring into Allegations of Scientific Misconduct* is published separately.[1] This booklet outlines the key elements of good research practice, setting out the principles that should be taken into account when planning and conducting research, and likewise when recording, reporting, and applying the results.

The seven principles of public life outlined by the Committee on Standards in Public Life (Nolan Committee) in 1995 provide a good starting point:
- selflessness
- integrity
- objectivity
- accountability
- openness
- honesty
- leadership

Other MRC guidance[2] sets out the scientific and ethical principles underpinning the conduct of research; this guide is about ensuring that these principles are achieved in practice.

The Department of Health's Research Governance Framework (in draft, publication expected in 2001) addresses the need to clarify responsibilities for initiation, conduct, and oversight of research conducted within the NHS at organisational as well as personal levels.

Although these guidelines are primarily for scientists supported by the MRC, we hope that other researchers, and those involved in reviewing or supervising research, will find them helpful.

2 Principles

2.1 General principles

Good Research Practice (GRP) is essentially an attitude of mind that becomes an attitude to work. It is about the way in which research is planned and conducted, the results are recorded and reported, and the fruits of research are disseminated, applied, and exploited. GRP will allow ready verification of the quality and integrity of research data, provide a transparent basis for investigating allegations of bad practice or fraud, and lead to better research. While the integrity and responsibility of individual researchers are of the utmost importance, research institutions, research funders, and the research community in general also share responsibility for promoting and verifying good practice, especially through their arrangements for training and supervision and through the ethos they create.

In clinical studies, the rights, safety, and wellbeing of participants must be safeguarded. Issues of consent and confidentiality are paramount. For clinical trials, the MRC has published separately *MRC Guidelines for Good Clinical Practice in Clinical Trials*, to which researchers should refer.[3]

For near-market projects sponsored by industry and some other funders, the more rigorous requirements of Good Laboratory Practice may be mandatory.[4] There must be adequate resources to accommodate these requirements and further advice should be sought from those with relevant expertise.

Investigational therapeutic products should be manufactured, handled, and stored in accordance with Good Manufacturing Practice[5] or other appropriate guidelines for the manufacture of medicinal products.

GRP can only be achieved if staff at all levels are trained and supervised properly in a research culture that encourages frank discussion and debate. Research team leaders are responsible for seeing that a constructive atmosphere prevails and must ensure that staff have the appropriate training and experience to carry our their duties as effectively as possible; this is especially important for new staff.

To ensure the quality of research practice, supervision and checking are an integral part of the process; a senior member of each research group should take personal responsibility for this. The steps that may be needed to supervise GRP include monitoring of training and supervision of new staff and of continuing professional development, regular checks on data recording and notebooks, and occasional checks on the day-to-day conduct of experiments. From time to time and randomly, experiments should be tracked back from conclusion to conception to ensure that all necessary paper/electronic "trails" are in place.

2.2 Conflicts of interest

Conflicts of interest happen in all walks of life; medical research is no exception. A conflict arises when a person's judgement concerning a primary interest, such as scientific knowledge, could be unduly influenced by a secondary interest, such as financial gain or personal advancement. There is nothing inherently unethical in finding oneself in a position of conflict of interest; what is required is to recognise the fact and deal with it accordingly.[6] Researchers must pay as much attention to *perceived* and potential conflicts of interest as to actual conflicts. How one is perceived to act influences the attitudes and actions of others, and the credibility of scientific research overall.

Conflicts of interest can occur at every stage of the research endeavour – from planning the research to disseminating and exploiting the results – and in many forms. Apart from financial interests, conflicts might, for example, be personal, academic, or political. Researchers should automatically ask themselves "Would I feel comfortable if others learnt about my secondary interest in this matter *or* perceived that I had one?" If the answer is no, the interest must be disclosed and addressed appropriately, for example according to the policy of an employer, a peer-review body, or a journal.

3 Planning the research

All research projects, both clinical and non-clinical, should be conceived, designed, and implemented according to the highest standards, including:

- Clear documentation of the rationale for the study and any subsequent modifications – typically in laboratory notebooks or, for more complex projects, in well-kept files. Each key document and any changes should be signed and dated by the researcher responsible to establish the provenance of the study and protect intellectual property rights.
- Adherence to current safety practices, ethical standards, and law.
- Securing all necessary ethical review and regulatory approvals in good time, for example from Local Research Ethics Committees or the Home Office.

- In clinical studies, identifying a health professional who will take overall responsibility for the well-being and interests of patients or healthy volunteers involved and for ensuring that their rights (eg, in terms of consent and confidentiality) are protected.
- Identifying the individual or group that will take ultimate responsibility for overseeing the scientific and ethical conduct of the study as the scientific plans are put into practice. This is especially important in projects affecting patients or volunteers and in other complex and collaborative programmes.
- Consultation with patients or other beneficiaries/ consumers wherever appropriate, especially in clinical and applied research.
- Consultation with statisticians at the planning stage, where relevant. The statistical power of a study should be an early consideration, and researchers should draw on professional statistical advice if needed. This is especially important for studies involving people or animals to avoid unnecessary or unproductive experiments.
- Ensuring that organisations responsible for the care of any patients involved are aware that the research is being planned.
- Assessment of resources needed (eg, space, staff, funding, biological resources, facilities, and clinical support) to ensure the study is viable within the available means.
- Economy in the use of resources, for example not purchasing more reagents than are needed for the planned sample size and regular review to determine when to stop experiments.
- Regular review of progress so that new findings can be taken into account and the project plan modified accordingly, especially if plans involve any risk to participants or use of animals.
- Agreement in advance on who will be writing any planned publications and the authorisation required to publish (see 6.1).
- Acknowledgement of formal or informal contributions to the work, including sponsoring organisations and scientific collaborators.

4 Conducting the research

4.1 Information and organisation

The legal and ethical requirements relating to human participants, animals, and personal information should be familiar to each person involved in the study, and they should know to whom to turn for advice. Since ethical issues, guidance, or requirements often change, research

teams and centres must have effective arrangements for disseminating knowledge and documents. Each person should also know when changes may call for new ethical/regulatory approval and should be able to recognise unforeseen results or incidents that need to be reported and discussed.

4.2 Use, calibration, and maintenance of equipment

Equipment used to generate data should be appropriately located, safe, suitable for the purpose, of appropriate design, and of adequate capacity. It should be calibrated and serviced regularly by trained staff so that performance is optimal and the results can be trusted. A designated person should be responsible for ensuring the proper use and maintenance of equipment and, where appropriate, for training staff in its use; when this is not possible, the users themselves should take on the responsibility. Records should be kept of calibration, servicing, faults, breakdowns, and misuse of equipment.

A standard operating procedure (see 4.4) should be maintained for each piece of equipment; in some cases this might be the manufacturer's instruction manual. There should be easily accessible instructions for the safe shutdown of equipment in case of emergency.

4.3 Hazardous processes and materials

Experiments should be conducted in accordance with MRC and/or local policies on training, and health and safety regulations and guidelines. Where appropriate, risk assessments complying with the regulations on Control of Substances Hazardous to Health (COSHH) should be prepared before the work is carried out. Where necessary, materials and equipment should be decontaminated according to specified health and safety practices including an approved risk assessment. Waste should be disposed of and recorded in accordance with these practices and the appropriate health, safety, and environmental regulations, and also in compliance with local rules for dealing with spillages. Where relevant, the appropriate authority should be notified. Staff should be properly trained and monitored so as not to endanger themselves, others, or the environment.

4.4 Standard operating procedures

Standard operating procedures (SOPs) should be documented for all routine methods and for individual items of equipment (see 4.2) to ensure that data are collected consistently and accurately. When there is more than one approved technique for any given procedure, all should be covered by SOPs. SOPs should be written in simple language, readily accessible, and ideally in a standardised format. They should be updated as necessary, and only the current version should be available.

Standard written protocols should also be available covering the process of seeking informed consent from patients or volunteers, to ensure clarity and consistency. Written protocols are likewise essential for ensuring strict adherance to regulations/licences, for example in research involving animals.

5 Recording the data

5.1 Gathering and storing data

- Confidentiality of personal data is essential,[7] including data associated with tissue and biological samples. A Local Research Ethics Committee, Multi-Centre Research Ethics Committee, or other appropriate ethics committee must approve all research involving identifiable personal information or anonymised data from the NHS. All personal information must be encoded or anonymised as far as is possible and consistent with the needs of the study, and as early as possible after collection; ciphers should be held separately. This applies to both paper and electronic records. Detailed guidance is given in separate MRC publications: *Personal Information in Medical Research*[8] *and Human Tissue and Biological Samples for Use in Research: operational and ethical guidelines.*[9]
- Data should be stored in a way that permits a complete retrospective audit if necessary.
- Data should be stored safely, with appropriate contingency plans.
- Data records should be monitored regularly to ensure their completeness and accuracy.
- Raw (original) data/images should be recorded and retained (see 5.3 and 5.4); this is especially important where data/images are subsequently enhanced. If possible, both original and enhanced data/images should be stored. Over-enhancement or over-interpretation of images must be resisted.
- Confidentiality is also important where there is potential for commercial exploitation (see 7.1).

5.2 Retaining data

Retention of accurately recorded and retrievable results is essential for research.

- Primary research data (and where possible/relevant specimens, samples, questionnaires, audiotapes, etc) must be retained in their original form within the research establishment that generated them for a minimum of ten years from completion of the project.
- Work that informs national policy-making should be archived.
- Research records relating to clinical or public health studies should be retained for 20 years to provide scope for longer follow-up if necessary; for detailed guidance see MRC guidelines on *Personal Information in Medical Research.*[8]
- Researchers who are leaving the establishment that generated the data and who wish to retain data/copies of data for personal use must get permission from their team leader or head of department to do so. Where personal data are involved, the request should be refused unless it is clear that future use will be consistent with the terms of the consent.
- Publication of the data (including data in Masters/Doctoral theses) does not negate the need to retain source data.

5.3 Notebooks and electronic records

The following basic policies apply:

- All raw data should be recorded and retained in indexed laboratory notebooks with permanent binding and numbered pages or in an electronic notebook dedicated to that purpose.
- Machine print-outs, questionnaires, chart recordings, autoradiographs, etc which cannot be attached to the main record should be retained in a separate ring-binder/folder that is cross-indexed with the main record.
- Records in notebooks should be entered as soon as possible after the data are collected. Recorded data should be identified by date of the record and date of collection if the two do not coincide. Subsequent modifications or additions to records should also be clearly identified and dated.
- Special attention should be paid to recording accurately the use of potentially hazardous substances (eg, radioactive materials) in both laboratory notebooks and any central logbooks.
- In clinical studies, consent forms should be kept securely with the raw data, and normally for the same period of time.
- Supervisors should regularly (monthly or as appropriate to the nature of the work) review and "sign-off" notebooks of researchers to signify that records are complete

and accurate. Queries should be discussed immediately with the individual who recorded the data and any resultant changes to the records should be signed by both. Authentication of data collected and recorded electronically requires special consideration.

5.4 Computer-generated data

Special procedures are necessary for electronically generated data.

- Data should be backed-up regularly; duplicate copies should be held on disc in a secure but readily accessible archive.
- Where feasible, a hard copy should be made of particularly important data.
- Copies of relevant software, particularly the version used to process electronic data, must be retained along with the raw data to ensure future access. Software updates must be logged and stored as new formats and media are adopted.
- Special attention should be paid to guaranteeing the security of electronic data.

More comprehensive guidance on the use of electronic systems for data recording and analysis is given in a Department of Health advisory leaflet.[10]

6 Reporting the results

Once any issues of confidentiality and ownership have been addressed (see 7), research findings should be disseminated so that they can be assessed by scientific peers and more widely. This is essential if scientific knowledge is to be used appropriately and effectively. Accordingly, researchers should publish their data in a timely fashion in a peer-reviewed journal or in other equally reputable publications and/or present their results at scientific meetings.

It is equally unethical not to report results, or to exaggerate the importance of results for medical practice or policy. Both are areas in which a researcher's desire for advancement or recognition may conflict directly with the public interest in a complete, balanced, and rigorous account of the scientific evidence.

6.1 Publication policy

- The person with overall responsibility for the research programme should authorise publication of results;

authorisation should cover both the content of the paper (integrity of results, adequacy of internal peer review, appropriate protection of intellectual property rights, appropriate authorship) and the intended place of publication.
- Research findings with substantial implications for clinical practice or which are likely to attract strong public interest should be drawn to the attention of the MRC and/or other research funders before publication.
- A written agreement should be negotiated with external sponsors before the research is initiated to cover the free dissemination of research findings; this is especially important where funding has been secured from industry.
- Published reports should normally contain basic information about the ethical acceptability of the work and/or its legality, as well as information about the scientific method.
- The leader of the research team should authorise any release of the results on the Internet. Releasing information in this way may well compromise intellectual property rights, so there should be a suitable mechanism to monitor information placed on the web.

6.2 Authorship

- Authorship of papers should include those individuals who have made a major contribution to the work and who are familiar with the entire contents of the paper. Authors should have participated sufficiently in the research to take public responsibility for the content. The MRC subscribes to the guidance of the International Committee of Medical Journal Editors,[11] to which researchers should refer.
- Other contributions to the work should be acknowledged formally, as should financial support from sponsors. Authors are responsible for obtaining written permission from persons acknowledged by name.

6.3 Methods of publication

- Work should normally be published as a coherent entity rather than a series of small parts, unless there is a legitimate need to demonstrate first discovery by publishing preliminary data.
- Quality rather than quantity is paramount; the proliferation of multi-author papers to increase quantity should be discouraged.

- Authors must not publish the same data in different journals.

6.4 Correction of errors and retraction of published findings

- If an error is found that degrades the worth of published findings, the principal author must immediately discuss the matter with the research leader, with a view to notifying co-authors and publishing a correction as soon as possible setting out the basis of the reservations.
- Where the findings are found to be in serious doubt, a retraction should be published speedily.
- Where fraud is suspected, the procedure set out in the *MRC Policy and Procedure for Inquiring into Allegations of Scientific Misconduct*[1] should be followed.

7 Applying and exploiting the results

The MRC's mission can only be fulfilled if the results of research are communicated effectively. The MRC therefore expects those it supports to play their part in disseminating balanced information on scientific advances and their potential implications for society to the health professionals and policy makers who will be involved in applying them, and to the wider public.

7.1 Commercial exploitation

Since part of the MRC's mission is to improve quality of life and economic competitiveness, MRC-funded researchers are expected to maximise the prospects of research being taken into practice through the commercial route by protecting intellectual property rights (IPR).

- Intellectual property can only be protected adequately if researchers keep thorough, accurate, and contemporaneous research records.
- Researchers who collaborate with industry should take special care to keep detailed records of their research.
- IPR should be considered before data are submitted for publication or presented at meetings.
- All intellectual property, know-how, reagents, or materials generated by MRC employees while on MRC premises, or in connection with MRC research activities, is the property of the MRC. This is usually also the case for visiting workers who use MRC research facilities.
- Data placed on the web are considered to be in the public domain and so cannot be protected.

- Material transfer agreements (MTAs) and confidentiality agreements are important for protecting resources that may potentially have great value. MTAs are agreements between sender (eg, MRC) and recipient organisations regarding provision of research materials; they set out the terms on which the provider is prepared to release its material to the recipient. Confidentiality agreements recognise the need for tentative research and/or development partners to share proprietary research findings and/or commercial technologies before making formal commitment to a partnership; they therefore bind and protect the parties by limiting use of exchanged information to the discussions in hand. Researchers should generally seek expert guidance before entering into these agreements.

REFERENCES

1 Medical Research Council. MRC policy and procedure for inquiring into allegations of scientific misconduct. London: Medical Research Council, 1997.

2 Medical Research Council. Principles in the assessment and conduct of medical research and publicising results. London: Medical Research Council, 1995.

3 Medical Research Council. MRC Guidelines for Good Clinical Practice in Clinical Trials. London: Medical Research Council, 1998.

4 Good Laboratory Practice Regulations 1999 (Statutory Instrument 1999, 3106). London: Stationery Office, 1999.

5 Medicines Control Agency. Rules and guidance for pharmaceutical manufacturers and distributors. London: Stationery Office, 1997. ISBN 0-11-321-995-4.

6 Lemmens T, Singer PA. Bioethics for clinicians: 17. Conflict of interest in research, education and patient care. *CMAJ*, 1998:**159**: 960-65.

7 General Medical Council. Confidentiality: protecting and providing information. London: GMC, 2000.

8 Medical Research Council. Personal Information in Medical Research. London: Medical Research Council, 2000.

9 Medical Research Council. Human Tissue and Biological Samples for Use in Research: operational and ethical guidelines. London: Medical Research Council, 2001.

10 United Kingdom GLP Monitoring Authority. The Application of Good Laboratory Practice Principles to Computer Systems. London: Department of Health, 1995.

11 International Committee of Medical Journal Editors. Uniform requirements for manuscripts submitted to biomedical journals. *Med Educ*, 1999; **3**(1): 66–78.

OTHER PUBLICATIONS IN THIS SERIES

Responsibility in the Use of Animals in Medical Research, July 1993.
Personal Information in Medical Research, October 2000.

Principles in the Assessment of Medical Research and Publicising Results, January 1995.

MRC Policy and Procedure for Inquiring into Allegations of Scientific Misconduct, December 1997.

The Ethical Conduct of Research on the Mentally Incapacitated, December 1991, Reprinted August 1993.

Human Tissue and Biological Samples for Use in Research: operational and ethical guidelines Available 2001.

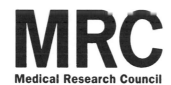

Medical Research Council

20 Park Crescent, London W1B 1AL
Telephone: 020 7636 5422   Facsimile: 020 7436 6179
Website: www.mrc.ac.uk

33

Research: the role and responsibilities of doctors

General Medical Council

February 2002

Good practice in research

This guidance sets out the standards expected of all doctors working in research in the NHS, universities and the private sector or other circumstances. It develops the general principles and standards on research set out in *our other guidance documents* and should be used in conjunction with them.

You must always follow the principles in this guidance and take note of other governance and good practice guidelines issued by the Departments of Health and other authoritative bodies. You must observe and keep up to date with the laws and statutory codes of practice which affect your work.

Contents

Introduction

1 Research involving people directly or indirectly is vital in improving care for present and future patients and the health of the population as a whole.

2 Doctors involved in research have an ethical duty to show respect for human life and respect peoples' autonomy. Partnership between participants and the health care team is essential to good research practice and such partnerships are based on trust. You must respect patients' and volunteers' rights to make decisions about their involvement in research. It is essential to listen to and share information with them, respect their privacy and dignity, and treat them politely and considerately at all times.

Scope of the guidance

3 Research in this document refers to any experimental study into the causes, treatment or prevention of ill health and disease in humans, involving people or their tissues or organs or data. It includes toxicity studies, clinical trials, genetic studies, epidemiological research including analyses of medical records, and other collections and analyses of data about health and illness, whether anonymised or not. It covers clinical research which may be therapeutic, that is of potential benefit to patients who participate, and non-therapeutic, where no immediate benefit to those patients or volunteers who participate is expected.

4 This guidance does not apply to clinical audit which involves no experimental study. Nor does it cover innovative therapeutic interventions designed to benefit individual patients. These activities are covered by the standards and principles set out in our other guidance.

Principles governing research practice

5 Because the benefits of the research are not always certain and may not be experienced by the participants, you must be satisfied that the research is not contrary to their interests. In particular:
  • you must be satisfied that, in therapeutic research, the foreseeable risks will not outweigh the potential benefits to the patients. The development of treatments and furthering of knowledge should never take precedence over the patients' best interests;
  • in non-therapeutic research, you must keep the foreseeable risks to participants as low as possible. In addition the potential benefits from the development of treatments and furthering of knowledge must far outweigh any such risks;
  • before starting any research you must ensure that ethical approval has been obtained from a properly constituted and relevant research ethics committee – such

committees abide by the guidance for local and multi-centre research ethics committees[1], whether they are within the NHS, the university sector, the pharmaceutical industry, or elsewhere[2].
  • you must conduct research in an ethical manner and one that accords with best practice;
  • you must ensure that patients or volunteers understand that they are being asked to participate in research and that the results are not predictable;
  • you must obtain and record the participants' consent; save in exceptional circumstances where specific approval not to obtain consent must have been given by the research ethics committee;
  • respect participants' right to confidentiality;
  • with participants' consent, keep GPs, and other clinicians responsible for participants' care, informed of the participants' involvement in the research and provide the GPs with any information necessary for their continuing care;
  • you must complete research projects involving patients or volunteers, or do your best to ensure that they are completed by others, except where results indicate a risk that participants may be harmed or no benefit can be expected;
  • you must record and report results accurately;
  • you must be prepared to explain and justify your actions and decisions.

6 If you undertake records based research which does not involve patients or volunteers directly you are still bound by the principles on which this guidance is based. You must be satisfied that you have appropriate authority to access any identifiable data; advice on access to, and use of, data is in paragraphs *30 to 42 below*.

7 The principles set out in our guidance *Good Medical Practice, Seeking patients' consent: the ethical considerations* and *Confidentiality: Protecting and Providing information* must be followed when undertaking research.

Putting the principles into practice

Protecting the autonomy and interests of participants

8 You must conduct all research with honesty and integrity and, in designing, organising and executing research, you must always put the protection of participants' interests first. You must:
  • not put pressure on patients or volunteers to participate in the research;
  • ensure that no real or implied coercion is used on participants who are in a dependent relationship to you, for

example, medical students, a junior colleague, nurse in your practice or employee in your company;

- keep to all aspects of the research protocol and make significant changes to, or deviations from, the protocol only with the agreement of the research ethics committee and the research funder.

9 If you have good reason to believe that participants are being put at risk by participating in the research or by the behaviour of anyone conducting the research, you should report your concerns to a senior colleague. If you remain concerned, you should inform the research ethics committee, and the research sponsor together with the employer or contracting body if appropriate.

10 You must report evidence of financial or scientific fraud or other contravention of this guidance to an appropriate person or authority, including where appropriate the GMC or other statutory regulatory body.

Research design

11 All research must be based on a properly developed protocol that has been approved by a research ethics committee[3]. It must be prepared according to the good practice guidelines given in this guidance and that of other relevant bodies, for example, the *Departments of Health*, *Royal College of Physicians of London* and the *Medical Research Council*, and where appropriate, the *International Conference on Harmonisation*.

12 You must ensure that:
- the aims, design and methodology of the project are justifiable, verifiable and scientifically valid;
- over-use of patient groups or individuals is avoided.

Conflicts of interest

13 You must always act in the participants' best interests when carrying out research. You must ensure that your judgement about the research is not influenced, or seen by others to be influenced, by financial, personal, political or other external interests at any stage of the process. You should always declare any conflicts that may arise to an appropriate person, authority or organisation, as well as to the participants.

Funding and payments

14 You must be open and honest in all financial and commercial matters relating to your research and its funding. In particular you must:

- declare to research ethics committees, prior to the research being approved, all financial interests and sums of money which you know, or estimate, will be paid for the research undertaken; accept only those payments and benefits approved by the research ethics committee;
- give participants information on how the research is funded, including any benefits which will accrue to researchers and/or their departments;
- respond honestly and fully to participants' questions, including inquiries about direct payments made to you and any financial interests you have in the research project or its sponsoring organisations;
- ensure that everyone in the research team, including nurses and non-medical staff, is informed about the way in which the research is being financed and managed;
- not offer payments at a level which could induce research participants to take risks that they would otherwise not take, or to volunteer more frequently than is advisable or against their better interests or judgement;
- not allow your conduct in the research to be influenced by payment or gifts.

Consent

15 Seeking consent is fundamental to research involving people.

Valid consent

16 Participants' consent is legally valid and professionally acceptable only where participants are competent to give consent, have been properly informed, and have agreed without coercion.

Consent for research

17 Obtaining consent is a process involving open and helpful dialogue, and is essential in clarifying objectives and understanding between doctors and research participants.

18 Effective communication is the key to enabling participants to make informed decisions. When providing information you must do your best to find out about participants' individual needs and priorities. For example, participants' current understanding of their condition and treatment, beliefs, culture, occupation or other

factors may have a bearing on the information they require. You must not make assumptions about participants' views, but discuss matters with them, and ask whether they have any concerns about the treatment or the risks involved in the research programme.

19 You must ensure that any individuals whom you invite to take part in research are given the information which they want or ought to know, and that is presented in terms and a form that they can understand. You must bear in mind that it may be difficult for participants to identify and assess the risks involved. Giving the information will usually include an initial discussion supported by a leaflet or sound recording, where possible taking into account any particular communication or language needs of the participants. You must give participants an opportunity to ask questions and to express any concerns they may have.

20 The information[4] provided should include:
- what the research aims to achieve, an outline of the research method, and confirmation that a research ethics committee has approved the project;
- the legal rights and safeguards provided for participants;
- the reasons that the patient or volunteer has been asked to participate;
- if the project involves randomisation, the nature of the process and reasons for it, and the fact that in double-blind research trials neither the patient nor the treatment team will know whether the patient is receiving the treatment being tested or is in the control group;
- information about possible benefits and risks;
- an explanation of which parts of the treatment are experimental or not fully tested;
- advice that they can withdraw at any time and, where relevant, an assurance that this will not adversely affect their relationship with those providing care;
- an explanation of how personal information will be stored, transmitted and published; what information will be available to the participant about the outcome of the research, and how that information will be presented;
- arrangements for responding to adverse events;
- details of compensation available should participants suffer harm as a result of their participation in the research.

21 You must allow people sufficient time to reflect on the implications of participating in the study, and provide any further information they request, including a copy of the protocol approved by the research ethics committee. You must not put pressure on anyone to take part in the research. You should make a record of the discussion and the outcome.

22 When seeking consent it is also important to consider the needs of particular groups of people and situations that require special consideration, advice is given in *paragraphs 43 to 58*.

Seeking consent to obtain organs, tissues or body fluids from living patients or volunteers

23 Samples of body fluids, tissues and organs can form a valuable archive for research purposes. You must obtain appropriate consent or authorisation before taking or retaining organs, tissues or body fluids, from patients or volunteers, for research purposes. This applies whether the material is obtained solely for research purposes or retained following a clinical or surgical treatment.

24 When seeking participants' consent, you must be satisfied that participants understand the amount and nature of tissues, organs or body fluids which will be taken. Where material is being obtained for a specific project, you must explain how the sample will be used; where a sample is to be stored and used in further research projects, this must be made clear. You must be prepared to respond honestly and sensitively to any questions which the participants may ask.

25 You must be open and honest about any financial transactions associated with the use of tissues, organs or body fluids (see *paragraph 14*). Financial remuneration for supplying such material to other organisations or individuals should be limited to administrative costs involved, and you should not be involved, directly or indirectly, in buying or selling human organs, tissues or body fluids.

26 Obtaining human organs, tissue and body fluids for use in research raises complex issues, and you must ensure that you take account of the relevant guidance. Professional guidance on post-mortem examinations, and the removal and retention of human material has been issued by a number of bodies; advice from the UK Health Departments is in preparation (see *Notes*).

Post-mortems

27 The legislation relating to post-mortems and retention of organs is currently being reviewed in the UK. You must keep up to date with and observe the law which governs this area of practice.

28 Different legal requirements arise in post-mortems undertaken at the direction of the coroner or procurator fiscal, from those undertaken at the instigation of the hospital. Nonetheless in all cases it is essential that the deceased's relatives are involved in the decision if it is planned to remove and retain any tissue, body fluids or organs for the purposes of research:

- where a child has died, the parental consent to the removal, storage and use of such material for research must be obtained;
- where an adult has died, reasonable efforts should be made to ascertain what the person would have wanted, for example by discussing the issues with their relatives or representatives, and reading any 'living will' or other statements made by that person.

29 It is essential that clear information is provided to the family or representatives of a deceased patient about the extent of the tissue and fluid or organs to be taken, and as far as possible, the nature of the research for which it will or may be used. You must be prepared to respond honestly and sensitively to any questions that they may ask and you should be considerate when giving information to and obtaining consent from them.

Confidentiality

30 Patients and people who volunteer to participate in research are entitled to expect that doctors will respect their privacy and autonomy. Where data is needed for research, epidemiology or public health surveillance you should:

1 Seek consent to the disclosure of any information wherever that is practicable;
2 Anonymise data where unidentifiable data will serve the purpose;
3 Keep disclosures to the minimum necessary;
4 Keep up to date with, and abide by, the requirements of statute and common law, including the Data Protection Act 1998 and orders made under the Health and Social Care Act 2001[5].

Use of existing records in research

Obtaining consent

31 Records made for one purpose, for example the provision of care, should not usually be disclosed for another purpose without the patient's consent. If you are asked to disclose, or seek access to, records containing personal information for research, you must be satisfied that express consent has been sought from the participant, wherever that is practicable.

32 Where it is not practicable for the person who holds the records either to obtain express consent to disclosure, or to anonymise records, data may be disclosed for research, provided participants have been given information about access to their records, and about their right to object. Any objection must be respected. Usually such disclosures will be made to allow a person outside the research team to anonymise the records, or to identify participants who may be invited to participate in a study[6]. Such disclosures must be kept to the minimum necessary for the purpose. In all such cases you must be satisfied that participants have been told, or have had access to written material informing them:

- that their records may be disclosed to persons outside the team which provided their care.
- of the purpose and extent of the disclosure, for example, to produce anonymised data for use in research, epidemiology or surveillance.
- that the person given access to records will be subject to a duty of confidentiality.
- that they have a right to object to such a process, and that their objection will be respected, except where the disclosure is essential to protect the patient, or someone else, from risk of death or serious harm.

33 Where you control personal information or records about patients or volunteers, you must not allow anyone access, unless the person has been properly trained and authorised by the health authority, NHS trust or comparable body and is subject to a duty of confidentiality in their employment or because of their registration with a statutory regulatory body.

Where consent cannot be obtained

34 Where it is not practicable to contact participants to seek their consent to the anonymisation of data or use of identifiable data in research, this fact should be drawn to the attention of a research ethics committee so that it can consider whether the likely benefits of the research outweigh the loss of confidentiality to the patient. Disclosures may otherwise be improper, even if the recipients of the information are registered medical practioners. The decision of a research ethics committee would be taken into account by a court if a claim for breach of confidentiality were made, but the court's judgement would be based on its own assessment of whether the public interest was served.

Projects which are not approved by research ethics committees

35 Some epidemiology, health surveillance and monitoring is, for good reason, undertaken without research ethics committee approval. Data can be used in these cases where there is a statutory requirement to do so, for example where the data relates to a known or suspected 'notifiable' disease, or where there is a relevant order under the Health and Social Care Act 2001[7].

36 Where there is no statutory duty to disclose information, disclosures must be made in accordance with the principles set out in *paragraph 30* above. Where it is not practicable to seek consent, nor to anonymise data, information may be disclosed or accessed where the disclosure is justified in the public interest.

Disclosures in the public interest

37 Personal information may be disclosed in the public interest, without the individual's consent, where the benefits to an individual or to society of the disclosure outweigh the public and the individual's interest in keeping the information confidential. In all cases where you consider disclosing information without consent from the individual, you must weigh the possible harm (both to the individual, and the overall trust between doctors and participants) against the benefits which are likely to arise from the release of information.

38 Before considering whether disclosure of personal information would be justified, you must be satisfied that:
   a. the participants are not competent to give consent; or,
   b. it is not practicable to seek consent, for example because:
      • the records are of such age and/or number that reasonable efforts to trace patients are unlikely to be successful;
      • the patient has been or may be violent;
      • action must be taken quickly (for example in the detection or control of outbreaks of some communicable diseases) and there is insufficient time to contact participants; or
   c. participants have been asked, but have withheld consent.

39 In considering whether the public interest in the research outweighs the privacy interests of the individual and society, you will need to consider the nature of the information to be disclosed, how long identifiable data will be preserved, how many people may have access to the data, as well as the potential benefits of the research project. A participant's wishes about the use of data can be overridden only in exceptional circumstances and you must be prepared to explain and justify such a decision.

40 Other circumstances in which disclosures may be made without consent are discussed below.

Records made during research

41 Records made during research should be kept securely and disclosed to people outside the research team only in accordance with the guidance in our booklet *Confidentiality: Protecting and Providing Information*.

Recording and reporting research results

42 When you are involved in a research project you must:
   • maintain complete and accurate records and retain them for purposes of audit;
   • record and report research results accurately and in a way that is transparent and open to audit;
   • report adverse findings as soon as possible to the research participants who are affected, to those responsible for their medical care, to the research sponsor and primary funder and to bodies responsible for protecting the public, such as the *Medicines Control Agency* or other licensing bodies;
   • make every effort to inform participants of the outcome of the research; or make the information publicly available if it is not practicable to inform individual participants;
   • ensure that claims of authorship are justified;
   • publish results whenever possible, including adverse findings, preferably through peer reviewed journals. You must always try to ensure that your research results appear in such journals before they are reported in other media, and if you are presenting your research findings to the non-medical press you should make every effort to ensure that your research findings are reported in a balanced way.
   • explain to the relevant research ethics committee if, exceptionally, you believe there are valid reasons not to publish the results of a study.

People and situations requiring special consideration

Vulnerable adults

43 Competent but vulnerable adults may find it difficult to withhold consent if they are put under implicit or explicit pressures from institutions or health care professionals. But the treatments being researched might be

of significant benefit to such people, and to exclude vulnerable groups could be a form of discrimination. Frail elderly people, people living in institutions and adults with learning difficulties or mental illness who remain competent should all be considered vulnerable. Pregnant women may also be subjected to hidden pressures to become involved in research, and their inclusion in a project may need special consideration.

44 Careful consideration should therefore be given to involving vulnerable adults in research, and particular attention should be given to the consent process, ensuring that they have sufficient information provided in a suitable format, and enough time to consider the issues. You should give consideration to their vulnerability and difficulties they may have in understanding or retaining information. You may need to encourage them to seek the help of a relative/close friend, support worker/advocate. You should proceed with the research only if you believe that the participant's consent is voluntary and based on an understanding of the information they have been given.

Assessing capacity

45 No one can give or withhold consent on behalf of an adult with mental incapacity[9]. Before involving participants who, by reason of mental disorder or inability to communicate, lack mental capacity, you must first assess their capacity to make an informed decision about participating in research.

Fluctuating capacity

46 Where participants have difficulty retaining information, or are only intermittently competent to make a decision, you should provide any assistance they might need to reach an informed decision. You should record any decision made while they were competent, including the key elements of the consultation. You should review any decision made whilst they were competent at appropriate intervals before the research starts, and at intervals during the study, to establish that their views are consistently held and can be relied on.

Adults who lack capacity

47 In England, Wales and Northern Ireland there is no legislation setting out the circumstances in which research involving adults with mental incapacity may be undertaken[10].

48 Research into conditions that are not linked to incapacity should never be undertaken with adults with incapacity if it could equally well be done with other adults. It should be limited to areas of research related to the participants' incapacity or to physical illnesses that are linked to their incapacity. If you involve this group of people in research you must demonstrate that:
- it could be of direct benefit to their health; or
- it is of special benefit to the health of people in the same age group with the same state of health; or
- that it will significantly improve the scientific understanding of the adult's incapacity leading to a direct benefit to them or to others with the same incapacity; and
- the research is ethical and will not cause the participants emotional, physical or psychological harm; and
- the person does not express objections physically or verbally.

49 You must also ensure that participants' right to withdraw from the research is respected at all times. Any sign of distress, pain or indication of refusal irrespective of whether or not it is given in a verbal form should be considered as implied refusal.

Advance statements

50 If you are involving adults who have lost capacity to consent to, or refuse to participate in research, for example through onset or progress of a mental disorder, you should try to find out whether they have previously indicated preferences in an advance statement ('advance directives' or 'living wills'). Adults can express their wishes about forms of treatment and about participation in research in an advance statement and their views should be taken into account. Any refusal to participate in a research trial or project, given when an adult patient was competent, which remains valid and clearly applicable, is legally binding and must be respected.

Research into treatment in emergencies

51 In an emergency where consent cannot be obtained, treatment can be given only if it is limited to what is immediately necessary to save life or avoid significant deterioration in the patient's health. This may include treatment that is part of a therapeutic research project, where the risks of the new treatment are not believed to exceed the known risks of standard treatment. If, during treatment, the patient regains capacity, the patient should be told about the research as soon as possible and their consent to continue should be sought.

52 If it is possible, you should discuss the situation with relatives and/or partners of the patient unless you have what you judge to be good reason to believe that the patient would wish otherwise.

53 You must always respect the terms of any valid advance refusal that you know about, or is drawn to your attention.

54 If there is time, you may want to seek the opinion or advice of another member of the research team to discuss the course of action you are intending to take.

Children and young people

55 Research involving children and young people is important in promoting their health and to validate in them the beneficial results of research conducted with adults. However, to the degree that they are unable to recognise their best interests, express their own needs, protect themselves from harm, or make informed choices about the potential risks and benefits of research, children and young people are vulnerable members of society.

56 When involving children and young people in research you must protect their ethical, physical, mental and emotional rights and ensure that they are not exploited. It is important to assess carefully the potential benefits and harm to them, at all stages of any research.

57 You must always ensure that you have obtained consent before undertaking any research on children and young people. If they are not competent, independently, to consent to treatment then they should not participate in research without the consent of someone with parental responsibility. GMC guidance *Seeking patients' consent: the ethical considerations* gives advice on consent.

58 A full exposition of the issues concerning research that involve children is contained in 'Guidelines for the ethical conduct of medical research involving children'[11].

Teaching, training and management

Teaching and supervision

59 All students should be introduced to the basic principles of good research practice as undergraduates. This should include the ethical importance of informed consent and the practical importance of related communication skills. It should also provide the basis for continuing, appropriate training at all stages of their education and professional development.

60 If you have special responsibilities for supervision of research or teaching[12] you must develop and demonstrate the skills, attitudes and practices of a competent teacher because you will be a significant role model. You must make sure that students and junior colleagues who undertake research are properly supervised. Junior staff and research students who are being trained or supervised should always be given clear information about the roles and responsibilities of supervisors, teachers and mentors.

Keeping up to date

61 As a researcher you should keep your knowledge and skills up to date throughout your working life. You should take part regularly in educational activities that develop you competence and performance in research methods[13].

Managerial responsibilities for research

62 If you have management responsibility in an organisation undertaking research, or are leading a research team or a research project, the management tasks you undertake will have to meet the standards set by the GMC[14].

63 If you have responsibility to act on concerns brought to your attention about the quality and integrity of the research including allegations of fraud or misconduct, you must ensure that systems are in place to deal with such concerns. Where such a concern is brought to your attention, you must take action promptly:
 • taking account of participants' safety;
 • establishing the facts as far as you are able, separating genuine concerns from those made mischievously or maliciously;
 • protecting the person who has made the allegations and the person about whom the allegation is made, from harmful criticisms or actions[15].

64 If you are leading a team, you must:
 • ensure the research plans are clearly explained to the appropriate ethics committee(s), the health care organisations in which the research will take place, and other bodies with supervisory or regulatory responsibilities;
 • ensure that all members of the team are competent and in a position to carry out their research responsibilities with integrity;

- take responsibility for ensuring that the team carries out the research in a manner which is safe, effective and efficient;
- do you best to make sure that the whole team understands the need to provide a polite, responsive and accessible service that respects the research participants' dignity and treats their information as confidential;
- ensure that research participants and colleagues understand your role and responsibilities in the team.

This booklet is not exhaustive. It cannot cover all the questions that may arise. You must therefore always be prepared to explain and justify your actions and decisions.

Other organisations issue guidance on issues of relevance to research and you will find details of where to obtain these at the *end of this guidance*.

GMC guidance and further information is available on our website www.gmc-uk.org To request publications please contact our publications department: tel 020 7915 3507, fax 020 7915 3685. or email publications@gmc-uk.org

NOTES

1 See Research Ethics Committees web site www.corec.org.uk
2 'A clinical trial with a medicinal product must receive authorisation for the supply of the product under Section 31 of the Medicines Act 1968 unless it is subject to an exemption. Applications are made to the Medicines Control Agency (MCA). The authorisation is subject to certain conditions including the requirement to report adverse reactions to the product to the MCA.
3 Department of Health Research Governance Framework for Health and Social Care, March 01.
4 *Consumers for Ethics in Research* (CERES) gives advice on providing information to research participants.
5, 7 In England and Wales
6 See our website for further guidance on Orders under the Health and Social Care Act 2001
8 See GMC website.
9, 10 In Scotland you must take account of the terms of the Adults with Incapacity Act 2000
11 *Guidelines for the ethical conduct of medical research involving children*, Royal College of Paediatrics and Child Health: Ethics Advisory Committee in Archives of Disease in Childhood, February 2000, Vol 82, No 2, p. 177–182.
12 General Medical Council guidance *The doctor as teacher* is of relevance to all doctors.
13 Details of organisations providing continuous professional development (CPD) from your employer and/or professional association.
14 *Management in Health Care: The Role of Doctors.*
15 Doctors should be aware of the terms of the Public Interest Disclosure Act 1998.

Organisations with guidance on research and some key legislation

Organisations

Association of the British Pharmaceutical Industry, 12 Whitehall, London SW1A 2DY: http://www.abpi.org.uk

British Medical Association, BMA House, Tavistock Square, London WC1H 9JR: http://www.bma.org.uk

Central Office for Research Ethics Committees, Room 78 Block, 40 Eastbourne Terrace, London W2 3QR: http://www.corec.org.uk

Child Bereavement Trust, Aston House, High Street, West Wycombe, High Wycombe, Buckinghamshire HP14 3AG: http://www.childbereavement.org.uk

Consumers for Ethics in Research (CERES), PO Box 1365, London N16 0BW: http://www.ceres.org.uk

Council for International Organisations of Medical Sciences, c/o World Health Organisation, Avenue Appia, 1211 Geneva 27, Switzerland: http://www.who.int

Council for Professions Supplementary to Medicine (CPSM), Park House, 184 Kennington Park Road, London SE11 4BU: http://www.cpsm.org.uk

Departments of Health

The Department of Health, Richmond House, 79 Whitehall, London, SW1A 2NS:
http://www.doh.gov.uk

Department of Health and Social Services Northern Ireland, Dundonald House, Upper Newtownards Road, Belfast BT4 3SF:
http://www.dhsspsni.gov.uk

National Assembly for Wales, Cardiff Bay, Cardiff CF99 1NA: http://www.wales.gov.uk

Scottish Executive Health Department, St Andrew's House, Regent Road, Edinburgh EH1 3DG:
http://scotland.gov.uk

European Agency for the Evaluation of Medicinal Products, ICH Technical Co-ordination, 7 Westferry Circus, Canary Wharf, London E14 4HB:
http://www.open.gov.uk/mca/mcahome.htm

Human Fertilisation and Embryology Authority, Paxton House, 30 Artillery Lane, London E1 7LS:
http://www.hfea.gov.uk

Human Genetics Commission:
http//www.hgc.gov.uk

International Conference on Harmonisation of Technical Requirements for Registration of Pharmaceuticals for Human Use: http://www.ifpma.org/ich1.html

Medical Research Council, 20 Park Crescent, London, W1B 1AL: http://www.mrc.ac.uk

Medicines Control Agency, Market Place, 1 Nine Elms Place, London SW8 5NQ: http://www.open.gov.uk/mca/mcahome.htm

National Childbirth Trust, Alexandra House, Oldham Terrace, Acton, London W3 6NH. http://www.nct-online.org

National Institute for Clinical Excellence: http://www.nice.org.uk

Nuffield Council on Bioethics, 28 Bedford Square, London WC1B 3EG: http://www.nuffield.org.uk/bioethics

Royal College of General Practitioners, 14 Princes Gate London SW7 1PU: http://www.rcgp.org.uk

Royal College of Paediatrics and Child Health. 50 Hallam Street London, W1N 6DE: http://www.rcpch.ac.uk

Royal College of Pathologists, 2 Carlton House Terrace, London SW1Y 5AF: http://www.rcpath.org.uk

Royal College of Physicians of Edinburgh, 9 Queen Street, Edinburgh, EH2 1JQ: http://www.rcpe.ac.uk

Royal College of Physicians of London, 11 St Andrew's Place, London, NW1 4LE: http://www.rcplondon.ac.uk

Royal College of Psychiatrists, 17 Belgrave Square London, SW1X 8PG: http://www.rcpsych.ac.uk

United Kingdom Central Council for Nursing, Midwifery and Health Visiting. 23 Portland Place, London W1N 4JT: http://www.ukcc.org.uk

World Association of Medical Editors: http://www.wame.org

World Medical Association: http://www.wma.net

Legislation

Available on HMSO website: http://hmso.gov.uk/acts

All legislation must be read against the Human Rights Act 1998 and the European Convention on Human Rights.

Anatomy Act 1984 and Anatomy Regulations 1988
Coroners Act 1988
Data Protection Act 1998
Health & Social Care Act 2001
Human Fertilisation and Embryology Act 1990
Human Tissue Act 1961
Human Rights Act 1998
Medicines Act 1968
Misuse of Drugs Act 1971
Mental Health Act 1983
Mental Health Act 1983 Revised Code of Practice
Public Interest Disclosure Act 1998

Northern Ireland

N Ireland Mental Health (N Ireland) Order 1986
Code of Practice Mental Health (N Ireland) Order 1986

Scotland

Adults with Incapacity (Scotland) Act 2000
Mental Health (Public Safety and Appeals) (Scotland) Act 1999

34

Guidelines for company-sponsored safety assessment of marketed medicines (SAMM)

Association of the British Pharmaceutical Industry

Introduction

It is well-recognised that there is a continuous need to monitor the safety of medicines as they are used in clinical practice. Spontaneous reporting schemes (e.g. the UK yellow card system) provide important early warning signals of potential drug hazards and also provide a means of continuous surveillance. Formal studies to evaluate safety may also be necessary, particularly in the confirmation and characterisation of possible hazards identified at an earlier stage of drug development. Such studies may also be useful in identifying previously unsuspected reactions.

Scope of guidelines

These guidelines apply to the conduct of all company-sponsored studies which evaluate the safety of marketed products. They take the place of previous guidelines on post-marketing surveillance which were published in 1988 (BMJ, 296: 399–400). Studies performed under those guidelines were found to have some notable limitations (BMJ, 1992, 304: 1470–1472) and these new guidelines have been prepared in response to the problems identified. The major changes may be summarised as follows:

1 The scope of the guidelines has been expanded to include all company-sponsored studies which are carried out to evaluate safety of marketed medicines. It should be emphasised that this includes both studies conducted in general practice and in the hospital setting. The name of the guidelines has been changed to reflect the emphasis on safety assessment rather than merely surveillance.

2 The guidelines have been developed to provide a framework on which a variety of data collection methods can be used to improve the evaluation of the safety of marketed medicines. Whilst it is recognised that the design used needs to be tailored to particular drugs and hazards, the guidelines define the essential principles which may be applied in a variety of situations. The study methods in this field continue to develop and therefore there will be a need to review regularly these guidelines to ensure that they reflect advances made in the assessment of drug safety.

The guidelines have been formulated and agreed by a Working Party which includes representation from the Medicines Control Agency (MCA), Committee on Safety of Medicines (CSM), Association of the British Pharmaceutical Industry (ABPI), British Medical Association (BMA) and the Royal College of General Practitioners (RCGP). Other guidelines exist for the conduct of 'Phase IV clinical trials' where the medication is provided by the sponsoring company (see section 2(b) below). Some of these studies will also meet the definition of a SAMM study (see below) and should therefore also comply with the present guidelines.

1 Definition of safety assessment of marketed medicines

(a) Safety assessment of marketed medicines (SAMM) is defined as 'a formal investigation conducted for the purpose of assessing the clinical safety of marketed medicine(s) in clinical practice'.

(b) Any study of a marketed drug which has the evaluation of clinical safety as a specific objective should be included. Safety evaluation will be a specific objective in postmarketing studies either when there is a known safety issue under investigation and/or when the numbers of patients to be included will add significantly to the existing safety data for the product(s).

Smaller studies conducted primarily for other purposes should not be considered as SAMM studies. However, if a study which is not conducted for the purpose of evaluating safety unexpectedly identifies a hazard, the manufacturer would be expected to inform the MCA immediately and the section of these guidelines covering liaison with regulatory authorities would thereafter apply.

In cases of doubt as to whether or not a study comes under the scope of the guidelines the sponsor should discuss the intended study plan with the MCA.

2 Scope and objectives of SAMM

(a) SAMM may be conducted for the purpose of identifying previously unrecognised safety issues (hypothesis-generation) or to investigate possible hazards (hypothesis-testing).

(b) A variety of designs may be appropriate including observational cohort studies, case-surveillance or case-control studies. Clinical trials may also be used to evaluate the safety of marketed products, involving systematic allocation of treatment (for example randomisation). Such studies must also adhere to the current guidelines for Phase IV clinical trials.

(c) The design to be used will depend on the objectives of the study, which must be clearly defined in the study plan. Any specific safety concerns to be investigated should be identified in the study plan and explicitly addressed by the proposed methods.

3 Design of studies

Observational cohort studies

(a) The population studied should be as representative as possible of the general population of users, and be unselected unless specifically targeted by the objectives of the study (for example a study of the elderly). Exclusion criteria should be limited to the contraindications stated in the data sheet or summary of product characteristics (SPC). The prescriber should be provided with a data sheet or SPC for all products to be used. Where the product is prescribed outside the indications on the data sheet, such patients should be included in the analysis of the study findings.

(b) Observational cohort studies should normally include appropriate comparator group(s). The comparator group(s) will usually include patients with the disease/indication(s) relevant to the primary study drug and such patients will usually be treated with alternative therapies.

(c) The product(s) should be prescribed in the usual manner, for example on an FP10 form written by the general practitioner or through the usual hospital procedures.

(d) Patients must not be prescribed particular medicines in order to include them in observational cohort studies since this is unethical (see section 15 of the 'Guidelines on the Practices of Ethics Committees in Medical Research involving Human Subjects', Royal College of Physicians, 1990).

(e) The prescribing of a drug and the inclusion of the patient in a study are two issues which must be clearly separated. Drugs must be prescribed solely as a result of a normal clinical evaluation, and since such indications may vary from doctor to doctor a justification for the prescription should be recorded in the study documents. In contrast, the inclusion of the patient in the study must be solely dependent upon the criteria for recruitment which have been specifically identified in the study procedures. Any deviation from the study criteria for recruitment could lead to selection bias.

(f) The study plan should stipulate the maximum number of patients to be entered by a single doctor. No patient should be prospectively entered into more than one study simultaneously.

Case-control studies

(g) Case-control studies are usually conducted retrospectively. In case-control studies comparison is made between the history of drug exposure of cases with the disease of interest and appropriate controls without the disease. The study design should attempt to account for known sources of bias and confounding.

Case-surveillance

(h) The purpose of case-surveillance is to study patients with diseases which are likely to be drug-related and to ascertain drug exposure. Companies who sponsor such studies should liaise particularly closely with the MCA in order to determine the most appropriate arrangements for the reporting of cases.

Clinical trials

(i) Large clinical trials are sometimes useful in the investigation of post-marketing safety issues and these may involve random allocation to treatment. In other respects, an attempt should be made to study patients under as normal conditions as possible. Exclusion criteria should be limited to the contraindications in the data sheet or SPC unless they are closely related to the particular objectives of the study. Clinical trials must also adhere to the current guidelines for Phase IV clinical trials (see 2(b) above). Studies which fulfil the definition of SAMM but are performed under a clinical trial exemption (CTX) or under the clinical trial on a marketed product (CTMP) scheme are within the scope of these guidelines.

4 Conduct of studies

(a) Responsibility for the conduct and quality of company-sponsored studies shall be vested in the company's medical department under the supervision of a named medical practitioner registered in the United Kingdom, and whose name shall be recorded in the study documents.

(b) Where a study is performed for a company by an agent, a named medical practitioner registered in the United Kingdom shall be identified by the agent to supervise the study and liaise with the company's medical department.

(c) Consideration should be given to the appointment of an independent advisory group(s) to monitor the safety information and oversee the study.

5 Liaison with regulatory authorities

(a) Companies proposing to perform a SAMM study are encouraged to discuss the draft study plan with the Medicines Control Agency (MCA) at an early state. Particular consideration should be given to specific safety issues which may require investigation.

(b) Before the study commences a study plan should be finalised which explains the aims and objectives of the study, the methods to be used (including statistical analysis) and the record keeping which is to be maintained. The company shall submit the study plan plus any proposed initial communications to doctors to the MCA at least one month before the planned start of the study. The MCA will review the proposed study and may comment. The responsibility for the conduct of the study will, however, rest with the sponsoring pharmaceutical company.

(c) The company should inform the MCA when the study has commenced and will normally provide a brief report on its progress at least every six months, or more frequently if required by MCA.

(d) The regulatory requirements for reporting of suspected adverse reactions must be fulfilled. Companies should endeavour to ensure that they are notified of serious suspected adverse reactions and should report these to the MCA within 15 days of receipt. Events which are not suspected by the investigator to be adverse reactions should not be reported individually as they occur. These and minor adverse reactions should be included in the final report.

(e) A final report on the study should be sent to the MCA within 3 months of follow-up being completed. Ideally this should be a full report but a brief report within 3 months followed by a full report within 6 months of completion of the study would normally be acceptable. The findings of the study should be submitted for publication.

(f) Companies are encouraged to follow MCA guidelines on the content of progress reports and final reports.

6 Promotion of medicines

(a) SAMM studies should not be conducted for the purposes of promotion.

(b) Company representatives should not be involved in SAMM studies in such a way that it could be seen as a promotional exercise.

7 Doctor participation

(a) Subject to the doctor's terms of service, payment may be offered to the doctor in recompense for his time and any expenses incurred according to the suggested scale of fees published by the BMA.

(b) No inducement for a doctor to participate in a SAMM study should be offered, requested or given.

8 Ethical issues

(a) The highest possible standards of professional conduct and confidentiality must always be maintained. The patient's right to confidentiality is paramount. The patient's identity in the study documents should be codified and only his or her doctor should be capable of decoding it.

(b) Responsibility for the retrieval of information from personal medical records lies with the consultant or general practitioner responsible for the patient's care. Such information should be directed to the medical practitioner nominated by the company or agent, who is thereafter responsible for the handling of such information.

(c) Reference to a Research Ethics Committee is required if patients are to be approached for information, additional investigations are to be performed or if it is proposed to allocate patients systematically to treatments.

9 Procedure for complaints

A study which gives cause for concern on scientific, ethical or promotional grounds should be referred to the MCA, ABPI and the company concerned. Concerns regarding possible scientific fraud should be referred to the ABPI.

They will be investigated and, if appropriate, referred to the General Medical Council.

10 Review of guidelines

The Working Party will review these guidelines as necessary.

Association of the British Pharmaceutical Industry (ABPI)
British Medical Association (BMA)
Committee on Safety of Medicines (CSM)
Medicines Control Agency (MCA)
Royal College of General Practitioners (RCGP)

35

Guidelines for medical experiments in non-patient human volunteers

Association of the British Pharmaceutical Industry

1 Introduction

1.1 The Association of the British Pharmaceutical Industry (ABPI) established a committee in 1969, under the Chairmanship of Sir Charles Stuart-Harris, to investigate and advise on medical experiments involving pharmaceutical company staff volunteers. The report of this Committee, issued in 1970, set a standard of practice for member companies to provide safeguards for staff volunteers in drug studies. These published guidelines also acted as a basis for volunteer studies organised outside the pharmaceutical industry. However, research practices and opinions have inevitably changed during the past eighteen years, and these are not fully reflected in the 1984 updated commentary on the 1970 Stuart-Harris report.

1.2 In October 1986 the Royal College of Physicians published a report entitled 'Research on Healthy Volunteers'. The Association subsequently set up a Working Party to reconsider its own position, to review current guidelines related to volunteer studies, and to draft new ones. These guidelines take account of the conclusions reached by the Royal College of Physicians. The membership of the Working Party is shown in Appendix D.

1.3 In its 1970 report and the 1984 Update, the ABPI referred to staff and human volunteers, but did not define the term volunteer. Key elements in the definition of a non-patient volunteer are that the individual cannot be expected to derive therapeutic benefits from the proposed study, is not known to suffer any significant illness relevant to the proposed study, and whose mental state is such that he is able to understand and freely give valid consent to the study. This definition embraces the term 'healthy volunteer'.

1.4 Volunteer studies must only be undertaken when the appropriate aims, objectives, and methodologies are clearly defined and set out in a written, approved protocol.

1.5 No reference was made in the 1970 or 1984 documents to the payment which may be required by investigators in non-patient volunteer studies. That was because the previous guidelines referred exclusively to medical experiments on staff volunteers. It is recognised that volunteer studies sponsored by industry are conducted outside the premises of member companies, and a statement is therefore included on payment to investigators. (6.3).

1.6 The previous ABPI guidelines (1970 and 1984) stated that only new experimental designs such as the administration of a new chemical entity required the programme of work envisaged to be submitted to and approved by an independent and properly constituted Ethics Committee. It is now strongly recommended that all volunteer study protocols be submitted to and approved by an independent and properly constituted Ethics Committee. The definitive report on Ethics Committees, supported by the ABPI, is the 1984 document entitled 'Guidelines on the Practice of Ethics Committees in Medical Research' published by the Royal College of Physicians of London.

1.7 Companies conducting in-house volunteer studies should follow these ABPI guidelines, and should require that all volunteer studies conducted on their behalf should also follow the guidelines.

2 Justification for volunteer studies, and the assessment of risk

2.1 Medical experiments on human subjects are necessary to obtain information on the effects of substances intended to be used for diagnostic, prophylactic or therapeutic purpose. The justification for testing any agent in healthy individuals depends upon not only the importance of the information that can be obtained by this means but also the risks involved in obtaining it.

2.2 The acquisition of knowledge of the safety, pharmacokinetics and pharmacodynamics of a new medicine in man is important for the design of clinical trials in patients. While tests on volunteers may be desirable at any stage in the development of a medicinal product and the elucidation of its mode of action, they are of particular importance during the initial stages of investigation in man. Prophylactic agents such as vaccines must be entirely evaluated in people who are apparently healthy, so the use of volunteers for such studies is unavoidable and the justification depends upon laboratory evidence of potential efficacy and safety. Different considerations arise with respect to therapeutic agents, the efficacy and related safety of which can only be evaluated in patients. Human volunteer studies nevertheless enable those responsible for the development of a new medicine to understand better the way it is absorbed and metabolised before beginning to study its clinical effect in patients.

2.3 Volunteer studies should only be conducted after appropriate pre-clinical biological studies (toxicology, pharmacology, and drug metabolism) and chemistry and pharmaceutical development have been undertaken. Where a new chemical entity is involved the toxicological work should normally be equivalent to that which would be undertaken in support of a CTX or CTC for studies involving patients at the same stage of a medicine's development (Ref: Guidelines on Data Needed to Support the Administration of New Chemical Entities to Non-Patient Volunteers, ABPI. May, 1985).

2.4 The value of pharmacological studies in healthy volunteers justifies their acceptance as a normal phase in the investigation of a medicine prior to its use in patients. Such studies are not mandatory and volunteer studies should not be performed if they involve medicines whose identifiable toxicity or lack of safety is only compensated for by their potential unique efficacy. Such substances must be evaluated after their initial pre-clinical pharmacological evaluation by observations on their therapeutic activity in patients.

3 Recruitment of volunteers

3.1 Volunteers must be recruited of their own free will. They should initially be made aware of the possibility of volunteering by means of a general notice, rather than by direct approach, so that the initiative for volunteering rests entirely with the individual. Widespread or public advertising, especially if it is aimed at the poor, needy or socially disadvantaged, is unacceptable. Neither payment, nor the level thereof, should be mentioned in a public notice. This principle should apply wherever studies are conducted. No member of staff, student or other persons should be made to feel under obligation to volunteer, nor should they be disadvantaged in any way by not volunteering. The principles ennshrined in the WMA Declaration of Helsinki as revised in 1975 (Tokyo) and 1983 (Venice) should be upheld.

3.2 No volunteer should be recruited unless capable of giving legally valid consent. All volunteers must be fully and properly informed so as to allow clear understanding of the nature and purpose of the proposed study. Any risks, either known or suspected, and any inconvenience, discomfort or pain likely to be experienced should be made clear to prospective volunteers, who must make their own decision on whether to participate or not. Volunteers should be informed verbally and in writing that they are free to withdraw from a study at any time and without explanation or reason, and that the registered medical practitioner in charge of the trial may withdraw them at any time if he considers it appropriate.

3.3 All establishments conducting volunteer studies must keep accurate records and avoid the excessive use of any volunteer. It is difficult to stipulate the maximum participation for any individual volunteer because of the variety of procedures and medicines involved; however, no person should take part in more than one study at a time, nor should any person receive a new chemical entity administered systemically at study intervals of less than four months. Account should taken of such facts as the total exposure to test substances in any one year, and the total volume of blood taken in the year.

4 Monitoring exposure

4.1 There are three ways in which study participation may be monitored and excess participation prevented: by contact with the general practitioner (in the United Kingdom); by counselling the volunteer and supplying the volunteer with a record card; and by maintaining a register within a department conducting volunteer studies.

4.2 Potential volunteers should sign a form prior to each study giving the name and address of their general practitioner consenting to any approach which is made and consenting to the provision of relevant information by the general practitioner. If contact is made by a pharmaceutical company it should be the registered medical practitioner responsible for the study who contacts the general practitioner.

4.3   Volunteers should themselves be given a record card which gives relevant details of the studies in which they have taken part and dosages of drugs and details of radioactive exposure for which there are safety limits which should be recorded. They should be counselled appropriately on the potential dangers of excessive volunteering.

4.4   It is the responsibility of the establishment to maintain its own register of volunteers who have participated in studies. The volunteer establishment should maintain full records of studies and volunteers for a minimum of five years after the study is completed.

5 Special groups

Pregnancy

5.1   Women of childbearing potential should not normally be accepted as volunteers in early studies. In studies which involve drugs likely to be used in the treatment of women, volunteers who are women of childbearing potential may be accepted subject to the approval of an independent ethics committee. In this situation adequate safeguards must be taken to ensure absence of conception of a pre-existing pregnancy. Satisfactory reproductive toxicology studies must have been performed.

Children

5.2   Children should not normally be used in volunteer studies of pharmaceutically active substances.

Elderly

5.3   As the elderly may be at special risk their use in volunteer studies should be generally avoided. When it is likely that a substance will be used extensively in elderly patients, however, or where the effects of a medicine and its metabolism may be different in the elderly, then the use of elderly volunteers may be justified.

Mentally handicapped

5.4   Volunteer studies in the mentally handicapped cannot be justified.

Prisoners

5.5   Prisoners should never be used in volunteer studies.

6 Financial and other inducements

Reward

6.1   Volunteers may be rewarded in cash or in kind, but the amount should be reasonable and related to the nature and degree of inconvenience and discomfort involved. Payment should never be offered for undergoing risk. Payment of excessive amounts is discouraged especially as this may lead to inappropriate repeated volunteering solely for financial gain. Attention is therefore drawn to paragraph 3.3 regarding the maximum participation by any individual.

Withdrawal

6.2   When a volunteer withdraws or is withdrawn from a study for medical reasons related to the study, full payments should be made. If the volunteer withdraws for other reasons, including non-related medical reasons, a proportional payment may be made at the discretion of the investigator.

Investigators

6.3   Payments to investigators and institutions must be seen to be at a reasonable level for the work involved.

7 Safeguards

7.1   Great care and precautions must be taken before experiments on volunteers are commenced. It is the responsibility of the investigator to confirm that a volunteer is healthy, and suitable for inclusion in the study against carefully pre-determined criteria.

7.2   Volunteers for studies should be screened by a clinician who should take an appropriate medical history including reference to allergies, smoking, alcohol or consumption of other medically active substances. This screening must take place shortly before the study begins. The medical examination should be appropriate to the study proposed including relevant blood, urine or other tests. If the history, examination, or tests show any abnormality that could be associated with an increased risk for the individual if he or she participated in the study, the volunteer should not take part. Any evidence of drug abuse including alcohol, should also preclude acceptance of the volunteer into the study.

7.3   All volunteer studies must be supervised by a medical practitioner fully registered in the United Kingdom, who is a fully paid up member of a recognised medical defence body. This practitioner should have appropriate facilities and experience to cope with any foreseeable medical contingency, should sign each protocol and consent form, and should be familiar with resuscitation techniques and capable of using the available equipment. He also has responsibility for the well being of the volunteers and may withdraw them at any time during the study.

7.4   All volunteers should be supervised during the administration of a medicine and for an appropriate period thereafter and advised to take appropriate precautions should the known or suspected effects of the medicine so demand. For example, any volunteer taking a medicine which is likely to cause drowsiness should not be allowed to drive or work with dangerous machinery or chemicals. (The volunteer should be advised of this in advance.) Details of any drug given to a volunteer must be recorded on a document to be carried by the volunteer, and this document must also give the telephone number(s) of the medical staff who can be contacted on a 24 hours a day basis in an emergency.

7.5   The initial dose in the first study of a new chemical entity should be well below the amount indicated as pharmacologically active in humans by previous animal studies, and only a small percentage of the no-toxic effect in animals.

7.6   Safeguards regarding communicable diseases must be taken to protect the volunteer, the investigator and all other staff involved including remote laboratory staff. Investigators should refer to the guidelines prepared by the ABPI Working Party on the handling of blood samples (1987). Volunteers found on initial examination to have medical contra-indications against participation in the study should be clearly advised of the reasons for their exclusion, and appropriately counselled. This will usually be by informing the volunteer's own general practitioner, with the consent of the volunteer.

7.7   Any adverse events occurring during a volunteer study should be followed up as appropriate.

7.8   The supervising doctor should pay particular regard to the possible need to follow up volunteers who withdraw from a study.

8 Suitability of facilities

8.1   Premises in which non-patient volunteer studies are conducted should be custom equipped and designed and be adequate for the purpose, including the provision of appropriate resuscitation equipment. Staff must have been properly trained in the use of this equipment. The facilities should be of the high standard expected for the involvement of healthy persons in experiments, and should be open to scrutiny by members of the independent Ethics Committee which considers the protocols for the studies conducted in each specific centre.

8.2   Member companies should satisfy themselves that studies conducted on their behalf by other establishments are conducted in premises which at minimum fulfil the above criteria.

8.3   Consideration will be given by ABPI to the compilation of a directory of centres conducting studies on volunteers, listing all the facilities available within each centre, as suggested by the Medicines Commission (advice to Health Ministers on Healthy Volunteer Studies, DHSS, June 1987).

8.4   This directory should include pharmaceutical companies, contract houses, academic departments, medical schools, and any hospitals conducting volunteer studies.

9 Design and protocol

9.1   Research involving non-patient volunteers should conform to the highest ethical and scientific standards which apply to all clinical research. Ethical standards should apply in accordance with the Guidelines on the Practice of Ethics Committees in Medical Research published by the Royal College of Physicians of London in 1984.

9.2   The protocol should define the experiment, and contain an account of the information that will be provided to the volunteer. References should also be made to the provision of a formal agreement and consent form. A model outline protocol is detailed in Appendix A. Every volunteer study protocol must be submitted to and approved by an independent Ethics Committee prior to the administration of the test substances.

9.3   Animal studies must have been carried out appropriate to the particular pharmaceutical form to be used in the volunteer study, except where the test substance is already a licensed product. These will be referred to in the protocol and have the following objectives:
   i) to determine the target organ and toxic effects in animals of relatively large doses, repeated at intervals depending on the test substance's biological and toxicological properties and the proposed human dosage and usage
   ii) to demonstrate that the preparation elicits the required pharmacological response in experimental animals

that are likely to be analogous to the desired effects in man

iii) to attempt to define the absorption, distribution, metabolism and excretion of the test compound.

10 Ethics committees

10.1 All studies involving the administration of substances to non-patient volunteers, must have a written protocol submitted to and approved in writing by an appropriate independent Ethics Committee before the study begins.

10.2 Pharmaceutical companies contracting outside establishments to conduct volunteer studies on their behalf must ensure that protocols have been submitted to and approved by an independent Ethics Committee.

10.3 Once ethical approval has been given for the study, the supervision of the study becomes the sole responsibility of the named registered medical practitioners sponsoring and supervising the study. However, major protocol amendments should be referred to the Committee or its Chairman, and no further test substances should be administered before approval is received.

11 Consent and study administration

11.1 All volunteers participating in a clinical study must sign a simple form of agreement that records the basis upon which they have agreed to participate in the study. This agreement may be either with the sponsoring pharmaceutical company or the outside research establishment depending upon which is primarily responsible for recruitment and supervision of the study. The sponsoring company should ensure that it is fully satisfied with any agreements to be used by the outside research establishment.

11.2 The agreement should

i) evidence the fact that the volunteer has consented to participate in the light of proper explanation from the investigator of the nature and purpose of the study and any foreseeable risks attaching to participation.

ii) record that the volunteer has been told he is free to withdraw without need to justify that decision.

iii) deal with the issue of confidentiality and the agreement of the volunteer to disclosure of information generated by the study.

iv) if the investigator deems it appropriate to do so, authorise the investigator to contact the volunteer's general practitioner and authorise the general practitioner to disclose any information concerning the volunteer's health relevant to participation of the study.

Any information arising during the course of the study which the investigator wishes to be conveyed to the general practitioner or occupational physician should be the subject of further authorisation by the volunteer.

All records containing information about volunteers should be treated as confidential and, for staff volunteers, should be kept separate from other personnel records (preferably in the Medical Department). It must be recognised that they may become subject to disclosure in any legal proceedings where they are relevant to the issues in those proceedings.

11.4 It is good practice for the investigator to sign a corresponding statement, incorporated into the agreement or attached to it, to the effect that he has counselled the volunteer on the study and given the volunteer the opportunity to question him on any points felt by the volunteer to require clarification.

11.5 The explanation given by the investigator to the volunteer should be witnessed and the witness may reasonably be asked to sign a statement confirming this fact.

11.6 The information document, provided to the volunteer in connection with the study, should be referred to in the agreement and copy attached. Companies should make every effort to ensure that the information document is comprehensible to the volunteer. The following points should be considered for inclusion in that document:

a confirmation of the principal features of the study;

b procedures to be used if assistance or advice is required;

c that the volunteer should at all times carry the personal record card giving details of the study;

d that the implications of his agreement to participate, in terms of any insurance cover that he may already have or may happen to be negotiating at the time, have been drawn to the volunteer's attention;

e that the study has been subject to review by an independent ethics committee;

and

f that the volunteer will disclose relevant medical information during the course of the study;

A model information document appears as Appendix C.

11.7 The agreement should clearly record the obligation the pharmaceutical company or research establishment has accepted in terms of financial rewards for participation and compensation in the event of injury. In particular, the volunteer should be given a clear commitment that in the event of bodily injury he will receive appropriate compensation without having to prove either that such injury arose through negligence or that the product was defective in the sense that it did not fulfil a reasonable expectation of safety. The agreement should not seek to remove that right of the volunteer, as an alternative, to pursue a claim on the basis of either negligence or strict liability if he is so minded.

11.8 Where pharmaceutical companies sponsor studies to be performed in outside research establishments, the responsibility for paying compensation would be clarified and reflected in the contractual documentation with the volunteer. Where the sponsor company is to provide the undertaking regarding compensation, it is recommended that the sponsor company enters into an unqualified obligation to pay compensation, it is recommended that the sponsor company enters into an unqualified obligation to pay compensation to the volunteer on proof of causation, having previously protected its rights to recourse against the research establishment in its agreement with that establishment, to cover the position where the negligence of its contractor may have caused or contributed to the injury by the volunteer. A volunteer can reasonably expect that compensation will be paid quickly and that any dispute regarding who will finally bear the cost of the compensation paid to him will be resolved separately by the other parties to the research.

11.9 It is recommended that a simple arbitration clause is included as part of the provisions concerning compensation for injury, whereby any difference or dispute in relation to the implementation of the compensation provisions may be resolved with a minimum of formality.

11.10 A model agreement, which is drawn on the basis that the pharmaceutical company is conducting the research in-house, appears as Appendix B. Where the research is performed elsewhere two documents may need preparation, the first dealing with the provisions relating to compensation for injury and the second dealing with all other matters relevant to the contractual relationship with the volunteer.

12 Conclusion

12.1 Medical experiments on non-patient volunteers constitute an essential step towards the development of many medicinal products. Information from such experiments is indispensible for the scientific assessment and development of most new medicines. These guidelines aim to provide a framework within which these studies can be conducted.

Amendments to ABPI guidelines for medical experiments in non patient human volunteers

Replacement for existing Paragraph 4.2

4.2 Potential volunteers should sign a form prior to each study giving the name and address of their general practitioner consenting to any approach which is made and consenting to the provision of relevant information by the general practitioner. In the case of staff volunteers, it would be good practice to treat the provision of such information as subject to the Access to Medical Reports Act 1988. Accordingly, applications to general practitioners should not be made without staff volunteers having first been informed of their rights under the Act. The Act is concerned with reports provided in connection with employment or insurance and, in summary, enables employees to see the report before it is passed on to the employer and to suggest appropriate amendments. If the medical practitioner refuses to amend it, the employee may:
  i) withdraw consent for the report to be issued;
  ii) ask the medical practitioner to attach to the report a statement setting out the employee's own views;
  iii) agree to the report being issued unchanged.
If contact is made by a pharmaceutical company it should be the registered medical practitioner responsible for the study who contacts the general practitioner.

Appendix B to the guidelines:

Replacement for existing Clause 4 of the Draft Provisions for the Volunteer Agreement and Consent Form.
4. I agree to Dr[   ] contacting my general practitioner [and teaching or university authority if appropriate] to make known my participation in the study and I authorise my general practitioner to report details of my relevant medical or drug history, in confidence. [For staff volunteers] I have been informed of and understand my rights under the Access to Medical Reports Act 1988.

May 1990

36

Facilities for non-patient volunteer studies

Association of the British Pharmaceutical Industry

Facilities for non-patient volunteer studies

Both the ABPI and the Royal College of Physicians have recently issued guidelines for the Conduct of Non-Patient Volunteer Studies. The ABPI proposals include a recommendation that a register of the units conducting these studies should be established. The ABPI Non-Patient Volunteers Working Party considered that registration would only be meaningful if criteria were established to ensure that the facilities provided by the units conducting Non-Patient Volunteer Studies were appropriate for the safe conduct of these studies. The document that follows sets out guidelines on standards which should be set for such facilities.

Guidelines on standards for the facilities in which studies on non-patient volunteers are conducted

The following proposals are intended to be read in conjunction with the ABPI Guidelines for the conduct of Non-Patient Volunteer Studies and are a standard towards which the ABPI would expect a volunteer facility to aim prior to the initiation of a full range of clinical pharmacology studies.

1 Facilities

1.1 The building should be purpose built or appropriately modified and must meet local planning requirements and safety (fire) requirements.

1.2 The unit should be large enough to allow the separation of ward, laboratory, administration, catering and toilet facilities.

© Association of the British Pharmaceutical Industry.

1.3 The unit must be easily accessible to emergency services and construction of doorways and corridors should allow the easy movement of a stretcher patient.

1.4 If not attached to a hospital, the unit should have easy road access for an ambulance.

1.5 The unit should be situated in reasonable proximity to a hospital with a casualty unit and intensive care facilities.

1.6 An overnight facility should be available for volunteers considered unfit to be sent home after a study, plus accommodation for doctors, nurses and any other necessary staff.

1.7 The facility should be so constructed or equipped that adequate monitoring of all volunteers can be achieved from at least one position.

1.8 To preserve confidentiality, visual and physical access to areas where volunteers are studied should be restricted to authorised personnel.

1.9 Emergency lighting should be available in the event of a failure of the electricity supply.

2 Staff

There should be a sufficient number of staff, appropriately qualified according to the number and nature of studies to be undertaken by the unit including the following:

2.1 A medically qualified practitioner (the Study Director) who should be responsible for all medical aspects of the study. This person should:

2.1.1 Be suitably qualified with relevant experience in the areas of work to be undertaken. The following requirements are preferred although not all are essential.

(a) Post graduate medical qualification, eg MRCP, FRCS.

(b) Three years post full registration experience.

(c) Experience of at least 2 years as a clinical pharmacologist in industry with maintained clinical contact and supervision by an experienced clinical pharmacologist

and/or

Specialist training and experience in specific therapeutic areas as registrar, consultant or lecturer in a recognised unit.

2.1.2 Be fully conversant with Good Laboratory Practice, Good Clinical Practice, local Regulatory Authority Guidelines, and the requirements of the Declaration of Helsinki as amended at Tokyo and Venice.

2.1.3 Be fully conversant with modern emergency and resuscitation procedures and attend refresher courses at least once per year in addition to regular practice sessions in his/her own particular unit.

2.2 At least one additional back-up medically qualified staff who should also meet the requirements of 2.1.1. to 2.1.3. above should be available and close at hand.

2.3 Where the size of the unit justifies, a medically qualified Unit Director should be appointed, ultimately responsible for all medical aspects of studies and who should have experience relevant to the kind of study being undertaken and a training exemplified by:

a) at least 2 years' experience as a clinical pharmacologist in industry,

and/or

b) experience of at least 2 years at registrar grade or above in a university-recognised clinical pharmacology or therapeutics department, and

c) a postgraduate medical diploma or qualification or accreditation in medicine or clinical pharmacology, and be conversant with emergency and resuscitation procedures.

2.4 One or more RGN qualified nursing staff, one of whom should be of a senior status (sister/charge nurse), ideally with intensive care unit experience. They should have responsibility for the general welfare of the volunteers and should carry out technical procedures as directed by the study physician. Each of the nursing staff should:

2.4.1 Be adequately qualified and experienced in this work which he/she will undertake.

2.4.2 Be fully conversant in modern emergency and resuscitation procedures and attend a refresher course at least every two years.

2.4.3 Participate in regular reviews of the unit resuscitation procedures at least every six months.

2.5 Sufficient adequately qualified laboratory staff in the areas listed in 4 (below) to ensure that studies are conducted and reported to standards required by the sponsor, guidelines on Good Laboratory Practice, and Good Clinical Research Practice, and various Regulatory Authorities.

3 Emergency procedures and equipment

The unit should have established procedures, have standard equipment and provide the staff with adequate training in order to deal with any emergency that arises during a volunteer study as follows:

3.1 Procedures

3.1.1 A standard operating procedure for dealing in the first instance, with the most likely emergency situations such as: cardiac arrest, anaphylaxis, hypotension.

3.1.2 A standard operating procedure for summoning additional help and transfer of the subjects to hospital facilities.

3.1.3 A standard operating procedure for providing adequate medical cover for the volunteers throughout the study period.

3.1.4 A standard operating procedure for 'Call-Out' so that volunteers may be in telephone contact with the supervising physician should problems arise outside normal working hours.

3.1.5 A standard operating procedure that ensures that adverse drug reactions and adverse events are reported without delay, so that other ongoing studies may be modified or discontinued as required.

3.1.6 A designated area where all study documentation including randomisation code is kept for emergency access.

3.1.7 A procedure which allows any doctor with clinical responsibility for the general medical care of the volunteer, and who is not familiar with the experimental drug, to get in contact with someone who is familiar with it.

Additionally, evidence that regular training is given and assessment of individuals made in the above procedures should be on record.

3.2 Emergency equipment

The following is a suggested list of equipment to provide basic and essential emergency cover:

1) Blood pressure monitoring and recording equipment.
2) Continuous multi-lead ECG monitor with facility for permanently recording any trace.
3) Defibrillator.
4) Cardiac pacer, unless this is always carried by the local cardiac arrest crash team.
5) Tilting beds, or blocks to enable beds to be tilted.
6) Alarm call system for summoning assistance, including nearby telephone with permanent access to a public line.
7) Emergency trolley carrying oxygen plus its delivery apparatus and instruments for procedures such as intubation, emergency tracheostomy and canullation.
8) Suitable fluids for IV infusion.
9) Equipment for immediate measurement of blood glucose levels, but only if studies are to be conducted using medicines likely to cause hypoglycaemia.
10) A procedure for regular testing of the above equipment and documenting the inspection should be implemented.
11) A back-up power supply for lighting and essential equipment expected to be required for an emergency.
12) Ambu bag, or equivalent, for assisted ventilation.
13) Aspiration equipment.

N.B. The ECG monitor/defibrillator should be operable by battery as well as mains; this is important if transferring a subject to hospital.

3.3 Emergency medicines

The unit should have a secure pharmacy area with adequate facilities for the correct and accurate preparation and storage of the test drug and standard medicines. In addition, one section of the pharmacy area should be devoted to medicines for emergency use, which should be secure but immediately accessible when required. The emergency area should contain:

3.3.1 A specific antidote for the medicine(s) being tested (when available).

3.3.2 The following medicines which will be kept in the ward area along with the equipment when a study is in progress:
(See Appendix I)

3.3.3 A list of the expiry dates or shelf life of the medicines, which should be checked regularly.

4 Supporting services

In order for the unit to conduct work to the standard required by the Sponsor, GLP, GCP, and Regulatory Authorities, the following are required:

4.1 Studies to be conducted by the unit will have been approved by an independent properly constituted Ethics Committee.

4.2 The Ethics Committee will have access to the unit to inspect.

4.3 Adequately equipped and staffed chemical pathology and haematology laboratories and assay facilities.

4.4 A specially designated, secure pharmacy area with appropriate medicine storage facilities, staff and equipment for preparing the correct does of the test substance and keeping precise records of the receipt, use and disposal of test medicines.

4.5 Access to legal advisers who will assist in relation to questions such as consent, compensation and insurance affecting the unit, its staff and volunteers.

4.6 Sufficient competent administrative, secretarial and domestic staff to ensure that study procedures and documentation and correspondence are complete, adequately recorded and filed.

4.7 An agreed contingency arrangement for the admission of volunteers to a local hospital should the need arise.

5 Records and archiving

The Unit and its staff have a responsibility to ensure that adequate records are kept of each study and that they are filed and kept for a specified period, and that on request they are easily retrievable. The unit should:

5.1 Assign a specific person(s) to the filing and archiving of clinical study data.

5.2 Assign a specific area of the unit as an archive where data are kept in secure, locked, fireproof metal cabinets.

37

Multi-centre research in the NHS – the process of ethical review when there is no local researcher

Supplementary operational guidelines for NHS research ethics committees – November 2000 (v2)

Central Office for Research Ethics Committees

1 Introduction

1.1 Many research projects undertaken in the NHS take place across numerous sites, sometimes clustered together, but often spread widely throughout the country. It is a requirement that all such multi-centre research has a named *"principal investigator"*, who has the prime ethical responsibility for the project and its implementation throughout the UK. This is the individual who applies to a Research Ethics Committee (REC) for ethical approval of the protocol, which includes the patient information sheet and the proposed arrangements for taking consent.

1.2 For much multi-centre research, especially where a modification of the standard patient treatment is involved (e.g. therapeutic research, clinical trials), there is a clear role for a *"local researcher"* at each research site. This person takes local responsibility for the research project, and there is thus a need for local scrutiny of the suitability of this individual and the local research facilities.

1.3 This is in direct contrast to some types of *non-therapeutic* research, where there is no need for a local individual to be formally part of the research team. In some of these cases there is no need for any direct contact with the patient or research subject. In others, further patient contact needs to be made only by the principal investigator or members of the specialist research team, once patient consent is obtained. This is particularly, but not exclusively, the case for much epidemiological and health services research. [Conversely some projects in these disciplines still retain a distinct need for a named local researcher, just as in the case of

therapeutic research, and therefore each project needs to be considered individually].

1.4 In many instances, although there is a need for further patient contact, this can be carried out very efficiently and safely, and much more conveniently for the patient, simply by using the technical *co-operation* of the patient's local clinician(s) without designating them as "local researchers".

2 Background

2.1 Experience by local and multi-centre research ethics committees (LRECs and MRECs) in reviewing research proposals has exposed the need for a more efficient way of undertaking the ethical review of projects where there is no need for someone to be designated as a local researcher. Many LRECs themselves have questioned the need for a local REC opinion in these cases, as long as sufficient safeguards are confirmed to be in place during the ethical review of the protocol by another REC in the NHS.

2.2 A working party was established to look at the complex issues and possible solutions. It was chaired by Dr Hugh Davies, Chairman of London MREC. The membership is shown in Annex A. A report from the Davies group was circulated to all LRECs and MRECs in the UK. From the report and the many helpful comments received, an operating system for ethical review of multi-centre research where there is no local researcher has now been formulated.

2.3 It is an operational modification to the existing system of ethical review described in HSG(91)5 for England, 1992(GEN)3 for Scotland and WHC(91)75 for Wales, which established Local Research Ethics Committees throughout the NHS; and in HSG(97)23 for England,

MEL(1997)8 for Scotland and DGM(98)25 for Wales, by which the MREC system was established.

3 Categories of research where there is no local researcher

These are considered under 5 headings:
- Data the use of which use does not require ethical review by RECs
- Use of data regarded as being in the public domain
- Establishment of a new disease or patient database for research purposes, and the use of such a database with no patient contact
- The use of such a database, with subsequent patient contact
- The use of an existing database, collected for previous research or other purposes.

A Data the use of which does not require ethical review by RECs

(i) It is currently well accepted that collection and analysis of some data does not require review by a NHS Research Ethics Committee. Examples would be the Adverse Drug Reaction reporting Scheme of the Committee on Safety of Medicines, Prescription Event Monitoring, National Morbidity Surveys and Post Market Surveillance of new medications.

B Use of data regarded as being in the public domain

(i) Investigators do not need to obtain informed consent to use publicly available information for epidemiological studies.

(ii) Use of many databases in the public domain (eg death certificates, ONS data) will usually fall outside the remit of MRECs/LRECs. Nevertheless, potential researchers should contact the guardians of any such databases to find out if ethical review is required, and if so whether an internal ethics committee is available. If not, an MREC will offer an ethical opinion on request.

C Establishment of a new disease or patient database for research purposes, and the use of such a database with no patient contact

(i) An example would be the attempt to ascertain the prevalence of a rare disease or medical complication. In order to collect the information, the principal investigator might wish to contact local NHS health care professionals through the appropriate professional networks.

(ii) The principal investigator should apply to the appropriate MREC for *ethical* approval. The MREC will consider, among other things
- whether consent is required
- the method used for collecting the information
- the nature of the information
- how it is to be stored
- its intended use
- who will have access to it

(iii) Ethical approval by an MREC will cover the entire UK and there is no requirement subsequently to apply to LRECs.

(iv) It remains the responsibility of the principal investigator to ensure that in undertaking the collection, storage or use of the data, he/she is not contravening the legal or regulatory requirements of any part of the UK in which the data are collected, stored or used.

D The use of such a database, but with subsequent patient contact

(i) An example might be a request to collect further data, or a sample of blood to be analysed at the principal investigator's laboratory for research purposes. The principal investigator should apply to the same MREC that approved the establishment of the database.

(ii) The MREC will review the ethical aspects of the research proposal, which include among other things
- issues relating to the establishment of the existing database
- the scientific quality and relevance of the proposal
- the reasons for, and nature of, the patient contact
- the methods of seeking and of obtaining consent
- the information to be made available to the research subject
- the nature of any procedures to be undertaken
- scrutiny of those who will undertake local tasks (the principal researcher and his/her team, and the type and grade of local clinician)
- issues concerning indemnity

(iii) All initial patient contact should only be made through channels approved by the MREC as ethical. In practice, this will almost invariably be by means of a local clinician with responsibility for the care of the patient, or by his/her approved staff on his/her behalf.

(iv) The information sheet about the research (as approved by the MREC) is subsequently made available to the research subject, either directly or via the local clinician. It should be comprehensive, and contain full information about the principal investigator (and if necessary his/her other research staff).

It should also contain contact details for the members of the central research team who will be available to answer further questions from the potential research subjects before they give consent, or at a later date.

(v) Consent of the research subject may be obtained either by members of the central research team or by the local clinician, using methods approved by the MREC as ethical.

(vi) After approval by the MREC, members of the central research team themselves may carry out the procedures that the MREC has approved, and for which consent has been given by the research subject. Where these procedures take place in NHS premises, the researcher must first obtain the agreement of the local NHS management, who will need to be assured that the researcher holds an appropriate NHS contract, and that indemnity issues have been adequately addressed.

(vii) The local clinician may also perform technical procedures or additional data collection as described in the MREC-approved protocol as long as:

- they are well within his/her routine professional competence (the MREC will review whether this is so), and
- adequate facilities for such procedures would be routinely available as part of his/her normal professional practice.

An example might be a doctor taking a blood sample.

(viii) The local clinician will provide the samples/data to the researchers but will play no other part in the research.

(ix) This limited technical involvement of the local clinician does not now require the opinion of the LREC. The LREC should be informed of the project, and the name and contact details of the local clinician involved. If (unusually) the LREC has any reason to doubt that the local clinician is competent to carry out the tasks required, it should inform both the clinician and the MREC that gave ethical approval.

(x) The local clinician must inform his/her NHS organisation of his/her co-operation in the research project and the nature of his/her involvement, just as would be the case if he/she were a local researcher. He/she should ensure with the NHS organisation that local indemnity arrangements are adequate.

(xi) It remains the responsibility of the principal investigator to ensure that in subsequently undertaking the collection, storage or use of the data or research sample, he/she is not contravening the legal or regulatory requirements of any part of the UK in which the data or research material are collected, stored or used.

(xii) If the research requires a change in therapy, more substantial data collection or monitoring, or the need for the local clinician to perform tasks possibly outside his routine competence, then he/she should be regarded as a "local researcher" and not a "technical co-operator". The reviewing MREC will regard the research as being outside this revised system of review, and the local researcher would require appropriate scrutiny – currently by the LREC – as in the current standard system for ethical review of multi-centre research.

E The use of an existing database, collected for previous research or other purposes

(i) The researcher should apply to an MREC. Where the database was established for research purposes, and previously approved by an MREC, application should be made to that same MREC.

(ii) The MREC will wish to review the *ethical* issues of researcher access to the existing database for new purposes.

(iii) It remains the responsibility of the principal investigator to ensure that in gaining access to or subsequently using the data, he/she is not contravening the legal or regulatory requirements of any part of the UK in which the data are collected, stored or used. He should do this in full and active collaboration with the guardian of the database.

(iv) Subsequent use of the database is governed by the same principles laid out above in Section D.

4 Communications

4.1 Standard MREC forms for communication must continue to be used, with correct version numbers and dates.

4.2 Standard format letters will be available for principal researchers and local clinicians to inform the necessary branches of the NHS (LRECs and NHS management). The MREC administrator will provide these.

5 Guidance notes for researchers

1 If you think that your research proposal falls into any of the categories that now allow exemption from application to an LREC after MREC approval, you should state this in the covering letter that accompanies your application to the MREC.

2 The MREC administrator and Chairman, or the staff of the Central Office for Research Ethics Committees (COREC), may be able to advise potential applicants in advance whether or not this is likely to be the case, but the final decision rests with the MREC.

3 The application to the MREC should be on the standard MREC form. Occasionally the MREC may require supplementary information prior to its consideration of your application.

4 Having studied your application, the MREC will make the decision about the need for subsequent scrutiny by LRECs. The MREC administrator will then provide you with the necessary standard paperwork, and further guidance about what to do next.

5 Researchers should consult and be guided by the MRC Guidelines on Personal Information in Medical Research, which can be found on the MRC web-site: http://www.mrc.ac.uk

38

Medical devices regulations and research ethics committees

Medical Devices Agency

To the Chairmen of all Multi-centre Research Ethics Committees and Local Research Ethics Committees in England, Scotland, Wales, Northern Ireland

June 2000

Dear Colleague

MEDICAL DEVICES REGULATIONS AND
RESEARCH ETHICS COMMITTES

Background

A series of three Medical Devices Directives, regulating the safety and marketing of medical devices throughout the European Community, started to come into effect from 1 January 1993. These Directives will eventually replace existing national systems in each Member State.

The Active Implantable Medical Devices Regulations 1992 (SI No 3146), which covers all implantable powered devices e.g. pacemakers, and which implements the provisions of the Active Implantable Medical Devices Directive 90/385/EEC, came into effect on 1 January 1993. The Medical Devices Regulations 1994 (SI No 3017), which covers most other medical devices with the exception of In Vitro Diagnostics and which implements the provisions of the Medical Devices Directive (93/42/EEC) came into effect on 1 January 1995. The In Vitro Diagnostic Medical Devices Regulations 2000 (SI No 1315), which covers any equipment or reagent intended to be used in vitro for the examination of substances derived from the human body, came into effect in the UK on the 7th of June 2000.

Regulatory Procedures

Under the provisions of these Regulations, no medical device with (with the exception of custom-made devices) may be placed on the market in the EC without a CE marking. In order to obtain this marking, the manufacturer must go through a conformity assessment procedure to confirm that the device in question complies with the relevant Essential Requirements relating to safety and performance.

In order to demonstrate this compliance satisfactorily, clinical data may be required, particularly in the case of higher risk devices. This data may be obtained from previous clinical experience with the device, or may be a compilation of scientific literature relating to the device or a similar device. If clinical data is not already available, however, e.g. in the circumstances of a new concept or device being produced, evidence from a specifically designed clinical investigation may be required in order to demonstrate that the device achieves its intended purpose as claimed by the manufacturer and does not comprise the clinical condition or safety of the patient or present a risk to the device user.

Under the provisions of the Devices Regulations, all such clinical investigations must be notified to the Competent Authority (Regulatory Body) of the Member State(s) in which the investigation(s) is(are) being performed. In the UK this is the Medical Devices Agency of the Department of Health. The Competent Authority then has 60 days in which to make an assessment of the information supplied as part of the notification and inform the applicant of any grounds for objection within that time period. Performance evaluation studies of in vitro diagnostic medical devices are dealt with differently. Manufacturers of such products which are to undergo performance evaluation are required simply to inform the Competent Authority in which they have their place of business, of the making available of such devices.

Relationship between the Competent Authority and Multi-centre/Local Research Ethics Committees

Until now, under the provisions of the Medical Devices Regulations, documentation required by the Competent Authority before it can make an assessment of the clinical investigation notification must contain a copy of the opinion of the relevant Multi-centre Research Ethics Committee (MREC) or Local Research Ethics Committee (LREC) from each participating centre. This has meant that, for the device investigations described above, the MREC/LREC opinion must always have been obtained prior to making a notification to the Competent Authority.

Since the introduction of the Medical Devices Regulations, however, the Competent Authority has received a number of complaints from both industry and clinicians about the time taken to obtain the MREC/LREC opinion and complete the Competent Authority system. This has often been considerable and has put the UK at a disadvantage in comparison to a number of other European countries where the systems for handling clinical investigations are different. It has also resulted in the fact that, in some instances, manufacturers have made a decision not to use UK centres for device clinical investigations in spite of the good reputation of the UK in carrying out research.

In order to address this problem, the Competent Authority has now amended the Regulations so that obtaining the MREC/LREC opinion and the Competent Authority notification can take place in parallel rather than in series. Under these circumstances, the manufacturer of the device proposed for investigation will be asked to submit the MREC/LREC opinion(s) as soon as it/these are obtained. This means that the Competent Authority, if it has no grounds for objection to the investigation proceeding, can inform the manufacturer that the clinical investigation may proceed at the UK centre(s) once the relevant Ethics Committee approval is obtained.

Because of the confidentiality requirements of the Regulations, no direct exchange of information can take place directly between the Competent Authority and a MREC/LREC. However, manufacturers are encouraged by the Competent Authority to inform MRECs/LRECs of the Competent Authority decision. MRECs/LRECs may also wish to contact the manufacturer directly, requesting a copy of the Competent Authority decision, although in the latter two instances the manufacturer has no legal obligation to comply.

Clinical investigations of CE marked devices do not require notification to the Competent Authority unless the manufacturer is proposing a use for the device in question other than that intended under its existing claims.

Yours faithfully

Dr Susanne M Ludgate
Medical Director
BSc MB ChB DMRT FRCR FRACR

Copies of the Regulations can be obtained from:

HMSO Books (Agency Section), HSMO Publication Centre, 51 Nine Elms Lane, London SW8 5DR
Tel: 020 7873 9090
Fax: 020 7873 8200

39

NHS indemnity
– arrangements for clinical negligence claims in the NHS

Department of Health

Purpose of this document

This document describes the arrangements which apply to handling clinical negligence claims against NHS staff (NHS Indemnity). It updates the guidance given in Health Circular HC(89)34.

GOOD PRACTICE

This document contains examples of and advice on good practice

Distribution	Directors and Chief Executives of NHS Trusts and Health Authorities
Author	Elizabeth Ryan, Complaints and Clinical Negligence Policy Unit, Quarry House, Leeds Tel 0113 2546377
Further copies from	Department of Health PO Box 410 Wetherby LS23 7LN
Catalogue number	96 HR 0024
Date of issue	October 1996
Other Relevant Publications	HSG (96)48

Contents

Executive summary

Introduction

This is a summary of the main points contained within *NHS Indemnity: Arrangements for clinical negligence claims in the NHS*, issued under cover of HSG 96/48. The booklet includes a Q&A section covering the applicability of NHS indemnity to common situations and an annex on sponsored trials. It covers NHS indemnity for clinical negligence but not for any other liability such as product liability, employers liability or liability for NHS trust board members.

Clinical negligence

Clinical negligence is defined as "a breach of duty of care by members of the health care professions employed by NHS bodies or by others consequent on decisions or judgements made by members of those professions acting in their professional capacity in the course of their employment, and which are admitted as negligent by the employer or are determined as such through the legal process".

The term health care professional includes hospital doctors, dentists, nurses, midwives, health visitors, pharmacy practitioners, registered ophthalmic or dispensing opticians (working in a hospital setting), members of professions allied to medicine and dentistry, ambulance personnel, laboratory staff and relevant technicians.

Main principles

NHS bodies are vicariously liable for the negligent acts and omissions of their employees and should have arrangements for meeting this liability.

NHS Indemnity applies where
(a) the negligent health care professional was:
  (i) working under a contract of employment and the negligence occurred in the course of that employment;
  (ii) not working under a contract of employment but was contracted to an NHS body to provide services to persons to whom that NHS body owed a duty of care.
  (iii) neither of the above but otherwise owed a duty of care to the persons injured.
(b) persons, not employed under a contract of employment and who may or may not be a health care professional, who owe a duty of care to the persons injured. These include locums; medical academic staff with honorary contracts; students; those conducting clinical trials; charitable volunteers; persons undergoing further professional education, training and examinations; students and staff working on income generation projects.

Where these principles apply, NHS bodies should accept full financial liability where negligent harm has occurred, and not seek to recover their costs from the health care professional involved.

Who is not covered

NHS Indemnity does not apply to family health service practitioners working under contracts for services, eg GPs (including fundholders), general dental practitioners family dentists, pharmacists or optometrists; other self employed health care professionals, eg independent midwives; employees of FHS practices; employees of private hospitals; local education authorities; voluntary agencies. Exceptions to the normal cover arrangements are set out in the main document.

Circumstances covered

NHS Indemnity covers negligent harm caused to patients or healthy volunteers in the following circumstances: whenever they are receiving an established treatment, whether or not in accordance with an agreed guideline or protocol; whenever they are receiving a novel or unusual treatment which, in the judgement of the health care professional, is appropriate for that particular patient; whenever they are subjects as patients or healthy volunteers of clinical research aimed at benefitting patients now or in the future.

Expenses met

Where negligence is alleged, NHS bodies are responsible for meeting: the legal and administrative costs of defending the claim or, if appropriate, of reaching a settlement; the plaintiff's costs, as agreed by the two parties or as awarded by the court; the damages awarded either as a one-off payment or as a structured settlement.

NHS indemnity clinical negligence – definition

1 Clinical negligence is defined as:
  "A breach of duty of care by members of the health care professions employed by NHS bodies or by others consequent on decisions or judgements made by members of those professions acting in their professional capacity in the course of employment, and which are admitted as negligent by the employer or are determined as such through the legal process."*
2 In this definition "breach of duty of care" has its legal meaning. NHS bodies will need to take legal advice in individual cases, but the general position will be that the following must all apply before liability for negligence exists:
  2.1 There must have been a duty of care owed to the person treated by the relevant professional(s);
  2.2 The standard of care appropriate to such duty must not have been attained and therefore the duty breached, whether by action or inaction, advice given or failure to advise;
  2.3 Such a breach must be demonstrated to have caused the injury and therefore the resulting loss complained about by the patient;

---

*The NHS (Clinical Negligence Scheme) Regulations 1996, which established the Clinical Negligence Scheme for Trusts, defines clinical negligence in terms of '. . . a liability in tort owed by a member to a third party in respect of or consequent upon personal injury or loss arising out of or in connection with any breach of a duty of care owed by that body to any person in connection with the diagnosis of any illness, or the care or treatment of any patient, in consequence of any act or omission to act on the part of a person employed or engaged by a member in connection with any relevant function of that member'.

2.4 Any loss sustained as a result of the injury and complained about by the person treated must be of a kind that the courts recognize and for which they allow compensation; and

2.5 The injury and resulting loss complained about by the person treated must have been reasonably foreseeable as a possible consequence of the breach.

3 This booklet is concerned with NHS indemnity for clinical negligence and does not cover indemnity for any other liability such as product liability, employers liability or liability for NHS trust board members.

Other terms

4 Throughout this guidance:

4.1 The terms "an NHS body" and "NHS bodies" include Health Authorities, Special Health Authorities and NHS Trusts but excludes all GP practices whether fundholding or not, general dental practices, pharmacies and opticians' practices

4.2 The term "health care professional" includes:

Doctors, dentists, nurses, midwives, health visitors, hospital pharmacy practitioners, registered ophthalmic or registered dispensing opticians working in a hospital setting, members of professions supplementary to medicine and dentistry, ambulance personnel, laboratory staff and relevant technicians.

Principles

5 NHS bodies are legally liable for the negligent acts and omissions of their employees (the principle of vicarious liability), and should have arrangements for meeting this liability. NHS Indemnity applies where:

5.1 the negligent health care professional was working under a contract of employment (as opposed to a contract for services) and the negligence occurred in the course of that employment; or

5.2 the negligent health care professional, although not working under a contract of employment, was contracted to an NHS body to provide services to persons to whom that NHS body owed a duty of care.

6 Where the principles outlined in paragraph 5 apply, NHS bodies should accept full financial liability where negligent harm has occurred. They should not seek to recover their costs either in part or in full from the health care professional concerned or from any indemnities they may have. NHS bodies may carry this risk entirely or spread it

through membership of the Clinical Negligence Scheme for Trusts (CNST – see EL(95)40).

Who is covered

7 NHS Indemnity covers the actions of staff in the course of their NHS employment. It also covers people in certain other categories whenever the NHS body owes a duty of care to the person harmed, including, for example, locums, medical academic staff with honorary contracts, students, those conducting clinical trials, charitable volunteers and people undergoing further professional education, training and examinations. This includes staff working on income generation projects. GPs or dentists who are directly employed by Health Authorities, eg as Public Health doctors (including port medical officers and medical inspectors of immigrants at UK air/sea ports), are covered.

8 Examples of the applicability of NHS Indemnity to common situations are set out in question and answer format in Annex A.

Who is not covered

9 NHS Indemnity does not apply to general medical and dental practitioners working under contracts for services. General practitioners, including GP fundholders, are responsible for making their own indemnity arrangements, as are other self-employed health care professionals such as independent midwives. Neither does NHS Indemnity apply to employees of general practices, whether fundholding or not, or to employees of private hospitals (even when treating NHS patients) local education authorities or voluntary agencies.

10 Examples of circumstances in which independent practitioners or staff who normally work for private employers are covered by NHS Indemnity are given in Annex A. The NHS Executive advises independent practitioners to check their own indemnity position.

11 Examples of circumstances in which NHS employees are not covered by NHS Indemnity are also given in Annex A.

Circumstances covered

12 NHS bodies owe a duty of care to healthy volunteers or patients treated or undergoing tests which they administer. NHS Indemnity covers negligent harm caused to these people in the following circumstances:

12.1 whenever they are receiving an established treatment, whether or not in accordance with an agreed guideline or protocol;

12.2 whenever they are receiving a novel or unusual treatment which in the clinical judgement of the health care professional is appropriate for the particular patient;

12.3 whenever they are subjects of clinical research aimed at benefitting patients now or in the future, whether as patients or as healthy volunteers. (Special arrangements, including the availability of no-fault indemnity apply where research is sponsored by pharmaceutical companies. See Annex B.)

Expenses met

13 Where negligence is alleged NHS bodies are responsible for meeting:

13.1 the legal and administrative costs of defending the claim and, if appropriate, of reaching a settlement, including the cost of any mediation;

13.2 where appropriate, plaintiff's costs, either as agreed between the parties or as awarded by a court of law;

13.3 the damages agreed or awarded, whether as a one-off payment or a structured settlement.

Claims management principles

14 NHS bodies should take the essential decisions on the handling of claims of clinical negligence against their staff, using professional defence organizations or others as their agents and advisers as appropriate.

Financial support arrangements

15 Details of the Clinical Negligence Scheme for Trusts (CNST) were announced in EL(95)40 on 29 March 1995.

16 All financial arrangements in respect of clinical negligence costs for NHS bodies have been reviewed and guidance on transitional arrangements (for funding clinical accidents which happened before 1 April 1995), was issued on 27 November 1995 under cover of FDL(95)56. FDL(96)36 provided further guidance on a number of detailed questions.

Annex A

Questions and answers on NHS Indemnity

Below are replies to some of the questions most commonly asked about NHS Indemnity.

1 Who is covered by NHS Indemnity?

NHS bodies are liable at law for the negligent acts and omissions of their staff in the course of their NHS employment. Under NHS Indemnity, NHS bodies take direct responsibility for costs and damages arising from clinical negligence where they (as employers) are vicariously liable for the acts and omissions of their health care professional staff.

2 Would health care professionals opting to work under contracts for services rather than as employees of the NHS be covered?

Where an NHS body is responsible for *providing* care to patients NHS Indemnity will apply whether the health care professional involved is an employee or not. For example a doctor working under a contract for services with an NHS Trust would be covered because the Trust has responsibility for the care of its patients. A consultant undertaking contracted NHS work in a private hospital would also be covered.

3 Does this include clinical academics and research workers?

NHS bodies are vicariously liable for the work done by university medical staff and other research workers (eg employees of the MRC) under their honorary contracts, but not for pre-clinical or other work in the university.

4 Are GP practices covered?

GPs, whether fundholders or not [and who are not employed by Health Authorities as public health doctors], are independent practitioners and therefore they and their employed staff are not covered by NHS indemnity.

5 Is a hospital doctor doing a GP locum covered?

This would not be the responsibility of the NHS body since it would be outside the contract of employment. The hospital doctor and the general practitioners concerned should ensure that there is appropriate professional liability cover.

6 Is a GP seeing a patient in hospital covered?

A GP providing medical care to patients in hospital under a contractual arrangement, eg where the GP was employed as a clinical assistant, will be covered by NHS Indemnity, as will a GP who provides services in NHS hospitals under staff fund contracts (known as "bed funds"). Where there is no such contractual arrangement, and the NHS body provides facilities for patient(s) who continue to be the clinical responsibility of the GP, the GP would be responsible and professional liability cover would be appropriate. However, junior medical staff, nurses or members of the professions supplementary to medicine involved in the care of a GP's patients in NHS hospitals under their contract of employment would be covered.

7 Are GP trainees working in general practice covered?

In general practice the responsibility for training and for paying the salary of a GP trainee rests with the trainer. While the trainee is receiving a salary in general practice it is advisable that both the trainee and the trainer, and indeed other members of the practice, should have appropriate professional liability cover as NHS indemnity will not apply.

8 Are NHS employees working under contracts with GP fundholders covered?

If their employing NHS body has agreed a contract to provide services to a GP fundholding practice's patients, NHS employees will be working under the terms of their contracts of employment and NHS Indemnity will cover them. If NHS employees themselves contract with GP fundholders (or any other independent body) to do work outside their NHS contract of employment they should ensure that they have separate indemnity cover.

9 Is academic General Practice covered?

The Department has no plans to extend NHS Indemnity to academic departments of general practice. In respect of general medical services, Health Authorities' payments of fees and allowances include an element for expenses, of which medical defence subscriptions are a part.

10 Is private work in NHS hospitals covered by NHS Indemnity?

NHS bodies will not be responsible for a health care professional's private practice, even in an NHS hospital. However, where junior medical staff, nurses or members of professions supplementary to medicine are involved in the care of private patients in NHS hospitals, they would normally be doing so as part of their NHS contract, and would therefore be covered. It remains advisable that health professionals who might be involved in work outside the scope of his or her NHS employment should have professional liability cover.

11 Is Category 2 work covered?

Category 2 work (eg reports for insurance companies) is by definition not undertaken for the employing NHS body and is therefore not covered by NHS Indemnity. Unless the work is carried out on behalf of the employing NHS body, professional liability cover would be needed.

12 Are disciplinary proceedings of statutory bodies covered?

NHS bodies are not financially responsible for the defence of staff involved in disciplinary proceedings conducted by statutory bodies such as the GMC (doctors), UKCC (nurses and midwives), GDC (dentists) CPSM (professions supplementary to medicine) and RPSGB (pharmacists). It is the responsibility of the practitioner concerned to take out professional liability cover against such an eventuality.

13 Are clinical trials covered?

In the case of negligent harm, health care professionals undertaking clinical trials or studies on volunteers, whether healthy or patients, in the course of their NHS employment are covered by NHS Indemnity. Similarly, for a trial not involving medicines, the NHS body would take financial responsibility unless the trial were covered by such other indemnity as may have been agreed between the NHS body and those responsible for the trial. In any case, NHS bodies should ensure that they are informed of clinical trials in which their staff are taking part in their NHS employment and that these trials have the required Research Ethics Committee approval. For non-negligent harm, see question 16 below.

14 Is harm resulting from a fault in the drug/equipment covered?

Where harm is caused due to a fault in the manufacture of a drug or piece of equipment then, under the terms of the Consumer Protection Act 1987, it is no defence for the producer to show that he exercised reasonable care.

Under normal circumstances, therefore; NHS indemnity would not apply unless there was a question whether the health care professional either knew or should reasonably have known that the drug/equipment was faulty but continued to use it. Strict liability could apply if the drug/equipment had been manufactured by an NHS body itself, for example a prototype as part of a research programme.

15 Are Local Research Ethics Committees (LRECs) covered?

Under the Department's guidelines an LREC is appointed by the Health Authority to provide independent advice to NHS bodies within its area on the ethics of research proposals. The Health Authority should take financial responsibility for members' acts and omissions in the course of performance of their duties as LREC members.

16 Is there liability for non-negligent harm?

Apart from liability for defective products, legal liability does not arise where a person is harmed but no one has acted negligently. An example of this would be unexpected side-effects of drugs during clinical trials. In exceptional circumstances (and within the delegated limit of £50,000) NHS bodies may consider whether an ex-gratia payment could be offered. NHS bodies may not offer advance indemnities or take out commercial insurance for non-negligent harm.

17 What arrangements can non-NHS bodies make for non-negligent harm?

Arrangements will depend on the status of the non-NHS body. Arrangements for clinical trials sponsored by the pharmaceutical industry are set out in Annex B. Other independent sector sponsors of clinical research involving NHS patients (eg universities and medical research charities) may also make arrangements to indemnify research subjects for non-negligent harm. Public sector research funding bodies such as the Medical Research Council (MRC) may not offer advance indemnities nor take out commercial insurance for non-negligent harm. The MRC offers the assurance that it will give sympathetic consideration to claims in respect of non-negligent harm arising from an MRC funded trial. NHS bodies should not make ex-gratia payments for non-negligent harm where research is sponsored by a non-NHS body.

18 Would health care professionals be covered if they were working other than in accordance with the duties of their post?

Health care professionals would be covered by NHS Indemnity for actions in the course of NHS employment, and this should be interpreted liberally. For work not covered in this way health care professionals may have a civil, or even, in extreme circumstances, criminal liability for their actions.

19 Are health care professionals attending accident victims ("Good Samaritan" acts) covered?

"Good Samaritan" acts are not part of the health care professional's work for the employing body. Medical defence organizations are willing to provide low-cost cover against the (unusual) event of anyone performing such an act being sued for negligence. Ambulance services can, with the agreement of staff, include an additional term in the individual employee contracts to the effect that the member of staff is expected to provide assistance in any emergency outside of duty hours where it is appropriate to do so.

20 Are NHS staff in public health medicine or in community health services doing work for local authorities covered? Are occupational physicians covered?

Staff working in public health medicine, clinical medical officers or therapists carrying out local authority functions under their NHS contract would be acting in the course of their NHS employment. They will therefore be covered by NHS Indemnity. The same principle applies to occupational physicians employed by NHS bodies.

21 Are NHS staff working for other agencies, eg the prison service, covered?

In general, NHS bodies are not financially responsible for the acts of NHS staff when they are working on an individual contractual basis for other agencies. (Conversely, they are responsible where, for example, a Ministry of Defence doctor works in an NHS hospital.) Either the non-NHS body commissioning the work would be responsible, or the health care professional should have separate indemnity cover. However, NHS Indemnity should cover work for which the NHS body pays the health care professional a fee, such as domiciliary visits, and family planning services.

22 Are former NHS staff covered?

NHS Indemnity will cover staff who have subsequently left the Service (eg on retirement) provided the liability arose in respect of acts or omissions in the course of their NHS employment, regardless of when the claim was notified. NHS bodies may seek the co-operation of former staff in providing statements in the defence of a case.

23 Are NHS staff offering services to voluntary bodies such as the Red Cross or hospices covered?

The NHS body would be responsible for the actions of its staff only if it were contractually responsible for the clinical staffing of the voluntary body. If not, the staff concerned may wish to ensure that they have separate indemnity cover.

24 Do NHS bodies provide cover for locums?

NHS bodies take financial responsibility for the acts and omissions of a locum health care professional, whether "internal" or provided by an external agency, doing the work of a colleague who would be covered.

25 What are the arrangements for staff employed by one trust working in another?

This depends on the contractual arrangements. If the work is being done as part of a formal agreement between the trusts, then the staff involved will be acting within their normal NHS duties and, unless the agreement states otherwise, the employing trust will be liable. The NHS Executive does not recommend the use of ad hoc arrangements, eg a doctor in one trust asking a doctor in another to provide an informal second opinion, unless there is an agreement between the trusts as to which of them will accept liability for the "visiting" doctor in such circumstances.

26 Are private sector rotations for hospital staff covered?

The medical staff of independent hospitals are responsible for their own professional liability cover, subject to the requirements of the hospital managers. If NHS staff in the training grades work in independent hospitals as part of their NHS training, they would be covered by NHS Indemnity, provided that such work was covered by an NHS contract of employment.

27 Are voluntary workers covered?

Where volunteers work in NHS bodies, they are covered by NHS Indemnity. NHS managers should be aware of all voluntary activity going on in their organizations and should wherever possible confirm volunteers' indemnity position in writing.

28 Are students covered?

NHS Indemnity applies where students are working under the supervision of NHS employees. This should be made clear in the agreement between the NHS body and the student's educational body. This will apply to students of all the health care professions and to school students on, for example, work experience placements. Students working in NHS premises, under supervision of medical academic staff employed by universities holding honorary contracts, are also covered. Students who spend time in a primary care setting will only be covered if this is part of an NHS contract. Potential students making preliminary visits and school placements should be adequately supervised and should not become involved in any clinical work. Therefore, no clinical negligence should arise on their part.

In the unlikely event of a school making a negligent choice of work placement for a pupil to work in the NHS, then the school, and not NHS indemnity, should pick up the legal responsibility for the actions of that pupil. The contractual arrangement between the NHS and the school should make this clear.

29 Are health care professionals undergoing on-the-job training covered?

Where an NHS body's staff are providing on-the-job training (eg refresher or skills updating courses) for health care professionals, the trainees are covered by NHS Indemnity whether they are normally employed by the NHS or not.

30 Are independent midwives covered?

Independent midwives are self-employed practitioners. In common with all other health care professionals working outside the NHS, they are responsible for making their own indemnity arrangements.

31 Are overseas doctors who have come to the UK temporarily, perhaps to demonstrate a new technique, covered?

The NHS body which has invited the overseas doctor will owe a duty of care to the patients on whom the technique is demonstrated and so NHS indemnity will apply. NHS bodies, therefore, need to make sure that they are kept informed of any such demonstration visits which are proposed and of the nature of the technique to be demonstrated. Where visiting clinicians are not formally registered as students, or are not employees, an honorary contract should be arranged.

32 Are staff who are qualified in another member state of the European Union covered?

Staff qualified in another member state of the European Union, and who are undertaking an adaptation period in accordance with EEC directive 89/48EEC and the European Communities (Recognition of Professional Qualifications) Regulations 1991 which implements EEC Directive 89/48/EEC) and EEC Directive 92/51/EEC, must be treated in a manner consistent with their qualified status in another member state, and should be covered.

Annex B

Indemnity for clinical studies sponsored by pharmaceutical companies

Section one

1 Clinical research involving the administration of drugs to patients or non-patient human volunteers is frequently undertaken under the auspices of Health Authorities or NHS Trusts.
2 When the study is sponsored by a pharmaceutical company, issues of liability and indemnity may arise in case of injury associated with administration of the drug or other aspects of the conduct of the trial.
3 When the study is not sponsored by a company but has been independently organised by clinicians, the NHS body will carry full legal liability for claims in negligence arising from harm to subjects in the study.
4 The guidance in Section 2 and the Appendix has three purposes:
   • to ensure that NHS bodies enter into appropriate agreements which will provide indemnity against claims and

proceedings arising from company-sponsored clinical studies;
   • to ensure that NHS bodies, where appropriate, use a standard form of agreement (Appendix) which has been drawn up in consultation with the Association of the British Pharmaceutical Industry (ABPI);
   • to advise Local Research Ethics Committees (LRECs) of the standard form of agreement.

Section two

1 A wide variety of clinical studies involving experimental or investigational use of drugs is carried out within NHS bodies. This includes studies in patients (clinical trials) and studies in healthy human volunteers. They may involve administration of a totally new (unlicensed) drug (active substance or 'NAS') or the administration of an established (licensed) drug by a novel route, for a new therapeutic indication, or in a novel formulation or combination.
2 Detailed guidance on the design, conduct, and ethical implications of clinical studies is given in:

HSG(91)5: Local Research Ethics Committees (with accompanying booklet). NHS Executive: 1991;

Guidelines for Medical Experiments in non-Patient Human Volunteers Research Involving Patients; Royal College of Physicians of London: 1990;

Guidelines in the Practice of Ethics Committees in Medical Research, 2nd edition; Royal College of Physicians of London: 1990;

Clinical Trial Compensation Guidelines ABPI: 1991

3 The Medicines Act 1968 provides the regulatory framework for clinical studies involving administration of drugs to patients. Drugs which are used in a sponsored* clinical study in patients will be the subject of either a product licence (PL), a clinical trial certificate (CTC), or clinical trial exemption (CTX) which is held by the company as appropriate. A non-sponsored study conducted independently by a practitioner must be notified to the Licensing Authority under the Doctors and Dentists Exemption (DDX) scheme. Studies in healthy volunteers are not subject to regulation under the Medicines Act and do not require a CTC, CTX, or

---

*A sponsored study may be defined as one carried out under arrangements made by or on behalf of the company who manufactured the product, the company responsible for its composition, or the company selling or supplying the product.

DDX. Further particulars of these arrangements are provided in Medicines Act leaflet *MAL 30: A guide to the provisions affecting doctors and dentists (DHSS: 1985)*.

4   Participants in a clinical study may suffer adverse effects due to the drug or clinical procedures. The appendix to this annex is a model form of agreement between the company sponsoring a study and the NHS body involved, which indemnifies the authority or trust against claims and proceedings arising from the study. The model agreement has been drawn up in consultation with the Association of the British Pharmaceutical Industry (ABPI).

5   This form of indemnity will not normally apply to clinical studies which are not directly sponsored by the company providing the product for research, but have been independently organised by clinicians. In this case, the NHS body will normally carry full legal liability for any claims in negligence arising from harm to subjects in the study.

6   The NHS body will also carry full legal liability for any claims in negligence (or compensation under the indemnity will be abated) where there has been significant non-adherence to the agreed protocol or there has been negligence on the part of an NHS employee, for example, by failing to deal adequately with an adverse drug reaction.

7   The form of indemnity may not be readily accepted by sponsoring companies outside the UK or who are not members of the ABPI. NHS bodies should, as part of their risk management, consider the value of indemnities which are offered and consider whether companies should have alternative arrangements in place.

8   Several health authorities and trusts have independently developed forms of indemnity agreement. However, difficulties have arisen when different authorities have required varying terms of indemnity and this has, on occasion, impeded the progress of clinical research within the NHS. Particular difficulties may arise in large multi-centre trials involving many NHS bodies when it is clearly desirable to have standardised terms of indemnity to provide equal protection to all participants in the study.

9   Responsibility for deciding whether a particular company-sponsored research proposal should proceed within the NHS rests with the Health Authority or Trust within which the research would take place, after consideration of ethical, clinical, managerial, financial, resource, and legal liability issues. The NHS body is responsible for securing an appropriate indemnity agreement and should maintain a register of all clinical studies undertaken under its auspices with an indication whether it is a company-sponsored study and, if so, with confirmation that an indemnity agreement is in place. If for any reason it is considered that the model form

of indemnity is not appropriate or that amendments are required, the NHS body involved should seek legal advice on the form or amendments proposed.

10   Even when the model form of indemnity is agreed, the NHS body should satisfy itself that the company sponsoring the study is substantial and reputable and has appropriate arrangements in place (for example insurance cover) to support the indemnity. The NHS body will carry full liability for any claims in negligence if the indemnity is not honoured and there is not supporting insurance.

11   Where a clinical study includes patients or subjects within several NHS bodies, for example in a multi-centre clinical trial, it is necessary for each Authority or Trust to complete an appropriate indemnity agreement with the sponsoring company.

12   Where independent practitioners, such as general medical practitioners, are engaged in clinical studies, Health Authorities should seek to ensure that such studies are the subject of an appropriate indemnity agreement. It is good practice for the GP to notify the Health Authority of his participation in any clinical study.

13   Clinical investigators should ensure that details of any proposed research study are lodged with the appropriate NHS body and should not commence company-sponsored research unless an indemnity agreement is in place.

14   Local Research Ethics Committees (LRECs) provide independent advice to NHS and other bodies and to clinical researchers on the ethics of proposed research projects that involve human subjects [HSG(91)5]. Clinical investigators should not commence any research project involving patients or human volunteers without LREC agreement. Acceptance of the ABPI guidelines and the terms of the model indemnity agreement should normally be a condition of LREC approval of any pharmaceutical company sponsored project.

Annex B: appendix

Form of indemnity for clinical studies

To: [Name and address of sponsoring company] ("the Sponsor")

From: [Name and address of Health Authority/ Health Board/NHS Trust] ("the Authority")

Re: Clinical Study No [   ] with [name of product]

1   It is proposed that the Authority should agree to participate in the above sponsored study ("the Study") involving

[patients of the Authority] [non-patient volunteers] ("the Subjects") to be conducted by [name of investigator(s)] ("the Investigator") in accordance with the protocol annexed, as amended from time to time with the agreement of the Sponsor and the Investigator ("the Protocol"). The Sponsor confirms that it is a term of its agreement with the Investigator that the Investigator shall obtain all necessary approvals of the applicable Local Research Ethics Committee and shall resolve with the Authority any issues of a revenue nature.

2 The Authority agrees to participate by allowing the Study to be undertaken on its premises utilising such facilities, personnel and equipment as the Investigator may reasonably need for the purpose of the Study.

3 In consideration of such participation by the Authority, and subject to paragraph 4 below, the Sponsor indemnifies and holds harmless the Authority and its employees and agents against all claims and proceedings (to include any settlements or ex-gratia payments made with the consent of the parties hereto and reasonable legal and expert costs and expenses) made or brought (whether successfully or otherwise):

(a) by or on behalf of Subjects taking part in the Study (or their dependants) against the Authority or any of its employees or agents for personal injury (including death) to Subjects arising out of or relating to the administration of the product(s) under investigation or any clinical intervention or procedure provided for or required by the Protocol to which the Subjects would not have been exposed but for their participation in the Study.

(b) by the Authority, its employees or agents or by or on behalf of a Subject for a declaration concerning the treatment of a Subject who has suffered such personal injury.

4 The above indemnity by the Sponsor shall not apply to any such claim or proceeding:

4.1 to the extent that such personal injury (including death) is caused by the negligent or wrongful acts or omissions or breach of statutory duty of the Authority, its employees or agents;

4.2 to the extent that such personal injury (including death) is caused by the failure of the Authority, its employees, or agents to conduct the Study in accordance with the Protocol;

4.3 unless as soon as reasonably practicable following receipt of notice of such claim or proceeding, the Authority shall have notified the Sponsor in writing of it and shall, upon the Sponsor's request, and at the Sponsor's cost, have permitted the Sponsor to have full care and control of the claim or proceeding using legal representation of its own choosing;

4.4 if the Authority, its employees, or agents shall have made any admission in respect of such claim or proceeding or taken any action relating to such claim or proceeding prejudicial to the defence of it without the written consent of the Sponsor such consent not to be unreasonably withheld provided that this condition shall not be treated as breached by any statement properly made by the Authority, its employees or agents in connection with the operation of the Authority's internal complaint procedures, accident reporting procedures or disciplinary procedures or where such statement is required by law.

5 The Sponsor shall keep the Authority and its legal advisers fully informed of the progress of any such claim or proceeding, will consult fully with the Authority on the nature of any defence to be advanced and will not settle any such claim or proceeding without the written approval of the Authority (such approval not to be unreasonably withheld).

6 Without prejudice to the provisions of paragraph 4.3 above, the Authority will use its reasonable endeavours to inform the Sponsor promptly of any circumstances reasonably thought likely to give rise to any such claim or proceeding of which it is directly aware and shall keep the Sponsor reasonably informed of developments in relation to any such claim or proceeding even where the Authority decides not to make a claim under this indemnity. Likewise, the Sponsor shall use its reasonable endeavours to inform the Authority of any such circumstances and shall keep the Authority reasonably informed of developments in relation to any such claim or proceeding made or brought against the Sponsor alone.

7 The Authority and the Sponsor will each give to the other such help as may reasonably be required for the efficient conduct and prompt handling of any claim or proceeding by or on behalf of Subjects (or their dependants) or concerning such a declaration as is referred to in paragraph 3(b) above.

8 Without prejudice to the foregoing if injury is suffered by a Subject while participating in the Study, the Sponsor agrees to operate in good faith the Guidelines published in 1991 by The Association of the British Pharmaceutical Industry and entitled "Clinical Trial Compensation Guidelines" (where the Subject is a patient) and the Guidelines published in 1988 by the same Association and entitled "Guidelines for Medical Experiments in non-patient Human Volunteers" (where the Subject is not a patient) and shall request the Investigator to make

clear to the Subjects that the Study is being conducted subject to the applicable Association Guidelines.

9 For the purpose of this indemnity, the expression "agents" shall be deemed to include without limitation any nurse or other health professional providing services to the Authority under a contract for services or otherwise and any person carrying out work for the Authority under such a contract connected with such of the Authority's facilities and equipment as are made available for the Study under paragraph 2 above.

10 This indemnity shall be governed by and construed in accordance with English/Scottish* law.

SIGNED on behalf of the Health Authority/Health Board/NHS Trust

....
Chief Executive/
District General Manager

SIGNED on behalf of the Company

....

Dated...

* Delete as appropriate

40

Clinical trial compensation guidelines

Association of the British Pharmaceutical Industry

Preamble

The Association of the British Pharmaceutical Industry favours a simple and expeditious procedure in relation to the provision of compensation for injury caused by participation in clinical trials. The Association therefore recommends that a member company sponsoring a clinical trial should provide without legal commitment a written assurance to the investigator – and through him to the relevant research ethics committee – that the following Guidelines will be adhered to in the event of injury caused to a patient attributable to participation in the trial in question.

1 Basic principles

1.1 Notwithstanding the absence of legal commitment, the company should pay compensation to patient-volunteers suffering bodily injury (including death) in accordance with these Guidelines.

1.2 Compensation should be paid when, on the balance of probabilities, the injury was attributable to the administration of a medicinal product under trial or any clinical intervention or procedure provided for by the protocol that would not have occurred but for the inclusion of the patient in the trial.

1.3 Compensation should be paid to a child injured in utero through the participation of the subject's mother in a clinical trial as if the child were a patient-volunteer with the full benefit of these Guidelines.

1.4 Compensation should only be paid for the more serious injury of an enduring and disabling character (including exacerbation of an existing condition) and not for temporary pain or discomfort or less serious or curable complaints.

© Association of the British Pharmaceutical Industry.

1.5 Where there is an adverse reaction to a medicinal product under trial and injury is caused by a procedure adopted to deal with that adverse reaction, compensation should be paid for such injury as if it were caused directly by the medicinal product under trial.

1.6 Neither the fact that the adverse reaction causing the injury was foreseeable or predictable, nor the fact that the patient has freely consented (whether in writing or otherwise) to participate in the trial should exclude a patient from consideration for compensation under these Guidelines, although compensation may be abated or excluded in the light of the factors described in paragraph 4.2 below.

1.7 For the avoidance of doubt, compensation should be paid regardless of whether the patient is able to prove that the company has been negligent in relation to research or development of the medicinal product under trial or that the product is defective and therefore, as the producer, the company is subject to strict liability in respect of injuries caused by it.

2 Type of clinical research covered

2.1 These Guidelines apply to injury caused to patients involved in Phase II and Phase III trials, that is to say, patients under treatment and surveillance (usually in hospital) and suffering from the ailment which the medicinal product under trial is intended to treat but for which a product licence does not exist or does not authorise supply for administration under the conditions of the trial.

2.2 These Guidelines do not apply to injuries arising from studies in non-patient volunteers (Phase I), whether or not they are in hospital, for which separate Guidelines for compensation already exist.[1]

2.3 These Guidelines do not apply to injury arising from clinical trials on marketed products (Phase IV) where a product licence exists authorising supply for administration under the conditions of the trial, except to the extent that the injury is caused to a patient as a direct result of procedures undertaken in accordance with the protocol (but not any product administered) to which the patient would not have been exposed had treatment been other than in the course of the trial.

2.4 These Guidelines do not apply to clinical trials which have not been initiated or directly sponsored by the company providing the product for research. Where trials of products are initiated independently by doctors under the appropriate Medicines Act 1968 exemptions, responsibility for the health and welfare of patients rests with the doctor alone (see also paragraph 5.2 below).

3 Limitations

3.1 No compensation should be paid for the failure of a medicinal product to have its intended effect or to provide any other benefit to the patient.

3.2 No compensation should be paid for injury caused by other licensed medicinal products administered to the patient for the purpose of comparison with the product under trial.

3.3 No compensation should be paid to patients receiving placebo in consideration of its failure to provide a therapeutic benefit.

3.4 No compensation should be paid (or it should be abated as the case may be) to the extent that the injury has arisen:
   3.4.1 through a significant departure from the agreed protocol;
   3.4.2 through the wrongful act or default of a third party, including a doctor's failure to deal adequately with an adverse reaction;
   3.4.3 through contributory negligence by the patient.

4 Assessment of compensation

4.1 The amount of compensation paid should be appropriate to the nature, severity and persistence of the injury and should in general terms be consistent with the quantum of damages commonly awarded for similar injuries by an English Court in cases where legal liability is admitted.

4.2 Compensation may be abated, or in certain circumstances excluded, in the light of the following factors (on which will depend the level of risk the patient can reasonably be expected to accept):
   4.2.1 the seriousness of the disease being treated, the degree of probability that adverse reactions will occur and any warnings given;
   4.2.2 the risks and benefits of established treatments relative to those known or suspected of the trial medicine.

This reflects the fact that flexibility is required given the particular patient's circumstances. As an extreme example, there may be a patient suffering from a serious or life-threatening disease who is warned of a certain defined risk of adverse reaction. Participation in the trial is then based on an expectation that the benefit/risk ratio associated with participation may be better than that associated with alternative treatment. It is, therefore, reasonable that the patient accepts the high risk and should not expect compensation for the occurrence of the adverse reaction of which he or she was told.

4.3 In any case where the company concedes that a payment should be made to a patient but there exists a difference of opinion between company and patient as to the appropriate level of compensation, it is recommended that the company agrees to seek at its own cost (and make available to the patient) the opinion of a mutually acceptable independent expert, and that his opinion should be given substantial weight by the company in reaching its decision on the appropriate payment to be made.

5 Miscellaneous

5.1 Claims pursuant to the Guidelines should be made by the patient to the company, preferably via the investigator, setting out details of the nature and background of the claim and, subject to the patient providing on request an authority for the company to review any medical records relevant to the claim, the company should consider the claim expeditiously.

5.2 The undertaking given by a company extends to injury arising (at whatever time) from all administrations, clinical interventions or procedures occurring during the course of the trial but not to treatment extended beyond the end of the trial at the instigation of the investigator. The use of unlicensed products beyond the trial period is wholly the responsibility of the treating doctor and in this regard attention is drawn to the advice provided to doctors in MAL 30[2] concerning the desirability of doctors notifying their protection society of their use of unlicensed products.

5.3 The fact that a company has agreed to abide by these Guidelines in respect of a trial does not affect the right of a patient to pursue a legal remedy in respect of injury alleged to have been suffered as a result of participation. Nevertheless, patients will normally be asked to accept that any payment made under the Guidelines will be in full settlement of their claims.

5.4 A company sponsoring a trial should encourage the investigator to make clear to participating patients that the trial is being conducted subject to the ABPI Guidelines relating to compensation for injury arising in the course of clinical trials and have available copies of the Guidelines should they be requested.

REFERENCES

1 Guidelines for Medical Experiments in Non-patient Human Volunteers, ABPI March 1988, as amended May 1990.
2 MAL 30 – A Guide to the Provisions affecting Doctors and Dentists, DHSS, (Revised June 1985).

The Association of the British Pharmaceutical Industry
12 Whitehall London SW1A 2DY

41

Research ethics: guidance for nurses involved in research or any investigative project involving human subjects

Royal College of Nursing

Standards of Care series
Royal College of Nursing of the United Kingdom
Research Society

Published by
The Royal College of Nursing of the United Kingdom
20 Cavendish Square
London WIM 0AB

Distributed by
RCN Publishing Company
Nursing Standard House
17–19 Peterborough Road
Harrow, Middlesex HA1 2AX

© This edition 1998 Royal College of Nursing

Revised edition 1998

ISBN 1 873853 01 7

Typesetting and Design by Helen Lowe, London W10 5UE

Foreword

The changing face of nursing over the past 20 years or so is seldom more clearly demonstrated than by the increased involvement, as supervisor, commissioner or participant, of the nurse in research. Both the nursing profession's expanding professional role and the status of research in health care in general have contributed to placing the nursing practitioner at the centre of a culture in health care which strives for progress and seeks to institutionalise evidence-based practice.

Although the shifting nature of the nurse's role is to be welcomed, it is vital that practitioners bear in mind fundamental principles which must inform all research. In order to do this, guidance is needed to ensure that the nurse, now an active and involved participant in health-care teams, can effectively safeguard the rights and interests of their patients, while at the same time contributing to the progress that research seeks to achieve.

This pamphlet seeks to clarify ethical problems in research and also to provide for nurses a set of standards of best practice against which they can measure their involvement in research projects. It is written with clarity and balance and will provide an excellent starting point for any nursing practitioner who is contemplating initiating or becoming involved in research. By identifying core values in a readable and intelligible way, this pamphlet should prove to be invaluable for nurses in the current health-care climate.

Sheila A.M. McLean, International Bar Association Professor of Law and Ethics in Medicine, Director, Institute of Law and Ethics in Medicine, Glasgow University

Contents

Introduction

The first RCN research guidance, *Ethics Related to Research in Nursing*, was published in 1977 when nursing research in the UK was in its infancy. It was not until 16 years later that this first edition was updated (RCN, 1993). During those years, research became a recognised and accepted part of professional nursing practice, in part due to the increased number of nurses who achieved graduate status in the 1980s and provided the foundation for the development of nursing research in the 1990s. The years since 1993 have seen nursing become fully integrated into the academic community and, while research has always played an important part in the activities of nurses in educational settings, increasingly many clinical nurses incorporate an element of research into their daily work. The fact that the guidelines need to be revised once more after only five years is a testimony to the way in which nursing has faced up to its new agenda and is prepared to be a full participant in the research community.

This revision of the booklet has been carried out by the Ethics Sub-group of the RCN Research Society. Membership of this group is listed in Appendix 4. Members were invited to participate because of their known interest in this area. Early drafts of the revised guidelines were then circulated to a wider group of nurses for comment and appraisal and changes made accordingly. These revised guidelines build upon the structure and work that was done for previous editions and we would like to pay tribute to the work done by our predecessors. Although the booklet has been written to address the needs and concerns of nurses who are involved in research, it may also be of interest to other researchers who work with nurses.

In Part 1 of the booklet, the ethical principles underpinning research have been updated to incorporate some of the latest thinking on the application of ethics to research. This work was largely that of Dr Paul Wainwright. In Part 2, three new sections have been added, reflecting the developing roles of nurses in research. These new sections give guidance for nurses who commission research, those who supervise research and those who utilise the findings of research. The importance of local research ethics committees and the new multicentre research committees is highlighted, and we have included a flow chart showing the relationship between these two committees, because nurses will increasingly be negotiating their way through their procedures. Both these committees are particularly concerned with 'informed consent' and we have produced a detailed explanation of this term in Appendix 3.

Confusion often surrounds the difference between research and audit but, from an ethical perspective, whether or not a particular investigative project is research or audit is often irrelevant, since the same ethical principles apply to both. Those who wish to increase their knowledge about the ethical issues and debates in research will find a short bibliography of useful texts in Appendix 5.

Finally, I would like to thank everyone who has participated in this revision of the guidelines. I hope that its readers will find them useful and informative. The RCN Research Society welcomes any comments, positive and negative, and we will take these into account when we carry our next revision.

Dr Claire Hale
Chair of the Ethics Sub-group

1 The ethical principles underpinning research

It has been suggested that the aims of nursing research are twofold (de Raeve 1996, p. 139):
• To understand what nursing is;
• To promote good nursing care and understand failures of practice with the aim of rectifying the situation.

The ethical imperative underpinning these two aims stems from the nature of the relationship between nurses and their patients or clients, a relationship based on trust. Patients and clients, who are by definition vulnerable and in a relationship with health care professionals in which there is an inherent imbalance of power in favour of the professional, trust nurses to provide the best possible nursing care based on up-to-date knowledge and research. Nurses, like all health professionals, have no right to intervene in the lives of those in their care, unless they have good reason to think that their interventions will be helpful. Nurses thus have an obligation to keep their knowledge and practice skills up to date by keeping abreast of the literature in their field. This may be achieved by developing the ability to read the literature critically and make balanced

Note: the terms 'nurses' and 'nursing' are used collectively in this booklet to refer to all branches of the nursing, midwifery and health visiting professions.

judgments about the quality and relevance of the work to their practice. This ability requires an understanding of research methods as well as technical knowledge.

The principle of accountability demands that practitioners who adopt new practices do so not because somebody else tells them to, but because they have formed their own opinion, based on the available evidence, as to the merit of a new procedure, dressing or drug. An equal, if not greater, burden of trust and accountability also rests on those nurses who conduct research and disseminate their results, positive and negative, by publication in peer-reviewed journals.

The ethical requirements of researchers can thus be considered under two broad headings. One concerns the quality of the research and the integrity and conscientiousness of the researcher, and the other relates in particular to research which involves humans as the subject of study.

Although responsibility for decisions about practice rests with individual practitioners, those who read research reports are entitled to place trust in the authors' integrity. Readers, whether practitioners, academics, or those who act as referees for peer-reviewed publications, must use their own skill and judgment to assess the quality of the work. However, in the final analysis, the reader has little option at present but to accept on trust the honesty and integrity of the researchers and to assume that their account of their methods, presentation of data and acknowledgment of any limitations in their study is complete and accurate. It could thus be argued that, among the qualities that make a good researcher, attributes such as honesty, courage, diplomacy and conscientiousness are important.

The protection of human research participants, whether healthy volunteers, patients, clients or members of staff, is the main concern of this pamphlet. Subsequent sections go into some detail about the practical steps to be taken by researchers in this regard. The starting point, once again, is the relationship of trust which researchers have with society generally and with research participants in particular.

All research involving humans is carried out at some cost to the participants. This cost may seem trivial, requiring no more than that participants give up a little of their time to complete a simple questionnaire, or it may be considerable, involving time-consuming invasive procedures that may carry real risks of harm to the participants. The use of humans as research participants, with the consequent costs and risks, is frequently justified by reference to what might loosely be called utilitarianism. This means that, while the participants may receive no direct benefit from their involvement, the research is likely to produce longer term gains from which many people will benefit. possibly including at some future date the research participants

themselves, Such an argument, from what Evans and Evans (1996) have called a colloquial and relaxed sense of utilitarianism, may be appealing. However, Evans and Evans go on to reject utilitarianism in the strict sense as a justification for the use of humans in research studies, arguing that human research participants should be seen as vulnerable volunteers and that this is sufficient reason for thinking that they "need and deserve appropriate respect and protection".

It is this vulnerability of human research participants and their need for respect and protection that form the basis for the ethical review of nursing research and against which the desirability and acceptability of any research must be weighed. There are many competing theoretical approaches to ethics, such as deontology, consequentialism, theories of rights, and virtue ethics, any and all of which might provide the basis for justifying an approach to nursing research. All have been the subject of an extensive literature and it must be for individual researchers to decide to which theoretical approach they would appeal when considering their own research projects.

One approach which has received some attention in health-care ethics in recent years, has been referred to as a principle-based approach (Beauchamp & Childress 1994, Edwards 1996). This attempts to identify some common ground between the various theoretical approaches. The four principles to which Beauchamp and Childress refer are:

• Beneficence;
• Non-maleficence;
• Respect for autonomy;
• Justice.

These are all necessarily quite broad concepts, leaving considerable scope for interpretation in their application. Although such an approach has its limitations, it can serve as a useful basis from which to consider the protection of human participants in research and can provide a helpful starting point for any discussion of research and the obligations of researchers.

The principle-based approach

This section offers a brief outline of the principles introduced above and their relevance for nursing research.

Beneficence

The principle of beneficence holds that we should try to do good. As already suggested, there is a general assumption that the participation of nurses in research is important and necessary because of the obligation they have to give the best possible care. It is partly from the generation of knowledge gained through research that we can have confidence that we understand the role of the nurse even while this role is evolving. Nurses involved in research can therefore be thought to have at least the potential to do good.

However, the benefit to a patient or client that results from research is most likely to become apparent only some time after the completion and publication of the work, often because of the time lag between the completion of even the most clinically relevant research and its adoption in practice. Moreover, for many reasons, research may not lead directly to changes in practice. This may be because, although the work in question is basic research which increases our knowledge and understanding, it is not always immediately apparent how this knowledge can be applied to practice, or it may be because the study did not produce a positive result, or that the work was carried out as part of an educational programme for practitioners undergoing research training. In this latter case, it is the improved intellectual development and critical and analytical skills of the nurse researcher, rather than the findings from the research, that can be immediately applied in practice. An important question in reviewing a proposed study or reporting a completed study, will be to ascertain the extent of the potential for good to result and how this compares with any financial and other costs to individuals and organisations.

Non-maleficence

If one cannot always do good, or as much good as one would hope, one can certainly try to avoid doing harm, as the principle of non-maleficence requires. Some research carries obvious risks of harm, whether through the experimental testing of a new drug or operative procedure, or through the exploration of emotionally sensitive material with, for example, patients with malignant disease. Clearly such research does take place; many patients have died in the course of the search for treatments for previously untreatable conditions and much is known about the experiences of patients suffering from distressing conditions, and the nurses who care for them. If the notion of harm is extended to a broader notion of cost, then many people have given their time and energy and have allowed access to their private thoughts and experiences in the course of research. The point for the researcher is not that such costs should never be incurred, but that any risk of harm or cost

to the patient must be in proportion to the likely benefits from the research.

Respect for autonomy

The principle of autonomy holds that one of the characteristics of personhood is the ability to make free choices about oneself and one's life – to be 'self-governing'. This principle is at the heart of the doctrine of informed consent in health care and the tort of assault and battery in civil law. As with any other intervention in, or restraint upon, another's life or freedom of action, researchers who wish to conduct research using humans as 'subjects' must consider and take steps necessary to safeguard the autonomy of these 'subjects'. Thus it is required that humans give free and informed consent to taking part in research and therefore become not so much 'subjects' as 'participants'. Free in this context would mean that there was no duress or coercion used to persuade people to take part in research when they did not want to and that those who do agree to take part retain the right to withdraw at any point during the study. Refusal to take part in a research study, or a decision to withdraw, must carry no threat of retribution; patients and clients should be assured that the standard of their treatment will not be affected, at that time or in the future. Informed consent means that those who participate in research studies give their consent while in possession of all the relevant information necessary to allow them to make a proper choice.

However, there are those who would argue that free and informed consent is impossible to obtain as there will always be an imbalance of power and knowledge between researcher and research participants. For example, understanding the methodological intricacies of a particular study may require specialist knowledge, or the constraints of the study may mean that it is not possible to fully inform potential participants without compromising the research. The challenge for all researchers is to find ways to overcome these difficulties and ensure that subjects are always 'informed participants'.

Confidentiality

A further point which follows from the principle of autonomy concerns the right of the individual to control access to information about themselves. We all have areas of our lives that we would prefer to keep private, but it is precisely these aspects which may be the subject of many research studies. We are used to divulging personal information, in the context of a professional relationship with a nurse, doctor, or solicitor, but such information is imparted on the understanding that it will be shared only with those who have a 'need to know' for professional purposes. This control over disclosure is an important consideration for the researcher, who must ensure that, when research participants are offered anonymity or confidentiality, they really are protected – if they cannot be, then the researcher must ensure that participants have given consent to access and are fully aware of the consequences.

Justice

Justice, in the sense used here, is about fairness. There is much concern in the health-care system about the just distribution of resources, so that people are treated fairly, although it is worth noting that fairness does not always mean equality. For example, few people would suggest that everyone should receive an equal amount of health care, when in fact some of us require more than others. What is important is that we are treated alike when the situation demands and that people have equal access to appropriate care. For the manager and policy maker, there may be broad issues of resource distribution, in the sense that resources spent on research cannot then be spent on other activities, such as patient care. There will also be questions about the extent to which participation in research studies results in some individuals receiving an inequitable share of resources, such as preferential treatment. The researcher who also has clinical or teaching responsibilities might also be accused of injustice if he/she were to neglect everyday activities and responsibilities in favour of research.

Conclusions

The management, supervision, conduct and utilisation of research raise many ethical issues for all involved. Those who commission research, those who work in areas in which research is undertaken, those who do research, those who supervise the process of research and those who utilise the findings of research all have the responsibility for ensuring that research in which they are involved is conducted in ways that are ethically sound. It is not sufficient, for example, to rely on the researcher or the research ethics committee to ensure this. The research is more likely to be designed, completed and used in an ethically sound way

if all nurses understand and have thought through the implications of ethical principles which are relevant to nursing research. The identification of the values which guide their actions and the relationship of these to ethical principles is a prerequisite. The specific issues that may confront nurses whose role in any way brings them into contact with research are discussed in more detail in the Part 2 of this booklet.

REFERENCES

Beauchamp, T.L., Childress, J.F. (1994) *Principles of Biomedical Ethics.* Oxford University Press, Oxford.

Edwards, S. (1996) *Nursing Ethics: A principles based approach.* MacMillan, Basingstoke.

Evans, D., Evans, M. (1996) *A Decent Proposal: Ethical review of clinical research.* John Wiley, Chichester.

de Raeve, L. (ed). (1997) *Nursing Research: An ethical and legal appraisal.* Baillière Tindall, London.

2 Ethical guidelines for nurses involved in research

The principles outlined in Part 1 provide a useful framework for understanding the ethical issues underpinning research. However, nurses involved in research must also abide by a large number of statutory ethical guidelines as well as professional and moral ethical codes. The guidelines presented here are designed to help nurses ensure that research, from the planning and commissioning stage to the dissemination and utilisation of findings, is conducted in an ethically acceptable way, consistent with current statutory ethical guidelines.

Guidelines are provided for:
- Nurses undertaking research;
- Nurses in positions of authority where research is to be carried out;
- Nurses practising in settings where research is being undertaken;
- Nurses commissioning research;
- Nurses supervising research;
- Nurses utilising the findings of research.

These guidelines, while comprehensive, do not provide an exhaustive list of all possible ethical implications of research but are intended to give information which will enable ethical research to be carried out and the findings utilised. Suggestion for wider reading are given in Appendix 5.

Research ethics committees

In 1991, the Department of Health Circular HSG (91) 5 required each health authority in England and Wales[1,2] to set up a local research ethics committee (LREC). These committees were given the authority to review and approve research proposals involving patients and healthy volunteers within the NHS. The committees are composed of a mixture of lay and professional members. Researchers are denied access to NHS patients without the approval of the relevant LREC and all nursing research proposals which involve or affect patients and/or healthy volunteers (including some projects which may be 'classed' as audit) should be submitted to the LREC.

In 1997, the Department of Health Circular HSG (97)23[3] authorised the setting up of multicentre research ethics committees (MRECs). These will be responsible for considering research which is to be conducted across five or more LREC geographical boundaries. Information about LRECs and MRECs can be obtained from health authority offices or regional NHS executive R&D offices. The working relationship between LRECs and MRECs is described in the flow chart in Appendix 2.

Guidelines for nurses undertaking research

Nurses undertake research in a number of capacities. This may be as principal investigator on a project they have been commissioned to carry out, as research student for an academic qualification, or as a member of a research team. All nurses involved in research should adhere to the following guidelines.

Integrity of the researcher

1 All nurses involved in research must possess relevant knowledge and skills, compatible with their involvement in the proposed investigation. Researchers must recognise the nature and limits of their research competence and should not accept or try to undertake work which they are not equipped to carry out.

2 Nurses who are learning to do research should work under the guidance and supervision of an experienced

researcher. This is a minimum requirement to safeguard the well-being of research participants and to maintain professional credibility.

3 Researchers have a responsibility to recognise and make known to sponsors, supervisors or commissioners of research any relevant personal prejudices, biases or conflicts of interest which may influence the investigation.

4 Researchers should ensure that ethical implications arising from the research are identified in their written plan of the proposed study, that ethical approval is obtained where appropriate and that all members of the research team are aware of these and of the general importance of ethical standards in research.

5 Researchers working in any setting must assure themselves that the arrangements for data management, storage, retrieval and ownership are constructed so as to protect participant confidentiality and avoid introducing bias into the data set. This includes collecting data according to a stated protocol, identifying and minimising potential sources of bias, recording data coding and analysis decisions, ensuring that data are reported accurately and that, if an error is discovered, it is corrected and made public. Principal investigators should be aware of their team's responsibilities under the Data Protection Act (1984) and, from October 1998, the Council of the European Union Directive on Data Protection (1995).

6 Nurses who are principal investigators should ensure that an audit trail is kept for independent inspection if necessary. This includes keeping primary data, field notes and an account of the basis on which decisions were made. This makes the entire process open, defensible and justifiable and could lead to an increase in the reliability and validity of the data collected.

7 Nurses who are principal investigators should ensure that the project team prospectively determines the responsibilities, obligations, degree of involvement and role of each member. The establishment of an advisory group for the project is recommended.

8 Researchers have a responsibility to indicate in their final report any ways in which their involvement, interactions or interventions may have affected the participants in the study and, in turn, the validity of the data, or resulted in limitations in the research.

9 Researchers have a responsibility to publish, or otherwise make available, the results of their research. This includes information about methods and research tools, all relevant data (including negative findings), any limitations of the research, and the extent to which results obtained can be generalised. These findings should be

---

[1] For Scotland, NHS Circ 1992(Gen)3.

[2] For current procedures in Northern Ireland contact the Information and Research Policy Branch, Dept of Health and Social Services, Belfast.

[3] For Scotland, NHS MEL(1997)8.

disseminated, if appropriate, locally, regionally, nationally and internationally. Ideally, such publications should be independently peer-reviewed to assure their quality.

10 Prior to publication of the research findings, it is the responsibility of the grant holder or principal investigator to ensure that consensus about the nature of the material to be published is reached by members of the research team and other stakeholders.

11 Formal agreement should be obtained before names are cited and copyright regulations should be strictly followed in relation to the use of quotations and references to published works.

12 Authors of research publications should be defined as the persons making a substantial contribution to the published work, including responsibility for:

(a) Conception and design, or analysis and interpretation of the data;

(b) Drafting the article or revising it critically for important intellectual content;

(c) Final approval of the version to be published.

These three conditions must all be met. Acknowledgment should be made of the contribution of others to any research study but these should not be deemed authors. Each author should have participated sufficiently in the work to take public responsibility for the content. The order of authorship should be a joint decision of the co-authors[4].

13 Nurses working as researchers on multidisciplinary research projects should receive proper recognition and acknowledgment for their contribution.

14 Researchers should take every available opportunity to promote the appropriate use of their research findings and should not ignore any apparent misuse.

Responsibility to research participants

1 Before undertaking any research, the researcher must be satisfied that the knowledge which is being sought is not already available and could not be acquired equally well by other means. A comprehensive literature review should have been carried out. However, replication

---

[4] These authorship guidelines are based on those of the International Committee of Medical Journal Editors. Uniform requirements of manuscripts submitted to biomedical journals (*Br Med J* 1991, **302:** 338–41). However, 'authorship' is frequently the subject of debate and, in case of doubt, researchers should always check with specific journal editors.

studies are sometimes necessary to test for generalisability and these may add to knowledge in the area being researched.

2 In all studies where NHS patients or clients are to be involved, the approval of the LREC is necessary prior to commencing the research. When the research is being carried out in more than five LREC areas, approval must be sought first from the appropriate MREC. Any amendments to a study protocol after permission has been granted should be submitted to the committee for approval. The MREC and/or LREC should be informed of any serious adverse events or deaths occurring in participants as a consequence of their involvement and should also be informed of any problems of an ethical nature which occur during the data collection. The MREC and/or LREC should be notified when any research study that they have approved is completed. Research on humans outside the NHS should, wherever possible, be referred for independent ethical review, for example to a university or departmental ethics committee where possible. Where research studies involve NHS staff as research participants, local NHS policy regarding ethical approval should be followed.

3 In research which involves human participants, there must be identifiable safeguards for their protection against physical, mental, emotional and social harm. If there is any foreseeable possibility of physical discomfort or emotional distress, then participants should be forewarned in order to take this into account when considering consent for their involvement.

4 It is the responsibility of the principal investigator to ensure that appropriate insurance indemnity has been obtained for the study, not only for participants but also for all personnel involved. It is also important to ensure that all team members are aware of and understand the terms of the indemnity.

5 Researchers are responsible for obtaining freely given and informed consent from each individual who is to be a participant in a study or personally involved in some other way in the research. This requires that the researcher explain as fully as possible, and in terms meaningful to each prospective participant, the nature and purpose of the study, how and why he/she was selected and invited to take part, what is required of participants and who is undertaking and financing the investigation. This information should be provided in written form at all times and the participant's written consent must be recorded. Ideally, the individual should be allowed time to consider taking part in the study and to discuss this with family and friends before making a decision (for

exceptions, see Guidelines 7 and 8 below). (See Appendix 3 for discussion of informed consent.)

6 In seeking voluntary informed consent, the researcher must emphasise that subjects have the absolute right to refuse to participate or to withdraw from the study at any time without the quality of their care or other rights being affected in any way. The rights of refusal and withdrawal must be respected by researchers.

7 Where individuals are incapable of giving informed consent (for example, if they are unconscious or unable to reason because of age or infirmity), in some cases it may be appropriate to seek consent by proxy (this is sometimes referred to as 'assent'). This may be given by an advocate who is concerned with the welfare of that individual, for example a parent or guardian. In addition, the consent of a child over seven years of age should usually be sought directly from the child. As a general principle, people who are mentally impaired or have a learning disability should not be participants in a research study if the research could equally be carried out on other adults. However, if the research is associated with their disability, they may be the most appropriate participants to be involved in the study, in which case those unable to give consent should only be involved in research into their condition and then usually only if there is direct therapeutic value to them.

8 In research studies involving patients who have an acute life-threatening condition (for example, acutely ill cardiac patients) it may be impossible to obtain consent prior to entry into a study. When gaining permission for such studies from the LREC/MREC, procedures for informing the patient or patient's family should be approved by the committee, which will normally expect that the individual's consent be obtained retrospectively if possible.

9 Researchers should be aware that personal health information, such as is held in medical records and nursing notes, is confidential; permission, consent and ethical approval are therefore required for its use in research. However, if a large number of records are involved it is not always possible or practical to seek the consent of each and every patient or client. In these cases consent for the transfer of information from records should be sought from the 'custodian of the record' who in most cases will be the doctor currently responsible for the patient's or client's care. Where possible and practical it is always good practice to obtain the consent from the individual patient or client. Some NHS trusts now give patients a document telling them that information recorded in their medical notes may be entered in computer files and used, in confidence, for medical purposes other than their immediate care, including research. In cases of uncertainty researchers should seek the advice of the LREC/MREC in advance.

10 If a research study involves the use of information, materials or specimens gathered for another purpose, separate consent must be obtained even if consent was obtained for the original use of the information, material or specimen. The exception to this is information which may be regarded as being within the ownership of an institution, such as information used for audit.

11 The nature of any promises of confidentiality or restriction on the use of data must be made clear to the research participants and subsequently strictly adhered to by the researcher and research team. This obligation continues through to the dissemination of research findings.

12 To safeguard the welfare of participants in research situations, researchers must decide at what point ethical requirements necessitate an intervention in order to maintain the safety of the patient or client, whatever the consequences for the research. This could include abandoning data collection in that area if the incident would influence data collected subsequently.

13 The researcher should be alert for and address any irregularities in patient compliance which may vitiate the findings from the research study (for example, patients reporting that they have taken medication when in fact they have not).

Relations with sponsors, employers and colleagues

1 Researchers should not undertake work beyond their competence and have an obligation to make this clear to employers and sponsors.

2 Researchers should decline requests to undertake research if resources (finance, time, personnel or equipment) are insufficient for the achievement of the research aims.

3 Researchers must make clear to sponsors, employers and colleagues that the research does not necessarily guarantee solutions to problems, and should make explicit the limitations and benefits that may arise as a result of the proposed research.

---

[5] For further guidance in this matter refer to the current ICH Harmonised Tripartite Guideline for Good Clinical Practice and the European Commission draft directive COM(97)369.

[6] Royal College of Physicians (1996) *Guidelines on the Practice of Ethics Committees in Medical Research Involving Human Subjects.* Royal College of Physicians, London.

4 The terms and conditions under which the research is to be carried out should be negotiated, documented and signed by the appropriate people so as to avoid later problems arising from misunderstandings or misgivings. A copy of the signed document should be kept with the study documentation and a copy sent to the contracting sponsor.

5 When the researcher is a member of staff of the organisation funding the research, it is important to clarify in advance the researcher's responsibilities within the organisation, how much autonomy he/she has, the lines of communication and the means of settling any problems or conflicts of interest which may arise. The setting up of an independent advisory group is advisable in these circumstances.

6 Researchers have a responsibility to be fully conversant with the terms and conditions attached to any grant awarded to support their research, and to recognise any consequent constraints on their activity or autonomy. Grant holders are responsible for the expenditure of the funds and must ensure that they can justify the way the funds are used. Proper financial records must be kept.

7 Researchers have a responsibility to notify and obtain approval from sponsors and/or employers of any proposed departure from the plan of investigation and conditions agreed at the outset.

8 Whether or not the aims of the research are achieved, the researcher has an obligation to provide the sponsor and/or employer and colleagues with a report on completion of the study. Sponsors and/or employers may request interim reports and may exercise the right to see the final report before its release and publication. Before accepting a research contract, the researcher should clarify any possible restrictions that may be placed by the sponsor and/or employer on the publication of findings.

9 Nurses who have a research role in a clinical area should seek clarification about the division between their research role and their professional obligations. It is unlikely that a nurse in a research role will have responsibility for the service, care, treatment or advice given to patients or clients other than that which is stipulated within the design of the research. Any intervention by the nurse in a professional capacity, other than that required by the study protocol, should therefore be confined to situations in which a patient or client requires to be protected or rescued from danger.

10 In a research project which is experimental in design, or which involves a new or altered form of practice, agreement must be reached in advance with those who are directly responsible for patient care and/or service provision, concerning the requirements for the research intervention, the process of its implementation and the respective responsibilities of the researcher and service staff.

11 A patient or client's involvement in a research project usually requires the prior permission of the medical consultant or general practitioner responsible for that individual's medical care. Even if permission is not required, the researcher should ensure that, where appropriate, the general practitioner or medical consultant concerned is aware of the individual's involvement in the study. Sometimes this may involve obtaining permission from the individual patient or client before informing the general practitioner or medical consultant. In some research studies, an individual's refusal to allow his/her general practitioner or medical consultant to be informed of his/her involvement would lead to that individual being excluded from participation in the study.

Guidelines for nurses in positions of authority where research may be carried out

The following guidelines are intended for nurses who have a managerial or professional responsibility for staff and/or patients in clinical areas where research may be carried out.

1 Nurses with the authority to sanction research within units or organisations for which they are responsible must satisfy themselves that:

(a) The research is worthwhile, achievable and ethical and, taking account of service demands, is a feasible proposition. In reaching these decisions, the advice of an independent experienced researcher and/or a research committee is likely to be valuable;

(b) There is a rigorous procedure by which voluntary informed consent will be obtained from participants. Particular attention should be given to situations in which the participants may be in a special or vulnerable relationship to the investigator (for example, students participating in a project where their teacher is the investigator);

(c) Clinical staff are in agreement with the granting of access and understand the implications of this;

(d) Clinical staff are not expected to carry out research activities beyond their competence without appropriate training;

(e) The interests of patients and clients are not compromised by the demands of the research, taking into account the manager's responsibility to facilitate research wherever possible.

2 Nurses employing or managing a research worker should ensure that the person employed has the necessary competences (or is prepared to be supervised while gaining them) to carry out the work. Nurses in a position of authority must also respect a researcher's right to refuse to undertake a project because he/she considers that it is beyond his/her competence, that it is is not feasible within the resources or timescale available, or that it involves practices to which the individual objects on grounds of conscience.

3 Any promises of anonymity or confidentiality given to the participants by the researcher must be respected by the relevant nurse manager. No attempt should be made to probe data or results in order to identify any individual, instance or place which has been concealed deliberately by the researcher.

4 Nurse managers who agree to a research study being carried out should do their best to ensure that, whatever the findings, the results are published and disseminated, critically appraised and appropriately used.

5 Research data or findings must not be used for purposes of disciplinary proceedings in connection with individuals' involvement in the study, the exception being instances of gross misconduct or fraud that require action to be taken.

Guidelines for nurses practising where research is undertaken

The higher profile of research activity in the NHS has meant that increased numbers of nurses are working in areas where research is being carried out by many different health professionals. The following guidelines are intended for clinical nurses practising in settings where research is being undertaken by other people.

Responsibilities as practitioners

1 In the course of their normal work, nurses may be involved in research studies. This involvement may comprise:
 • Caring for patients who are participants in a study;
 • Acting as witness that informed consent has been given by the patient/client or his/her representative (see also 'Responsibility to research participants', Guideline 5, page 15, and Appendix 3);
 • Collecting data for the research study;
 • Carrying out procedures or activities which are the topic of research.

This involvement in research carries with it two major responsibilities – to ensure that informed consent has been given and to be satisfied that the research is being conducted in an ethically acceptable way. To comply with these responsibilities the nurse should always:
 (a) Check the content of any information sheet to ensure that it contains relevant and accurate information;
 (b) Check that a patient (and/or the patient's relative or guardian) who is involved in a research study understands the aims of the study, the degree of involvement expected (for example, documentation to keep, medication to take, tests to be carried out) and that he/she can withdraw at any time without detriment to present or future care;
 (c) Know from whom further information can be obtained;
 (d) Understand the nature of his/her own involvement, if any, in the research study.

2 A primary or named nurse has a responsibility to be satisfied that studies involving patients in his/her care are being conducted in an ethically acceptable way. In practice, this might mean that the nurse obtains confirmation that the study has LREC approval. In the event of the nurse considering the research to be unethical or to be having any unnecessary adverse effect on subjects or on the service, the nurse concerned should convey his/her anxieties to the researcher and/or to the appropriate person in authority (his/her line manager). Concerns can also be directed to the chairperson of the LREC.

Responsibilities as data collectors

1 Nurses asked to participate in research as data collectors in addition to their usual duties have an obligation to make it known if this extra responsibility might be, or has become, detrimental to their normal work.

2 Nurses agreeing to assist with data collection must adhere to the ethical principles incumbent on all researchers. Integrity and accuracy are essential requirements of anyone involved in data collection.

3 Nurses acting as data collectors must recognise the implications of this dual role and, in particular, those which relate to confidentiality of data. Information about research participants, which is confidential to them as nurses, should not be made available to the research team unless agreed as part of the approved research plan. Likewise, data collected for research purposes are confidential to the research team and should not be used by the nurse in the course of his/her normal work, or for any other

purpose, without permission of the principal investigator, who in turn requires the consent of the research participant.

4 Nurses invited to participate in research studies must ensure that they are competent to carry out the required procedures.

5 Nurses invited to participate in research trials of commercial products must satisfy themselves that the research design is sound and that the study is based on ethical principles. If these trials involve patients or clients within the NHS then, as with all such studies, they should be approved by the LREC/MREC. In participating in commercially sponsored research, nurses should avoid any association with the advertisement or promotion of a particular product and should be aware of and adhere to any workplace guidelines on this subject.

Guidelines for nurses commissioning research

With the increased profile being given to evidence-based practice and the changes in research funding in the NHS, nurses in executive positions may now wish to commission research studies. The following guidelines have been designed to help with this process.

1 Nurses with the authority to commission research within the units or organisations for which they are responsible must satisfy themselves that the research is worthwhile, achievable and ethical. In reaching these decisions, the nurse may wish to invite a reputable organisation to organise/manage the commissioning process on his/her organisation's behalf.

2 Nurses who are in a position to manage their own commissioning process should ensure that the procedures are fair and transparent.

3 Nurses commissioning research or employing a research worker must respect the researcher's right to refuse to undertake a project which, in the researcher's opinion, is beyond their research competence or is not feasible within the resources or timescale available.

4 Nurses commissioning research should satisfy themselves that, in accordance with the above guidelines for nurses undertaking research, there is a sound procedure by which voluntary informed consent will be obtained from subjects. Particular attention should be given to situations in which the subjects may be in a special or vulnerable relationship to the investigator (for example, students participating in a research project where their teacher is the investigator).

5 A nurse who has commissioned a study must respect any promises of anonymity or confidentiality given to the participants by the researcher. No attempt should be made to probe data or results in order to identify any individual, instance or place which has been concealed deliberately by the researcher.

6 Nurses who commission a research study should ensure that the results of the work are critically appraised, disseminated and appropriately used, whatever the findings.

Guidelines for nurses supervising research

The increased educational opportunities which have been available to nurses over recent years have meant that many now have research skills and are in a position to supervise less experienced researchers. These guidelines are designed for nurses who work in educational or service organisations and who may be required to supervise research.

1 Nurses supervising research and those they supervise should agree guidelines for their relationship at the start of the project. The nature of these guidelines will depend on several factors, including the time commitment of the supervisor, the experience of the researcher and whether or not the project forms part of an academic award. This can avoid later problems arising from misunderstandings and misgivings.

2 Nurses supervising research should be aware of the ethical principles underpinning research and should provide guidance to ensure that those they supervise are also aware of these.

3 Nurses supervising research must ensure that all the researchers for whom they are responsible are aware of, understand and abide by the guidelines for the 'Integrity of the researcher' outlined in this booklet (page 10) and 'Responsibility for research participants' (page 12).

4 Nurses supervising research should help those conducting the research to articulate the ethical issues arising from their project and provide guidance as to how these can be addressed.

5 Nurses supervising research should ensure that the research proposal is in an acceptable format for submission to any internal and external committees.

6 Nurses supervising research should ensure that the research proposal has been approved by all the appropriate university or service committees prior to the start of the project.

7 When a project involves patients and clients within the NHS, nurses supervising the research should ensure that the researcher has obtained ethical approval from the appropriate LREC/MREC prior to the start of the project.

8 Nurses supervising research should abide by the guidelines for 'Integrity of the researcher' outlined in this booklet (page 262) and should not exploit their relationship with researchers under their supervision.

9 Nurses supervising research should provide training, mentorship and fair and constructive appraisal of the researcher's performance. This should include the allocation of sufficient time for the supervisory process.

Guidelines for nurses utilising research findings

The increased emphasis on clinical effectiveness and evidence-based practice has meant that nurses should base their practice and teaching on sound research evidence where available, introducing change where necessary. The following guidelines should be observed.

1 Nurses need to be equipped to appraise the scientific value of this evidence, because it is unethical to implement the findings of research the validity of which is questionable. Nurses who do not as yet have the skills of critical appraisal should ensure that any research findings that they wish to incorporate into their practice have been appraised by suitably skilled colleagues.

2 From an ethical perspective, when carrying out critical appraisals, nurses should pay particular attention to the following:
   (a) The competence of the researchers;
   (b) The funding body;
   (c) That the study has had ethical approval from an appropriate body;
   (d) That sufficient information is available about the methods of the study to make judgements about its scientific value.

3 When considering implementing changes in practice which are based on research findings, nurses should:
   (a) Be aware of the financial implications and any effect that these may have on available resources;
   (b) Be alert to any possibility that the care of other patients or clients might be compromised by the implementation of the changes.

4 Nurses should be aware that it is unethical to be carrying out practices when substantial evidence exists confirming that these practices are detrimental to patient care.

42

Ethical principles for conducting research with human participants

The British Psychological Society

Introduction to the revised principles

The Standing Committee on Ethics in Research with Human Participants has now completed its revision of the Ethical Principles for Research with Human Subjects (British Psychological Society, 1978). The new 'Ethical Principles for Conducting Research with Human Participants' (q.v.) have been approved by the Council.

The Standing Committee wishes to highlight some of the issues that concerned it during the drawing up of the Principles published below. In the forefront of its considerations was the recognition that psychologists owe a debt to those who agree to take part in their studies and that people who are willing to give up their time, even for remuneration, should be able to expect to be treated with the highest standards of consideration and respect. This is reflected in the change from the term 'subjects' to 'participants'. To psychologists brought up on the jargon of their profession the term 'subject' is not derogatory. However, to someone who has not had that experience of psychological research it is a term which can seem impersonal.

Deception

The issue of deception caused the Committee considerable problems. To many outside the psychology profession, and to some within it, the idea of deceiving the participants in one's research is seen as quite inappropriate. At best, the experience of deception in psychological research

can make the recipients cynical about the activities and attitudes of psychologists. However, since there are very many psychological processes that are modifiable by individuals if they are aware that they are being studied, the statement of the research hypothesis in advance of the collection of data would make much psychological research impossible. The Committee noted that there is a distinction between withholding some of the details of the hypothesis under test and deliberately falsely informing the participants of the purpose of the research, especially if the information given implied a more benign topic of study than was in fact the case. While the Committee wishes to urge all psychologists to seek to supply as full information as possible to those taking part in their research, it concluded that the central principle was the reaction of participants when deception was revealed. If this led to discomfort, anger or objections from the participants then the deception was inappropriate. The Committee hopes that such a principle protects the dignity of the participants while allowing valuable psychological research to be conducted.

Debriefing

Following the research, especially where any deception or withholding of information had taken place, the Committee wished to emphasise the importance of appropriate debriefing. In some circumstances, the verbal description of the nature of the investigation would not be sufficient to eliminate all possibility of harmful after-effects. For example, an experiment in which negative mood was induced requires the induction of a happy mood state before the participant leaves the experimental setting.

Risk

Another area of concern for the Committee was the protection of participants from undue risk in psychological research. Since this was an area in which the Principles might be looked to during an investigation following a complaint against a researcher, the Committee was concerned to seek a definition that protected the participants in the research without making important research impossible. Risks attend us every moment in life, and to say that research should involve no risks would be inappropriate. However, the important principle seemed to be that when participants entered upon a psychological investigation they should not, in so doing, be increasing the probability that they would come to any form of harm. Thus, the definition of undue risk was based upon the risks that individuals run in their normal lifestyle. This definition makes possible research upon individuals who lead a risk-taking or risk-seeking life (e.g. mountaineers, cave divers), so long as the individuals are not induced to take risks that are greater than those that they would normally encounter in their life outside the research.

Implementation

The Council of the Society approved the Principles at its meeting in February 1990. There followed a two-year period during which the new Principles were provisionally in operation. In Spring 1992 the Council reviewed the Principles, in the light of experience of their operation. During this period researchers were unable to identify problems in the working of the Principles. Following minor amendment the Principles were formally adopted in October 1992.

The Council urges all research psychologists to ensure that they abide by these Principles, which supplement the Society's Code of Conduct (q.v.) and thus violation of them could form the basis of disciplinary action. It is essential that all members of the psychological profession abide by the Principles if psychologists are to continue to retain the privilege of testing human participants in their research. Psychologists have legal as well as moral responsibilities for those who help them in their study, and the long-term reputation of the discipline depends largely upon the experience of those who encounter it first-hand during psychological investigations.

Ethical principles for conducting research with human participants

1 Introduction

1.1 The principles given below are intended to apply to research with human participants. Principles of conduct in professional practice are to be found in the Society's Code of Conduct and in the advisory documents prepared by the Divisions, Sections and Special Groups of the Society.

1.2 Participants in psychological research should have confidence in the investigators. Good psychological research is possible only if there is mutual respect and confidence between investigators and participants. Psychological investigators are potentially interested in all aspects of human behaviour and conscious experience. However, for ethical reasons, some areas of human experience and behaviour may be beyond the reach of experiment, observation or other form of psychological investigation. Ethical guidelines are necessary to clarify the conditions under which psychological research is acceptable.

1.3 The principles given below supplement for researchers with human participants the general ethical principles of members of the Society as stated in The British Psychological Society's Code of Conduct (q.v.). Members of The British Psychological Society are expected to abide by both the Code of Conduct and the fuller principles expressed here. Members should also draw the principles to the attention of research colleagues who are not members of the Society. Members should encourage colleagues to adopt them and ensure that they are followed by all researchers whom they supervise (e.g. research assistants, postgraduate, undergraduate, A-Level and GCSE students).

1.4 In recent years, there has been an increase in legal actions by members of the general public against professionals for alleged misconduct. Researchers must recognise the possibility of such legal action if they infringe the rights and dignity of participants in their research.

2 General

2.1 In all circumstances, investigators must consider the ethical implications and psychological consequences for the participants in their research. The essential principle is that the investigation should be considered from the standpoint of all participants; foreseeable threats to their psychological well-being, health, values or dignity should be eliminated. Investigators should recognise that, in our multi-cultural and multi-ethnic society and where investigations involve individuals of different ages, gender and social background, the investigators may not have sufficient knowledge of the implications of any investigation for the participants. It should be borne in mind that the best judge of whether an investigation will cause offence may be members of the population from which the participants in the research are to be drawn.

3 Consent

3.1 Whenever possible, the investigator should inform all participants of the objectives of the investigation. The investigator should inform the participants of all aspects of the research or intervention that might reasonably be expected to influence willingness to participate. The investigator should, normally, explain all other aspects of the research or intervention about which the participants enquire. Failure to make full disclosure prior to obtaining informed consent requires additional safeguards to protect the welfare and dignity of the participants (see Section 4).

3.2 Research with children or with participants who have impairments that will limit understanding and/or communication such that they are unable to give their real consent requires special safe-guarding procedures.

3.3 Where possible, the real consent of children and of adults with impairments in understanding or communication should be obtained. In addition, where research involves any persons under 16 years of age, consent should be obtained from parents or from those in loco parentis. If the nature of the research precludes consent being obtained from parents or permission being obtained from teachers, before proceeding with the research, the investigator must obtain approval from an Ethics Committee.

3.4 Where real consent cannot be obtained from adults with impairments in understanding or communication, wherever possible the investigator should consult a person well-placed to appreciate the participant's reaction, such as a member of the person's family, and must obtain the disinterested approval of the research from independent advisors.

3.5 When research is being conducted with detained persons, particular care should be taken over informed consent, paying attention to the special circumstances which may affect the person's ability to give free informed consent.

3.6 Investigators should realise that they are often in a position of authority or influence over participants who may be their students, employees or clients. This relationship must not be allowed to pressurise the participants to take part in, or remain in, an investigation.

3.7 The payment of participants must not be used to induce them to risk harm beyond that which they risk without payment in their normal lifestyle.

3.8 If harm, unusual discomfort, or other negative consequences for the individual's future life might occur, the investigator must obtain the disinterested approval of independent advisors, inform the participants, and obtain informed, real consent from each of them.

3.9 In longitudinal research, consent may need to be obtained on more than one occasion.

4 Deception

4.1 The withholding of information or the misleading of participants is unacceptable if the participants are typically likely to object or show unease once debriefed. Where this is in any doubt, appropriate consultation must precede the investigation. Consultation is best carried out with individuals who share the social and cultural background of the participants in the research, but the advice of ethics committees or experienced and disinterested colleagues may be sufficient.

4.2 Intentional deception of the participants over the purpose and general nature of the investigation should be avoided whenever possible. Participants should never be deliberately misled without extremely strong scientific or medical justification. Even then there should be strict controls and the disinterested approval of independent advisors.

4.3 It may be impossible to study some psychological processes without withholding information about the true object of the study or deliberately misleading the participants. Before conducting such a study, the investigator has a special responsibility to
(a) determine that alternative procedures avoiding concealment or deception are not available;

(b) ensure that the participants are provided with sufficient information at the earliest stage; and
(c) consult appropriately upon the way that the with holding of information or deliberate deception will be received.

5 Debriefing

5.1 In studies where the participants are aware that they have taken part in an investigation, when the data have been collected, the investigator should provide the participants with any necessary information to complete their understanding of the nature of the research. The investigator should discuss with the participants their experience of the research in order to monitor any unforeseen negative effects or misconceptions.

5.2 Debriefing does not provide a justification for unethical aspects of any investigation.

5.3 Some effects which may be produced by an experiment will not be negated by a verbal description following the research. Investigators have a responsibility to ensure that participants receive any necessary debriefing in the form of active intervention before they leave the research setting.

6 Withdrawal from the investigation

6.1 At the onset of the investigation investigators should make plain to participants their right to withdraw from the research at any time, irrespective of whether or not payment or other inducement has been offered. It is recognised that this may be difficult in certain observational or organisational settings, but nevertheless the investigator must attempt to ensure that participants (including children) know of their right to withdraw. When testing children, avoidance of the testing situation may be taken as evidence of failure to consent to the procedure and should be acknowledged.

6.2 In the light of experience of the investigation, or as a result of debriefing, the participant has the right to withdraw retrospectively any consent given, and to require that their own data, including recordings, be destroyed.

7 Confidentiality

7.1 Subject to the requirements of legislation, including the Data Protection Act, information obtained about a participant during an investigation is confidential unless otherwise agreed in advance. Investigators who are put under pressure to disclose confidential information should draw this point to the attention of those exerting such pressure. Participants in psychological research have a right to expect that information they provide will be treated confidentially and, if published, will not be identifiable as theirs. In the event that confidentiality and/or anonymity cannot be guaranteed, the participant must be warned of this in advance of agreeing to participate.

8 Protection of participants

8.1 Investigators have a primary responsibility to protect participants from physical and mental harm during the investigation. Normally, the risk of harm must be no greater than in ordinary life, i.e. participants should not be exposed to risks greater than or additional to those encountered in their normal lifestyles. Where the risk of harm is greater than in ordinary life the provisions of 3.8 should apply. Participants must be asked about any factors in the procedure that might create a risk, such as pre-existing medical conditions, and must be advised of any special action they should take to avoid risk.

8.2 Participants should be informed of procedures for contacting the investigator within a reasonable time period following participation should stress, potential harm, or related questions or concern arise despite the precautions required by the Principles. Where research procedures might result in undesirable consequences for participants, the investigator has the responsibility to detect and remove or correct these consequences.

8.3 Where research may involve behaviour or experiences that participants may regard as personal and private the participants must be protected from stress by all appropriate measures, including the assurance that answers to personal questions need not be given. There should be no concealment or deception when seeking information that might encroach on privacy.

8.4 In research involving children, great caution should be exercised when discussing the results with parents, teachers or others acting in loco parentis, since evaluative statements may carry unintended weight.

9 Observational research

9.1 Studies based upon observation must respect the privacy and psychological well-being of the individuals studied. Unless those observed give their consent to being observed, observational research is only acceptable in situations where those observed would expect to be observed by strangers. Additionally, particular account should be taken of local cultural values and of the possibility of intruding upon the privacy of individuals who, even while in a normally public space, may believe they are unobserved.

10 Giving advice

10.1 During research, an investigator may obtain evidence of psychological or physical problems of which a participant is, apparently, unaware. In such a case, the investigator has a responsibility to inform the participant if the investigator believes that by not doing so the participant's future well-being may be endangered.

10.2 If, in the normal course of psychological research, or as a result of problems detected as in 10.1, a participant solicits advice concerning educational, personality, behavioural or health issues, caution should be exercised. If the issue is serious and the investigator is not qualified to offer assistance, the appropriate source of professional advice should be recommended. Further details on the giving of advice will be found in the Society's Code of Conduct.

10.3 In some kinds of investigation the giving of advice is appropriate if this forms an intrinsic part of the research and has been agreed in advance.

11 Colleagues

11.1 Investigators share responsibility for the ethical treatment of research participants with their collaborators, assistants, students and employees. A psychologist who believes that another psychologist or investigator may be conducting research that is not in accordance with the principles above should encourage that investigator to re-evaluate the research.

These Guidelines are reproduced by permission of the British Psychological Society and form part of its Code of Conduct on research with human participants. The full Code of Conduct can be obtained from the Society or found on its website at www.bps.org.uk

43

Statement of Ethical Practice

British Sociological Association

Guidance notes

The British Sociological Association gratefully acknowledges the use made of the ethical codes produced by the American Sociological Association, the Association of Social Anthropologists of the Commonwealth and the Social Research Association.

Styles of sociological work are diverse and subject to change, not least because sociologists work within a wide variety of settings. Sociologists, in carrying out their work, inevitably face ethical, and sometimes legal, dilemmas which arise out of competing obligations and conflicts of interest. The following statement aims to alert the members of the Association to issues that raise ethical concerns and to indicate potential problems and conflicts of interest that might arise in the course of their professional activities. While they are not exhaustive, the statement points to a set of obligations to which members should normally adhere as principles for guiding their conduct. Departures from the principles should be the result of deliberation and not ignorance. The strength of this statement and its binding force rest ultimately on active discussion, reflection, and continued use by sociologists. In addition, the statement will help to communicate the professional position of sociologists to others, especially those involved in or affected by the activities of sociologists.

The statement is meant, primarily, to inform members' ethical judgements rather than to impose on them an external set of standards. The purpose is to make members aware of the ethical issues that may arise in their work, and to encourage them to educate themselves and their colleagues to behave ethically. The statement does not, therefore, provide a set of recipes for resolving ethical choices or dilemmas, but recognises that often it will be necessary to make such choices on the basis of principles and values, and the (often conflicting) interests of those involved.

Professional integrity

Members should strive to maintain the integrity of sociological enquiry as a discipline, the freedom to research and study, and to publish and promote the results of sociological research. Members have a responsibility both to safeguard the proper interests of those involved in or affected by their work, and to report their findings accurately and truthfully. They need to consider the effects of their involvements and the consequences of their work or its misuse for those they study and other interested parties.

While recognising that training and skill are necessary to the conduct of social research, members should themselves recognise the boundaries of their professional competence. They should not accept work of a kind that they are not qualified to carry out. Members should satisfy themselves that the research they undertake is worthwhile and that the techniques proposed are appropriate. They should be clear about the limits of their detachment from and involvement in their areas of study.

Members should be careful not to claim an expertise in areas outside those that would be recognised academically as their true fields of expertise. Particularly in their relations with the media, members should have regard for the reputation of the discipline and refrain from offering expert commentaries in a form that would appear to give credence to material which, as researchers, they would regard as comprising inadequate or tendentious evidence.

Relations with and responsibilities towards research participants

Sociologists, when they carry out research, enter into personal and moral relationships with those they study, be they individuals, households, social groups or corporate entities. Although sociologists, like other researchers are committed to the advancement of knowledge, that goal does not, of itself, provide an entitlement to override the rights of others. Members must satisfy themselves that a study is necessary for the furtherance of knowledge before embarking upon it. Members should be aware that they have some responsibility for the use to which their research may be put. Discharging that responsibility may on occasion be difficult, especially in situations of social conflict, competing social interests or where there is unanticipated misuse of the research by third parties.

1 Relationships with research participants

[a] Sociologists have a responsibility to ensure that the physical, social and psychological well-being of research participants is not adversely affected by the research. They should strive to protect the rights of those they study, their interests, sensitivities and privacy, while recognising the difficulty of balancing potentially conflicting interests. Because sociologists study the relatively powerless as well as those more powerful than themselves, research relationships are frequently characterised by disparities of power and status. Despite this, research relationships should be characterised, whenever possible, by trust. In some cases, where the public interest dictates otherwise and particularly where power is being abused, obligations of trust and protection may weigh less heavily. Nevertheless, these obligations should not be discarded lightly.

[b] As far as possible sociological research should be based on the freely given informed consent of those studied. This implies a responsibility on the sociologist to explain as fully as possible, and in terms meaningful to participants, what the research is about, who is undertaking and financing it, why it is being undertaken, and how it is to be promoted.

   (i) Research participants should be made aware of their right to refuse participation whenever and for whatever reason they wish.

   (ii) Research participants should understand how far they will be afforded anonymity and confidentiality and should be able to reject the use of data-gathering devices such as tape recorders and video cameras. Sociologists should be careful, on the one hand, not to give unrealistic guarantees of confidentiality and, on the other, not to permit communication of research films or records to audiences other than those to which the research participants have agreed.

   (iii) Where there is a likelihood that data may be shared with other researchers, the potential uses to which the data might be put may need to be discussed with research participants.

   (iv) When making notes, filming or recording for research purposes, sociologists should make clear to research participants the purpose of the notes, filming or recording, and, as precisely as possible, to whom it will be communicated.

   (v) It should also be borne in mind that in some research contexts, especially those involving field research, it may be necessary for the obtaining of consent to be regarded, not as a once-and-for-all prior event, but as a process, subject to renegotiation over time. In addition, particular care may need to be taken during periods of prolonged fieldwork where it is easy for research participants to forget that they are being studied.

   (vi) In some situations access to a research setting is gained via a 'gatekeeper'. In these situations members should adhere to the principle of obtaining informed consent directly from the research participants to whom access is required, while at the same time taking account of the gatekeepers' interest. Since the relationship between the research participant and the gatekeeper may continue long after the sociologist has left the research setting, care should be taken not to disturb that relationship unduly.

[c] It is incumbent upon members to be aware of the possible consequences of their work. Wherever possible they should attempt to anticipate, and to guard against, consequences for research participants which can be predicted to be harmful. Members are not absolved from this responsibility by the consent given by research participants.

[d] In many of its guises, social research intrudes into the lives of those studied. While some participants in sociological research may find the experience a positive and welcome one, for others, the experience may be disturbing. Even if not exposed to harm, those studied may feel wronged by aspects of the research process. This can be particularly so if they perceive apparent intrusions into their private and personal worlds, or where research gives rise to false hopes, uncalled for self-knowledge, or unnecessary anxiety. Members

should consider carefully the possibility that the research experience may be a disturbing one and, normally, should attempt to minimise disturbance to those participating in research. It should be borne in mind that decisions made on the basis of research may have effects on individuals as members of a group, even if individual research participants are protected by confidentiality and anonymity.

[e] Special care should be taken where research participants are particularly vulnerable by virtue of factors such as age, social status and powerlessness. Where research participants are ill or too young or too old to participate, proxies may need to be used in order to gather data. In these situations care should be taken not to intrude on the personal space of the person to whom the data ultimately refer, or to disturb the relationship between this person and the proxy. Where it can be inferred that the person about whom data are sought would object to supplying certain kinds of information, that material should not be sought from the proxy.

2 Covert Research

There are serious ethical dangers in the use of covert research but covert methods may avoid certain problems. For instance, difficulties arise when research participants change their behaviour because they know they are being studied. Researchers may also face problems when access to spheres of social life is closed to social scientists by powerful or secretive interests. However, covert methods violate the principles of informed consent and may invade the privacy of those being studied. Participant or non-participant observation in non-public spaces or experimental manipulation of research participants without their knowledge should be resorted to only where it is impossible to use other methods to obtain essential data. In such studies it is important to safeguard the anonymity of research participants. Ideally, where informed consent has not been obtained prior to the research it should be obtained post-hoc.

3 Anonymity, privacy and confidentiality

[a] The anonymity and privacy of those who participate in the research process should be respected. Personal information concerning research participants should be kept confidential. In some cases it may be necessary to decide whether it is proper or appropriate even to record certain kinds of sensitive information.

[b] Where possible, threats to the confidentiality and anonymity of research data should be anticipated by researchers. The identities and research records of those participating in research should be kept confidential whether or not an explicit pledge of confidentiality has been given. Appropriate measures should be taken to store research data in a secure manner. Members should have regard to their obligations under the Data Protection Act. Where appropriate and practicable, methods for preserving the privacy of data should be used. These may include the removal of identifiers, the use of pseudonyms and other technical means for breaking the link between data and identifiable individuals such as 'broadbanding' or micro-aggregation. Members should also take care to prevent data being published or released in a form which would permit the actual or potential identification of research participants. Potential informants and research participants, especially those possessing a combination of attributes which make them readily identifiable, may need to be reminded that it can be difficult to disguise their identity without introducing an unacceptably large measure of distortion into the data.

[c] Guarantees of confidentiality and anonymity given to research participants must be honoured, unless there are clear and overriding reasons to do otherwise. Other people, such as colleagues, research staff or others, given access to the data must also be made aware of their obligations in this respect. By the same token, sociologists should respect the efforts taken by other researchers to maintain anonymity. Research data given in confidence do not enjoy legal privilege, that is they may be liable to subpoena by a court. Research participants may also need to be made aware that it may not be possible to avoid legal threats to the privacy of the data.

[d] There may be less compelling grounds for extending guarantees of privacy or confidentiality to public organisations, collectivities, governments, officials or agencies than to individuals or small groups. Nevertheless, where guarantees have been given they should be honoured, unless there are clear and compelling reasons not to do so.

4. During their research members should avoid, where they can, actions which may have deleterious consequences for sociologists who come after them or which might undermine the reputation of sociology as a discipline.

Relations with and responsibilities towards sponsors and/or funders

A common interest exists between sponsor, funder and sociologist as long as the aim of the social inquiry is to advance knowledge, although such knowledge may only be of limited benefit to the sponsor and the funder. That relationship is best served if the atmosphere is conducive to high professional standards. Members should attempt to ensure that sponsors and/or funders appreciate the obligations that sociologists have not only to them, but also to society at large, research participants and professional colleagues and the sociological community. The relationship between sponsors or funders and social researchers should be such as to enable social inquiry to be undertaken as objectively as possible. Research should be undertaken with a view to providing information or explanation rather than being constrained to reach particular conclusions or prescribe particular courses of action.

1 Clarifying obligations, roles and rights

[a] Members should clarify in advance the respective obligations of funders and researchers where possible in the form of a written contract. They should refer the sponsor or funder to the relevant parts of the professional code to which they adhere. Members should also be careful not to promise or imply acceptance of conditions which are contrary to their professional ethics or competing commitments. Where some or all of those involved in the research are also acting as sponsors and/or funders of research the potential for conflict between the different roles and interests should also be made clear to them.

[b] Members should also recognise their own general or specific obligations to the sponsors whether contractually defined or only the subject of informal and often unwritten agreements. They should be honest and candid about their qualifications and expertise, the limitations, advantages and disadvantages of the various methods of analysis and data, and acknowledge the necessity for discretion with confidential information obtained from sponsors. They should also try not to conceal factors which are likely to affect satisfactory conditions or the completion of a proposed research project or contract.

2 Pre-empting outcomes and negotiations about research

[a] Members should not accept contractual conditions that are contingent upon a particular outcome or set of findings from a proposed inquiry. A conflict of obligations may also occur if the funder requires particular methods to be used.

[b] Members should try to clarify, before signing the contract, that they are entitled to be able to disclose the source of their funds, its personnel, the aims of the institution, and the purposes of the project.

[c] Members should also try to clarify their right to publish and spread the results of their research.

[d] Members have an obligation to ensure sponsors grasp the implications of the choice between alternative research methods.

3 Guarding privileged information and negotiating problematic sponsorship

[a] Members are frequently furnished with information by the funder who may legitimately require it to be kept confidential. Methods and procedures that have been utilised to produce published data should not, however, be kept confidential unless otherwise agreed.

[b] When negotiating sponsorships members should be aware of the requirements of the law with respect to the ownership of and rights of access to data.

[c] In some political, social and cultural contexts some sources of funding and sponsorship may be contentious. Candour and frankness about the source of funding may create problems of access or co-operation for the social researcher but concealment may have serious consequences for colleagues, the discipline and research participants. The emphasis should be on maximum openness.

[d] Where sponsors and funders also act directly or indirectly as gatekeepers and control access to participants, researchers should not devolve their responsibility to protect the participants' interests onto the gatekeeper. Members should be wary of inadvertently disturbing the relationship between participants and gatekeepers since that will continue long after the researcher has left.

4 Obligations to sponsors and/or funders during the research process

[a] Members have a responsibility to notify the sponsor and/or funder of any proposed departure from the terms of reference of the proposed change in the nature of the contracted research.

[b] A research study should not be undertaken on the basis of resources known from the start to be inadequate, whether the work is of a sociological or interdisciplinary kind.

[c] When financial support or sponsorship has been accepted, members must make every reasonable effort to complete the proposed research on schedule, including reports to the funding source.

[d] Members should be prepared to take comments from sponsors or funders or research participants.

[e] Members should, wherever possible, spread their research findings.

[f] Members should normally avoid restrictions on their freedom to publish or otherwise broadcast research findings.

At its meeting in July 1994, the BSA Executive Committee approved a set of Rules for the Conduct of Enquiries into Complaints against BSA members under the auspices of this Statement, and also under the auspices of the BSA Guidelines on Professional Conduct. If you would like more details about the Rules, you should contact the BSA Office at the address/phone number given at the end of this statement.

APPROVED AGM 92; AMENDED AGM 93 (draft amendments added December 1996).
bsamisc\ethgu2.doc

British Sociological Association
Units 3F/G, Mountjoy Research Centre, Stockton Road, Durham DH1 3UR [UK]
telephone +44 (0) 191 383 0839, facsimile +44 (0) 191 383 0782
e-mail: britsoc@dial.pipex.com, Home page: http://dspace.dial.pipex.com/britsoc/
The BSA is a charity registered in England, number 213577

(B) Tissue and genes

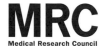

Human tissue and biological samples for use in research
Operational and Ethical Guidelines

Medical Research Council, 2001

Foreword

Several factors led the MRC to decide that there was a need to develop guidance for researchers on ethical, legal and management issues relating to the use of samples of human biological material for research. Technical advances, for instance in the ability to extract genetic material, meant that the potential to use old samples for research was increasing. We were regularly being asked for advice on what should happen to potentially useful sample collections when a research team disbanded or a lead researcher retired, and on what research would be permissible using stored samples originally collected for another purpose. Also it was clear that, following on from rapid developments in knowledge of the human genome sequence, large numbers of well documented human DNA samples would be essential for the research needed to translate this knowledge into real benefits for public health and health care.

In view of widespread concern about informed consent, confidentiality and ethical issues relating to genetic research, we felt it was essential to establish the general principles that could govern the use of all human biological material in research, including DNA.

The use of human biological material is critical for medical research. Consequently, the public and research participants should have confidence that researchers will handle and use such material sensitively and responsibly. It is likewise important to the MRC to ensure that collections of human biological material can be used optimally for research to benefit health. Since our responsibility as a public body is to ensure that our funds are used wisely, we do not want to fund the unnecessary collection of new material. Also, it is unethical to ask people to donate new samples when the research questions could be addressed using existing samples.

These guidelines were developed by a Working Group that included members with expertise in law and ethics as well as medical research. They, along with their interests, are listed at the front of the document. Working drafts of the guidelines were sent out for consultation to a wide range of organisations and individual scientists with an interest in the use of human material in research. Their comments were taken into account in developing an interim version, which was then published, together with a more detailed report of the working group's discussions, for wider public consultation and input. Comments were received from Research Ethics Committees, from researchers, patient and consumer groups, and from the MRC's Consumer Liaison Group.

Safety and protection from potential biological hazards are clearly important issues for researchers handling samples of human material, but were not within the remit of the group and are not addressed in these guidelines.

The guidelines are intended to be short and easily readable: the aim is therefore to set out general principles that can be applied in most situations rather than to cover every possible eventuality. It became clear from the consultation that views vary widely, and MRC will keep this guidance under review in the light of ongoing public debates about some of the key issues, and the work of the Human Genetics Commission, the Nuffield Council on Bioethics and the Council of Europe. This guide, as with other MRC ethics guides, is available on MRC's website at www.mrc.ac.uk, and changes will be highlighted there as they arise.

Glossary

Anonymised samples or data have had any identifying information removed, such that it is not possible for the researcher using them to identify the individual to whom they relate. The term is used in these guidelines to refer to both linked and unlinked anonymised data and samples.

- Linked anonymised samples or data are fully anonymous to the people who receive or use them (e.g. the research team) but contain information or codes that would allow others (e.g. the clinical team who collected them or an independent body entrusted with safekeeping of the code) to link them back to identifiable individuals.
- Unlinked anonymised samples or data contain no information that could reasonably be used by anyone to identify the individuals who donated them or to whom they relate.

Coded samples or data have a coded identification to protect the confidentiality of the individual during routine use, but it is possible for the user to break the code and thus identify the individual from whom they were obtained.

Custodianship: Responsibility for safe keeping of samples and control of their use and eventual disposal in accordance with the terms of the consent given by the donor. Custodianship implies some rights to decide how the samples are used and by whom, and also responsibility for safeguarding the interests of the donors.

Genetic research: Investigation of variation in the nuclear or mitochondrial DNA that forms the genome of an individual and may be inherited from parent to child. This may involve direct analysis of DNA or analysis of gene products.

Genetic testing: Tests to detect the presence or absence of, or alteration in, a particular gene, chromosome or gene product, in order to provide diagnostic or predictive information in relation to a genetic disorder. (Such testing does not necessarily require the use of genetic technology.)

Human material: All biological material of human origin, including organs, tissues, bodily fluids, teeth, hair and nails, and substances extracted from such material such as DNA or RNA.

Human tissue or sample collection: Any samples of human biological material to be kept for reference, teaching or future research use.

Existing collections: collections comprising samples that were collected and stored before these guidelines came into operation.

Personal information: all information about individuals, living or dead. This includes written and electronic records and information obtained from samples.

Summary of key principles

Much medical research depends on the use of samples of human biological material. This material often provides the best way of studying human biology and human disease, and appropriate use of such material reduces the need to use animals in research. Material for research may be from healthy people, from patients or from people who have died. Researchers may ask volunteers to donate material (e.g. blood samples) specifically for research, or may use material left over after diagnostic testing or surgery. Samples stored for one purpose may later prove useful for research that was not envisaged at the time the samples were taken.

The following principles should guide all MRC funded research using samples of human biological material.

Research should only go ahead if the potential benefits outweigh any potential risks to the donors of the samples. The physical risks involved in donating samples for research will usually be minimal, but the risk that information from laboratory tests on a sample might harm the donor or their interests must not be forgotten.

The human body and its parts should be treated with respect. Researchers should ensure that they are aware of cultural or religious differences in the meaning and significance attached to the body or specific parts of it before approaching potential donors.

Samples of human biological material obtained for use in research should be treated as gifts. Researchers have a responsibility to ensure the donors' wishes are respected when using the material.

The human body and its parts shall not, as such, give rise to financial gain. Researchers may not sell for a profit samples of human biological material that they have collected as part of MRC funded research, and research participants should never be offered any financial inducement to donate samples. Payment of reasonable expenses or costs is however acceptable. Donors should be informed if their samples might be used in commercial research. Intellectual property rights (IPR) arising from research using human samples may be sold or licensed in the same way as other IPR.

Informed consent is required from the donor (or the next of kin, if the donor has died) whenever a new sample is taken wholly or partly for use in research. Donors should understand what the sample is to be used for and how the results of the research might impact on their interests.

Consent must also be obtained for storage and potential future use of samples.

Patients should always be informed when material left over following diagnosis or treatment (described as surplus to clinical requirements) might be used for research. Wherever practicable, and always when the results of the research could affect the patient's interests, consent should be obtained to the use of such surplus material.

All research using samples of human biological material must be approved[1] by an appropriately constituted research ethics committee. This is an important way of ensuring that the interests of the donors are safeguarded.

Researchers should treat all personal and medical information relating to research participants as confidential. This applies as much to the results of laboratory tests done as part of the research project as to information obtained directly from donors or from their medical records. People who donate samples for research must be told what personal or medical information about them will be used in the research, who it might be shared with, and what safeguards are in place to protect their confidentiality.

Research participants have a right to know individual research results that affect their interests, but should be able to choose whether to exercise that right. Researchers must decide at the beginning of a project what information about the results of laboratory tests done on samples should be available to the participants, and agree these plans with the Research Ethics Committee. If research results have immediate clinical relevance, there is a clear duty of care to ensure the participant is informed.

1 Introduction

1.1 Purpose

The Medical Research Council is committed to the highest ethical standards in medical research, and to ensuring that optimum use is made of the public funds it administers. These guidelines draw attention to the practical, ethical and legal issues that should be considered when collecting and using samples of human biological material for research, and address how such material should best be used to increase scientific understanding for the benefit of human health.

These guidelines should be followed by:
- Those preparing research proposals for support by the MRC that include the collection of new samples of human biological material.
- Those planning, undertaking or collaborating in research funded by the MRC, using stored samples of human biological material, whether the samples were collected by themselves or by others.
- Those managing collections of human materials made with MRC funding, or research using such collections.

We hope they might also be of interest to others collecting or using human material for research, as well as to research ethics committees, to research participants and to members of the public.

This guidance applies to the use of samples of human biological material for research purposes. It is not intended to cover the use (or re-use) of human samples for clinical diagnostic purposes, clinical audit, disease surveillance or quality control of existing diagnostic testing procedures[2].

The principles in these guidelines must be applied to all new samples of human material obtained wholly or partly for use in medical research, whether to be used immediately or to be stored for future use. However, it is acknowledged that it will not always be possible to apply them retrospectively to samples stored before the guidelines were issued. MRC recognises that many existing collections of human material are immensely valuable for research, and that using these collections may be ethical, and in the interests of both patients and the public. Research Ethics Committees have a crucial role in ensuring that they are used in a responsible and ethically acceptable way that is not against the donors' interests.

1.2 Ethical principles

The general ethical principles for research involving human participants are set out in the Council's booklet "Responsibility in investigations on human participants and material and on personal information." The known and potential risks and benefits of the research to the participants and the potential benefits to others must be evaluated and research should only proceed if the potential benefits outweigh any associated risks. The interests of research participants should always take precedence over those of science and society. In most circumstances research can only be done with the full and informed consent of the

---

[1] Although Research Ethics Committees are advisory bodies, they do have to come to a favourable view of each research project before it can begin; we therefore adopt the commonly used term ethics committee approval in these guidelines.

[2] See Guidelines on the practice of ethics committees in medical research involving human subjects 3rd edition, (1996, Royal College of Physicians of London) Section 6, for a discussion of the distinction between research, clinical practice and audit.

individual participants, and confidentiality of participants must be maintained. An important principle underlying use of any human material for research should be respect for the human body and for the known wishes of the donor of the material. Researchers must always ensure that their use of human material will not compromise the interests of the donor.

1.3 Special issues relating to collections of human material

Human biological material is very important in medical research. Efficient and well coordinated use of such material can promote scientific advance and reduce both the research demands on patients and the need to use animals. The MRC wishes to promote better use of valuable material by ensuring that it is easier for other scientists to use it, where appropriate. There are, however, special issues in relation to samples of human material:

- Samples can be stored for a long time, and may be of considerable value for research that was not, and could not have been, envisaged at the time the material was obtained.
- Using material for studies not specifically foreseen at the time it was obtained raises difficult ethical issues in relation to consent.
- It is often either not possible or not practicable to go back to the donors for new consent.
- Information obtained from research using biological samples can have implications not only for the individual donor but also for their relatives, and may sometimes have the potential to lead to discrimination in employment or other areas of life, if disclosed.

In addition, the value of many samples of human material for research depends upon the related clinical or personal information; respect for the confidentiality of information about the donor is therefore important. A parallel booklet in the MRC Ethics Series "Personal Information in Medical Research" gives more detailed guidance on this issue.

1.4 Different types of human biological material used in research

Samples of human material for use in research may be obtained from healthy volunteers, from patients or from people who have died. There are also many types of human material used in medical research, ranging from whole organs or large pieces of tissue, such as surgically removed tumours, to very small samples of blood or urine. The importance and meaning people attach to the donation and use of such samples, and the ethical and practical considerations may differ widely in different circumstances. The main distinctions drawn in these guidelines are between:

- Research on new collections and research re-using stored samples
- Material obtained from living donors and material taken from people who have died
- Human material donated solely or partly for research and material left over following diagnosis or treatment (described as 'surplus to clinical requirements' in these guidelines).

General issues applying to the collection and use of all types of human material are considered first, followed by sections dealing with specific issues. This guide does not give detailed advice on the use of human sperm, eggs or embryos. Use of such material is subject to the Human Fertilisation and Embryology Act (1990) and must be approved by the Human Fertilisation and Embryology Authority.

2 Ownership and Custodianship

2.1 The legal position in relation to uses of human tissue was discussed in detail in the Nuffield Council on Bioethics Report "Human Tissue: Ethical and Legal Issues" (1995). In the UK it is not legally possible to own a human body. The law is unclear as to whether or under what circumstances anyone can legally "own" samples of human biological material or whether donors of biological material have any property rights over "their" samples. For human material used in research, the important consideration is not legal ownership, per se, but who has the right to control the use made of samples or their transfer to a third party. Therefore in these guidelines we use the term "custodianship" rather than ownership, to imply responsibility for safe storage of samples, for safeguarding the donors' interests, and for the control of use or disposal of the material.

2.2 We recommend that tissue samples donated for research be treated as gifts or donations, although gifts with conditions attached. This is preferable from a moral and ethical point of view, as it promotes the "gift relationship" between research participants and scientists, and underlines the altruistic motivation for participation in research. It also provides a practical way of dealing with the legal uncertainty over ownership, in that any property rights that the donor might have in their donated sample would be transferred, together with the control of use of the sample, to the recipient of the gift. Gifts may be conditional (that is, a donor may specify what the recipient can do with a gift), and it is very important that the donor understands and agrees to the proposed uses of the donated material. The assumption by the donor is that nothing will be done that would be detrimental to his or her interests, or bring harm to him or her.

2.3 If samples taken for research are to be treated as gifts, there must be a recipient, to whom formal responsibility for custodianship of a donated sample of material is transferred. While the principal investigator should have day-to-day responsibility for management of a collection of human material, the MRC considers that it is more appropriate for formal responsibility for custodianship of collections of human material to rest with institutions rather than with individual researchers. This provides greater security for valuable collections, provides better assurance that donors' rights will be protected and makes it easier to deal with changes in individual circumstances of the principal investigator(s). The university, hospital or other host institution where the principal investigator is based will usually be the most appropriate body to have formal responsibility for custodianship of human material donated for research, but occasionally the MRC will wish to retain custodianship of collections that it funds (see 2.6 below). When central banking facilities are available, there may be a requirement for the investigator to split the sample and provide a portion to the bank as a condition of research funding. Valid consent from the donor will of course be required to share a sample with other researchers in this way.

2.4 **When consent is obtained, the donor (or the person giving consent in the case of material obtained after death) needs to understand that he/she is making a donation of the sample for use in research. They must be clear who will be responsible for custodianship of the sample and of any personal or confidential data related to the sample, and what it will be used for.**

2.5 The Council of Europe Convention on Human Rights and Biomedicine states that "The human body and its parts shall not, as such, give rise to financial gain", and the MRC fully supports this principle: the sale of human biological samples for research is not ethically acceptable. Therefore, **while reasonable expenses (e.g. travel expenses) may be reimbursed, research participants should never be offered any financial or material inducement to donate biological samples for research. Also, researchers may not sell for profit (in cash or in kind) samples that they have collected with MRC funding. Recovery of reasonable costs, based on a standard accounting system is, however, acceptable.** A clear distinction can be drawn between samples of human material and intellectual property rights arising from research making use of such samples. Such intellectual property may be sold or licensed in the usual way.

2.6 For all new collections of human biological materials funded by the MRC, researchers and their host institutions must reach agreement with the MRC on specific arrangements for the custodianship and control of use of sample collections (both while the project is ongoing and after it is finished) before funding is released. For large sample collections with contributions from many clinical centres, and for collections set up with the intention from the outset of providing a research resource, the MRC may wish to retain formal responsibility for custodianship of the collection. In the case of jointly funded collections, arrangements for custodianship will be negotiated with the other funding organisations. We understand that custodianship brings with it the right to determine what happens to a collection after the original project funding is finished, but also the responsibility for its subsequent maintenance. The MRC will normally delegate day-to-day responsibility for management of sample collections to the principal investigator of the research project and their host institution.

3 Use of human material surplus to clinical requirements for research

3.1 Tissue or organs removed in the course of surgical treatment or excess human material left over after diagnostic testing can be of considerable value for research and teaching and are widely used for such purposes. However, there is currently little public awareness of this practice, nor indeed of what normally happens to such material if it is not used for research. In a legal analysis, such human material might be considered to have been "abandoned" by the patient and therefore available for use however the surgeon or pathologist sees fit. There is some evidence that people do view use of such material in a rather different light from samples donated specifically for research purposes, adopting the position that it is better that the material should serve some useful purpose than simply be disposed of. However, it would be wrong to assume that such a view is universal, and MRC recommends that wherever practicable individual consent should be obtained for the use for research of human material surplus to clinical requirements. At the very least, for example, patients should be made aware in any surgical consent form that they sign that surplus material may be used for research, and be given the opportunity to refuse. Patients need sufficient information to understand how (if at all) the research might affect their interests, and how their confidentiality will be protected. Where surplus material is to be used in a way that allows research results to be linked to the individual patient, individual informed consent *must* be obtained if there is any possibility that such results might affect the patient's interests.

3.2 It is acceptable to use human material surplus to clinical requirements for research without consent if it is anonymous and unlinked. An example is the use of surplus diagnostic samples for screening to establish the prevalence of an infectious disease such as hepatitis or HIV. Information from such studies is very valuable not only for research but also for public health or health service planning purposes, and provided there is no possible way to link the results of tests to identifiable individuals their interests cannot be compromised. While it is not necessary to obtain individual written consent for anonymised unlinked research, it is good practice to ensure that patients are informed that their samples may be used for research once all clinical requirements have been fulfilled, for example by a clearly displayed notice to that effect.

3.3 All research using human material surplus to clinical requirements must be approved by an ethics committee, whether or not the samples can be linked to identifiable individuals. This is an important way of ensuring that patients' interests are safeguarded.

3.4 There must always be explicit separation of the consent to the treatment or diagnostic test from the consent to the use of surplus tissue for research. It should be clear to patients that refusal to allow surplus material to be used for research will not affect their treatment in any way. It is also important to make clear to patients what will happen to the surplus material if they do not give consent for its retention for research or teaching.

3.5 If individual written consent cannot be obtained, research using samples of material surplus to clinical requirements is only acceptable if the results cannot affect the patient's or their family's interests. The patient must also have been informed at the time the sample was taken that their material might be used for research, for example by clearly displayed notices, by distribution of leaflets, or on the clinical consent form itself.

4 Use of human material for commercial research

4.1 The MRC's mission is to support research that will ultimately benefit human health. The development of new drug therapies, and diagnostic and screening tests, to the point where they can be made sufficiently widely available to benefit human health, is crucially dependent on commercial involvement. Therefore access by the commercial sector to samples of human material collected in the course of MRC-funded research should be facilitated, where this is consistent with our mission. **However, it is NOT appropriate for any one company to be given EXCLUSIVE rights of access to a collection of samples made with the benefit of public funds,** nor is it acceptable for any individual to profit financially from providing samples of human material to a third party.

4.2 One of the major concerns in allowing commercial access to human material originally collected for research projects funded by the public or charity sectors is the potential to damage the gift relationship between scientists and research participants. Research participants may be particularly sensitive to the idea of a company or an individual making a profit out of research material that they have freely donated. It is important that research participants are made aware of the potential benefits of allowing commercial access, and that the role of any one individual's sample in the generation of future profits is likely to be minimal as well as impossible to quantify. Given the possible sensitivities, **it is essential that research participants know that their sample or products derived from it may be used by the commercial sector, and that they will not be entitled to a share of any profits that might ensue.**

4.3 It is important to distinguish between the samples themselves and the data or intellectual property derived from research using them. Exclusive access to data arising directly from a company's experiments for sufficient time to secure patent protection or other commercial advantage is acceptable, as is ownership by a company of any intellectual property rights arising from their own research using samples of human material.

4.4 Patenting of inventions based on, or using, biological material of human origin is covered by the EU Directive on the Legal Protection of Biotechnological Inventions. To comply with the Directive, a person from whose body the material used for an invention is taken must have had an opportunity of expressing free and informed consent (Recital 26). This should be borne in mind when there is a possibility that human material collected for research may be used *directly* in making a biotechnology product. For instance, if a cell line is to be made and used for commercial purposes the donor must be consulted and consent obtained.

4.5 Custodians of collections of human biological material should ensure that a written agreement covering access to data and ownership of intellectual property rights is secured before allowing access to samples by either commercial companies or academic researchers.

5 Confidentiality

5.1 In many cases the use of human material in research also involves the use of personal or clinical information related to the individual who donated the sample. Tests done on the material may also give rise to information about the individual donor. Doctors and researchers should treat any information about an individual, however derived, as confidential. This is what the public expects, and is underpinned by the duty of confidentiality in Common Law, and in Data Protection legislation. Both the data collected from individuals or their medical records to characterise samples in a collection, and data derived from experiments done on those samples, are covered by the Data Protection Act (1998), so long as they can be linked to an identifiable individual. Researchers must ensure that their registration under the Act covers all their uses of data related to samples.

5.2 Detailed guidance on confidentiality is available in the MRC booklet "Personal information in medical research" (see box for a summary of the key points) and in the General Medical Council guidelines on confidentiality. People who donate samples for research must be told what information about their medical history or other personal details will be used in the research, who it might be shared with, and what safeguards are in place to preserve confidentiality. They should give explicit consent to these arrangements.

Key principles of the MRC guidance on personal information in medical research

- Personal information provided for health care or medical research is confidential. Wherever possible people should know how information about them is used. Researchers should normally have each person's explicit consent to obtain, store and use information about them.
- All medical research using identifiable personal information or anonymised data from the NHS that is not already in the public domain must be approved by a Research Ethics Committee.
- All personal information must be coded or anonymised as far as is possible and as early as possible in the data processing.
- Each individual entrusted with patient information is personally responsible for their decisions about disclosing it. Personal information should only be handled by health professionals or staff with an equivalent duty of confidentiality.
- Principal investigators have personal responsibility to ensure that procedures and security arrangements are sufficient to prevent breaches of confidentiality.
- At the outset researchers must decide what information about the results should be available to the people involved, and agree these plans with the Ethics Committee.

5.3 Data that have not been anonymised should not be transferred without informed consent. The responsibility lies with the custodian to ensure that all data related to samples of human material are unidentifiable before release to other researchers or inclusion in a common database. It is good practice to store, process and analyse personal data in a form that does not allow individuals to be identified. Personal information should only be accessible to staff who have a formal duty of confidence to the research participants. Researchers handling personal information should have a duty of confidence to research participants included in their contract of employment. In addition, identifiable data should not be transferred to a country outside the European Economic Area unless it has an equivalent data protection regime.

5.4 Users of anonymised samples of human material must undertake not to attempt to identify individual research participants, and individuals, families or groups should not be identifiable from published data. Any renewed contact with donors not specified in the original research protocol (for example, if it is necessary to collect additional information) requires further ethics committee approval. This contact must be via the original researcher responsible for making the collection or the current custodian of the samples, and at their discretion.

5.5 The value of a collection for research will usually be significantly increased if all the data relating to the samples are stored together and made available in an anonymised form to all users. Custodians of collections of human material are encouraged to make it a condition of access to the samples that copies of all data generated by other users are provided to the custodian for inclusion in a common database. A suitable period of exclusive access may be allowed, to give sufficient time to analyse the data and prepare publications. The requirements of confidentiality and data protection must of course be met. This sharing of data is an essential requirement where sample collections are being managed as a resource for multiple users.

6 Consent

6.1 The General Medical Council guidelines "Seeking patients' consent: the ethical considerations" include general advice on seeking consent for research. When obtaining consent to take a sample of biological material for research, it is important that donors have sufficient understanding not only of the process involved in obtaining the sample and any associated physical risks, but also of what the sample is to be used for and how the results of the research might impact on their interests. Written evidence of consent must normally be obtained, as stated in the GMC guidelines. Written consent is not a substitute for careful explanation. It is simply a means of providing documentary evidence that an explanation of the research has been provided and consent has been sought. In some countries verbal consent is acceptable. There must however always be a written record that consent has been obtained even when the person giving consent is not able to write or when verbal consent is the accepted practice. Signed consent forms or documentary evidence of consent, together with copies of patient information materials, must always be kept for future reference. If the information leaflets are revised in the course of a study, all the new versions must be numbered and kept and details of when the changes were introduced should be recorded.

6.2 When obtaining consent to take a sample of human material for research, it is important to allow for the fact that it might subsequently be useful for new experiments that cannot be foreseen. Therefore, unless a sample will be fully used up for the initial project or cannot be stored, **a two-part consent process is recommended, the donor being first asked to consent to the specific experiment(s) already planned, and then to give consent for storage and future use for other research.** Unless the sample is to be anonymised and unlinked prior to storage (in which case this should be explained to donors), it is not acceptable to seek unconditional blanket consent, for example using terms such as 'all biological or medical research'.

If samples may be stored or used in a form that allows them to be linked to individuals, possible future research should be explained in terms of the types of studies that may be done, the types of diseases that could be investigated, and the possible impact of the research on them personally. The benefits of enabling more efficient use of valuable samples should be explained to donors. For example, a researcher collecting samples from patients with diabetes might seek consent to store the samples for future research into the biological basis and treatment of diabetes and related complications, on the basis that researchers using the sample for secondary research cannot identify the donor. Researchers undertaking a broader epidemiological study might seek consent to store samples for future research into biological or genetic factors affecting the risk of developing a range of common medical conditions, on the understanding that results of tests done for research purposes will not have direct clinical implications for the donor. Similarly, donors must be made aware that other researchers might use their samples, including scientists working for commercial companies (if appropriate). Participants must be given the reassurance that all secondary use will require approval by an ethics committee, and that no tests of known clinical value for diagnosing or predicting disease on samples that can be linked to them individually will be done without their consent. Information for participants should include an explanation of how any surplus material will be disposed of when it is no longer required.

Where a two-part consent process is used, donors must always be given the option of specifying that their sample may only be used for the research project already planned. If consent is obtained to use a newly collected sample for one specific study only, the only purpose for which it can be re-used is to verify the results of that study. When no longer required for that purpose it should be destroyed. **It is the responsibility of the custodian to ensure that all uses of a sample are in accordance with the consent obtained from the donor.**

6.3 If research using samples will require the collection of information from the donor's medical records, then consent must be obtained. It must be clear who will access the records, what information will be obtained, and how the patient's confidentiality will be protected.

6.4 The special sensitivity of the public with regard to genetics research should always be taken into account. If there is the possibility that secondary use may include genetic research, this must be included in the explanation of possible future research when consent is obtained. There are certain types of genetics research which currently give rise to particular concern, for instance that relating to personality, behavioural characteristics, sexual orientation or intelligence. It is particularly important that specific consent is obtained to use samples in these or other areas of research likely to cause special concern to the donors, even if the samples are to be anonymised and unlinked.

6.5 When seeking consent for research, information for potential participants must be presented in a form that they can understand. Where lack of ability to understand written information may be a problem, the use of audio taped information is recommended. If potential participants do not speak English, interpreters should have sufficient understanding of scientific and medical issues to explain adequately the aims of a research protocol. These interpreters should preferably be patient advocates or NHS interpreters rather than relatives. If relatives must be involved, they should be competent adults who are themselves fluent in English. Information leaflets should be translated by people with a technical knowledge of the field. Researchers should be aware that members of some ethnic or religious groups might find some types of research, or donation of certain types of human material, unacceptable.

6.6 Particular considerations apply in the case of research involving children (see 12.3) and people who, as a result of permanent or temporary mental incapacity, cannot give valid consent (see 12.4). The Council's guidance on the latter situation is set out in a separate

publication[3] and there are also guidelines for Research Ethics Committee and guidelines issued by the Royal College of Physicians and by the Royal College of Paediatrics and Child Health (see Appendix 1). A summary of all the issues to be addressed in the process of obtaining consent is at Appendix 3 and a model consent form is at Appendix 4.

7 Ethics committee review

Ethics committee approval must be obtained to collect samples of human material for research, and for all research projects using samples of human material. New ethics committee approval is required for all research projects not specifically mentioned when consent was originally obtained or in previous ethics committee submissions. This is an important means of safeguarding the interests of the donors. Ethics committee approval must also be obtained if there is a need to access patients' medical records without their specific consent. This may be justified under certain circumstances: if the study is of sufficient importance, if there are no practicable alternatives, if the infringement of confidentiality is kept to a minimum, and if there is no intent to make future contact with the patient.[4]

8 Feedback of information

8.1 Tests done on samples of human material in the course of research may reveal information that has implications for the donors' future health or healthcare, or otherwise impacts on their interests. It is important to decide before the start of a research project what will be done if this arises. Researchers should be cautious about assuming that they, rather than the individuals concerned, are best placed to judge what information is of interest to donors on a case-by-case basis. For instance, some researchers may take the view that information should only be fed back if there is a treatment or preventive intervention available. However, research participants might wish to know predictive information about their future health, even if there is no treatment available, for example to take it into account when making important life decisions, such as

---

[3] The Ethical Conduct of Research on the Mentally Incapacitated MRC Series, December 1991.

[4] See the MRC Ethics booklet "Personal Information in Medical Research" for more detailed guidance.

whether to have children. Researchers should assume that participants have a right to know information that may affect their interests, but that they might choose not to exercise that right. When participants are asked to make a decision on whether or not they want results to be fed back to them they must be given sufficient information to allow them to decide what their interests are and to make any refusal meaningful. Researchers must decide at the outset what their strategy will be with regard to feeding back information and whether any linkage of research results to individuals will be possible or alternatively whether the unlinked anonymous technique is appropriate. This must be set out in their submission to the ethics committee, and the policy adopted must be explained clearly to research participants before they consent to take part in the research.

8.2 Research results obtained on anonymised unlinked samples cannot have any impact on the interests of an individual donor, and cannot be fed back. Much research can be done using anonymised unlinked samples, and indeed in many instances this is the most appropriate technique. For example, it has been used successfully in research into the spread of HIV infection.

However, irreversibly breaking the link between a sample and the individual donor can undoubtedly reduce its value for some types of research, for instance by making it impossible to add follow-up data or to audit fully the research results. In deciding whether to use anonymised unlinked samples, researchers should take into account the nature of the foreseeable research findings, the importance of obtaining follow-up information on participants, the initial consent obtained and the feasibility of obtaining further consent. The ability to provide feedback linked to counselling and clinical care must also be considered. There are various possible strategies for unlinking: samples can be irreversibly unlinked from the outset, or they can be unlinked after the initial study is done, either before being used for any secondary studies or before use in specific studies only.

8.3 Incidental clinical findings

Where a result that can be linked to an individual has immediate clinical relevance (for example, if it reveals a serious condition for which treatment is required), the clinician involved has a clear duty of care to inform the research participant, either directly or via the clinician responsible for his or her care. The clinician responsible for care should always be notified, and participants should be informed that this will occur. A research result should not be relied on as the sole basis for diagnosis, since quality control standards in research laboratories generally differ from those used for clinical testing. Research participants or their clinicians should be advised to seek a repeat or confirmatory test by a clinical diagnostic laboratory where possible. Where a confirmatory test is not available via the NHS the diagnosis might need to be verified by the research laboratory using a new sample.

8.4 Research results

There is currently no consensus on whether, or under what circumstances, it is appropriate to feed back research results to participants on an individual basis[5]. Often the clinical relevance or predictive value of a research result is unclear, at least initially, and there will be no individual data of value to be fed back. It will always be difficult to define the point at which a research hypothesis becomes a clinical fact. Where consent is being sought for a specific research project at the time a sample is collected, the potential relevance, if any, of the results for the participant should be explained and the opportunity to receive feedback of individual results should be offered where appropriate. There should be a mechanism in place for participants to change their minds (for instance, a contact telephone number). If feedback is requested, they should be given appropriate instructions about how to notify researchers of a change in their address. Researchers feeding back individual results must be prepared to explain their significance to the participant and to advise on access to counselling or treatment where indicated.

It is good practice to offer research participants the opportunity to be kept informed about the general results of research projects done using the samples they have donated, though this may not be appropriate in all circumstances. Participants could be informed by posting information on research outcomes on a website, or by offering them the opportunity to receive a newsletter. Where the clinical relevance of research results becomes clear some time after the sample was obtained, or where the results obtained from secondary research may impact on the donors' interests,

---

[5] The MRC will be monitoring the debate in this contentious area and expects that the position will evolve as a result of ongoing consultation and research

these routes should be used to inform donors that results of potential interest may be available and offer them the opportunity to receive individual feedback or advice if they wish. Similarly, when new predictive tests of clinical value become available as a result of the research, participants can be informed how to access these tests if they wish.

Where samples may subsequently be used for secondary studies, a mechanism should be put in place to allow participants the opportunity to seek individual results that might impact on their interests. It is acceptable for the onus to be on the participant to seek the information rather than on the researcher to be pro-active in providing it. The research protocols for secondary studies and the arrangements (if any) for feeding back results to participants must be reviewed by an ethics committee, preferably the committee that oversaw the making of the collection. If samples from a collection are shared with other researchers, the custodian of the collection is responsible for all contacts with donors, including providing any information on research results with a possible impact on individuals.

8.5 Specific issues related genetic research

Much genetic information obtained for research purposes is of unknown or uncertain predictive value. Genetic tests of known clinical or predictive value should not be done on samples that can be linked to an individual without their specific consent, and appropriate counselling should be available if consent for such a test is sought. Participants should be advised of the possible implications of genetic information for other family members and the potential impact on family relationships, and also of the implications of genetic risk information for employment or their ability to obtain insurance, before they decide whether to give consent to the test or whether they want to know the result. The feeding back of other genetic information, the significance of which is currently unknown, could also have similar implications in the future. The Advisory Committee on Genetic Testing guidance to Research Ethics Committees gives more detailed advice on feedback in relation to genetic information (see Box).

Summary of ACGT guidance on feeding back genetic information.

- Whenever practical there should be a clear distinction between diagnostic testing and research.

If a research participant later requests a test for clinical purposes a new sample should be taken.

- Genetic testing should not be added to an existing research study without consent.
- Unless samples are anonymous and unlinked, prior consent must be obtained for each genetic test carried out for research purposes.
- If genetic test results are to be disclosed to research subjects or added to their medical record, then informed consent is required for the tests. It must be clear what use may be made of test results and subjects must be fully informed of potential adverse consequences for insurance, employment and effects on family members.
- The fundamental issues of information, consent and confidentiality are the same for research involving multiple gene tests, such as genotyping. Researchers should establish suitable methods by which complex information about the research can be explained to participants.

9 Management of collections of human material

9.1 The MRC reserves the right to specify the arrangements for management and access of sample collections as a condition for awarding funding. In the case of jointly funded collections, these arrangements would be negotiated with the other funders. This will allow us to ensure that collections are managed appropriately to maintain their usefulness, and to ensure that optimum use is made of them.

9.2 The MRC wishes to promote sharing of useful collections with bona-fide academic researchers undertaking high-quality research, provided that appropriate consent has been obtained and that such use is not against the interests of the donor. Use of samples by third parties must be on terms that do not disadvantage those involved in making and maintaining the collection or unnecessarily hamper or restrict future uses. The onus is on the custodian of a collection of human material to facilitate optimum usage; this will usually mean undertaking to provide access to other researchers once the requirements of the original project have been satisfied. In the case of collections made for a specific research project, it will usually be appropriate for the investigators making the collection to have priority access and the right to control use of the collection for the duration of the initial study.

9.3 For large collections, and those set up specifically to provide a resource for multiple users, requests for access should usually be dealt with by a management committee, which should have an independent chair and some independent membership. Criteria for access should be agreed at the outset. For example, proposed research should be subject to peer review as a means of ensuring scientific quality, samples and associated data should only be used for purposes approved by the committee, and researchers should agree to put all new data into a common dataset. Where supplies of samples are limited, transparent arrangements for prioritising requests for access are essential. Proper records of sample distribution must be kept and users must agree to return or destroy material surplus to their requirements and not use it for additional studies or pass it on to others. The management committee should also be given copies of all papers describing research using the collection before publication (but should not have the right to delay or veto publication).

9.4 Custodians of samples of human biological material are responsible for keeping proper records of all uses that have been made of the material, whether by themselves or by others. They must also ensure that all uses have appropriate ethics committee approval, and keep copies of such approvals for reference. Where linked anonymous samples are provided to a third party, the custodian is responsible for safe keeping of the code enabling samples to be linked to individual donors.

10 Established collections

10.1 Custodianship, management and access

It is important to assess periodically whether old samples of human material should be kept, taking into account both their scientific value and ethical issues. If samples are no longer of value, they should be disposed of safely and sensitively. For many old collections, no specific arrangements for custodianship of samples and management of access will have been put in place. This can present problems when researchers retire or move to a different job, or when there is disagreement over who should be allowed to use the samples. When a researcher wishes to move samples to a new location, the agreement of the current and the future host institution must be sought, and contributors to the collection must be consulted where possible. When a researcher retires and sample collections are to be retained, the institution or department should ensure arrangements are put in place for future maintenance and management, and that a new person is identified to take on responsibility for the collection. Custodians of established collections are encouraged to ensure that they are used optimally, and to allow access to other researchers wherever practicable, provided this is consistent with the consent that was obtained and confidentiality is not breached.

10.2 What research can be done using old samples?

There are many potentially valuable collections of human samples for which consent was only obtained for a single research project, or for which information on the parameters of the consent obtained has not been adequately recorded. Generally, established collections can be used for research when samples have been anonymised, and there is no potential harm to the donors of the material, individually or as a group[6]. Researchers should satisfy themselves that the samples were not obtained in an unethical or improper way and that there was valid consent to the taking. The HUGO Ethics Committee "Statement on DNA sampling: control and access" specifies the circumstances under which it is acceptable to do genetics research on archived samples. This suggests that such research is permissible on coded samples. The MRC believes that where a genetic test is of known predictive value, or gives reliable information about a known heritable condition, samples must be anonymised and unlinked before testing unless specific consent is obtained[7]. Even when a donor has died, genetic test results can have implications for surviving relatives. If the predictive value of the genetic information to be obtained is not known, research on anonymised linked samples is permissible, provided there is a strong scientific justification for not irreversibly anonymising the samples (for example, the need to link new information on clinical outcomes to genetic information).

---

[6] "Research based on archived information and samples" 1999 Royal College of Physicians, London

[7] This principle has been set out in the Advisory Committee on Genetic Testing Guidance to Research Ethics Committees

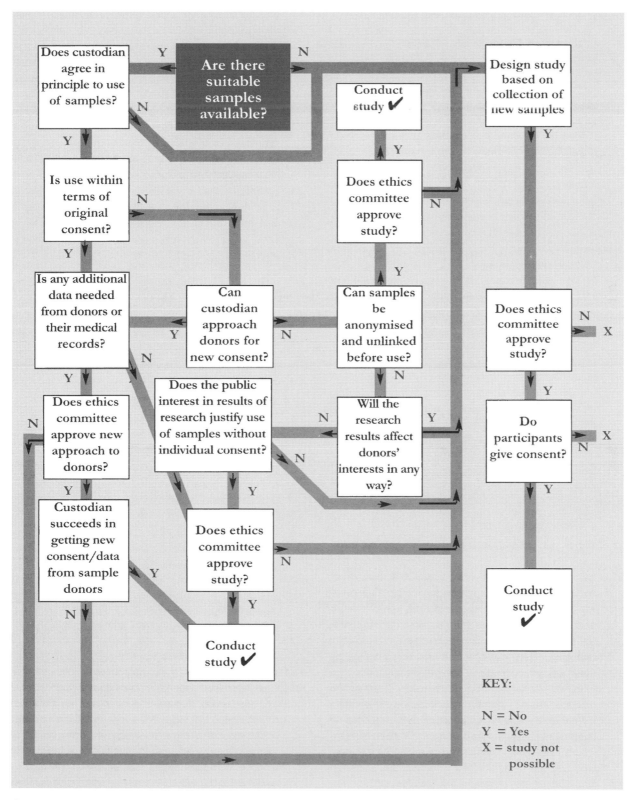

Figure 1 Using established collections in research – a decision tree

10.3 When is it necessary to seek new consent?

It is of course necessary to seek new consent when collecting new data from research participants. Consent should also be obtained to access participants' medical records if this was not done when the sample was originally collected. Where samples can be anonymised and unlinked before use, no new consent is required. In some rare circumstances research on linked samples originally taken for another research purpose may be permissible without consent. An example would be epidemiological research where the only practicable approach is to use stored samples and identifiers are needed to link samples and different types of health records. Before stored samples are used in this way researchers must demonstrate that contacting donors to seek consent is not possible or not practicable. Old samples of material surplus to clinical requirements may be used for linked research without specific consent if there is no possibility that the research could affect the patients' interests in any way and if obtaining individual consent is not practicable. Ethics committee approval is essential for all new research using stored samples of human material. Detailed guidance on the circumstances under which access to medical records without specific consent may be acceptable can be found in the Ethics booklet "Personal Information in Medical Research". In NHS institutions, the designated "Caldicott Guardian" must approve the use of confidential information.

11 Samples obtained after death

11.1 As with other research using human material, ethics committee approval is required for research involving the collection or use of material obtained after death. Before removing and retaining human material for research at a post-mortem examination, all reasonable steps must be taken to ascertain that the deceased would not have objected (for example, for religious reasons). Informed consent to the retention of material for research must normally be obtained from the surviving spouse, partner or next of kin. The person asked to give consent should be given clear information about what tissue/organ will be retained, who will be custodian, how long the sample will be kept, what types of research it may be used for and how it will be disposed of when no longer required.

Since this consent is being sought at a particularly stressful time, relatives should wherever possible, be given time to reflect before making their decision, and it is particularly important that written information is provided for later reference. Contact details of the research team must be provided in case relatives have further questions or change their minds later. While in this situation there is clearly no possibility of harming the person from whom the material is obtained, some research results (e.g. from genetic studies) may have implications for the surviving family members. The potential implications for relatives of any research to be done using linked samples must be discussed, and they must be given the opportunity to learn about any research results that might impact on their interests.

11.2 In the case of post-mortems required by law, the Coroner (or Procurator Fiscal in Scotland) cannot authorise the retention of tissue for research, but can prohibit it, even if consent has been obtained from a relative. Therefore the Coroner or Procurator Fiscal must be consulted before tissue is retained for research.

11.3 If no surviving relatives can be traced, and a post-mortem examination is required to establish the cause of death, the person legally in possession of the body (usually the hospital authority or Trust if death occurred in hospital) may authorise the removal and retention of tissues or organs to establish the cause of death. Once the cause of death of that person has been established, the person legally in possession of the body may at present legally authorise the retention of surplus material already removed from the body for research or teaching purposes. However, MRC recommends that tissue or organs should not be removed and retained solely for research purposes (i.e. if not required to establish the cause of death) if it is not possible to obtain consent from a relative or other appropriate person.

11.4 In some situations, the request for material will have been discussed with the deceased prior to death and informed consent obtained directly from them. In this instance it is not necessary to seek the consent of the next of kin, but it is important to make sure that they know what material will be retained, by whom and for how long. If they have strong objections these should be respected in spite of the wishes of the deceased.

12 Special circumstances

12.1 Samples obtained from abroad

When obtaining samples of human material from abroad, researchers must be satisfied that they have been ethically obtained. The researcher should obtain from the clinician providing samples written assurance that they were obtained with proper consent in accordance not only with these guidelines but also with guidelines applicable in the country of origin. The recent Nuffield Council on Bioethics discussion document on "Research in Developing Societies" highlights the ethical issues and the report of their ongoing enquiry should be available in 2001.

12.2 Fetal and embryonic tissue

Fetal tissue must be obtained and used in accordance with recommendations of the Polkinghorne report[8]. This specifies that, where tissue is obtained from therapeutic abortions, there must be clear separation between the decision to induce abortion and any decision concerning use. The decision to terminate a pregnancy must not be influenced by consideration of the possible use to which the tissue may be put, and the Polkinghorne report states that no specific references should be made to any particular research use when consent is obtained. This is therefore one situation where consent must be obtained for general research use and not for a particular project. To ensure proper separation is maintained, MRC recommends that researchers needing to use fetal tissue obtain it from one of the established tissue resources that the Council funds. The placenta and other contents of the uterus are not considered fetal tissue, and consent should be obtained from the mother in the same way as for the use of any other human material. Any research on pre-implantation embryos created as a result of in vitro fertilisation must be approved by the Human Fertilisation and Embryology Authority.

12.3 Children

There are several sources of detailed ethical guidance on research in children (see Appendix 1). Parents with parental responsibility may legally give consent on behalf of a child. When children have sufficient understanding and intelligence to understand what is proposed, they themselves should consent to participation in the research, and it is good practice to seek parental consent also. Where a sample of biological material has been obtained from a young child on the basis of consent from their parent and stored for subsequent research use, and there is ongoing contact (e.g. in longitudinal studies), the child should be asked for consent to continued use of that sample once they are old enough to understand. Tests of known predictive value for adult onset diseases should not be done for research purposes on individually identifiable samples from children[9].

12.4 Adults not able to give consent

The Council's booklet "The ethical conduct of research on the mentally incapacitated" sets out the conditions that must be satisfied for inclusion of those unable to consent in research. The person must not object or appear to object, and an informed independent person acceptable to the Local Ethics Committee must agree that the individual's welfare and interests have been properly safeguarded. Risk of harm must be negligible (for non-therapeutic research) or must be outweighed by the likely benefits, and the research must not be against the individual's interests.

Researchers should seek the agreement of carers or relatives when seeking the involvement in research of adults that cannot themselves give valid consent, but should be aware that there is no provision in English law for anyone to give consent on behalf of another adult. In Scotland, following the implementation of the Adults with Incapacity (Scotland) Act (2000), it will be legally possible for a guardian or person with power of attorney to give consent to medical treatment or research on behalf of an adult unable to consent for themselves.

When seeking consent, it is important for the researcher to ascertain whether the potential participant has the capacity to consent. There will be individuals who, while not suffering from mental illness as such are, through grave illness or stress, in a state of altered consciousness or reduced comprehension when samples are obtained. The validity

---

[8] Review of the Guidance on the Research Use of Fetuses and Fetal Material HMSO July 1989

[9] Advisory Committee on Genetic Testing Report on Genetic Testing for Late Onset Disorders 1998

of consent obtained under these circumstances is questionable. If taking samples cannot be delayed, participants must be given full information about the research and the opportunity to withdraw when capacity to give valid consent is regained. If they do not wish to participate in the research their sample and all related data must be destroyed.

Bibliography • Appendix 1

Nuffield Council on Bioethics. Human Tissue, Ethical and Legal Aspects. London: Nuffield Council on Bioethics, 1995.

Medical Research Council. Responsibility in investigations on human participants and material and on personal information. London: Medical Research Council, 1992.

Statement from the Royal College of Physicians Committee on Ethical Issues in Medicine. Research based on archived information and samples. Journal of the Royal College of Physicians of London, 33:264–6:1999.

Royal College of Pathologists. Consensus statement of Recommended Policies for uses of Human Tissue in Research, Education and Quality Control – with notes reflecting UK law and practices. London: Royal College of Pathologists, 1999.

Advisory Committee on Genetic Testing. Advice to Research Ethics Committees. London: Department of Health, 1998.

Advisory Committee on Genetic Testing. Report on Genetic Testing for Late Onset Disorders. London: Department of Health, 1998.

The Human Genome Organisation Ethics Committee. Statement on DNA Sampling: Control and Access. London: Human Genome Organisation, 1998.

Royal College of Pathologists. Guidelines for the retention of tissues and organs at post-mortem examination. London: Royal College of Pathologists, 2000.

Royal College of Paediatrics and Child Health. Guidelines for the Ethical Conduct of Medical Research Involving Children. London: Royal College of Paediatrics and Child Health, 1999.

Medical Research Council. The Ethical Conduct of Research on the Mentally Incapacitated. London: Medical Research Council, 1991.

The Wellcome Trust. Guidelines for Issues to be Addressed When Considering Support for Collections of Human Samples. London: The Wellcome Trust, 1998.

General Medical Council. Seeking patients' consent: the ethical considerations. London: General Medical Council, 1998.

General Medical Council. Confidentiality: protecting and providing information. London: General Medical Council, 2000.

Nuffield Council on Bioethics. Mental disorders and genetics: the ethical context. London: Nuffield Council on Bioethics, 1998.

Review of the Guidance on the Research Use of Fetuses and Fetal Material. London: Stationery Office, 1989.

Grubb A. I, Me, Mine: Bodies, Parts and Property. Medical Law International; 3:299: 1998.

The Inquiry into the management of care of children receiving complex heart surgery at the Bristol Royal Infirmary: Interim Report. Removal and retention of human material. http://www.bristolinquiry. org.uk, 2000.

The Royal Liverpool Children's Inquiry: Summary and Recommendations. http://www.rlcinquiry.org.uk, 2001.

Doyal L, Tobias J S. Informed consent in medical research. BMJ Books, London, 2000. ISBN 0-7279-1486-3.

Checklist for research based on samples of human material • Appendix 2

Source of samples

- If new samples are to be collected for this research, will appropriate measures be taken to minimise any risks of physical harm? Could the approach to potential donors cause distress?
- If samples are to be collected from patients temporarily unable to give consent (e.g. during emergency surgery), are there appropriate arrangements to consult next of kin to obtain informed consent later and for patients to opt out if they wish?
- If the research is using samples originally collected for another research project, is the research covered by the consent already obtained? If not, can new consent be obtained from the donors or can the samples be anonymised and unlinked?
- If the research will use material surplus to clinical requirements, are the patients aware that their material might be used in this way and of their right to object? Would it be practicable to obtain individual consent?
- If samples are to be obtained after death, is it possible to discuss the study with potential donors and obtain consent before death? If not, are appropriate arrangements in place to get consent from the next of kin?

Justification for the study

- Could information obtained in the course of the research bring harm or distress to the donors, individually or as a group, or to members of their family?
- Do the potential benefits of the research outweigh the risks?

Conduct of the research

- Are adequate measures in place to protect the confidentiality of personal information required for or revealed by the research[10]?

---

[10] See Personal Information in Medical Research (2000, MRC Ethics Series) for a more detailed checklist regarding protection of confidentiality.

- Is it clear to donors who will have access to their samples or personal information about them?
- What will happen to the samples after the research is finished? Will appropriate consent be obtained if they will be stored for future use?

Feedback of information

- Could tests done on the samples as part of the research reveal information of immediate relevance to a donor's health or healthcare? If so, will the donors be made aware of this possibility and are the arrangements for feeding back this information appropriate? Have the arrangements been agreed with the people responsible for the donors' clinical care?
- Could tests done on the samples as part of the research reveal predictive or other information that might affect the interests of the donor or their family? If so, are arrangements in place to make that information available to donors, and will they have adequate information to make a decision as to whether they want the information? Would it be better if the samples were anonymised and unlinked before testing?
- Is it clear to participants where they can get information about the outcome of the research?

Summary of issues to address when obtaining consent • Appendix 3

General guidance on the production of patient information leaflets has been prepared by a working group on behalf of Multi-Centre Research Ethics Committees and is provided to all MREC applicants. This indicates general issues that must be covered for all research studies. In addition, the following specific issues should be covered in the process of obtaining informed consent and in the patient information leaflet for studies in which samples of biological material will be taken from participants. Information leaflets should always meet basic criteria for good quality information provision.

1 For all samples

- The sample will be treated as a gift.
- The donor has no right to a share of any profits that might arise from research using the sample.
- Who will be responsible for custodianship of the sample (host institution/funding body)?
- What personal information will be used in the research?
- The arrangements for protecting the donor's confidentiality.
- If the research might reveal any information of immediate clinical relevance, this will be fed back.
- Arrangements for feeding back or obtaining access to individual research results, if any, and for informing participants of the outcome of the research.
- Consent to access medical records, if required.
- Specific consent for any genetic tests, if required.

2 If the sample is to be stored for possible secondary use

- The types of studies the sample may be used for and the diseases that may be investigated.
- Possible impact of secondary studies on the interests of donors and their relatives.
- Means of accessing information on secondary studies, if appropriate.
- Secondary studies will have to be approved by an ethics committee.
- Consent to share samples with other users.
- Consent to commercial use, and an explanation of the potential benefits of commercial involvement, if appropriate.

Model consent form for research involving new samples of human biological material • Appendix 4

This form is a model, to be adapted as appropriate to suit particular studies. Sections not required should be omitted, and other sections may be needed if the project involves more than simply collecting a sample.

> ┌─────────────────────┐
> │ Host hospital/institution │
> │   headed paper   │
> │   │
> └─────────────────────┘

Thank you for reading the information about our research project. If you would like to take part, please read and sign this form.

Centre number:
Study number:
Patient identification number for this study:

Title of project: ....

Name of researcher: ....

Contact details for research team: ....

Please initial boxes

1. I have read the attached information sheet on this project, dated ....(version............), and have been given a copy to keep. I have been able to ask questions about the project and I understand why the research is being done and any risks involved. ☐

2. I agree to give a sample of (blood-afterbirth-tissue-other, as appropriate) for research in this project. I understand how the sample will be collected, that giving a sample for this research is voluntary and that I am free to withdraw my approval for use of the sample at any time without giving a reason and without my medical treatment or legal rights being affected. ☐

3. I give permission for someone from the research team to look at my medical records to get information on (complete as appropriate). I understand that the information will be kept confidential. ☐

4. I understand that (my doctor and/or I, as appropriate) will be informed if any of the results of the medical tests done as a part of the research are important for my health. ☐

5. I understand that I will not benefit financially if this research leads to the development of a new treatment or medical test. ☐

6. I know how to contact the research team if I need to, and how to get information about the results of the research ☐

7 Consent for storage and use in possible future research projects
I agree that the sample I have given and the information gathered about me can be stored by (name of custodian) at the (name of host institution/host institution on behalf of MRC) for possible use in future projects, as described in the attached information sheet[11]. I understand that some of these projects may be carried out by researchers other than (name of study team) who ran the first project, including researchers working for commercial companies. ☐

[11] Participants must be given written information to keep on possible future research – its goals, the types of tests that are to be done, the diseases that might be investigated, and how the results might affect their interests. The written information should also include an explanation of the safeguards in place to protect their interests, including information on ethical review and how their confidentiality will be protected.

8 Consent for genetic research[12]

A: For genetic tests of known clinical and/or predictive value:

I give permission for (name of genetic test) to be carried out on the sample I give, as part of this project. I have received written information about this test and I understand what the result could mean to me and/or members of my family.

I want/do not want (delete as applicable) to be told the results of this test.
I understand I can change my mind about this later.

B: For other genetic research:

I understand that (the project/future research, as appropriate) using the sample I give may include genetic research aimed at understanding the genetic influences on (complete as appropriate) but that the results of these investigations are unlikely to have any implications for me personally.

....
Name of patient   Date   Signature
(BLOCK CAPITALS)

....
Name of person taking consent   Date   Signature
(if different from researcher)

....
Name of researcher   Date   Signature

Would you like to be sent information about the progress of this project?   ☐   ☐

                                                                     Yes   **No**

Form version and date
Thank you for agreeing to participate in this research

[12] If genetic research may be carried out on the sample then specific consent is required. One or both sections A, or B, should be included in the consent form.

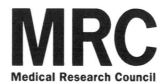

MRC
Medical Research Council

20 Park Crescent, London W1B 1AL
Telephone: 020 7636 5422   Facsimile: 020 7436 6179
Website: www.mrc.ac.uk

Transitional guidelines to facilitate changes in procedures for handling 'surplus' and archival material from human biological samples

June 2001

Royal College of Pathologists

The Royal College of Pathologists
2 Carlton House Terrace
London
SW1Y 5AF

Registered Charity No. 261035

Summary of the main recommendations

1 Procedures should be put in place to allow patients to control the use of surplus tissues* left over after diagnostic and therapeutic procedures are complete. In implementing such procedures, care must be taken to minimise disruption to NHS services.

2 The overall aim of these recommendations should be to seek the explicit consent of all patients to the ethically regulated use of surplus tissues for the benefit of other patients and society as a whole. The system developed for this purpose could also be used to record patients' opinions on a variety of other subjects and hence increase the autonomy of patients, especially for those who subsequently are unable to express an opinion through ill health. However, the implementation of such a system has major resource implications and will take time. These recommendations establish a coherent route towards this goal, which will produce rapid

---

* The word 'tissue' has led to misunderstandings in the past. In this document it is used to include the full range of human biological samples, including whole organs, small biopsies, cytological specimens, serum and blood samples, since all these can be used to extract DNA or produce other information of relevance to the tissue donor. In some circumstances, depending on the use to which the material is being put, in may be appropriate to include other samples including other body fluids, urine and faeces.

---

improvements in patient choice and will avoid blocking work which is important to the NHS during the transitional period.

3 There should be rapid implementation of methods to inform patients of how their surplus tissues may be used, the benefits to society from such use, and the limits and safeguards in place to prevent misuse. Appropriate information sheets should be developed.

4 This information could be delivered in a variety of ways, each of which has strengths and weaknesses:
   • an additional section on surgical consent forms
   • notice on the walls of phlebotomy rooms and GP surgeries
   • information sheets provided at each contact with the NHS
   • advertisements in the media or a 'mailshot' to all homes.

These options are not mutually exclusive. Sources of more detailed information should be made available for those who request it.

5 'Generic consent' for use of surplus tissue in laboratory quality control, teaching and research should be sought from all patients who use the NHS.

6 Generic consent is valid for the use of surplus and archival tissue for teaching, laboratory quality control and research work only if the work is ethically acceptable, if it is not in a controversial area and if it poses no risk of any adverse effect on the tissue donor.

7 Oversight of these safeguards will fall to local ethics committees. However, a central body should be created (or an existing body given powers) to:
   • oversee all uses of human tissues
   • guide research ethics committees in the oversight of such use
   • devlop and/or approve documentation and information sheets

- define protocols for routine work where individual review by an ethics committee is not necessary
- decide (with guidance from public consultation) which areas of research are too controversial to proceed without specific consent.

8 To implement these changes rapidly, and to avoid blocking essential work, it will initially be necessary to invite objections to the use of surplus and archival tissues, rather than to seek positive consent from all patients. The absence of such objections from adequately informed patients will represent *implied consent* rather than *explicit consent*. This is not ideal, but it is a considerable improvement on the present position where there is an assumption of implied consent which is not justified. *This will represent a transitional phase pending implementation of procedures to seek explicit consent from every NHS patient.* We anticipate that a move to recording positive consent, rather than absence of objection, should be made as soon as possible, but only after successful trials of the necessary procedures.

9 NHS databases should be modified to allow patients' opinions to be recorded as part of their records, not with each sample. In this way, an opinion expressed and recorded once will influence the use of all samples from that patient, including those already in existing archives. Secure, efficient access to this information should be available to those responsible for the management of tissues and tissue archives.

It may be appropriate to record the views of patients in relation to other aspects of health care as part of this process.

10 Work that uses surplus or archival tissues should not proceed without first checking that each patient involved has not recorded an objection to such use. The validity of such checks will increase as mechanisms to inform patients/record objection/obtain consent are implemented.

11 The use of surplus tissues for teaching or laboratory quality control need not be considered by an ethics committee unless there are unusual or controversial aspects to the work.

12 Research projects that use human tissue should be considered by a research ethics committee, with the possible exception of very simple projects that follow a previously approved protocol. This is a new task for ethics committees, so there is an urgent need for clear central guidance. We provide suggestions and ethical arguments for the content of such guidance.

13 The project submission form and the procedures of research ethics committees should be revised and streamlined (under central guidance) to facilitate this task.

14 Laboratories should comply with requests from patients for the return of their tissues. Protocols should be established to achieve this safely.

15 Paraffin blocks and microscope slides are of potential importance to a patient's future medical care and may be of importance to their relatives, even long after death. We recommend that they should not be given to patients. However, if this recommendation is rejected they should be given to patients only after a clear explanation of the potential importance of this material has been provided.

16 To make an unjustified assumption of consent is unethical, but to block work that is of benefit to patients is also unethical. There is therefore a need to implement these proposals as rapidly as possible. The Departments of Health may need to impose a deadline by which time NHS trusts must have implemented appropriate changes.

Introduction

1 It is in the vital interests of society that human tissues* can be used in NHS hospital laboratories, not only for biomedical research, but also in teaching medical and other NHS staff, and as part of audit and quality control procedures. These are essential to maintain the standards of medical laboratory services and the NHS as a whole.

2 A series of recent events has led to an urgent reappraisal of the ways in which human tissues are used in the health service and in biomedical research. Considerable distress has been suffered by relatives of the deceased by the retention of specimens removed at post-mortem examination, especially from children.[1,2] In this field, it is clear that some practices in pathology departments were out of date. Urgent changes have been made and are ongoing, continuing the trend we have seen throughout medicine to put greater emphasis on the value of individual autonomy.

3 In many hospitals, we have seen parallel changes being applied to 'surplus' human tissue. This has mainly taken the form of a requirement for consent from the tissue

---

* The word 'tissue' has led to misunderstandings in the past. In this document it is used to include the full range of human biological samples, including whole organs, small biopsies, cytological specimens, serum and blood samples, since all these can be used to extract DNA or produce other information of relevance to the tissue donor. In some circumstances, depending on the use to which the material is being put, it may be appropriate to include other samples including other body fluids, urine and faeces.

donor. Restrictions have been applied in an inconsistent manner in different institutions. They have been applied retrospectively, to samples taken and stored in archives under procedures considered perfectly acceptable at the time the samples were obtained. Restrictions designed for controversial subjects such as testing for inherited disease have been applied to other, much less contentious uses. Furthermore, restrictions have been applied immediately, before there has been any opportunity to implement mechanisms to obtain, record and retrieve information about consent.

4 In institutions where the most severe restrictions have been applied, there has been considerable disruption of research, staff training and laboratory quality assurance. These effects are contrary to the 'common good'; such indiscriminate restrictions are damaging the healthcare of the very individuals whose rights they are intended to protect.

5 **The consideration of using 'surplus' tissue needs separation from the consideration of post-mortem tissue, for several reasons.**

6 After death, the tissues of the deceased are often regarded by relatives as precious – as they are all that remains after a grievous loss. Even a lock of hair may be treasured. In contrast, surveys of public opinion[3,4] indicate that most patients are pleased to get rid of diseased tissue when it is removed for the good of their own health. They consider it to be 'waste' and support its being used for the common good if that is possible.

7 The use of surplus tissue was the subject of a detailed ethical review as recently as 1995.[5] This review concluded that, in the absence of evidence to the contrary, it was reasonable to assume that a patient's consent to the removal of the tissue implied consent to its subsequent use for any ethically acceptable purpose.

8 Consideration of basic ethical principles also suggests a distinction between the use of surplus tissues and post-mortem tissues. Surplus tissues invariably are produced as a by-product of a medical procedure. It can be argued that, having chosen to avail themselves of the right to such treatment, patients have a responsibility to facilitate the smooth running and development of the system they have chosen to benefit from, unless they have a reason to do otherwise.

9 One approach to defining an unethical act argues that, if the principle underlying an act cannot be 'universalised' (i.e. if we cannot will that the principle of the act be acted upon by everyone), then the act is unethical. (This is the Kantian 'categorical imperative'.)[6] In the present context, if everyone (without specific reason) refused to allow their tissues to be used for teaching, quality

assurance and research, the health services they need and have benefited from, and which produced the samples, could not exist. The act cannot be universalised, which indicates that to act this way is immoral. An act is morally unworthy if the principle underlying it cannot be shared.

10 Recent events demonstrate that in the UK, society has chosen not to follow these arguments. Nevertheless, their existence serves to emphasise the point that the wishes of a single individual cannot invariably be assumed to be paramount: such wishes cannot take precedence over the rights of large groups of individuals without reason. A balance needs to be found which invites and respects reasonable individual objections but which allows work for the common good to continue.

11 The aim of this document is threefold:

   i. to outline briefly the standards to which we aspire in the handling of human tissues, which we hope will be implemented in the near future (Section 1)

   ii. to suggest a practical route by which we can move as rapidly as possible towards this position, but in a planned way and with minimum disruption (Section 2)

   iii. to define procedures which we believe are acceptable at the present, which will as far as possible maximise the rights of patients to control how their tissue samples are used but which will permit the NHS, its diagnostic laboratories and its biomedical research projects to continue to function (Section 3).

Section 1

Where we should be in the near future

12 At the time of writing, a fundamental review of all uses of human tissue is being undertaken by the Department of Health. This review is likely to result in changes in the legislation. It is impossible to predict precisely the outcome of that review, but it seems certain that there will be considerable emphasis on obtaining the consent of tissue donors. In the context of major research projects, it is likely that the position will be similar to that recommended by the MRC in its publication, *Human tissue and biological samples for use in research.*[7]

13 However, *this MRC document cannot be applied to all uses of human tissue in the NHS.* The most obvious reason is that it was drafted with only research in mind, whereas the NHS also uses tissue for diagnosis, treatment, audit, teaching and to maintain the quality of its diagnostic laboratories. Furthermore, it was drafted

with large, carefully pre-planned research projects in mind. It did not consider the sort of 'micro-research' project which is common in the NHS, where a chance observation may lead laboratory staff merely to review a few samples to test whether an idea may be worth further investigation. Such 'micro-research' can have important results (such as the discovery of *H. pylori* as the cause of peptic ulceration) but would be blocked if complex procedures designed for much larger projects were universally applied.

The need for 'generic' consent for the use of human tissue

14 If tissue samples are to remain useful for future projects, unplanned at the time of sampling, it is logically impossible to obtain consent which is specific to the project in question at the time of sampling. If we do not accept some form of 'generic' consent for research use it would be necessary to re-contact each tissue donor for renewed consent before each new project. This has serious disadvantages for the tissue donor, the researcher and for society. It would often be impossible.[7]

15 The validity of generic consent was recently considered in detail by the House of Lords Select Committee on Science and Technology, in the relatively contentious context of using tissue samples and other data for genetic research.[8] The conclusion of that report was that generic consent to the use of human tissues (and personal information) *must* be accepted, though with appropriate safeguards. The MRC has recently stressed that consent for future, unforeseen projects should be requested whenever tissue samples are taken.[7] We support this conclusion.

16 If such generic consent is to be valid, certain safeguards must apply.

- When generic consent is obtained, the donor must understand, in general terms, the positive and negative consequences of giving or withholding consent and the mechanisms which are in place to control future use of the samples (outlined below).
- Confidentiality must be maintained, as with any use of medical information.
- The work must have an ethically acceptable purpose.[5] It must serve 'the common good' and satisfy the basic ethical principles of respect for autonomy, beneficence, non-maleficence and justice. Some projects (such as the development of biological weapons) would obviously be excluded by this requirement. Others (such as research into contraception or assisted reproduction, or the involvement of commercial organisations) are more difficult to judge. Such

judgements would have to be made on a case-by-case basis. Guidance in making such decisions should be sought from intermittent surveys of public opinion on the use of 'surplus' tissues in potentially controversial areas.

- The work must be designed so that there is no risk of adverse consequences for the tissue donor. This can be achieved by a variety of means. Irreversible anonymisation of samples is one approach, but will be impossible in some projects and could be unethical in others, as discussed below. Alternative approaches such as a secure coding system or 'linked anonymisation' may produce similar benefit with fewer disadvantages. Some projects by their nature pose no conceivable possibility of adverse consequences for the tissue donor. The best way to prevent adverse consequences for the tissue donor should be decided on a project-by-project basis, with ethics committee approval.

The need to seek consent from everyone

17 One of the main strengths of research using human tissue in the NHS is that the existence of large archives permits the identification of groups of similar cases. This is often essential to design studies of adequate power, especially if the conditions being studied are relatively rare. The coverage of the whole population also permits meaningful epidemiological work – if enough of the relevant specimens are available. It is rarely possible to identify in advance which specimens will be of value. Consequently, if such studies are to continue it will be necessary to seek generic consent from all NHS patients.

18 Seeking generic consent from all NHS patients is a considerable logistic challenge, because it must include recording the decisions and development of methods for data retrieval. Appropriate methods for providing the necessary information for patients will have to be developed (as discussed below). It is likely that eventually a record of each patient's opinions will be held as part of the unified electronic NHS record. This may eventually include numerous other items. A list of such items could potentially include:

- using surplus tissues (including blood) for laboratory quality control
- using surplus tissues for teaching
- using surplus tissue for biomedical research which is ethically controlled and has no possibility of adverse consequences for the donor (as discussed above).
- any specific exceptions to the above
- an answer to the question 'if a research project produces information which is relevant to your

health – positive or negative – would you want to be told?' (This complex question raises problems, but has been proposed elsewhere in the context of genetic information.)[8, paragraph 7.65c]

- access to case notes for purposes of medical audit
- access to case notes for purposes of ethically controlled biomedical/epidemiological research
- transfer of data to disease registries
- providing lists of patients with a specific diagnosis to epidemiological researchers
- permission to send postal questionnaires or surveys relating to health matters
- permission to send postal invitations to participate in a research project
- access of medical students; to take a history, to perform an examination, to carry out minor procedures under supervision.

More contentious items might include:

- attitudes to organ donation
- transfer of surplus tissue to commercial companies (on a not for profit basis, in accordance with ethical guidelines, and relinquishing any share in the commercial organisation's profits)
- do not resuscitate orders, advance directives ('living wills')
- consent to post mortem examination.

19 Much of this information would be very valuable if a patient is subsequently brought into hospital unconscious or otherwise without the capacity to give consent.

20 Inevitably, some research projects that need to use human tissue will not satisfy the requirements for using generic consent. If such projects are to proceed, it will be necessary to re-contact the tissue donors to seek specific consent. This poses different problems, especially with old samples where donors may have changed address or died; the ethics committee would have to agree the most appropriate course of action.

The need for oversight

21 The requirements for judgement in the above paragraphs demonstrate the need for an external review mechanism. The House of Lords Select Committee on Science and Technology suggested the establishment of a single, central 'Medical Data Panel' specifically for this purpose,[8] but it seems likely that in most cases the task will have to be devolved to local clinical or research ethics committees.

22 Most research projects will need individual review by a research ethics committee, but this would be unnecessarily bureaucratic for some other uses of human tissue, such as medical audit, routine laboratory quality control

and most teaching applications. Here it will be necessary to approve general procedures. A project would then require specific review only if variation from the agreed general procedure is envisaged.

23 To avoid inhibiting curiosity-driven 'micro-research' it may also be possible to use approval of a standard procedure for some types of very simple research. An example might be where a pathologist merely wishes to review systematically a group of previously reported histological sections, and no new processing of tissue is involved.

Section 2

Transitional guidelines: changes which need to be implemented

24 A large number of changes must be implemented, locally and nationally, before we reach the above position.

Providing appropriate information

25 If consent (either implied or explicit) is to be valid, it must be given by a competent individual, in the absence of coercion and with appropriate information. The Department of Health has recently issued a *Reference guide* to consent for examination and treatment, which explains these requirements in some detail.[9] It also discusses the evaluation of competence and what to do when (because of youth or illness) an individual is not competent to make a decision.

26 In the context of consent to use of surplus tissues, there is a problem in providing appropriate information, since in most cases the person in contact with the patient may have little or no experience of laboratory procedures. It is therefore necessary to provide sources of information.

27 For the patient, the information needed if consent is to be valid will include a summary of the positive and negative consequences of a decision to give or refuse consent, a description as far as is practical of the ethical uses to which tissue may be put, and an outline of the system for ethical oversight and regulation. The mechanisms by which the patient's opinions are recorded will need to be explained.

28 Those who discuss these matters with the patient will also need this information; in addition they should be familiar with the principles underlying informed consent, as explained in the Department of Health *Reference guide.*[9]

29 Information leaflets should be developed to provide the necessary information, for NHS staff as well as patients.

A single information leaflet cannot answer all possible questions, so it must provide routes to more detailed information for those who want it. This may be a direction to an individual, perhaps in the local hospital laboratory, or to more detailed information sheets on specific topics.

30 It seems inevitable that initial steps in the implementation of consent procedures will have to be taken by individual hospitals. It would be much more cost-effective, and it would help to harmonise procedures, if 'model' information sheets, notices, consent forms etc. could be provided and maintained centrally.

31 To this end, the Patient Liaison Group of the Royal College of Pathologists has agreed to develop a basic set of patient information sheets. The text will be made available over the Internet from the College website (www.rcpath.org). The leaflets will explain:

- why samples are sent to NHS laboratories
- what usually happens to any material remaining after tests are complete
- how surplus material and archival material may be alternatively be of benefit in maintaining the quality of laboratory services, training NHS staff, and in biomedical research
- the controls imposed on such uses, including an explanation of the role of the ethics committee, mechanisms used to ensure that there is no adverse impact on the tissue donors, mechanisms to protect confidentiality and avoidance of controversial research topics (with examples)
- that specific consent will be sought for any proposed projects which do not satisfy these requirements
- how patients can control or limit such uses of their tissues
- the fact that a refusal to permit use of surplus tissues will not influence the patient's medical care
- sources of more information.

These leaflets will be accessible directly by patients and staff. The College will renounce copyright on the information leaflets. They may be downloaded by healthcare organisations which may then edit the text as necessary, inserting locally relevant information, such as local contacts for further information, information about the local ethics committee and brief details of active research projects in local hospitals.

32 Suggestions for improvement of the central resource will be welcomed, but the initial project will of necessity be limited. Patient information sheets may need to be made available in several languages. They need to be carefully constructed, avoiding medical terminology and checked for the clarity of the language. They

need periodic maintenance to keep them up to date. This has significant resource implications and it may ultimately be necessary for the College to obtain funding or transfer responsibility for this work to another body.

Seeking consent, recording objections

33 The ideal outcome, as noted above, would be for all citizens to record their wishes, positive or negative, on a suitably secure national database. This would allow individuals the ongoing possibility of changing their consent in the light of new information. It would be available if the patient was incapacitated or – as in the case of archival tissue samples – not readily contactable. An opportunity to record or change opinions could be offered repeatedly throughout life, for example, at every contact with the health service, as children reach an appropriate age, and at any time on request. We believe that the Departments of Health should consider implementing such a scheme, but this would obviously require considerable resources and will take time. Interim procedures are required more urgently.

34 *There are several ways in which NHS Trusts could rapidly implement such interim procedures, which inform patients of how their tissues may be used and which seek consent or invite objections. All the following suggestions should be considered.* None is ideal. Most represent 'absence of objection' rather than positive consent, but it should be recognised that this is a transitional process. Most do not cover all sample types, but they are not mutually exclusive.

i. A section may be added to the surgical consent form. This should include information stating that:

- any tissue removed will be sent to the hospital laboratory for diagnostic examination
- small fragments and microscope slides may be retained in the laboratory as part of the patient's hospital record
- any larger samples will be safely disposed of, usually by incineration
- as an alternative to incineration, in some cases such 'surplus' tissue may be used for teaching, checking the quality of laboratory testing procedures, or research, under the control of a research ethics committee.

It should be stressed that no more tissue will be removed than is required to achieve the diagnostic or therapeutic purpose. Patients who object to any of these procedures should be asked to instruct the person who is seeking consent to record this objection in the notes, *and* to inform the pathology laboratory of their wishes. (It must be remembered that laboratory staff do not have free access to patients' case notes).

    ii. A notice may be placed on the wall of any phlebotomy room explaining that, although no more blood will be taken than is thought to be necessary, if any blood is left over after testing is complete it may be used for teaching, laboratory quality control or ethically regulated research. Patients who object should instruct the phlebotomist to record their objection on the pathology request form. A similar notice or leaflet for patients could be made available to those who take blood samples in other situations, such as on hospital wards.

    iii. An information sheet may be provided to patients, when they are sent an invitation to attend hospital, on arrival in Accident and Emergency, in GP surgeries and so on. This could not only explain the potential uses of surplus samples, it could also be used to satisfy other requirements, such as consent to transfer of data to disease registries. A mechanism would have to be identified by which those who wish to object may register their views.

    iv. The Departments of Health may wish to consider an advertising campaign, to explain how the NHS uses human tissue (and personal information) for the common good, and to indicate a route by which objections can be recorded. The recent media interest in post-mortem organ retention has distorted public understanding, making such a campaign particularly desirable at the present. One may hope that the moral reasons for agreeing to such use, to help the communal health services, would be emphasised. A publicity campaign would require considerable planning and support in case it produced a very large number of enquiries and calls in a short time.

35 *The above proposals are framed to record objections rather than positive consent. This is a compromise, but we argue that for the moment it is acceptable as a rapidly attainable transitional position pending implementation of a scheme which will record positive consent.* It can also be supported by the arguments given above (paragraphs 5–10) suggesting that most members of the public regard tissues which have been removed for a therapeutic purpose as being much less emotionally valuable than post mortem tissues.

36 The experience of hospitals which have already introduced a 'tissue consent' clause on their surgical consent forms indicates that objections are likely to be relatively infrequent, so recording objections rather than positive consent will reduce the resource implications of implementing a new scheme. This approach will also facilitate a smooth transition from the present arrangements, as outlined below. The present position is an unjustified assumption of absence of objection, so it is unavoidable that we must start from this position and seek gradual improvement.

37 We recognise that it is preferable to move to positive recording of consent, but this should be regarded as the next step.

38 Unfortunately, direct experience of the level of diligence with which pathology request forms are completed leads us to doubt whether positive consent would be transmitted reliably to the pathology laboratory through a 'check box' on a pathology request form. Transmission of an unusual event (such as an objection) is likely to be much more reliable, particularly as receipt of one objection would be taken to indicate that the patient holds the same objection for all samples of a similar type.

39 Using mechanism (34 iii) above, positive consent could be sought if a specific member of staff were given the responsibility to seek answers as part of the admission/booking in procedure. This has resource implications. Furthermore, in view of the logistic problems we anticipate if other staff are required to inform the laboratory about consent, *we recommend that prior to national implementation, small-scale trials should be carried out to ensure that protocols for obtaining, recording and retrieving positive affirmation of consent are reliable, efficient and cost effective.*

Recording and retrieving consent data

40 Tissue samples in the NHS are held in very large numbers, almost exclusively in hospital laboratories. If patients' wishes are to be respected without disrupting health laboratory work, it follows that laboratory staff will need rapid, easy access to information about each patient's recorded opinions on the use of their tissue and blood samples. This implies electronic data storage, with suitable security procedures.

41 A decision has to be made whether the patient's opinions should be stored with the record of each sample or with the record of each patient. The structure of modern relational databases indicates that *information about consent to tissue use should be stored with the patient record, rather than the sample record*, for the following reasons:

- the record of each sample will automatically be linked to the patient's record, so the consent status will be available whenever a sample record is accessed
- this provides a 'failsafe' mechanism; if a patient has recorded one objection to the research use of one

blood sample, it is reasonable to assume in the absence of information to the contrary that the same will apply to all blood samples

- each patient will generate many samples, so linking to the patient record will minimise data entry
- when patients change their mind, a single change to the database will influence the use of all samples from that patient. Similarly, the act of recording a patient's opinion once will control the use of all samples from that patient already in the hospital archive.

42 For each patient, *we suggest that as a minimum it should be possible to record consent or objection to 'generic' research use, as outlined above and to teaching and quality control. Consent or objection should be assumed to apply to all samples from that patient, unless otherwise specified.* We may anticipate that some patients who are content for blood samples to be used may object to the use of whole organs or products of conception, and it should be possible to record this distinction. To facilitate the next move, to recording explicit consent, the database record should permit three options:

  i. no opinion recorded
  ii. objection recorded
  iii. explicit consent recorded.

43 We understand that most of the commercial database systems used in NHS laboratories can be amended at relatively little expense to record and retrieve this sort of information. However, *it may be appropriate to consider recording this information in the hospital patient administration system database rather than in the laboratory.* This could facilitate direct recording of consent data by ward staff, which will probably become necessary with a move to recording positive consent. It would also tie in with the need to record patient opinions on other matters, such as research access to case notes, advance directives and so on.

44 It will be necessary for the databases involved to provide suitable search and display algorithms for retrieval of consent data, together with suitable security measures to control access and prevent disclosure of unnecessary information.

Oversight

45 We support the suggestion of the Select Committee on Science and Technology that a 'medical data panel' should be set up to oversee the use of medical data, including tissue samples, where generic rather than specific consent for use has been obtained. We anticipate that such a body would be responsible for establishing guidelines whereby samples may be used for audit, teaching and quality control, and possibly for some very simple research projects, without the need for specific consideration by an ethics committee.

46 Most or all research projects which use human tissue will need to be reviewed by a local research ethics committee. We anticipate that a central 'medical data panel' or equivalent will be responsible for providing detailed guidance to local ethics committees on the review of projects which use 'generic' consent. However, two urgent developments are required.

  i. Research ethics committees are at present taking inconsistent and contradictory decisions. They need to be issued with detailed guidance on how they should handle proposals for research projects that use surplus or archival human tissue in the present situation, before any 'generic consent' procedures have been implemented. Our suggestions for such an approach are provided in the following section.

  ii. The present application form for ethical approval is a centrally imposed, complex multi-page document which was designed principally for randomised controlled clinical trials. The form was designed at a time when most laboratory-based projects would not have been deemed to require ethics committee approval. Much of it is irrelevant to laboratory studies, especially those using archival material. There is an urgent need for a research ethics approval form which is specifically designed for such studies. Consideration should also be given to streamlining the process. At present, it is not unusual for obtaining approval to take much longer than carrying out the work.

Implementation

47 Three aspects of these recommendations need to be emphasised.

  i. The changes have resource implications.
  ii. Changes are urgently required if the function of NHS pathology departments is not to be compromised.
  iii. Most of the changes must be carried out at a hospital or NHS-wide level. Pathology departments cannot implement them, even though such departments are best placed to identify problems and are most motivated to achieve a solution.

48 *These points leave us gravely concerned about implementation, and the speed at which it will occur. We believe it highly unlikely that NHS Trusts will act with sufficient urgency merely on the basis of recommendations from the Royal College of Pathologists. We therefore urge the Departments of Health to distribute appropriate instructions concerning the implementation of these*

or similar procedures, with reasonable deadlines for the date of implementation throughout the NHS.

Section 3

What is acceptable now?

49 Audit, teaching, laboratory quality control and biomedical research are all activities carried out for the common good. We have identified changes which are needed to facilitate the proper use of human tissues in support of such work, but such changes will take a little time to implement. *We argue that it is unethical to block such work while new procedures are being developed and implemented.*

50 Hence, where in the following proposals we indicate that workers should first check that the patient from whom the surplus tissue originated has not recorded an objection to its use, in most cases it will initially be unavoidable to assume – as in the past – that there is no objection, as there has been no systematic mechanism by which such objections can be recorded. As systems to record objections and consent are implemented, this check will gradually become more meaningful.

Primary diagnosis

51 Laboratory staff should continue to assume that the removal of a tissue or blood sample, and its transfer to the laboratory accompanied by a request form, indicate the existence of consent to carry out the requested investigation. Where the results of the initial tests indicate the desirability of further investigation ('reflex testing'), senior laboratory staff should decide whether the clinical staff or the patient should first be contacted to confirm consent before the further test is carried out. In most cases, this will not be necessary, and rapid performance of a reflex test is good laboratory practice. However, if it is possible that it may be in the patient's best interests (broadly interpreted) *not* to carry out a reflex test, renewed consent should be sought. The most obvious situation where such consent is mandatory is HIV testing.

Returning specimens to patients

52 At present, very few patients request the return of resected organs or other samples. When patients are specifically informed of what happens to such specimens, it is likely that such requests will increase in frequency, especially in relation to larger samples including whole organs, the disposal or retention of which

may have emotional implications. Laboratories should have established protocols to permit compliance with such requests while minimising any risk to the patient or others from infection or toxic chemicals.

53 Advice is needed from the Departments of Health on how to respond to requests for the return of paraffin blocks and microscope slides, which are in effect part of the patient record. In the past, having been 'substantially modified' by NHS laboratories they have been regarded as the property of the Secretary of State, but this position has not recently been reaffirmed. The importance of this material to the future healthcare of patients (and their relatives) is such that we recommend that blocks and slides should not be given to patients. However, if this recommendation is rejected, patients should be warned of the potential importance of this material for future medical care.

Audit

54 Reviewing results or repeating a test to confirm the accuracy of the original result is essential to good laboratory practice. Provided that confidentiality is maintained, consent and external oversight should not be required.

55 Clinical teams may request data from pathology laboratories in a form which facilitates their own clinical audit. Collation and transfer of such data is acceptable as long as it is provided to the team with responsibility for the care of the patient, and appropriate controls are in place to maintain confidentiality.

56 In some situations, it may be debatable whether a project should be regarded as 'audit' or 'research'. If the work involves any new manipulation of a sample, beyond that required for the primary diagnostic purpose, it should for this purpose be regarded as research. Any project which generates new data, or which could have any adverse effect on the patient, should be regarded as research.

Laboratory quality assurance

57 Laboratories should assume that surplus tissue is available for quality assurance procedures (internal quality control and external quality assessment) unless an objection has been received from the patient. Precautions should be taken to ensure confidentiality. In many cases this will be most readily done by irreversible anonymisation of the samples. However, in some situations this will be inappropriate; for example, in interpretive histopathology external quality assurance schemes it is possible that use of a sample will demonstrate that the original diagnosis was incorrect. It will then be

necessary to inform the relevant clinical team of this error: to fail to do this would be indefensible.[10] In such situations, a secure coding system should be used to maintain confidentiality.

58 When work is being done to achieve the successful local implementation of a new laboratory technique which has previously been established elsewhere, or to improve of an existing technique, the use of surplus tissue should be preceded by a check that an objection to such use has not been recorded. It should not require oversight by an ethics committee. Confidentiality should be preserved and wherever possible irreversibly anonymised samples should be used. The development of a completely new technique should be regarded as research.

59 Where samples for quality assurance purposes are taken specifically for that purpose and are not 'surplus' to diagnostic requirements, as in some large clinical chemistry schemes, the approach to obtaining consent should parallel that for taking samples specifically for research, as set out by the MRC.[7]

Teaching

60 Where teaching is carried out on an 'apprenticeship' basis, such as in histopathology departments, an attempt to exclude cases where a patient objects to the use of their sample in teaching would be disruptive to the point of being impossible to implement. This would be equivalent to a patient demanding that he is only treated by the senior consultant and the ward sister, a demand which would not be possible to accommodate in the NHS. Such teaching must therefore continue as before. As noted above, it is reasonable to assume those who wish to use the services of trained staff should not put obstacles in the way of training without reason.

61 However, when cases are to be used for more formal teaching sessions (such as slide seminars or presentation at clinico-pathological case conferences) then those preparing such material should check that an objection to use in teaching has not been received from the patient. Steps must be taken to preserve patient confidentiality.

62 The preservation of surgical resection specimens as 'museum pots' for teaching purposes should parallel guidance for the retention of post-mortem specimens for the same purpose, with the obvious exception that the consent of the patient rather than the relatives should be sought.

63 These considerations also apply to preparing study material for medical students. Here it is also necessary to remember that some methods of dissemination of teaching material (e.g. distribution on the Internet) effectively represent publication. The GMC has indicated that consent is needed before publication of images of patients,[11] although consent is not required for images of microscopic preparations.[12] It is required for any macroscopic images of the external surface of the body, even if the patient is not identifiable from the image. It is required for images from an operation, radiographs and arguably for recognisable whole organs.[11]

64 We believe that the procedures for recording generic consent for teaching use described above will be sufficient to permit most material entering pathology laboratories to be used for most teaching purposes, with the exception of publication of macroscopic images and the preservation of whole organs.

Research

65 In the past, research projects which used exclusively 'surplus' material and which did not require any direct patient contact were usually conducted without referral to a research ethics committee (REC). We believe that in the future, all research projects which use human tissue should be considered by a suitable REC, and tested against national guidelines. Given the current modes of operation of most RECs, this will cause considerable delay and disruption, and we have noted the need for new procedures to facilitate this process, but we believe such a conclusion to be unavoidable. For simple 'micro-research' projects which have no potential for adverse impact on the donor (such as a review of old slides) it may be possible to define generic protocols where the project can proceed merely with a requirement to inform the REC. Problems with the distinction between research, audit and laboratory development are noted above.

66 We have already seen considerable variation in way RECs have responded to such requests, presumably because RECs have not previously been required to consider projects of this type. There is a real danger that the NHS will be fragmented if there is not uniformity of approach. Guidelines should be developed centrally by the 'medical data panel' or equivalent, but *in the absence of such guidelines we suggest that the following factors should be considered when research projects that use 'generic' consent are reviewed by a research ethics committee.*

67 **Impact on the tissue donor.** If a project is to use 'generic' consent for research use, it is part of the agreement with the donor that there should be no possible adverse consequences for the donor, and the review process must ensure this. The simplest way to ensure that research

data are not fed back inappropriately to the donor is irreversible anonymisation of the samples. Some have argued that anonymisation is *invariably* a requirement for the use of 'generic' consent – although the word 'anonymisation' is sometimes used loosely, to include securely coded samples. Such arguments are often promoted in the context of genetic studies which may reveal susceptibility to an incurable genetic disease, where the risk of producing distressing and damaging information is obvious. Most biomedical research carries little or no such risk. Irreversible anonymisation can cause serious problems, for the donor and the research.

- Anonymisation vastly reduces the possibility of investigating unexpected results. It makes it impossible to contact the donor to request consent for further studies. Hence either the follow-up study is never done – which wastes information – or the original study has to be repeated – which wastes resources.
- It has been argued that this problem should be avoided by assembling a mass of data at the start of a project 'just in case' it is needed, before anonymisation of the samples. To collect volumes of personal data without clear purpose is itself morally objectionable and is arguably contrary to the Data Protection Act 1998.
- Anonymisation eliminates any possibility of obtaining further information about the patient's subsequent course, which may have added to the value of the study. The MRC has expressed the view that '...there had to be some means of linking data back to the individual in many kinds of research...'.[8, paragraph 7.26]
- Anonymisation makes it impossible for donors to change their minds and remove samples from an archive.
- Anonymisation makes it impossible to provide any information to the donor, whether harmful or beneficial. It is difficult to see why producing information which may cause damage is inherently worse than failing to give information which may cause good. Research results are not invariably damaging; it is quite possible that a research project might identify information (such as an idiosyncratic drug reaction) which could be life-saving. The MRC has recognised that there are some circumstances where it is essential to return research data to tissue donors, though careful ethical oversight is necessary.[7, section 8]
- If a product with potential for commercial development (such as a cell line) is generated directly from a human sample, the consent of the donor must first be sought. Anonymisation would make this impossible,

thus prohibiting dissemination of a useful product. (This argument does not apply to intellectual property rights.)

68 Hence, rather than insisting on irreversible anonymisation of samples, we argue that *each research project should be considered individually against the requirement that, if 'generic' consent is to be used, there should be no risk of adverse consequences for the donor.* The ideal method by which this is achieved will vary in different circumstances.

Nature of the project

69 Some projects cannot use generic consent because of their nature. If human tissues are to be used it is essential that the purpose is ethically acceptable, that the project aims to produce some benefit for humanity, and that it has a reasonable prospect of achieving that aim. If generic consent is to be used it is also important to avoid 'controversial' subjects, where a significant number of donors may have undeclared objections.

70 In most cases, this distinction will be clear: work which seeks to alleviate suffering will be acceptable, the production of weapons of mass destruction will not. The basic ethical principles of respect for autonomy, beneficence, non-maleficence and justice must be respected. However, if 'generic' consent to research use is to be used we must recognise those areas where there is public debate and concern. For example, at the present we must assume that generic consent cannot be taken to infer consent to therapeutic cloning. For the same reasons it seems unlikely that research into improving contraception or infertility treatment can be carried out using generic consent.

71 The boundary of which areas can be supported by generic consent is a subject for ethical debate, but it is heavily influenced by public opinion. The boundary will have to be defined by the 'medical data panel' or equivalent. This should be subjected to periodic review. In the future, it may be appropriate for the Panel to carry out surveys of public opinion to illuminate this debate. Initially this decision will fall to local research ethics committees, which will presumably be obliged to take a relatively conservative view of what is 'controversial'.

72 There may be individuals who for personal reasons have a specific and unusual aversion to involvement in some type of research which most members of the public consider to be non-controversial. We believe that such individuals may reasonably be expected to recognise that their objections are unusual, and therefore they will be aware of the need to make their objections known.

Obtaining specific consent

73 Re-contacting the patient to seek specific consent has potential disadvantages for donor as well as researcher.[8] If an REC decides that, for any of the above reasons, it is desirable that the tissue donors should be contacted to obtain specific consent for use of their samples, the REC should first consider any possible adverse consequences for the donors of such a decision. They should also consider whether it is practical, bearing in mind that some donors may have died or changed address, and it may not be possible for the research workers to identify the cases where this applies. The REC should then define what sort of contact and consent is required; an instruction to 'obtain consent' is insufficiently specific. The options that may be considered include:

- posting an information sheet to the patient, inviting objections. Where none are received within a specified time, the samples may be used; hence samples from patients who cannot be contacted may be used
- posting an information sheet to the patient, requesting the return of a form giving consent; hence samples from patients who cannot be contacted (or are apathetic) cannot be used. The position in relation to patients who have died would need to be defined, if these can be identified
- establishing personal contact, and providing explanation to standards equivalent to those used in taking samples specifically for research.

74 It should be noted that as these options give progressively greater weight to the requirement for consent, they simultaneously become more intrusive and potentially distressing for the patient, and they run a progressively greater risk of making the project impractical.

The use of existing archival material

75 The NHS currently holds large archives of human samples which have vast potential for future research. The exact direction of such research cannot be predicted, for example, the existence of archives of human tissue permitted retrospective study of the epidemiology of 'new' diseases such as AIDS and new variant CJD.

76 It has been recognised that if there is a requirement to seek consent from donors before existing tissue archives can be used for any ethically legitimate purpose this would, in effect, prohibit almost all use of the archives. The MRC has recommended that such archives should remain available for research without a requirement for such consent provided each project is approved by an appropriate ethics committee.[7] The REC would have to be satisfied that there is no potential for any adverse consequence for the tissue donor, as discussed above.

77 One advantage of recording consent or objection to tissue use as part of the patient record is that whenever an opinion is recorded, the database should automatically link this opinion to all older samples from the same patient. In this way the problem of consent to the use of old archival samples will gradually diminish.

78 Archives are also of great value in teaching, especially in providing educational examples of rare conditions. Here the archives are represented not only by tissue samples and microscope slides but also by large numbers of photographs. Many of these are photographs of whole organs or of the external surface of patients, but as many are quite old and most have been irreversibly anonymised it is no longer possible to go back to the patient to seek consent. *We see no useful purpose in prohibiting the use of such anonymised images in teaching, but we note the GMC's guidance that (excepting photomicrographs) they should not be published without consent.*[11]

The Data Protection Act 1998

79 The Data Protection Act 1998[13] is relevant to the use of tissue samples. We have received a detailed explanation from the Office of the Information Commissioner that, in most circumstances, the analysis of 'identifiable' samples is covered by the requirements of this Act. Although there are some exceptions, the Act usually requires consent for the processing of data, but we are assured that this does not necessarily require the signature of a consent form; if consent is obtained in a way that is ethically acceptable (as discussed above) then this requirement of the Act is satisfied. The MRC has recently expressed the opinion that implied consent (as explained above) is ethically acceptable for the research use of surplus tissue if there is no possibility of the research affecting the patient's interests.[7, section 3] This indicates that in this context, implies consent satisfies the requirements of the Act.

80 Irreversible anonymisation (or the death of the patient) takes the matter outside the scope of the Act. This may also be achieved by some secure methods of coding; the issues are complex and are discussed in more detail elsewhere (http://www.rcpath.org/news/data_act.html).

81 If identifiable samples from old archives are to be studied, there is a potential conflict between the requirements of the Act and the view[7,14] that it is ethical to allow access (within defined constraints) to existing archival samples without invariably re-contacting the donors. Here, until such time as we can reasonably assume that patients are aware that their samples may be used in research and that they have the right to object,

the law appears to demand more than is ethically required. The Information Commissioner has indicated that it is 'unlikely' that proceedings will be instituted in relation to archival samples taken before the Act came into force. It is good practice to take samples outside the scope of the Act by anonymisation or secure coding wherever possible. In some studies, the exceptions provided by the Act may be invoked. In others, especially those which use relatively recent samples, it may be necessary to inform the tissue donors and invite objections.

Continuation of existing projects

82 In a few instances, we have heard of research projects which have been given approval by an ethics committee in the past but which on review do not meet current standards. In at least one case, a postgraduate student was warned just before submission that a research thesis might not be admissible on this basis.

83 It is clearly inappropriate to suggest that the ethical approval of research projects should never be reconsidered. However, in the case of time-limited projects it seems reasonable to suggest that wherever possible they should be judged by the standards prevailing at the time of their initial assessment, and that if ethical review subsequently becomes essential every consideration should be given to finding ways in which the project may be brought to a satisfactory conclusion.

Taking tissue before diagnostic procedures are complete

84 This discussion has concentrated on archives and tissues which are surplus after diagnostic procedures are complete. However, some procedures (notably the evaluation of gene expression) require fresh tissue, and/or cannot be applied to formalin fixed material. Here there is a need for rapid sampling of tissues which have to be removed as part of the therapeutic procedure, but where it is possible to identify in advance that their use will not in any way prejudice the diagnostic examination which follows. Examples might include sampling uninvolved kidney from a nephrectomy for carcinoma, or taking fragments of a tumour which is removed piecemeal, but where routine laboratory processing would only examine a small proportion of the tissue fragments, chosen at random.

85 We believe that such sampling is ethically acceptable, but only if the subsequent pathological examination is completely unaffected. This means that a protocol to ensure this must be agreed between the pathologist responsible for the examination and the researcher, and the agreed protocol must be part of the ethics committee review of the project.

86 Whether such sampling can be performed with only 'generic consent' is debatable. Where the sample removed for research is small and the absence of any adverse effect on the patient is incontestable we suggest that it can.

REFERENCES

1 *The inquiry into the management of care of children receiving complex heart surgery at the Bristol Royal Infirmary.* 2000. http://www.bristol-inquiry.org.uk/

2 *The Report of The Royal Liverpool Children's Inquiry* (the 'Richards Report'). 2001. http://www.rlcinquiry.org.uk/

3 Start RD, Brown W, Bryant RJ, *et al.* Ownership and uses of human tissue: does the Nuffield bioethics report accord with opinion of surgical inpatients? *BMJ* 1996; 313: 1366–1368.

4 *Public perceptions of the collection of human biological samples.* Medical Research Council, London. 2001. http://www.mrc.ac.uk/publicperceptions.htm

5 *Human tissue: ethical and legal issues.* Nuffield Council on Bioethics, London. 1995. http://www.nuffieldfoundation.org/bioethics/

6 Kant I. From ordinary rational knowledge of morality to philosophical. In: *Groundwork of the metaphysics of morals* (1797; translated Paton HJ, 1948). New York: Harper & Row, 1964: 69–71.

7 *Human tissue and biological samples for use in research: operational and ethical guidelines.* Medical Research Council, London. 2001. http://www.mrc.ac.uk/PDFs/Tissue%20Guidelines_final.pdf

8 Select Committee on Science and Technology Fourth Report; *The opportunities and challenges arising from the use of human genetic databases.* House of Lords, London. 2001. http://www.parliament.the-stationery-office.co.uk/pa/ld200001/ldselect/ldsctech/57/5701.htm

9 *Reference guide to consent for examination or treatment.* Department of Health, London. 2001.

10 *Recommendations for the development of histopathology/cytopathology External Quality Assessment Schemes.* Royal College of Pathologists, London. 1998. http://www.rcpath.org/activities/publications/eqawg.html

11 *Confidentiality: protecting and providing information.* General Medical Council, London. 2000.

12 *Making and using visual and audio recordings of patients.* General Medical Council, London. 1997.

13 Data Protection Act. HM Stationery Office, London. 1998. http://www.hmso.gov.uk/acts/acts1998/19980029.htm

14 *Statement on DNA sampling: control and access. Report of the Human Genome Organisation Ethics Committee.* Human Genome Organisation, London. 1998.

Code of practice on the use of fetuses and fetal material in research and treatment (extracts from the Polkinghorne Report)

The Stationery Office/Department of Health

The guidance in this Chapter is taken from the Review of the Guidance on the Research Use of Fetuses and Fetal Material ("The Polkinghorne Report") CM 762, HMSO 1989 and the figures in brackets refer to the relevant paragraph in the text of the Report.

In this Code fetus means the embryo or fetus from implantation until gestation ends and, unless qualified by the words in utero, includes the fetus outside the womb. (1.5)

1 Treatment of the fetus

1.1 Two categories of fetus are recognised:

   a. The live fetus, whether in utero or ex utero, which should be treated on principles broadly similar to those which apply to treatment and research conducted with children and adults. (2.4, 3.2).

   b. The dead fetus. The determination of death shall be by reference to the absence of vital functions, as indicated by the absence of spontaneous respiration and heartbeat after consideration of possibly reversible factors, such as the effects of hypothermia in the fetus, or of drugs or metabolic disorders in the mother. This determination shall be made or confirmed by a doctor responsible for the clinical management of the mother and the fetus and not involved with the subsequent unconnected use of fetal tissue. (3.7).

   Only tissue from the dead fetus is ethically available for use in therapy.

1.2 It is unethical to administer drugs or carry out any procedures during pregnancy with the intent of ascertaining whether or not they might harm the fetus. (3.3)

1.3 In the case of nervous tissue only isolated neurones or fragments of tissue may be used for transplantation. (3.11)

2 Contents of the uterus other than the fetus

The contents of the uterus resulting from pregnancy other than the fetus (ie the placenta, fluid and membranes) may be used for research or therapeutic purposes subject to the conditions relating to screening at section 4.5 of this Code and those relating to finance at section 7(3.12).

3 Separation of the supply of fetal tissue from the practice of research and therapy

3.1 The decision to carry out an abortion must be reached without consideration of the benefits of subsequent use. The generation or termination of pregnancy to produce suitable material is unethical. (4.1).

3.2 The management of the pregnancy of any mother should not be influenced by use of the fetus in research or therapy. In this context, management of the pregnancy should be taken to include:

   a. the method and timing of an abortion;

   b. the clinical management of a mother whose fetus dies in utero or who has a spontaneous abortion.

3.3 No inducements, financial or otherwise, should be put to the mother or to those who are in a position to influence her decision to have her pregnancy terminated, or to allow fetal tissue to be used. (4.4).

3.4 The mother should not be informed of the specific use which may be made of fetal tissue, or whether it is to be used at all. (4.2, 4.6).

3.5 Those involved in the process of abortion and responsible for the clinical care of the mother should not knowingly be involved in research on the fetus or fetal tissue collected. Dissection of the dead fetus, research on it, or transplantation of fetal tissue should, when practicable, be on separate premises and certainly not in the same room. However, ethically acceptable exceptions to this degree of separation occur when research is concerned with the investigation of cases of fetal death in utero, or spontaneous abortion or analogous post-mortem concerns arising from previous medical history. (5.7).

3.6 The source must keep records indicating the next destination of any fetal tissue which is released for purposes of research or therapy, and it should have a means of satisfying itself that anyone to whom tissue is sent has satisfied the requirements of this Code. The mother's identity should not be revealed when fetal tissue is released, although some coding will be necessary which will enable her to be traced by those responsible for her clinical management, should relevant information come to light through examination of the fetal tissue. (5.3).

3.7 Any intermediary or tissue bank which receives or passes on fetal tissue must keep a record of the destination and origin of all tissue and not reveal details of the identity of the source to the user and vice versa. (5.4).

3.8 On the same principle the user should be able to satisfy itself that any material it receives has been procured in accordance with the requirements of this Code. It must keep records indicating the proximate source of any fetal tissue and the use to which it is put, but should not reveal details of the use to the source. (5.5).

3.9 Details about a fetus (eg gestational age) which might be of significance for research but could not be used for identification may be released by the source, but it is not acceptable for the source to be approached with requests for fetuses with particular characteristics. (5.6).

4 Consent

4.1 The written consent of the mother must be obtained before any research or therapy involving the fetus or fetal tissue takes place. Sufficient explanation should be offered to make the act of consent valid. (6.3).

4.2 Consent to the termination of pregnancy must be reached before consent is sought to the use of fetal tissue, and without reference to the possibility of that use. Provided the question of use is not introduced until consent to the termination of pregnancy has been obtained, it is permissible to deal with the two issues on the same occasion. (6.5).

4.3 It may be desirable to consult the father since, for example, tests on fetal tissue may reveal a finding of potential significance to him, and because he may have knowledge of a transmissible or hereditary disease, but his consent shall not be a requirement nor should he have the power to forbid research or therapy making use of fetal tissue. (6.7).

4.4 In the case of spontaneous abortions (or where death of the fetus has occurred in utero) consent to use fetal tissue should preferably be sought only after the fetus has died. (6.4).

4.5 Consent should be obtained from the mother to tests if any screening is to take place for transmissible disease or if any procedure is contemplated which could have similar consequences for the mother and affect her clinical management. Any such tests, and the counselling to accompany them, should be conducted according to the best current practice and guidance, in a manner which ensures that the principles of separation are maintained. (6.9).

5 Conscientious objection

No member of the medical or nursing staff should be under any duty to participate in research or therapy involving the fetus or fetal tissue if he or she has conscientious objection. This right of non-participation does not extend to the prior or subsequent care of a patient thus treated. (2.11).

6 Ethics committees

All research or therapy of an innovative character involving the fetus or fetal tissue should be described in a protocol and be examined by an ethics committee. Projects should be subject to review until the validity of the procedure has been recognised by the committee as part of routine medical practice. The ethics committee has a duty to examine the progress of the research or innovative therapy (eg. by receiving reports). It should have access to records and be able to confirm that the material is in fact being used for the purpose set out in the protocol. It should also be able to examine the record of any financial transactions involving fetal tissue. Before permitting research the ethics committee must satisfy itself: (7.4).

a. of the validity of the research or use proposed;
b. that the objectives of the proposed use cannot be achieved in any other way;
c. that the researchers or clinicians have the necessary facilities and skill.

Taken from Appendix B of Local Research Ethics Committees HSG(91)5, 1991

7 Finance

There should be no monetary exchange for fetuses or fetal tissue. Profit from any dealing in fetal tissue or the other contents of the uterus is unethical (8.1, 8.3).

47

Guidance on the supply of fetal tissue for research, diagnosis and therapy

Department of Health

Background and general principles

A fundamental ethical principle in the Polkinghorne Report ("Review of the guidance on the research use of fetuses and fetal material", Cm 792,1989 HMSO) is that the decision to terminate a pregnancy and the method and timing of the abortion must not be influenced by consideration of the possible use which may be made of the tissue. That principle operates and can be seen to operate when fetal tissue required for research, diagnosis or therapy is obtained from a tissue bank rather than supplied direct from centres which perform abortions.

At present the only national facility for providing fetal tissue for research or other use is the MRC Fetal Tissue Bank at the Hammersmith Hospital. In many circumstances this tissue bank will be able to supply the needs of research workers and diagnostic laboratories. However, there will be some circumstances in which it will be essential for tissue to be obtained locally. This note sets out the factors that will need to be taken into account in deciding whether tissue should be obtained from the MRC Fetal Tissue Bank or through local arrangements. Whatever supply arrangements are appropriate must comply with the Polkinghorne principle of separation of supplier from user.

In accordance with current good practice all tissue of human origin should be regarded as potentially infectious. This is the case whether or not the donor source or tissue itself has been screened for evidence of infection. In any event the users of fetal tissue should be advised of whether screening was performed and if so the nature of that screening. The question of the woman's consent to testing in considered in paragraph 6.9 of the Polkinghorne Report.

Local research ethics committees

Research or innovative therapy involving fetal tissue must be assessed on the merit of the individual proposal and the ethical issues involved. Local research ethics committees need to examine all such proposals, having regard to the principle that the decision to perform an abortion should be separated from decisions on the subsequent use of tissue. They should be assisted by the following guidelines on supply of tissue.

GUIDELINES

These guidelines provide a code of practice for the arrangements for supplying fetal tissue for research, diagnosis and therapy which take account of the need to separate the user from the source of supply.

1 Tissue banks

For research and diagnostic investigations that can be done using tissue which has been frozen, the fetal tissue required should be obtained from the MRC Fetal Tissue Bank. The tissue bank is able to supply centres anywhere in the UK. Therefore geographical considerations should not normally determine whether tissue should be obtained from a local source.

2 Fresh tissue

For many research and diagnostic investigations requiring fresh, non-frozen tissue, it would be feasible to obtain the fetal tissue from the MRC Fetal Tissue Bank. However, some research and diagnostic investigations will require that fetal tissue is available as soon as possible after the termination of pregnancy and without having been frozen. The transfer of the fetus to the MRC Fetal Tissue Bank will not be appropriate in these circumstances. Examples of research in which fresh tissue may be required are biochemical assays and structural studies where the integrity of the fetal tissue must be as close as possible to that found in life. The justification for using fresh fetal tissue and the local arrangement to separate supplier from use must be described in any submission to a local research ethics committee.

3 Transplantation of fetal tissue

There may be occasions when fetal tissue is to be used in innovative therapy and there will be advantages in using the tissue as soon as possible. The delays involved in transferring tissue to and from the MRC Fetal Tissue Bank might prejudice the outcome of the therapeutic intervention. For such work the local research ethics committee must be given information on the proposed local arrangements to ensure separation of the termination of the pregnancy from the subsequent use of the tissue.

4 Import and export of fetal tissue

As the Polkinghorne Report stated (paragraph 8.5), the Committee's recommendations will be of little value if they can be circumvented by the import and export of fetal tissue. Important ethical and safety issues arise which are not easily resolved because it will not always be possible to know with confidence what arrangements apply in the country from which the tissue came or to which it is to be supplied. In the circumstances the MRC Fetal Tissue Bank does not propose generally to export or import tissue. Those involved in termination of pregnancy, research or in other uses of fetal tissue, are advised to adopt the same policy. Where it is considered that, exceptionally, such traffic is justified, the Department of Health should be consulted before any decision is made.

5 Research on the fetus *in utero*

The requirements of these guidelines do not apply where research has taken place on the fetus *in utero*, e.g. to investigate the effects of particular procedures undertaken during that pregnancy. These circumstances are considered in paragraphs 3.2 and 3.3 of the Polkinghorne Report. Specific consent from the woman herself will be required because she is involved in the research, so the principle of separation cannot be applied.

48

Guidance on making proposals to conduct gene therapy research on human subjects

(seventh annual report – section 1)

Gene Therapy Advisory Committee

Introduction

1 This document gives guidance on the procedures that should be followed in the United Kingdom when proposals are made to conduct gene therapy research on human subjects. It details the information that should be submitted in order to enable the Gene Therapy Advisory Committee (GTAC) to assess the acceptability of gene therapy research proposals.

2 Some guidance is also given on the requirements of other regulatory bodies or committees, including Local Research Ethics Committees, the Medicines Control Agency, the Health and Safety Executive and the Department of Environment, Transport and the Regions.

3 The guidance should be read in addition to general guidance on clinical trials and research governance in the NHS (see Further Reading).

4 Supplementary guidance and reports have been issued by GTAC in relation to monitoring of patients enrolled in adenoviral gene therapy studies and *in utero* gene therapy. Both can be obtained as stand-alone documents from the GTAC web-pages. (www.doh.gov.uk/genetics/gtac.htm).

GTAC review process

5 GTAC reviews proposals to conduct gene therapy research and provides advice in related areas. GTAC reviews are in addition to those of local research ethics committees (LREC), whose roles and responsibilities are unchanged.

6 GTAC approval should be obtained before NHS personnel conduct any gene therapy research on human subjects, whether conducted on NHS or other premises, in the UK. GTAC approval should also be sought where any part of gene therapy research on human subjects takes place in the UK. This would include enrolment, monitoring, follow-up and other study related procedures. NHS personnel who conduct gene therapy research overseas are encouraged to submit protocols to GTAC for information (this should include any information that will be given to prospective participants).

7 GTAC expects applicants to provide a full account of what is proposed. This should place particular emphasis on the ethical aspects, including an assessment of the scientific merit and safety of the proposed work.

8 In conducting such reviews, GTAC continues to reflect the principles established by the Clothier committee, namely that:

- gene therapy is research and not innovative treatment;
- only somatic therapy should be considered. Germ line interventions are considered to pose unacceptable safety and ethical concerns;
- patients should take part in gene therapy research trials only after a full explanation of the procedures, risks and benefits and after they have given their informed consent, if they are capable of doing so; and
- therapeutic research involving patients must not put them at disproportionate risk. For this reason gene therapy should be restricted to patients with serious disorders where current alternative treatments are not wholly effective.

Definition of gene therapy

9 GTAC has reviewed and revised the 1994 definition of gene therapy in the light of experience and of definitions

established by other countries and international bodies. GTAC wishes to maintain a wide definition of gene therapy in order not to exclude certain novel approaches from GTAC oversight. Within the context of GTAC's terms of reference, gene therapy can be defined as:

The deliberate introduction of genetic material into human somatic cells for therapeutic, prophylactic or diagnostic purposes.

---

10 This definition is intended to include studies involving the use of most of the established techniques for delivering genes into cells. A non-exhaustive list of examples includes genetically modified viral vectors, liposome-encapsulated DNA, anti-sense techniques, naked DNA injection, DNA-mismatch repair, GM stem cell therapy, and xenotransplantation of genetically modified animal cells (but not solid organs).

11 GTAC *does not* normally wish to consider any study which may be deemed to fall within the general definition, but which is adequately reviewed by other national or local ethics committees. Such research includes, for example:
- transplantation or transfusion of organs or cells, from whatever human source, provided that they have not been genetically modified;
- xenotransplantation of solid animal organs;
- vaccine studies, involving the use of genetically attenuated viruses intended to raise a prophylactic immune response to that virus (provided that the virus does not express any heterologous proteins);
- *ex vivo* fusion of autologous cells and other cells, for example dendritic cells, for the treatment of cancer.

12 In cases of doubt, researchers are invited to contact the GTAC Secretariat for an informal discussion prior to submitting a research proposal.

Germ line gene therapy

13 In line with the Clothier committee report and relevant international Instruments, research aimed at modifying the Germline of subjects will not be considered at this stage. The possibility of inadvertent targeting or modification of germ cells should be carefully assessed during pre-clinical studies. GTAC will need to be satisfied that measures are in place to ensure that patients do not conceive a child during or shortly after the study.

Relationship between GTAC and other agencies

Local research ethics committees

14 Any proposal to carry out gene therapy research on human subjects must comply with the established system of review by a local research ethics committee (LREC). LRECs must be consulted about any research proposal involving NHS patients, their records or NHS premises. A new web-site containing details of LRECs will be launched shortly: http://www.doh.gov.uk/research/recs.

15 Where a research project is to be carried out within five or more LRECs' geographical boundaries and hence would normally be referred to a multi-centre research ethics committee (MREC), GTAC acts as the MREC for gene therapy research.

16 The timing of LREC reviews will vary depending on the local arrangements and on the nature of the research. Researchers are advised for reasons of practicality to submit applications to GTAC in advance of the LREC.

Medicines control agency

17 The MCA is required by legislation to assess the safety and quality of medicinal products to be used in clinical trials. Before testing gene therapy products in patients, sponsors or investigators must apply to the Medicines Control Agency for a Clinical Trial Certificate (CTC), a Clinical Trial Exemption (CTX), or a Doctors and Dentists Exemption (DDX), or claim the "named-patient" exemption in writing.

18 Further details of MCA's role in regulating gene therapy medicinal products can by obtained by contacting the MCA Clinical Trials Unit (Tel: 020 7273 0327) and be found at: http://www.open.gov.uk/mca/mcahome.htm

Medical devices agency

19 Some forms of gene therapy may involve the use of medical devices, for example novel delivery systems. Details of the regulation of medical devices and the role of the MDA can be found at: http://www.medical-devices.gov.uk/

UK Xenotransplantation regulatory authority (UKXIRA)

20 UKXIRA is responsible for approving proposals to conduct xenotransplantation on human subjects. If a gene therapy proposal involves the transfer of viable animal tissue to patients, the GTAC Secretariat will discuss with

the UKXIRA Secretariat how to consider the application. In some cases UKXIRA will consider a proposal in parallel with GTAC. The xenotransplantation process would require UKXIRA to make a recommendation to UK Government Ministers who would then make the final decision. Further information can be found at: http://www.doh.gov.uk/ukxira.htm

Genetically modified organisms regulations

21 Proposals to conduct gene therapy research, where they involve the use of live genetically modified organisms (for example, a genetically modified viral vector delivery system), must comply with the relevant regulations controlling the contained use or deliberate release of genetically modified organisms. These are concerned with the protection of human health and the environment. Contained use is where control measures are used to limit contact of the GMOs with people and the environment. Where contact cannot be appropriately limited the activity is likely to constitute a deliberate release.

22 Further details on contained use legislation may be found in, "A guide to the Genetically Modified Organisms (Contained Use) Regulations 1992", as amended in 1996 (ISBN 0-7176-1186-8). This Guide will be replaced by "A guide to Genetically Modified Organisms (Contained Use) Regulations 2000" once expected new legislation has been produced (ISBN 0-7176-1758-0). Detailed technical guidance in matters such as risk assessment and containment measures can be found in the Advisory Committee on Genetic Modification's Compendium of Guidance which is available on the HSE web site: http://www.hse.gov.uk/.

23 For further advice about contained use legislation and technical guidance contact the Health and Safety Executive, GM Notifications Unit, Technology Division 6, Magdalen House, Stanley Precinct, Bootle, Merseyside, L20 3QZ. Tel: 0151 951 4722, Fax: 0151 951 3474.

24 For further details on deliberate release legislation contact the Department of Environment, Transport and the Regions: http://www.detr.gov.uk/

Method of working

25 In order to develop experience of the issues raised by gene therapy, GTAC has previously sought comments from external reviewers and held discussions with the proposers in full committee. However, increasing experience of gene therapy proposals allows a case-by-case approach to the review process.

26 GTAC therefore intends to move towards a more graded system of review, based on the novelty and complexity of the proposal and the extent to which it clearly falls within GTAC's remit.

27 In general, full GTAC review will be appropriate for studies that involve novel delivery systems, that extend the use of known agents to a different disease, raise new ethical issues, pose significant risks to subject's health or raise wider safety issues for the patient, staff or public health or are proposed by groups with no prior experience of clinical gene therapy research.

28 In all cases it is recommended that those contemplating gene therapy research submit a completed GTAC application form at an early stage. The Secretariat will then be in a position to provide informal advice on the need for a full GTAC application and the likely route of review.

Decisions of the committee

29 The outcome of the above review process will be sent to the lead applicant, the LREC, the host institution and the MCA. This might take the form of unconditional approval; conditional approval; deferral with recommendations for changes before the proposal is reconsidered or rejection. In all cases where further information is sought, the Committee will give its reasons to the applicants in writing and encourage dialogue via the Secretariat.

Disclosure of information

30 Applications to GTAC will be considered to be in confidence and treated as such throughout the review process, including the external review stage. However, care should be taken to ensure that information that might serve to identify individual patients or groups of patients is not included. This is particularly relevant to studies that involve rare diseases or small patient groups.

31 Some elements of a proposal may be considered to be commercially confidential. Such information should be clearly marked and supported by a reasoned justification for the claim. This will enable the Secretariat to determine how to handle the proposal during review. It should be stressed that failure to provide sufficient information at the initial stages will inevitably lead to delay in the GTAC review process.

32 A summary of the discussions at GTAC is placed in the public domain after each meeting. This is normally via a summary of the meeting posted to the GTAC web pages (www.doh.gov.uk/genetics/gtac.htm).

Reporting requirements

Adverse event reporting

33 Researchers are required by law to report all serious unexpected adverse reactions[1] (SARs) in gene therapy studies to the MCA in accordance with their requirements. In addition all serious adverse events[2] (SAE) should be reported to GTAC within 14 days (7 for death) regardless of whether the event is deemed related or unrelated to the gene therapy and whether unexpected or expected. In the case of a subject's death, a more detailed report, including, where appropriate, findings at post mortem, additional studies and a statement on the cause of death should be submitted as soon as possible.

34 Summaries of all Adverse Events should be reported to GTAC on an annual basis as part of the annual progress report (see paragraph 40). Adverse events should also be notified to the relevant LREC in accordance with their requirements.

35 The report should use the standard format for reporting adverse reactions to medicinal products, however GTAC's reporting arrangements are in addition to those for reporting severe adverse reactions to the MCA.

Long-term flagging project

36 GTAC has advised that there should be arrangements for the long-term monitoring of the subject and for monitoring any subsequent children born to those who have taken part in gene therapy research. This will in future be possible via the GTAC Flagging Project involving the NHS Central Registry and the Office of National Statistics (for those living in England and Wales) or the General Register Office for Scotland (for those living in Scotland). This study has been approved by an independent MREC.

37 Proposers are asked to seek informed consent from all subjects capable of giving it (or otherwise on behalf of the subject) at the time of their enrolment for monitoring of their long-term health and on behalf of any children that the patient may conceive following participation in the study.

38 For the purposes of clinical audit, subject's NHS records will be flagged indicating that they have taken part in a gene therapy research study. Investigators will be asked to provide directly to the Office for National Statistics (or General Register Office for Scotland) the NHS numbers of each subject along with a cipher specific to the study and one to identify the subject within that study. Submissions to the ONS will be on a six-monthly basis using the supplied electronic pro-forma for the purpose of emailing returns.

39 Clinical records and specimens from gene therapy patients should be stored indefinitely to enable follow-up. The storage of DNA samples needs special consideration and appropriate consent.

Progress reports

40 All investigators with active studies will be asked to provide an annual progress report to GTAC. A format for this will be supplied by the Secretariat each year, covering matters such as progress with the recruitment of subjects, observed adverse events and any relevant clinical findings. These progress reports will not be released by GTAC, however, the data provided, for example on the total number of gene therapy patients, may be incorporated into the GTAC annual report. No information will be released that may identify individual patients.

41 GTAC also expect to see reports on completion of the study and would encourage prompt publication in peer-reviewed journals as a means of promoting wider dissemination of research findings.

Information to be included in GTAC applications

GTAC must be given sufficient information to make a judgement about the ethical acceptability of the study.

Proposals for gene therapy research submitted to GTAC should normally consist of:
- √ A GTAC application form;
- √ The clinical protocol;
- √ Patient information material and consent forms;
- √ Information about relevant qualifications and experience of the principal investigator(s);
- √ Details supporting the suitability of the research centre.
- √ Supporting technical appendices.

42 GTAC has developed an application form to provide a common framework for an overview of the design of the study and the issues that it raises. The application form

---

[1] A serious noxious and unintended response to a medicinal product.
[2] A serious untoward medical occurrence which does not necessarily have to have a causal relationship to the medicinal product.

is available on the web, by email from the Secretariat or as a hard copy.

43 For full proposals, the clinical protocol and a succinct summary of relevant pre-clinical and safety data (possibly including that prepared for other regulatory bodies) should support the application form.

44 Proposers should aim to strike a balance between giving sufficient information to enable the committee and external referees to understand the study whilst keeping the documents accessible to the lay members of the committee.

45 The following headings are suggested to structure the proposal. In some cases the information may be adequately conveyed in the study protocol, in others it may be necessary to provide additional supporting information in the application form or technical appendices.

A Objectives and rationale

46 There should be a brief introductory statement that provides the background to the proposed research. It should refer to the disease to which the study relates, its prevalence, severity and health burden; their natural history and biology; the available therapies, what is to be learnt from the research and the potential for improving the subject's health.

B Patient population

47 The proposal should describe and justify the proposed study population, bearing in mind GTAC's key principles (paragraph 8).

Risk/benefit

48 The proposal should include an appraisal of the risks to the subject and the possible benefits. This should include a summary of the alterations to normal clinical care that will arise as part of the research, especially any invasive procedures and those that may be uncomfortable or inconvenient for the subject (such as procedures that involve lengthy or frequent attendance as outpatients or inpatients or requirements to remain in an isolation room).

49 The patient's disease should also be relatively stable with a predictable likely clinical progression. In cases where there is rapid progression, GTAC will need to be convinced that the clinical management of the patient will not be impaired by the requirements of the trial.

C The gene construct and delivery system

50 The proposal must include details of the genetic material and its manufacture to enable an assessment of the safety and likely benefit. Technical information such as sequence data, derivation of vectors and producer cell lines may be provided as part of the supporting technical appendices.

51 The proposal should describe the nature and structure of the genetic material that is to be administered and the rationale for its use. It should include:
- an overview of the therapeutic gene construct and its regulatory elements;
- the methods used to produce it, including any producer cell lines;
- the method of delivery, and;
- the form in which the material will be administered to the patient.

Manufacture

52 The proposal should summarise the arrangements for the manufacture and handling of the therapeutic product. The detailed arrangements for achieving compliance with the requirements of the MCA are not normally required, but may be appended as part of the supporting technical material.

D Prior studies

53 The proposal should describe the evidence relating to the safety and likely efficacy of the proposed gene construct and delivery system. Wherever possible the data presented should relate to the proposed construct and delivery system in the most appropriate *in vitro* or animal model of the disease. Where this is not possible there must be a full account of how the data is extrapolated to the intended disease and construct. In some cases available data may also be extrapolated to avoid excessive animal studies, especially in non-human primates.

54 The proposal should provide a reasoned justification for the choice of construct and delivery system. In particular, GTAC will be looking for evidence that the safety of the proposed study has been considered in depth at the pre-clinical and clinical stages. This should include consideration of the stability of safety features in any viral vectors used and tests to assess the presence of contaminants.

55 Where possible, reference should be made to any previous applications to GTAC, to published studies and to

guidance from GTAC or others on the safety and tolerance of the vector system in human subjects.

Pre-clinical studies

56 The evidence provided from pre-clinical studies should normally include:
- Studies of the gene delivery system;
- Studies demonstrating gene transfer and expression and biological effect;
- Studies to demonstrate target specificity;
- Studies relating to the route of entry;
- Studies related to the safety of the genetic material and the delivery system. In some cases this may be supported by material elsewhere in the proposal, such as on the delivery system and manufacture.

Distribution to non-target organs

57 The proposal should provide evidence of the target specificity of the therapeutic product and, where appropriate, the absence of accumulation/retention on non-target tissues or organs, especially the gonads.

Previous clinical experience

58 A summary of relevant data from previous clinical trials, including peer-reviewed publications, should be submitted to support the safety and likely efficacy of the proposed study.

E Study protocol

59 The detailed arrangements for the clinical and technical procedures involved in the research should be specified in the study protocol. This should include an outline of the clinical procedures and the tests used to monitor the patient.

Study design

60 The type of study being proposed, the size of the study population and other relevant factors should be detailed. There should be some consideration of whether the procedures and requirements are reasonable and equitable.

Criteria for inclusion/exclusion

61 The inclusion and eligibility criteria should be detailed. The number of subjects should be given, along with a comment on the likelihood of recruiting sufficient subjects. There must be careful characterisation of the specific patient population for the studies regarding not only their disease, its stage, and previous standard treatments, but also the expected prognosis.

62 The proposal should set out what other options would be available to such patients in clinical practice or current clinical research. Specific inclusion and exclusion criteria by virtue of disease, abnormal tests or treatment, should be justified explicitly in relation to the treatment and/or its evaluation.

63 Where subjects are to be HIV tested for the purpose of excluding HIV positive patients from the gene therapy study, consent for the test should be explicitly sought and the appropriate provision made for counselling.

64 The eligibility criteria should take account of the need to minimise the risk of unintended transfer of genetic material to germ cells or the fetus. If conception is possible, it should normally be a condition that subjects or their partners use an effective form of birth control during and for at least 3 months after the study. Fertile women should have a negative pregnancy test shortly before commencing the study.

65 Children should be the subject of research only when it is essential and the information could not be obtained from adult subjects or in any other way. Where children are to be the subjects of such research, then the presumption must normally be that there is some possibility of therapeutic benefit for the child. The child's parents or legal guardian must be fully informed and consent obtained. The minimum age for entry into an adult trials should be set at 18 years.

Dose escalation studies

66 Particular attention should be given to the design of dose escalation studies to ensure that early indications of dose limiting toxicity can be identified. Investigators should set the initial dose to be administered to patients at least two logs lower than the maximum safe dose predicted by pre-clinical studies.

67 GTAC will normally wish to see details of the arrangement for assessing toxicity and considering progression to the next dose level. This might include details of the parameters to be used in assessing adverse effects and toxicity. Where there is a reference to standard criteria, e.g. the NCIC toxicity criteria, it is not necessary to reproduce these in full.

68 For certain protocols raising particular safety issues, GTAC may wish to be provided with safety data for each dose level before giving permission to proceed to a higher dose. A case-by-case assessment will be

made by GTAC when reviewing proposals to determine whether investigators should seek approval for progression between doses. No unnecessary delay in granting approval for to proceed to the next dose level is anticipated.

69 In any Phase I study, no further patients should be dosed following an unexpected, clinically meaningful grade IV toxicity until the investigator has adequately reviewed the monitoring and safety data. Procedures for review in this event should be detailed in the protocol. Any necessary amendments to the protocol and patient information material should be approved by GTAC before the trial recommences.

Additional clinical procedures

70 The protocol should detail the clinical procedures, particularly those that are in addition to or differ from normal patient care. This should include details of any preliminary treatments, for example surgery or chemotherapy to remove or reduce the number of abnormal cells.

71 The procedures and regime for administering the gene therapy material should be given, including the nature and timing of administration and monitoring.

72 If cells are to be removed and treated *ex-vivo* details should be provided of the type of cells and the procedures to be used.

Monitoring

73 Screening tests used solely for the purpose of the study should be explained and justified. Arrangements should be set out for explaining to patients, and performing those that are not part of standard care, but which result from participation in the study.

74 The arrangements for monitoring subjects before and after the administration of the genetic material should be given. It should specify the frequency and duration of monitoring, the biochemical, physiological, pathological tests to be done, the clinical endpoints of the study and whether special post-mortem studies will be requested if a patient dies.

75 The monitoring procedures should be designed with a view to identifying at an early stage the possible side effects so that action can be taken to prevent or mitigate such events. The relevance of tests used in monitoring the study should be set out, together with sufficient detail on those that are not standard practice to enable their assessment. The way in which such tests are to be analysed in relation to study end-point should be made clear, including the validation of novel techniques where appropriate. If material is to be stored and/or transported long distances, evidence should be provided to show that the process of storage and/or transport and any consequential delay, do not adversely or unpredictably affect the results obtained.

76 There should also be some consideration of the methods used to determine whether the gene sequences are inserted and expressed in the subjects. This might include, where available, tests to determine any non-target effects, such as expression in other tissues or cells or shedding of vector into the wider environment.

77 A reference sample of the material injected should be stored to allow for retrospective analysis. Where possible, it is also recommended that serum (and, if feasible, cell) samples should be taken at suitable intervals and stored to provide for retrospective analysis in the event of adverse reactions.

78 GTAC has prepared separate guidance on monitoring of studies involving adenovirus vectors (see references).

F Information for patients and consent

Patient information leaflets

79 The application should detail the arrangements for informing prospective subjects, or their parents or guardians in the case of children, about the research before seeking consent to take part in the study. The application to GTAC will need to include copies of the patient information sheet that subjects will receive, as well as any wider promotional material about the research team or unit (including any material available on the Internet) if this mentions gene therapy.

80 There should be a simple introductory document that explains, in non-technical language, what is proposed. This should be supported by arrangements for further oral and/or written information. Advice on preparing clear patient information material is at Annex 1.

81 GTAC is sensitive to the hopes and motives of potential participants who have a life-threatening disease, and it is imperative that they understand clearly when a trial offers them no prospect of clinical benefit. It is also important to make clear whether or not participation in the initial non-therapeutic stages of a research programme influences their eligibility for future therapeutic studies.

82 GTAC also advocates appropriate independent counselling for research subjects, and details of the arrangements should be clear from the proposal and the patient information leaflet.

Consent

83 Research subjects should take part in gene therapy research trials only after a full explanation of the procedures, risks and benefits and after they have given their consent, if they are capable of doing so.

84 Consent should also be sought for each participant's NHS number, in an anonymised form, to be sent to GTAC and to be recorded on the central NHS register. In order to obtain consent to the flagging arrangements, two standard paragraphs should be inserted into the patient information leaflet (see Annex 1).

Insurance

85 The proposal should confirm that appropriate insurance or indemnities are in place to cover the participants in the trial.

Payments

86 Subjects should have their travel and other out of pocket expenses fully reimbursed. The patient information sheet should make clear that they will not be expected to meet the costs of any clinical procedures (material, tests or medical care) related to the study.

G Details of investigator(s) and nature of the research site

87 GTAC wishes to be satisfied that gene therapy is only conducted in centres of excellence, until it can be considered to be a normal part of clinical research. Therefore, the proposal should provide details of the staff (especially the Principal Investigator) and the facilities in which the research will take place (the Host Institution). In particular this information should demonstrate that there is:
- a substantial multidisciplinary team of clinical researchers,
- a suitable infrastructure of facilities in clinical and laboratory environments,
- on-site support in a range of disciplines, including microbiology/infection control, immunology, and;
- a proven track record of high-grade clinical research.

88 The proposal should be supported by a summary of the relevant training and experience (in the form of a brief CV) of the principal investigator (PI). The names and qualifications of junior clinical and research staff should also be provided. There should be appropriate arrangements to ensure adequate supervision of junior

staff and access for the patients to the PI in the event of problems or queries.

89 Arrangements should be in place to ensure that there is no untoward conflict of interest, financial or otherwise, between the trial sponsor and those individuals responsible for enrolling and caring for the patients.

90 It is strongly recommended that the proposal identifies an individual with day-to-day responsibility for overall co-ordination, including liaison with GTAC. This might not be the same person as the PI, recognising that such people are often involved in a number of trials and other activities.

Containment

91 The arrangements to safeguard people other than the research subject, including clinical and non-clinical staff, relatives and visitors and the wider public will normally form part of requirements of the Health and Safety Executive. The GTAC proposal should, however, include information on the anticipated hazards of the proposed research and the proposed control measures. In particular it should highlight any measures over and above those required for normal clinical care, such as keeping the subject in isolation during the study, handling of any dressing and any restrictions on visitors.

Writing information leaflets for those participating in gene therapy research   Annex 1

92 The following section is based on guidance first issued in 1995. It provides more detailed advice for those with clinical responsibility for participants and those with responsibility for the design of gene therapy trials.

93 This guidance should be read with the sources of general advice on patient information and consent (see Bibliography).

Informing patients

94 Enabling the potential subjects of research to make a decision whether or not they might participate is one of the most important aspects of the ethical acceptability of research. They must be well informed about the procedures and risks of the protocol and the responsibilities that they are being asked to take on. This is true of all medical research which involves human subjects, but is especially so in the field of gene therapy. Not only is the topic unusually complex, but there is likely to be a need for long term follow up.

95 Although information can be given in a number of ways, the written information leaflet is particularly important and should always be provided. It is a permanent record of the key points of any research trial, to which the patient can refer, and therefore a critical element in informing consent. The document also provides a source of reference for families and friends. In addition it gives both Local Research Ethics Committees (LREC's) and GTAC an opportunity to assess this aspect of the research protocol.

General principles

96 There is no single correct way of writing information for patients. The aim must be to present sufficient but not excessive information in a form that is understandable. This calls for thoughtful and tested use of language, vocabulary and presentational techniques.

97 Understanding, and recall, of what to many patients will seem to be complex information, are reduced by:
- anxiety
- poor presentation
- complex language, technical terms and jargon.

98 Conversely, understanding and recall are enhanced by:
- keeping the format simple, so that it can be read and re-read at leisure; use of plain English;
- ensuring that other modes of communication, such as counselling, reinforce and amplify the written information, but do not contradict it.

99 Patients must be encouraged to ask questions about the research. Time must be set aside for the investigator to go over the information with patients to ensure that they understand all the implications. Patients will often only remember important questions after the first counselling.

100 The advice contained in this guidance covers three aspects of preparing information leaflets:
- The information to be included
- How to present the information
- How to evaluate its effectiveness

What to include

101 It is important to anticipate common concerns. Below are listed some common questions.
- Why have I been chosen for the study?
- Is the treatment really likely to cure me or not? The answer should be unambiguous.
- There should be no false hope.
- Are there any risks or disadvantages for me?
- What will the treatment entail? How, when, where and how often will it be administered and monitored?
- What will the side effects be? Will it be painful or uncomfortable?
- What costs or inconveniences may I incur?
- What are the responsibilities placed upon me for follow-up?
- What will the trial help to demonstrate?
- What action should be taken if I become unwell?
- Who can I talk to about this study?

102 The following points should be covered in addressing these concerns.

Why the research programme is being undertaken

103 Explain the purpose of the study. This needs to cover:
   a. The research questions being asked:
   - Why are they important?
   - How might they be answered?
   - Why has gene manipulation been chosen?
   - How the study has been designed:
   - Increasing dosage. Why is this necessary?
   - Use of placebo controls and what this means.
   - Does the study involve more than one centre?
   - Evaluation of results.
   b. The implications of the research for the individual.

Research procedures

104 Describe and explain the procedure(s) and commitment of participants in terms of time, costs, and how data will be collected (such as blood tests, x-rays, interviews). Describe any restrictions the research might place on the patient, particularly the use of isolation rooms and restrictions on visiting.

Consequences of participating

105 The predictable consequences of participating in the study should be explained.
   a. State whether or not there are possible benefits of participating in the proposed study. For research trials which are not reasonably expected to provide a therapeutic benefit to participating patients the information leaflet should clearly state that no direct clinical benefit is expected to occur as a result of participation in the study, although knowledge may be gained that may benefit others.
   b. Describe the nature and likelihood of risks, pain, injury or other harm, that may occur.
   c. Where it is appropriate to the patient, describe alternative therapies, including those being assessed in other research trials.

Non-participation or withdrawal from the study

106 Emphasise that participation in any study is voluntary. The decision to take part or not, should not influence any present or future treatment or care. Patients should know that they can withdraw from the study at any time without having to give a reason for doing so. Draw attention to any additional risks that might be associated with an incomplete course of treatment.

Use of contraception

107 It is important to avoid the possibility that any of the reagents used in gene transfer research could harm a fetus. Advise women that they should not become pregnant before or during the course of their participation in the study. Inform both men and women when effective contraception or abstinence is required during the active phase of their participation in the study and also for at least 3 months afterwards. Depending upon the nature of the research trial the information sheet might advise any woman not to participate if she thinks she may wish to become pregnant.

Confidentiality/Privacy

108 Affirm that confidentiality of personal information of trial participants will be protected. State who might have access to their anonymised research records and why this is necessary. In trials where personalised data needs to be reviewed, the patient's agreement must be obtained and this aspect of the research should be clearly explored in the information leaflet.

Long-term follow-up

109 It is important to evaluate the long term safety and efficacy of gene transfer. This requires co-operation of participants in follow-up beyond the active phase of the study. Explain the need for this commitment from the outset. The information leaflet or consent form should include a list of persons who can be contacted during the follow-up period.

110 Patients participating in gene therapy studies will be subject to clinical audit via the NHS central records system. In addition they will be invited to participate in the GTAC Flagging Project involving the NHS Central Registry and the Office of National Statistics. Proposers are asked to seek informed consent from all subjects at the time of their enrolment for monitoring of their long-term health and on behalf of any children that the patient may conceive following participation in the study.

111 The following paragraphs should be inserted into the patient information leaflet.

"Gene Therapy is a new development. Every effort is made to be sure it is safe but we need to watch out for any unexpected effects. To make this possible, all people who have gene therapy are flagged by the NHS records system. Accordingly, your NHS number and details of the trial in which you are participating will be provided to the Department of Health (DH) so that your participation in this trial can be recorded on the National Health Service Central Register. This information will be used for purposes of long-term follow-up. You will not be contacted by DH directly but your GP may be asked to provide information on your health on occasion.

In theory, gene therapy could affect the next generation. To cover this possibility, any children born to a person who had gene therapy will be flagged also and followed through until they are 16 years old. This system is subject to the same protection of confidentiality as all medical records. Any studies of these medical records will be under the supervision of the Gene Therapy Advisory Committee of the Department of Health who will make sure confidentiality is respected."

Further support

112 The information leaflet should make clear to potential participants who can be approached for:
a. further information
b. counselling.

How to write it

113 Experience has shown that it is best to:
- keep sentences short
- make only one point in each sentence
- use simple words
- avoid technical terms whenever possible. When they cannot be avoided, explain what the terms mean in simple language
- repeat important points in different ways
- avoid crowding pages with too much information
- summarise the key points.

Evaluation of a patient information leaflet

114 To determine how well an information leaflet will be understood it needs to be evaluated. Asking people not acquainted with the area to read the leaflet is the best way. They might include administrative or clerical staff in the hospital, or non-medical friends. The

management of your hospital may be able to assist in "piloting" the leaflet. Patient groups and other voluntary organisations are an important source of advice on both design and piloting leaflets.

115 The two most common ways in which written information is evaluated formally involve using readability formulae and through formal assessments by patients.

116 The "readability" of any text can be estimated by the application of standard formulae. Most modern word processing software can derive these figures automatically. The table below gives an interpretation of the Flesch reading ease score. A reading ease score for patient information leaflets of between 80 and 90 is desirable.

Reading ease	Verbal description	Typical text	Estimated Percentage who would understand
90–100	Very easy	Comics	97
80–90	Easy	Tabloids	95
70–80	Fairly easy	Popular	90
60–70	Standard	Magazine	90
50–60	Fairly hard	Broadsheet	77
30–50	Difficult	Academic	31
0–30	Very hard	Scientific	7

117 Assessments of leaflets by patients might include measures of understanding and satisfaction with the information provided.

Special issues

118 Potential subjects need time to make a decision about their participation in the research. They should have an opportunity to consider the information provided, seek further information and to consult with a named independent counsellor.

119 Where the study involves children who are not capable of giving consent, an information sheet for parents or guardians should be prepared according to the principles above. In addition, information should be provided to the child which is appropriate to the understanding ability of that child.

120 Additional consideration should be given to the needs and requirements of subjects whose first language is not English. The importance of written information is often greater in such circumstances. Special care should be taken to have information leaflets in other languages checked for accuracy, and to ensure cultural and ethnic sensitivities are properly handled.

121 Every effort should also be made to ensure that individuals who have difficulty reading are not disadvantaged through lack of information.

Report on the potential use of gene therapy in utero

Gene Therapy Advisory Committee

Background

1 Since gene therapy was first attempted in 1989, there have been over 300 clinical protocols approved world wide. 30 research trials in patients have been considered in the UK by the Gene Therapy Advisory Committee (GTAC) established in 1993 to review such work [1].

2 There is a wide consensus that, at present, gene therapy should be restricted to attempts to modify somatic (body) cells so that changes will not be passed to successive generations. GTAC has confirmed that its view remains that gene modification of the germ line, where effects could be transmitted to offspring, should not yet be attempted.

3 To date, all but two of the trials of somatic gene therapy considered by GTAC have been intended to be performed in adults or young persons over 16 years. The two exceptions were in young children born with inherited single gene disorders, Hurlers Disease and Severe Combined Immuno-Deficiency (SCID), where it may be possible to correct the gene deficiency before serious or life threatening symptoms develop.

4 However in many genetic disorders it may not be possible to use such potential therapies after birth. In some disorders the damage is already done before birth and there may be good clinical reasons to intervene in utero to try and correct the genetic damage.

5 Interventions in utero are not new. Surgical procedures are used to correct the accumulation of fluid in the bladder or chest; steroid drugs can be infused into the developing fetus and transfusion of blood or platelets directly into the fetus are established procedures.

Stem cell transplantation

6 To the list above, we must now add stem cell transplantation. There is considerable scientific and clinical interest in pluripotent haematopoietic stem cells (PHSC) – those cells that can self renew and which produce all lineages of blood cell formation. The potential to use PHSC before birth to treat congenital disease in theory offers a number of possible advantages.

   i. Because the fetal immune system has not yet developed, it will not reject foreign cells. Unlike bone marrow transplantation post-birth there is no need to match donor cells.

   ii. The fetus will become "tolerant" to the foreign cells allowing for further treatment after birth, again without the risk of rejection.

   iii. Intervention in utero will permit "correction" of a disorder before clinical manifestations have developed.

7 There is already a considerable body of evidence, from animal models and from a small number of in utero transplantations of unmodified bone marrow progenitor cells in human fetuses, that there is a "window of opportunity" that technically permits and favours engraftment of transplanted PHSC in utero.

8 There have already been a small number of such trials during human pregnancies involving such disorders as X-linked SCID, (alpha)thalassaemia, sickle cell anaemia and (beta)thalassaemia.

9 Possible sources of human PHSC include cord blood, fetal liver, adult bone marrow and adult peripheral blood. The use of cells derived from another fetus raises both practical and ethical issues, and to date much work has concentrated upon the use of adult derived cells as a renewable, low risk and ethically acceptable source of PHSC.

10 The technical aspects of in utero cell transplantation may be less complex than one might at first imagine. The fetal circulation can be accessed transabdominally under ultrasound from 17 weeks gestation. This technique is well established, in standard practice and the risks associated with it are well documented. The experimental technique of coelocentesis which accesses the exolcoelomic cavity by transvaginal puncture, may offer the possibility of stem cell engraftment much earlier in gestation (10+ weeks). Such very early interventions do not raise the issue of fetal awareness and pain (The Royal College of Obstetricians and Gynaecologists Working Party Report on Fetal Awareness, October 1997 [2], concluded that it is not possible for the fetus to be aware of events before 26 weeks' gestation).

The potential use of gene therapy in utero

11 A second approach will build on the PHSC trials described above and will apply genetically modified cells in utero – ie in utero gene therapy. It has been argued that two key issues need to be addressed before such an intervention is considered;

   i. that there must be a clear advantage over post-natal gene therapy;

   ii. that there must be an advantage over therapy with unmodified cells.

12 Pre-natal gene therapy has been proposed as most appropriate in disorders which result in irreversible illness or death in the pre or neonatal period. Examples may include Type 2 Gaucher's Disease, Krabbe's disease, Hurler's Disease etc. Considerable interest in the possibilities of gene therapy in utero was also stimulated by a letter to the "Lancet" in March 1997 in which an adenovirus vector was used in utero to correct the cystic fibrosis phenotype in mice [3].

Action by GTAC

13 At its September 1997 meeting GTAC agreed to establish a subgroup on New and Emerging Technologies (NETS).

14 The remit of the subgroup is to aid GTAC to fulfil one of its terms of reference "to advise UK Health Ministers on developments in gene therapy research and their implications". The subgroup's function was to report to GTAC on areas of any new technology that may have implications for gene therapy research or techniques.

15 The subgroup was asked to look at the potential of gene therapy in utero. Members were provided with the Minutes of the December 1994 meeting of the US Recombinant DNA Advisory Committee (RAC), which discussed this subject and a review based upon papers and posters presented at the "Second International meeting on in utero stem cell transplantation and gene therapy" held in September 1997 in Nottingham.

16 NETS met to consider this subject in November 1997 and presented its report to GTAC in February 1998.

NETS Report on in utero gene therapy

17 In considering the principles that should apply to in utero gene therapy, NETS first revisited and reaffirmed the six key elements currently employed by GTAC when considering gene therapy for adults and children. These were developed by GTAC upon the recommendations of the Clothier Committee Report of 1992 [4]. NETS concluded that these principles should also apply to in utero gene therapy.

18 These six principles state that;

   a. gene therapy is research and not innovative treatment;

   b. only somatic therapy should be considered;

   c. in view of safety and ethical difficulties germ line interventions are off limits at present;

   d. gene therapy should be restricted to life threatening disorders where no current alternative effective treatments are available;

   e. patients should take part in gene therapy research trials only after a full explanation of the procedures, risks and benefits and after they have given their informed consent, if they are capable of doing so; and

   f. recognising that some people, including young children, may not be able to give such consent, therapeutic research involving such patients must not put them at disproportionate risk.

19 The subgroup kept these principles in mind as they discussed in utero therapy issues, considered the papers prepared by RAC and heard presentations from relevant experts. The subgroup considered some of the key issues raised by both stem cell transplantation (SCT) using PHSC and gene therapy interventions in utero. The group considered both the scientific validity and the potential treatment advantages of such therapies.

20 The group considered that SCT in utero offered therapeutic opportunities for a wide range of genetic disorders, and that such techniques were much more likely to be used in the short term than in utero gene therapy.

21 Fetal liver cells were identified as the transplant of choice with discrete scientific advantages over either

cord blood or cells derived from adults. The subgroup noted that SCT with fetal liver cells is not a "new" technique having been first attempted in the UK over thirty years ago.

22 The subgroup agreed that there are ethical issues involved in the use of fetal tissues – those identified in the Polkinghorne Report "Review of the Guidance on the Research Use of Fetuses and Fetal Material" [5]. The NETS subgroup endorsed the code of practice recommended by the Polkinghorne Committee. Particular consideration should be given to those who might decline the use of fetal tissue whilst consenting to SCT using other donor tissue.

23 In considering in utero gene therapy the subgroup agreed that it was unlikely to be feasible in the short term. Reasons included the lack of a strong list of candidate disorders for potential therapy, and that at this stage, SCT offered better prospects for success.

24 The subgroup concurred with RAC's concern that in utero gene therapy may give rise to germ line effects. It was noted that in a sheep model it had been possible to transmit a gene insert in utero into multiple organs and tissues and to have the foreign gene(s) pass to subsequent generations.

25 The subgroup considered that there were particular concerns about the risk of germ line involvement in the use of a direct, or vector, mediated gene therapy in vivo. Such interventions are unacceptable in view of the safety and ethical difficulties that remain at present.

26 In contrast, the subgroup considered that the use of genetically modified stem cells in SCT was a possibility. Such ex vivo modification would be unlikely to carry with it any higher risk to the germ line than the trials of post natal somatic gene therapy which have already been approved. They agreed that ex vivo genetic modification prior to in utero SCT does not raise any new ethical concerns and could be considered by GTAC in the same manner as somatic gene therapy.

Conclusions

27 Following their discussion, the subgroup concluded that:

a. they did not consider that there were any new ethical issues raised by in utero gene therapy that were not already recognised in other interventions in utero, or in the use of gene therapy in other situations. The issue of consent remains a matter solely for the pregnant woman.

b. In order to be ethical, the risks of the physical procedures would need to be known.

c. The disorder or disease treated would need to be life threatening, or associated with severe disability, and for which no suitable treatment is available after birth, in order to justify intervention in utero.

d. Existing concerns with regard to gene therapy, in particular regarding the potential for germ line transmission, remain. Such concerns would need to be fully answered in the event of any protocols proposing in utero gene therapy being presented to GTAC.

e. With this in mind, GTAC believes that the use of a direct, or vector, mediated gene therapy in utero are unlikely to be acceptable for the foreseeable future, in view of the safety and ethical difficulties.

f. Somatic gene therapy protocols which involve ex vivo genetic modification of stem cells prior to bone marrow transplantation in infants have already received approval from GTAC. The Committee believes that stem cell transplantation in utero would be unlikely to carry with it significantly higher risk to the germ line than such post natal somatic gene therapy.

g. Such interventions could be considered by GTAC in the same manner as somatic gene therapy, ie subject to the strict criteria already established by the Committee.

November 1998

REFERENCES

[1] Department of Health. GTAC Fourth Annual Report.

[2] The Royal College of Obstetricians and Gynaecologists. Fetal Awareness. Report of a Working Party (October 1997). Published by the RCOG Press. ISBN 1 900364 07 7.

[3] Larsen JE et al (1997). Reversal of cystic fibrosis phenotype in mice by gene therapy in utero. The Lancet 349 (9052). p619.

[4] Department of Health. Report of the Committee on the Ethics of Gene Therapy. London HMSO, 1992; Cm 1788.

[5] Review of the Guidance on the Research Use of Fetuses and Fetal Material. (July 1989). Published by Her Majesty's Stationary Office. ISBN 0 10 107622 3.

GLOSSARY

Genes
  The biological units of heredity.
Gene therapy
  The genetic modification of body cells of an individual patient, directed to alleviating disease in that patient.

Germ-line
   The cells which transmit genetic information to the next generation.
   They are the sperm in males and the egg cells in females.
In utero
   In the womb.
Peripheral blood
   Blood circulating around the body in veins and arteries.
Stem cells
   A type of cell that can self renew and produce all types of blood cells.
Somatic cells
   The cells which make up the body of an individual excluding the egg
   or sperm cells.

GTAC Members of the New and Emerging Technologies (NETS) group.

Canon Keith Denison (Chairman).

Mrs Rosemary Barnes

Dr Brenda Gibson

Mrs Ann Hunt

Mrs Irene Train

Professor Ian Hart

Professor Michael Steel

Co-opted individuals taking part in discussion of in utero gene therapy in November 1997.

Dr Colin Casimir
Department of Haematology
St Mary's Hospital Medical School, London.

Dr David Liu
Department of Obstetrics and Gynaecology
City Hospital, Nottingham.

Human fertilisation and embryology authority
– code of practice (extracts)
5th edition 2001

Human Fertilisation and Embryology Authority

Part 7 Consent

General

Consent to examination and treatment

7.1 People generally have the right to give or withhold consent to examination and treatment. Centres' attention is drawn to the general guidance given in "A Guide to Consent for Examination and Treatment" by the Department of Health.

Treatment without consent

7.2 Centres may examine or treat people without first obtaining their consent only in exceptional circumstances. The only circumstances likely to arise in the course of infertility treatment services are where the procedure is necessary to save the person's life, cannot be postponed, and they are unconscious and cannot indicate their wishes.

Consent to the presence of observers

7.3 If a member of the centre's team wishes an observer to be present when a person is being examined, treated or counselled, they should explain, preferably beforehand, who the observer is and why this is desirable, and ask the person whether there is any objection. If the person objects, the observer should not attend.

General obligations

7.4 Centres should allow people seeking treatment, people considering donation and those seeking storage sufficient time to reflect on their decision, before obtaining

written consent. A copy of the consent form should be given to the person giving consent.

7.5 Centres should ensure that people do not feel under any pressure to give their consent.

7.6 In all cases, people giving consent may specify additional conditions subject to which their gametes or embryos may be used or stored, and may vary or withdraw their consent at any time provided that the gametes, or embryos created from them, have not been used in treatment services or a project of research.

7.7 Gametes must not be taken from anyone who is not capable of giving a valid consent or who has not given a valid consent to examination and treatment and an effective consent to the use or storage of those gametes.

Children and Gillick Competence

7.8 The General Medical Council describes Gillick Competence in their guidelines 'Seeking patients' consent: the ethical considerations' (GMC, November 1998).

7.9 In these guidelines they state the following: "You must assess a child's capacity to decide whether to consent or refuse proposed investigation or treatment before you provide it. In general, a competent child will be able to understand the nature, purpose and possible consequences of the proposed investigation or treatment, as well as the consequences of non-treatment."

7.10 Centres are also directed to the guidance issued by the British Medical Association. Centres are advised that if they are in doubt they should seek their own legal advice.

Consent to storage

7.11 Anyone consenting to the storage of their gametes, or of embryos produced from them, must:

a. specify the maximum period of storage (if this is to be less than the statutory storage period);

b. state what is to be done with the gametes or embryos if they die, or become incapable of varying or revoking their consent.

Statutory storage period

7.12 The normal storage period for gametes is usually 10 years, extension of this storage period is detailed in paragraphs 7.34–7.35, below.

7.13 In the case of sperm that was already in store on 1 August 1991, the written consent of the person who provided the sperm is not needed in order for storage to continue legally. However, there is no obligation on a centre to continue to store sperm where there is no written agreement to do so.

7.14 The normal storage period for embryos is usually five years, extension of this storage period is detailed in paragraphs 7.36–7.39, below.

Consent to use

7.15 If the intention is to create an embryo outside the body, the person giving consent to the use of an embryo produced from their gametes must specify the purpose or purposes for which it may be used, namely one or more of:

a. to provide treatment for themselves, or themselves and a named partner;

b. to provide treatment for others;

c. for research.

7.16 If consent to use sperm was given before 1 August 1991, that consent must be in writing and remain effective (i.e. not have been subsequently withdrawn).

7.17 If no written consent has been given before or after 1 August 1991, no use can be made of the sperm unless and until a consent to use is obtained.

7.18 It follows that where a person providing sperm has died and there is no written consent in existence no use can be made of the sperm.

7.19 If it is proposed that embryos are to be used, the terms of the consent of a person storing embryos produced using her eggs must be compatible with the consent of the man who provided the sperm.

Consent to export

7.20 The specific consent of people providing gametes must be obtained to the export of those gametes or of embryos produced using them (see also paragraph 9.32, below).

Posthumous use

7.21 Insemination of a woman at a licensed centre using her late husband's or partner's sperm is regulated under the HFE Act. For this to take place the man must have given consent to the posthumous use of his sperm to treat the woman.

7.22 People seeking treatment should be informed that the Human Fertilisation and Embryology Act states that if the sperm of a man is used after his death in treatment services i.e. for insemination, IVF or embryo transfer, he is not to be regarded in law as the father of any offspring produced from that treatment.

7.23 Similarly, if an embryo produced using the egg of a woman who has since died is used in treatment, the woman who provided the egg is not to be regarded in law as the mother of the child.

7.24 If donation of an embryo is being considered in the event of death or mental incapacity both partners should undergo screening as outlined in paragraphs 4.10–4.18.

People seeking treatment

Additional information

7.25 As well as considering the requirements of paragraphs 7.1–7.24 above, no licensed treatment should be given to any woman without her written consent to that particular treatment. The written consent should explain the nature of the treatment and the steps that are to be taken, and indicate that she has been given all the information referred to in paragraph 6.1–6.6 above. The woman should be given the opportunity to decide whether she wishes to consent to all stages of her IVF and GIFT treatment before it begins, or whether she would prefer to consider the number of eggs or embryos to be replaced after they have been retrieved. If she is to undergo frozen embryo replacement she should be asked to consider the number of embryos to be replaced at that stage. Examples of consent forms appear in Annex E. A copy of the consent form should be given to the person giving consent.

7.26 If it is possible that the question of treatment with donated gametes or embryos derived from them may arise, the centre should raise the matter with the person(s) seeking treatment beforehand. The centre should allow persons sufficient time to reflect before asking for consent to treatment with donated material.

Consent of the husband or male partner and legal fatherhood

7.27 As well as the general advice given above (paragraphs 7.1–7.24), centres should adopt the procedures described in the following paragraphs in the interests of preventing or resolving a dispute at a later stage about the fatherhood of a child (paragraph 3.15a).

7.28 A woman's husband will be the legal father of a child born as a result of treatment using donated sperm, unless they are judicially separated or he can prove that he did not consent to the treatment. If a married woman is being treated with donated sperm, centres should explain the position and ask her whether her husband consents to the treatment. If he does, the centre should take all practicable steps to obtain his written consent. If the woman does not know, or he does not consent, centres should, if she agrees, take all practicable steps to ascertain the position and (if this is the case) obtain written evidence that he does not consent.

7.29 If a woman is being treated together with a male partner, using donated sperm, and she is unmarried or judicially separated or her husband does not consent to the treatment, her male partner will be the legal father of any resulting child. Centres should explain this to them both and record at each appointment whether or not the man was present. Centres should try to obtain the written acknowledgement of the man both that they are being treated together and that donated sperm is to be used. Centres should also explain that when a child is born to an unmarried couple the male partner may not have parental responsibility for that child. Unmarried couples concerned about how parental responsibility affects their legal rights should seek their own legal advice.

People providing gametes and embryos for donation

Additional information

7.30 As well as considering the requirements of paragraphs 7.1–7.24 above, if the intention is to donate gametes for the treatment of others, including the creation of an embryo for that purpose, the person considering donation must consent in writing to their use for that purpose.

7.31 The centre does not have to obtain the consent of the donor's partner to the donation of the gametes. However, if the donated gametes are to be used for treatment, and the person providing the gametes is married or has a long-term partner, centres should encourage people providing gametes for donation to ask their partner to consent in writing to the use of the gametes for treatment.

7.32 The centre should be prepared to accept the financial loss if the woman withdraws after preparation for egg recovery has begun.

People seeking long term storage of gametes and embryos

Additional information

7.33 As well as considering the requirements of paragraphs 7.1–7.23 above, people seeking long term storage of gametes may give consent to storage separately from consent to use.

7.34 In addition to the requirements of paragraphs 7.12–7.13 above centres should be aware that, the normal storage period for gametes is 10 years, although gametes may be stored for more than 10 years where the person seeking storage was under 45 years of age when the gametes were placed in storage and providing the other conditions for an extended storage period have been satisfied.

7.35 Centres should ensure that anyone wanting to store gametes for more then 10 years satisfies all the conditions for an extended storage period before their consent is obtained.

7.36 As well as the requirements of paragraph 7.14 above centres should be aware that, the normal storage period for embryos is usually five years, although embryos may be stored for more than five years where the woman who would be treated by the embryos was under 50 years when the embryos were placed in storage and providing the other conditions for an extended storage period have been satisfied .

7.37 Centres should ensure that anyone wanting to store an embryo for more then five years satisfies all the conditions for an extended storage period before their consent is obtained.

7.38 People storing embryos produced using their eggs must specify the purpose for which they may be used, namely to provide treatment for themselves, or themselves and a named partner.

People involved in an egg sharing arrangement

Additional information

7.39 As well as considering the requirements of paragraphs 7.1–7.7; 7.11 and 7.14–7.31 above, statutory HFEA consent forms should be completed and signed as follows:

    a. The egg provider should complete a HFEA(00)7 for the use of the eggs and the storage of the embryos created for her own use. This HFEA(00)7 should be completed as though the egg provider was an IVF patient in accordance with HFEA guidance for the completion of HFEA (00)7.

    b. The egg provider should also complete a SEPARATE HFEA(00)7 for the use of the donated eggs and the embryos created for use by the recipient couple. This second HFEA (00)7 should be completed as though the egg provider was an egg donor in accordance with HFEA guidance for the completion of HFEA(00)7.

7.40 This arrangement allows different conditions to be placed on the storage of any spare embryos that may be created and cryopreserved. Using only one (00)7 does not allow consent to be varied in this way. It should be emphasised that, in accordance with the HFE Act, the provider may withdraw or vary her consent up to the time an embryo containing her gametes is used in treatment services or research, including cryopreserved embryos.

7.41 Any implications that may result from the withdrawal of consent should be made clear to all parties prior to treatment commencing. This should be fully detailed in the information given to the egg provider and the egg recipient. It should also be included in the written agreements.

7.42 The male partner of the egg provider and of the egg recipient should complete HFEA (00)6 in accordance with HFEA guidance as necessary.

Part 9   Use of gametes and embryos

General

Obtaining gametes and embryos

9.1 Centres may only import and export gametes and embryos in accordance with Directions made by the HFEA.

9.2 Centres may only transport gametes and embryos between licensed premises in accordance with Directions made by the HFEA.

9.3 Where any part of treatment services is to take place in premises not covered by a licence (a satellite centre), the law requires the licensed centre intending to carry out the subsequent embryo transfer to ensure that all the requirements of the HFE Act, the Code of Practice and any Directions made by the HFEA are complied with before any part of the treatment begins. These requirements cover information, counselling, the welfare of the child and confidentiality. Copies of the HFE Act and the Code of Practice should be supplied by the licensed centre to the satellite centre.

Clinical use

9.4 Eggs or sperm that have been subjected to procedures that carry an actual or reasonable theoretical risk of harm to their developmental potential, and embryos created from them, should not be used for treatment. Treatment centres should satisfy the HFEA that sufficient scientific evidence is available to establish that any procedures used do not prejudice the developmental potential of the gametes or embryos.

9.5 Similarly, embryos that have themselves been subject to procedures that carry an actual or reasonable theoretical risk of harm to their developmental potential should not be used for treatment. Treatment centres should satisfy the HFEA that sufficient scientific evidence is available to establish that any procedures used do not prejudice the developmental potential of the embryos.

9.6 Attempts to produce embryos in vitro should not be made if there is no intention to store or use the resulting embryo(s), unless there is a specific reason why it is necessary to do so in connection with the provision of treatment services for a particular woman. On each such occasion, the reason should be explained to the woman, implications counselling should be offered and the written consent of each person providing the gametes must have been obtained.

9.7 Frozen embryo transfer is a regulated activity. When a woman who has stored an embryo and wishes to have the embryo transferred in treatment, the centre must consider her for treatment in the normal way, taking into account the welfare of the potential child.

9.8 Gametes or embryos that have been exposed to a material risk of contamination that might cause harm to recipients or to any resulting children should not be used for treatment. If there is any doubt, centres should seek expert advice.

9.9 Centres should not select the sex of embryos for social reasons.

9.10 Centres should not use sperm sorting techniques in sex selection.

9.11 Centres should not attempt to produce embryos in vitro by embryo splitting for treatment purposes.

Termination and disposal

9.12 The special status of the human embryo is fundamental to the provisions of the HFE Act. The termination of the development of a human embryo and the disposal of the remaining material are sensitive and delicate issues. Centres should take full account of this when considering how the development of an embryo is to be brought to an end, and what is to happen thereafter. The approach to be adopted will depend on whether the embryos are being stored for treatment or to be used for research.

9.13 Where an embryo is no longer to be kept for treatment, the centre should decide how it is to be allowed to perish, and what is to happen to the perished material. The procedure should be sensitively devised and described, and should be communicated to the people for whom the embryo was being stored if they so wish.

9.14 In the case of embryos used for research, the centre should decide at the outset the duration of the culture period, the method that is to be used to terminate development, and the procedure which will ensure that embryos do not continue to develop after fourteen days or (if earlier) the appearance of the primitive streak.

People seeking treatment

Additional information

9.15 As well as considering the requirements of paragraphs 9.1–9.14, centres may allow a man to provide sperm produced at home in exceptional circumstances. Normally sperm should be produced in a licensed centre. If a centre does allow a man to provide sperm produced at home the centre should take all reasonable steps to satisfy itself that the sperm has been produced by that man, not more than two hours previously, and that it has not subsequently been interfered with. That the sperm has been produced at home, and that the centre is satisfied the above conditions have been met, should be formally noted in patient records.

9.16 Centres should ensure that facilities as detailed in Paragraph 2.5 are still available to patients if required.

9.17 Where embryos have been created using partner sperm produced at home and donation is being considered, the fact that the sperm was not produced at a licenced centre should be taken into account.

9.18 No more than, either, three eggs or three embryos should be placed in a woman in any one cycle, regardless of the procedure used.

9.19 Women should not be treated with the gametes or with embryos derived from the gametes of more than one man or woman during any treatment cycle.

9.20 Before donor insemination treatment begins, there should be discussion with the client about the number of treatment cycles to be attempted before further investigation into the causes of lack of success (if this arises). This matter should be reviewed at regular intervals.

9.21 Centres may supply sperm for home insemination if, but only if, there are exceptional circumstances making it impracticable or undesirable for the woman to be inseminated at the centre, and the procedures set out in paragraphs 9.22–9.26 are followed.

9.22 Where sperm is supplied for home insemination this should always be noted and the exceptional circumstances explained in the treatment records.

9.23 As with all other donor insemination treatment, the giving of information, assessment of the client, consideration of the welfare of the child and an offer of counselling are required in accordance with the HFE Act and other Code of Practice guidelines. If it is decided to offer home insemination, centres should obtain an undertaking in writing from the woman to be offered treatment that the sperm will be used by her alone.

9.24 Before supplying sperm for home insemination a centre should obtain an undertaking in writing from the woman to supply information to the centre about the outcome of the treatment.

9.25 The HFE Act forbids the supply of frozen sperm to a person not covered by a licence, and centres may therefore only supply sperm in the process of thawing. Provided that the woman has attended the clinic for assessment purposes, the sperm may be supplied to either, her in person or by courier.

9.26 The use of a dry shipper, or any other containment vessel that would keep the sperm in a frozen or preserved state after leaving the licensed centre is strictly prohibited by the HFE Act.

9.27 Centres should complete DI treatment cycle form (96)2 in the normal way, entering the date of supply or posting as the date of insemination and noting on the form that the sperm was supplied for home insemination.

People providing gametes and embryos for donation

Additional information

9.28 As well as considering the requirements of paragraphs 9.1–9.14, centres should only allow a donor to provide sperm produced at home in exceptional circumstances. Normally sperm should be produced in a licensed centre. If a centre does allow a donor to provide sperm produced at home the centre should take all reasonable steps to satisfy itself that the sperm has been produced by that man, not more than two hours previously, and that it has not subsequently been interfered with (so as to ensure that the screening procedures outlined in paragraphs 4.10–4.18 remain effective). That the sperm has been produced at home, and that the centre is satisfied the above conditions have been met, should be formally noted in patient records.

9.29 Where embryos have been created using partner sperm produced at home and donation is being considered, the fact that the sperm was not produced at a licenced centre should be taken into account.

9.30 Donated gametes or embryos should not be used for treatment once the number of live birth events that have occurred as a result of donations from that donor has reached 10. It is the responsibility of the supplier and of the user to agree an appropriate procedure for ensuring that the limit is not exceeded.

9.31 This limit of 10 may be exceeded only in exceptional cases, e.g. where a recipient wishes to have a subsequent child from the same donor. The HFEA should be notified whenever the limit is exceeded. If the person providing gametes for donation has specified a limit, this must never be exceeded.

9.32 Centres must not export gametes from donors who have produced 10 live birth events in the UK (see paragraphs 9.30 and 9.31, above).

People seeking long term storage of gametes and embryos

Additional information

9.33 As well as considering the requirements of paragraphs 9.1–9.14, insemination of a woman at a licensed centre using her late husband's or partner's sperm is regulated under the HFE Act (see paragraphs 7.21–24).

Part 11   Research

General

General standards

11.1 All research that involves the creation, keeping or using of human embryos outside the body must be licensed by the HFEA. A centre must apply to the HFEA for a separate licence for each research project.

11.2 The HFEA may grant licences for research projects for the following purposes only:

a. to promote advances in the treatment of infertility;

b. to increase knowledge about the causes of congenital disease;

c. to increase knowledge about the causes of miscarriages;

d. to develop more effective techniques of contraception;

e. to develop methods for detecting the presence of gene or chromosome abnormalities in embryos before implantation.

f. increasing knowledge about the development of embryos;

g. increasing knowledge about serious disease; or

h. enabling any such knowledge to be applied in developing treatments for serious disease.

11.3 The HFEA cannot grant a licence unless it is satisfied that the use of human embryos is necessary for the purposes of the research.

Prohibitions

11.4 The following activities are prohibited by law:

a. keeping or using an embryo after the appearance of the primitive streak or after 14 days, whichever is the earlier;

b. placing an embryo in a non-human animal;

c. replacing a nucleus of a cell of an embryo with a nucleus taken from the cell of another person, another embryo, or a subsequent development of an embryo;

d. altering the genetic structure of any cell while it forms part of an embryo.

11.5 Embryos that have been appropriated for a research project must not be used for any other purposes.

11.6 Centres should refer each research project to a properly constituted ethics committee for approval before applying for a research licence.

11.7 Centres within the NHS should refer research projects to the relevant Multiple Centre Research Ethics Committees (MREC) and/or Local Research Ethics Committee (LREC) of the relevant Health Authority. Centres outside the NHS may also refer projects to the LREC by prior arrangement, or may wish to set up their own committee. If so this should be an independent body of not fewer than five members. The chairman should be independent of the centre. No more than one third of its members should be employed by or have a financial interest in the centre. Membership of the ethics committee should be approved by the HFEA. For further information on the establishment and operation of a research ethics committee, centres should contact the Department of Health.

11.8 Proposals for research projects involving the use of embryos will be submitted for peer review to appropriate academic referees chosen by the HFEA.

11.9 Centres' attention is drawn to paragraphs 7.4–7.19 on consent to storage and use of gametes and embryos, paragraphs 9.4–9.11 on the use of gametes and embryos that have been subject to procedures that might prejudice their developmental potential, and paragraphs 9.12–9.14 on the termination and disposal of embryos that have been used for research.

Fifth Edition
Revised April 2001

The full Code of Practice can be read on
http://www.hfea.gov.uk

Human Fertilisation and Embryology Authority
Paxton House
30, Artillery Lane
London E1 7LS

Tel: 0207 377 5077
Fax 0207 377 1871

Protecting the interests of research participants
(A) General principles

51

Guidelines for researchers – patient information sheet and consent form

Central Office for Research Ethics Committees

The guidance which follows applies primarily to multi-centre pharmaceutical studies and encompasses the ICH Good Clinical Practice guidelines. However, the principles and much of the content will be of use to researchers writing information sheets in their particular fields, for trials involving patients, patient volunteers and healthy volunteers. You will find it helpful to refer also to other guidelines produced for writing patient information sheets.

Potential recruits to your research study must be given sufficient information to allow them to decide whether or not they want to take part. An Information Sheet should contain information under the headings given below where appropriate, and in the order specified. It should be written in simple, non-technical terms and be easily understood by a lay person. Use short words, sentences and paragraphs. 'The readability' of any text can be roughly estimated by the application of standard formulae. Checks on readability are provided in most word processing packages.

Consumers for Ethics in Research (CERES) publish a leaflet entitled 'Medical Research and You'. This leaflet gives more information about medical research and looks at some questions potential recruits may want to ask. You may obtain copies from CERES, PO Box 1365, London N16 0BW.

Use headed paper of the hospital/institution where the research is being carried out. Patient Information Sheets submitted to an MREC should be headed simply 'Hospital/Institution/GP Practice headed paper'. **If you are a local researcher for an MREC approved study, the Patient Information Sheet should be printed on local hospital/surgery paper with local contact names and telephone numbers before it is submitted to the LREC.** Unheaded paper is not acceptable.

© Central Office for Research Ethics Committees.

1 Study title

Is the title self explanatory to a lay person? If not, a simplified title should be included.

2 Invitation paragraph

This should explain that the patient is being asked to take part in a research study. The following is a suitable example:

'You are being invited to take part in a research study. Before you decide it is important for you to understand why the research is being done and what it will involve. Please take time to read the following information carefully and discuss it with others if you wish. Ask us if there is anything that is not clear or if you would like more information. Take time to decide whether or not you wish to take part.

Thank you for reading this.'

3 What is the purpose of the study?

The background and aim of the study should be given here. Also mention the duration of the study.

4 Why have I been chosen?

You should explain how the patient was chosen and how many other patients will be studied.

5 Do I have to take part?

You should explain that taking part in the research is entirely voluntary. You could use the following paragraph:-

'It is up to you to decide whether or not to take part. If you do decide to take part you will be given this information sheet to keep and be asked to sign a consent form. If you decide to take part you are still free to withdraw at any time and without giving a reason. A decision to withdraw at any time, or a decision not to take part, will not affect the standard of care you receive.

6 What will happen to me if I take part?

You should say how long the patient will be involved in the research, how long the research will last (if this is different), how often they will need to visit a clinic (if this is appropriate) and how long these visits will be. You should explain if the patient will need to visit the GP (or clinic) more often than for his/her usual treatment and if travel expenses are available. What exactly will happen e.g. blood tests, x-rays, (over and above those involved in standard diagnosis and treatment), interviews etc.? Whenever possible you should draw a simple flowchart or plan indicating what will happen at each visit. What are the patient's responsibilities? Set down clearly what you expect of them.

You should set out simply the research methods you intend to use – the following simple definitions may help:

Randomised trial

Sometimes because we do not know which way of treating patients is best, we need to make comparisons. People will be put into groups and then compared. The groups are selected by a computer which has no information about the individual – i.e. by chance. Patients in each group then have a different treatment and these are compared.

You should tell the patients what chance they have of getting the study drug/treatment e.g. a one in four chance.

Blind trial

In a blind trial you will not know which treatment group you are in. If the trial is a double blind trial, neither you nor your doctor will know in which treatment group you are (although, if your doctor needs to find out he/she can do so).

Cross-over trial

In a cross-over trial the groups each have the different treatments in turn. There may be a break between treatments so that the first drugs are cleared from your body before you start the new treatment.

Placebo

A placebo is a dummy treatment such as a pill which looks like the real thing but is not. It contains no active ingredient.

7 What do I have to do?

Are there any lifestyle restrictions? You should tell the patient if there are any dietary restrictions. Can the patient drive?, drink?, take part in sport? Can the patient continue to take their regular medication? Should the patient refrain from giving blood? What happens if the patient becomes pregnant?

Explain (if appropriate) that the patient should take the medication regularly.

8 What is the drug or procedure that is being tested?

You should include a short description of the drug or device and give the stage of development.

You should also state the dosage of the drug and method of administration. Patients entered into drug trials should be given a card (similar to a credit card) with details of the trial they are in. They should be asked to carry it at all times.

9 What are the alternatives for diagnosis or treatment?

For therapeutic research the patient should be told what other treatments are available.

10 What are the side effects of any treatment received when taking part?

For any new drug or procedure you should explain to the patients the possible side effects. If they suffer these or any other symptoms they should report them next time you meet. You should also give them a contact name and number to phone if they become in any way concerned. The name and number of the person to contact in the event of an emergency (if that is different) should also be given.

The known side effects should be listed in terms the patient will clearly understand (e.g. 'damage to the heart' rather than 'cardiotoxicity'; 'abnormalities of liver tests' rather than 'raised liver enzymes'). For any relatively new drug it should be explained that there may be unknown side effects.

11 What are the possible disadvantages and risks of taking part?

For studies where there could be harm to an unborn child if the patient were pregnant or became pregnant during the study, the following (or similar) should be said:

'It is possible that if the treatment is given to a pregnant woman it will harm the unborn child. Pregnant women must not therefore take part in this study, neither should women who plan to become pregnant during the study. Women who are at risk of pregnancy may be asked to have a pregnancy test before taking part to exclude the possibility of pregnancy. Women who could become pregnant must use an effective contraceptive during the course of this study. Any woman who finds that she has become pregnant while taking part in the study should immediately tell her research doctor.'

Use the pregnancy statement carefully. In certain circumstances (e.g. terminal illness) it would be inappropriate and insensitive to bring up pregnancy.

There should also be an appropriate warning and advice for men if the treatment could damage sperm which might therefore lead to a risk of a damaged fetus.

If future insurance status e.g. for life insurance or private medical insurance, could be affected by taking part this should be stated (if e.g. high blood pressure is detected.) If the patients have private medical insurance you should ask them to check with the company before agreeing to take part in the trial. They will need to do this to ensure that their participation will not affect their medical insurance.

You should state what happens if you find a condition of which the patient was unaware. Is it treatable? What are you going to do with this information? What might be uncovered?

12 What are the possible benefits of taking part?

Where there is no intended clinical benefit to the patient from taking part in the trial this should be stated clearly.

It is important not to exaggerate the possible benefits to the particular patient during the course of the study, e.g. by saying they will be given extra attention. This could be seen as coercive. It would be reasonable to say something similar to:

'We hope that both (all) the treatments will help you. However, this cannot be guaranteed. The information we get from this study may help us to treat future patients with (name of condition) better.'

13 What if new information becomes available?

If additional information becomes available during the course of the research you will need to tell the patient about this. You could use the following:

'Sometimes during the course of a research project, new information becomes available about the treatment/drug that is being studied. If this happens, your research doctor will tell you about it and discuss with you whether you want to continue in the study. If you decide to withdraw your research doctor will make arrangements for your care to continue. If you decide to continue in the study you will be asked to sign an updated consent form.

Also, on receiving new information your research doctor might consider it to be in your best interests to withdraw you from the study. He/she will explain the reasons and arrange for your care to continue.'

14 What happens when the research study stops?

If the treatment will not be available after the research finishes this should be explained to the patient. You should also explain to them what treatment will be available instead. Occasionally the company sponsoring the research may stop it. If this is the case the reasons should be explained to the patient.

15 What if something goes wrong?

You should inform patients how complaints will be handled and what redress may be available. Is there a procedure in place? You will need to distinguish between complaints from patients as to their treatment by members of staff (doctors, nurses etc.) and something serious happening during or following their participation in the trial i.e. a reportable serious adverse event.

Where there are no Association of the British Pharmaceutical Industry (ABPI) or other no-fault compensation arrangements, and the study carries risk of physical or significant psychological harm, the following (or similar) should be said:

'If you are harmed by taking part in this research project, there are no special compensation arrangements. If you are harmed due to someone's negligence, then you may have grounds for a legal action but you may have to pay for it. Regardless of this, if you wish to complain, or have any concerns about any aspect of the way you have been approached or treated during the course of this study, the normal National Health Service complaints mechanisms should be available to you.'

Where there are ABPI or other no-fault compensation arrangements the following (or similar) should be included:

'Compensation for any injury caused by taking part in this study will be in accordance with the guidelines of the Association of the

British Pharmaceutical Industry (ABPI). Broadly speaking the ABPI guidelines recommend that 'the sponsor', without legal commitment, should compensate you without you having to prove that it is at fault. This applies in cases where it is likely that such injury results from giving any new drug or any other procedure carried out in accordance with the protocol for the study. 'The sponsor' will not compensate you where such injury results from any procedure carried out which is not in accordance with the protocol for the study. Your right at law to claim compensation for injury where you can prove negligence is not affected. Copies of these guidelines are available on request.'

16 Will my taking part in this study be kept confidential?

You will need to obtain the patient's permission to allow restricted access to their medical records and to the information collected about them in the course of the study. You should explain that all information collected about them will be kept strictly confidential. A suggested form of words for drug company sponsored research is:

'If you consent to take part in the research any of your medical records may be inspected by the company sponsoring (and/or the company organising) the research for purposes of analysing the results. They may also be looked at by people from the company and from regulatory authorities to check that the study is being carried out correctly. Your name, however, will not be disclosed outside the hospital/GP surgery.'

or for other research:

'All information which is collected about you during the course of the research will be kept strictly confidential. Any information about you which leaves the hospital/surgery will have your name and address removed so that you cannot be recognised from it.'

You should always bear in mind that you, as the researcher, are responsible for ensuring that when collecting or using data, you are not contravening the legal or regulatory requirements in any part of the UK. This is not the responsibility of the REC.

You should explain that for studies not being conducted by a GP, the patient's own GP will be notified of their participation in the trial. This should include other medical practitioners not involved in the research who may be treating the patient. You should seek the patient's agreement to this. In some instances agreement from the patient that their GP can be informed is a precondition of entering the trial.

17 What will happen to the results of the research study?

You should be able to tell the patients what will happen to the results of the research. When are the results likely to be published? Where can they obtain a copy of the published results? Will they be told which arm of the study they were in? You might add that they will not be identified in any report/publication.

18 Who is organising and funding the research?

The answer should include the organisation or company sponsoring or funding the research (e.g. Medical Research Council, Pharmaceutical Company, charity, academic institution).

The patient should be told whether the doctor conducting the research is being paid for including and looking after the patient in the study. **This means payment other than that to cover necessary expenses** such as laboratory tests arranged locally by the researcher, or the costs of a research nurse. You could say:

'The sponsors of this study will pay (name of hospital department or research fund) for including you in this study' or

'Your doctor will be paid for including you in this study.'

19 Who has reviewed the study?

You may wish to give the name of the Research Ethics Committee(s) which reviewed the study (you do not however have to list the members of the Committee).

20 Contact for further information

You should give the patient a contact point for further information. This can be your name or that of another doctor/nurse involved in the study.

Remember to thank your patient for taking part in this study!

The patient information sheet should be dated and given a version number.

The Patient Information Sheet should state that the patient will be given a copy of the information sheet and a signed consent form to keep.

(Form to be on headed paper)

Centre Number::
Study Number:
Patient Identification Number for this trial:

CONSENT FORM

Title of Project:

Name of Researcher:

Please initial box

1. I confirm that I have read and understand the information sheet dated ....
    (version ....) for the above study and have had the opportunity to ask questions.

2. I understand that my participation is voluntary and that I am free to withdraw at any time,
    without giving any reason, without my medical care or legal rights being affected.

3. I understand that sections of any of my medical notes may be looked at by responsible
    individuals from [company name] or from regulatory authorities where it is relevant to my taking
    part in research. I give permission for these individuals to have access to my records.

4. I agree to take part in the above study.

_____   _____   _____
Name of Patient   Date   Signature

_____   _____   _____
Name of Person taking consent Date   Signature
(if different from researcher)

_____   _____   _____
Researcher   Date   Signature

1 for patient; 1 for researcher; 1 to be kept with hospital notes

52

ABPI Guidance note
– patient information and consents for clinical trials

Association of the British Pharmaceutical Industry

This guidance provides a checklist as to the items which ought to be covered when a Member Company is designing (for use in connection with a company-sponsored clinical trial in the United Kingdom) (a) an information leaflet to be provided to patients as candidates for inclusion in a clinical trial and (b) the form of consent for signature by patients prior to inclusion. Both forms should be provided separately and be approved by an appropriate Ethics Committee. It is not intended to recommend any particular format for these purposes. Some sponsoring companies prefer most information to be in the information leaflet, and the consent form merely to recite that consent has been given. Although this note suggests recitation of key matters in the Consent Form this is not critical provided the relevant information is drawn to the patient's attention in the leaflet. Obviously it is desirable that whatever the format, it is 'user friendly' and as comprehensive as possible for lay readers.

In preparing this guidance consideration has been given to legal, medical and ethical principles, the requirements of the Declaration of Helsinki, and to other relevant texts including the Report of the Royal College of Physicians of London entitled 'Research Involving Patients' (January 1990) ('the RCP Report'); CPMP/ICH guidelines on 'Good Clinical Practice'; (CPMP/ICH/135/95).

Compliance with the recommendations in this guidance note does not obviate the need to add to or adjust any documents to take account of any unusual features in a trial. Moreover, it is always important to ensure that all other aspects of 'Good Clinical Practice' are followed.

This guidance is designed for patients proposed for entry into a clinical trial as distinct from volunteers for a Phase 1 Study.

The checklists follow, (words in italics are ancillary notes to each main item):

©Association of the British Pharmaceutical Industry.

(a) Patient Information (to be provided to candidates for inclusion in a clinical trial)

(i) Identify main items and describe the purpose of the study
Link with reference to the Protocol Number. Always state the study concerns 'a medicine, audit or device under research'. Provide the name and contact details of the study doctor and refer to the name of the sponsor on whose behalf the study is being conducted.

(ii) Explain participation in voluntary **but why invitation has been issued**.

(iii) Explain who is involved in the study
Indicate how many patients in the study. ***Some ethics committees have apparently wanted to know in addition how many patients have received the study drug so far and generally want this communicated in the patient information. This would only be relevant in Phase II and III trials***.

(iv) Explain what is involved (for the patient) by participation in the study
If, in addition to treatment, the patient has to undergo other procedures (e.g. blood tests), this must be explained also. If the study involves a placebo or comparison treatments, this must be clearly stated. Indicate number of times visits must be made to doctor, hospital and/or elsewhere, and what will be involved.

(v) State the expected duration of the study.

(vi) Provide any instruction about record-keeping.

(vii) Indicate where and how further information can be obtained *(Note that the patient will be informed of new information material to the consent if this becomes known during the progress of the study).*

(viii) Describe possible side-effects and what to do if concerned
Explain what to do about unexpected side-effects.

(ix) Provide any instructions relating to consumption of other medicines, food, drinks etc whilst in the study.

(x) Provide any instructions relating to any restrictions on driving, using machinery, sport or other activities whilst in the study.

(xi) **In exceptional circumstances, where it is applicable to the patient population, instructions should be provided for pregnant patients or patients who might become pregnant.**
Such patients are normally excluded from clinical trials.

(xii) Explain benefits of and risks (as reasonably foreseen) of participating in the study
Benefit can be for the patient, society at large or both. Refer to potential benefits and risks of alternative therapies, if applicable. Inform the patient of the physical and psychological risks both in terms of the magnitude of the risk (chance of it arising) and its potential seriousness.

(xiii) Explain rights to withdraw from study without giving a reason and without any prejudice to continuing rights to treatment and alternative therapy
*Explain that the doctor may also decide to withdraw a patient from the study and why. **If possible patients should be told what the alternative treatments are.***

(xiv) Explain how data is recorded and who may have access to it **and the source documentation.**
Record that the patient's general practitioner will be informed about the patient's participation in the study. Access may be available to Doctors, Study monitors and clinical trial auditors, ethics committees and regulatory authorities.
The study results may be publicised. The patient's identity will not be disclosed in publication.

(xv) Explain that compensation may be available for **any injury attributable to administration of a medicinal product within the trial or any clinical intervention or procedure provided for by the protocol that would not have occurred but for the inclusion of the patient in the trial.**
Record that compensation will be considered in accordance with the 'Clinical Trial Compensation Guidelines' issued by ABPI (1991, reprinted 1994), where applicable, and inform the patient that a copy of the guidelines can be made available on request.

(xvi) Explain if travel or other costs will be reimbursed and, if so, to what extent and how, and specify any other payment made to patients who participate.

Other information may be included if appropriate. Updates should be provided when necessary.

As a final note, the following extract is re-produced from the RCP Report.

'It is unreasonable to ask a patient to agree on the spot to take part in research which either involves more than minimal risk or involves extended inconvenience or discomfort. Time should be allowed for the patient to consider the position, to read the Information Sheet in unhurried circumstances and to discuss it with a friend or relative. The time required for this will depend on what seems appropriate in the circumstances. For research which is low risk or undemanding it might, for example, be quite acceptable for a patient attending a hospital clinic or a general practitioner to have a cup of tea and to reach a decision within a few minutes. In other circumstances it might seem appropriate for the decision to be declared at a different visit on a different day.'

(b) Patient consent form (to be signed by patients prior to inclusion within a clinical trial)

(i) Refer to the Study by name and the Protocol by number as well as the name of the patient.

(ii) Confirm the patient has read **and understood** the Patient Information Leaflet which should be attached to the Consent Form for identification purposes.

(iii) Confirm name, address and phone number of the Study Doctor for the patient.

(iv) Confirm discussion of the patient's possible participation with study (or other nominated) Doctor.

(v) Confirm the patient's duties to report possible side-effects, other health changes, and/or changes to medical treatment.

(vi) Confirm (when Study Doctor is not the patient's GP) that Study Doctor may contact General Practitioner to obtain medical records.

(vii) Confirm the patient's understanding about access to data.

(viii) Confirm the patient has had an opportunity to ask questions and has received satisfactory answers.

(ix) Confirm the patient has received enough information about the Study to ensure the patient appreciates what the research entails.

(x) Confirm the patient's right to withdraw from the trial at any time, without having to give a reason, and without any prejudice to continuing treatment.

(xi) Confirm the patient is agreeing to participate on a voluntary basis.

(xii) Confirm the retention of all legal rights for the patient and, where applicable, eligibility for compensation in accordance with the 'Clinical Trial Compensation Guidelines' issued by ABPI (1991).

The patient should sign and date the consent form personally to be followed by a signature and date from the doctor who has conducted the discussion about participation in the study to confirm that proper counselling has taken place and the consent was freely given. For patients who cannot read, or have intellectual or other difficulties in speech or understanding, an impartial witness should also sign and date the form to confirm that (s)he was present when the counselling took place and that in the opinion of the witness the consent of the patient was based upon a reasonable understanding of what the research involved. Further guidance (eg the RCP Report) should be sought and followed where the patient is a child or suffering from incapacity. The patient should be given a copy of the patient information and consent form when signed for future reference.

The Association of the British Pharmaceutical Industry
12 Whitehall London SW1A 2DY

53

The protection and use of patient information
(HSG(96)18/LASSL(96)5)

Department of Health

Executive

Health Service Guidelines

HSG(96)18
LASSL(96)5

The protection and use of patient information

Date 7 March 1996

DA(80)14 is cancelled.

Addresses

For action:
Regional Health Authorities
District Health Authorities
Special Health Authorities
Special Hospitals Services Authority
Family Health Services Authorities
National Health Service Trusts
Directly Managed Units

For information:
Directors of Social Services
Community Health Councils

© Department of Health.

From:

Health Promotion Division
Room 123
Wellington House
133–155 Waterloo Road
London SE1 8UG
Tel: 0171-972 4925

Further copies of this document and booklet may be obtained by writing to:
Department of Health
PO Box 410
Wetherby
LS23 7LL
Tel 01937 840 250
Fax 01937 845 381

Please quote serial number appearing at the top of this column.

Crown copyright 1996

Protection and use of patient information

1 The accompanying booklet offers guidance on the protection and use of patient information. It is being issued following consultation with a wide range of organisations, including those representing the NHS, the health professions and patients.

Status of the guidance

2 The guidance is based on two fundamental considerations:

i patients' expectation, set out in the *Patient's Charter*, that information about them will be treated as confidential;

ii the importance of making patients fully aware that NHS staff and sometimes staff of other agencies need to have strictly controlled access to such information, anonymised wherever possible, in order to deliver, plan and manage services effectively.

3 Patient information is currently protected by the common law duty of confidence and, in the case of computerised information, by the **Data Protection Act 1984**. There are some other specific statutory provisions (for example, relating to information about sexually transmitted diseases), as well as professional ethical duties of confidence.

4 The recently adopted **EC Directive on Data Protection** must be implemented by October 1998. The present guidance acknowledges this, but further specific guidance may be necessary once detailed consideration has been given to its provisions.

5 The guidance is consistent with the Code of Practice on Openness in the NHS. Subject to the duty of confidence to patients, the guidance does not affect the rights of staff to raise concerns about the delivery of care or other matters: see NHS Executive (1993) *Guidance for staff on relations with the public and the media.*

6 In support of the action called for in this circular the Executive will be reviewing all uses of person identifiable health data for purposes other than direct care and clinical research, to ascertain the extent to which identifying details are justified and to ensure that where person identified data is justified it is adequately protected.

7 Some relevant publications by the NHS Executive and the Data Protection Registrar are mentioned in the guidance. EL(95)108 required all NHS bodies to review their information management and technology security measures prior to connecting to the NHS-wide networking system. A computer security manual will be issued shortly. Recent Audit Commission reports, obtainable from HMSO, have also addressed some of the issues: *For Your Information: A Study of Information Management and Systems in the Acute Hospital* (1995) and *Setting the Record Straight: A Study of Hospital Records* (1995).

Action

8 Each NHS body, including all separate NHS data users under the Data Protection Act, must adopt clear policies and procedures on the use and protection of patient information. These should be drawn to the attention of all staff and must:

i be consistent with the enclosed guidance;

ii include locally agreed arrangements for ensuring that patients are personally made aware of the purposes to which information about them may be put, as well as ways in which they can exercise choice;

iii be drawn to the attention of other bodies providing or working in conjunction with NHS services, and, where necessary, discussed or agreed with them;

iv be subject to monitoring and audit.

9 All NHS organisations (including the new authorities set up in April 1996) should therefore review their security arrangements against the requirements of this guidance by end July 1996. FHSAs should ensure that appropriate action is taken in GP practices. The NHS Executive's Medical Director will be writing to all GPs on the subject shortly. All necessary remedial action should be implemented by November 1996 when Regional Offices will be seeking assurance from Trust and Health Authority Chief Executives that all actions has been completed.

10022 HP 7K Feb97 SA (0)

Contents

Chapter 1

Introduction

1.1. This guidance is based on:

   i patients' expectation that information about them
will be treated as confidential; and

   ii the importance of making patients fully aware that
NHS staff and sometimes staff of other agencies
need to have strictly controlled access to such information, anonymised wherever possible[1].

1.2. It is in everyone's interests that the NHS functions
efficiently and effectively and makes best use of the resources available to it. To that end personal information
about patients is not only essential for the prime task of
delivering personal care and treatment. It is necessary for
a number of other purposes:

   i **assuring and improving the quality of care and treatment** (*eg* through clinical audit);

   ii **monitoring and protecting public health;**

   iii **coordinating NHS care with that of other agencies** (*eg*
local authority, voluntary and independent services);

   iv **effective health care administration**, in particular:

     - managing and planning services;

     - contracting for NHS services, including the payment

---

[1] See paragraphs 1.3 and 4.5.

of staff and health care units for services and the authorisation of extra-contractual referrals[2];

   - auditing NHS accounts (including the work of external auditors appointed by the Audit Commission) and
accounting for NHS performance;

   - risk management (*eg* health and safety);

   - investigating complaints and notified or potential
legal claims;

  v **teaching;**

  vi **statistical analysis and medical or health services
research** to support (i)–(v).

1.3. As a consequence, patient information will be seen
and used by a number of NHS professional and administrative staff, as well as staff of other agencies contributing
to a patient's care. Most patients would be unlikely to trust
staff with detailed information about themselves and their
clinical condition if they thought this might be passed on
to others without proper controls. It is therefore a central
tenet of the NHS that, in the words of the *Patient's Charter
and you* (1995), **"everyone working for the NHS is under a
legal duty to keep your records confidential"**. In addition
the present guidance makes clear that personal information should be anonymised wherever possible.

EC Directive on Data Protection

1.4. The Directive on Data Protection, adopted by the
Council of the European Union in October 1995, has implications for personal information generally, not only that
relating to health. Member states must give effect to its
provisions by 24 October 1998.

1.5. One of the Directive's main purposes is to safeguard
"the fundamental rights of individuals". As with our existing
domestic law, the Directive:

   • establishes a set of principles with which users of personal information must comply (*eg* fair and lawful
"processing"[3] of information; information to be

---

[2] See EL(92)60: NHS Executive, *Handling confidential information
in contracting: A Code of Practice*; EL(95)75: NHS Executive, *Handling
Confidential Patient Information in Contract Minimum Data Sets*

[3] Under Article 2(b) of the **EC Directive**, "processing" is "any operation or set of operations which is performed upon personal data,
whether or not by automatic means". In relation to the **Data Protection
Act 1984** (see paragraph 4.2), which is concerned only with automatic
processing, the term means "amending, augmenting, deleting or rear-
ranging the data or extracting the information constituting the data and,
in the case of personal data, means performing any of those operations
by reference to the data subject . . . The definition does not specifically
refer to operations such as transmission, display or printing of the information contained in the data. However, in order to perform any of these
operations, extraction of the information must occur and, therefore, the
data have been processed" (Data Protection Registrar *Guideline 2*, 1994).

collected and processed only for specific purposes; information to be accurate and up to date, and retained in a form which identifies the subject only for as long as is necessary for the purpose);

- gives individuals the right to gain access to information held about them; and
- provides for a supervisory authority to oversee and enforce the law.

The Directive also:

i permits the **processing of health information** where this is required "for the purposes of preventive medicine, medical diagnosis, the provision of care or treatment or the management of health care services, and where those data are processed by a health professional subject under national law or rules established by national competent bodies to the obligation of professional secrecy or by another person also subject to an equivalent obligation of secrecy" *(Article 8, paragraph 3)*;

ii requires certain information to be provided to individuals whose personal information is processed;

iii applies both to computerised and manual records, and to some existing records as well as those made after implementation.

Purpose of the guidance

1.6 The Directive reflects many of the practices already established in the NHS and confirmed in this guidance. In the meantime, the guidance sets out:

- **the basic principles governing the use of patient information** *(section 2)*;
- **informing patients why information is needed, how it is used and their own rights of access to it** *(section 3)*;
- **safeguarding information required for NHS and related purposes** *(section 4)*;
- **the circumstances in which information may be passed on for other purposes or as a legal requirement** *(section 5)*.

Chapter 2

Basic principles

2.1 In general – and in all walks of life – any personal information given or received in confidence for one purpose may not be used for a different purpose or passed to anyone else without the consent of the provider of the information. This **duty of confidence** is long-established at common law, but with proper safeguards, need not be construed so

rigidly that, when applied to the NHS or related services, there is a risk of its operating to a patient's disadvantage or that of the public generally. Indeed, as a number of inquiry reports have shown, the prompt flow of accurate information in sensitive areas such as mental health and child care can often be for the benefit and safety of all concerned.

2.2 Personal information held on a computer system is safeguarded by the **Data Protection Act 1984**: see paragraph 4.2. This places obligations on those who record or use information, while at the same time giving specified rights to people about whom information is held. The **Computer Misuse Act 1990** provides criminal sanctions against unauthorised access ("hacking") or damage to computerised information[4].

2.3 In addition health professionals have **ethical duties of confidence**[5].

Patient information

2.4 In this guidance the term, "patient information", applies to all personal information about members of the public held in whatever form by or for NHS bodies or staff[6].

---

[4] Under the **Copyright, Designs and Patents Act 1988** it is illegal to copy computer software without the copyright owner's (or software developer's) permission.

[5] See paragraph 4.1 (iii). In this guidance generally "health professionals" refers to staff contributing to health care and to other professional staff, such as microbiologists, who have access to relevant patient information. The extent of their personal involvement in decisions relating to the use and protection of information will depend on a number of factors, including the particular circumstances of a case and locally agreed policies and practice. For the specific purposes of **access to health records** legislation and the **Data Protection Act 1984** "health professional" includes the following: registered medical practitioner, dentist, optician (*ie* optometrist or ophthalmic medical practitioner) or pharmaceutical chemist; registered nurse, midwife or health visitor; registered chiropodist, dietician, occupational therapist, orthoptist or physiotherapist; clinical psychologist, child psychotherapist or speech therapist; art or music therapist employed by an NHS body; or scientist employed by such a body as head of a department.

[6] The guidance thus applies to NHS patients receiving care within or outside the NHS, as well as private patients being cared for in NHS units. "Patient" should be taken where necessary to include "client" (*eg* a blood donor or a social services client to whose care the NHS is contributing) and others, such as research volunteers or people assessed psychiatrically at magistrates' courts, who may not always be patients as such. "NHS bodies" include health authorities, special health authorities, Trusts, general practices, hospitals and other units providing services: in fact, all parts of the NHS which handle patient information. They include also bodies such as the Prescription Pricing Authority, Dental Estimates Boards, Public Health Laboratory Service and the Department of Health. In addition the Office for National Statistics and other contractors handle some patient information on behalf of the NHS.

As well as obvious material such as medical records, it includes personal "non-health" information (*eg* a patient's name and address or details of his or her financial or domestic circumstances). In most instances such information will have been provided by the patient or added by NHS staff, but sometimes a relative or other person will be the source.

The relationship with patients

2.5 It is neither practicable nor necessary to seek a patient's (or other informant's) specific consent each time information needs to be passed on for a particular purpose. The public expects the NHS, often in conjunction with other agencies, to respond effectively to its needs; it can do so only if it has the necessary information. **Therfore, an essential feature of the relationship between patients and the NHS is the need for patients to be fully informed of the uses to which information about them may be put**: see section 3 and paragraph 4.4.

When information may be passed on

2.6 In summary, information may be passed to someone else:
- **with the patient's consent** for a particular purpose; *or*
- **on a "need to know" basis** if the following circumstances apply:
  i *for NHS purposes* (*including where services are either provided under contract to the NHS or are being planned or provided with other agencies*[7]):
  a **the recipient needs the information because he or she is or may be[8] concerned with the patient's care and treatment** (or that of another patient whose health may be affected by the condition of the original patient, such as a blood or organ donor)[9]; or
  b **the use of the information can be justified for the sort of wider purposes described at paragraph 1.2;** or

---

[7] See paragraphs 4.12 (iv) and 4.14–17.

[8] For example, when a number of cases, some not currently concerning a particular member of staff, are discussed within a multi-professional team or when a nursing team hands over charge of a ward to another team.

[9] **Carers** are often regarded as members of the care team: see paragraph 5.1. Under current guidance (HSG(92)2) **hospital chaplains** (or other religious representatives who are NHS staff) are also regarded as members of the team and may therefore be given information about a patient unless the patient has indicated otherwise. However, it is good practice to ask the patient on registration if he or she has a religious affiliation. *Information many not be passed to a religious organisation or its representatives outside the NHS without the patient's consent.*

ii **the information is required by statute or court order;** or
iii **passing on the information can be justified for other reasons,** usually for the protection of the public: see section 5.

Chapter 3

Keeping patients informed

Providing advice on how patient information is used

3.1 **All NHS bodies must have an active policy for informing patients of the kind of purposes for which information about them is collected and the categories of people or organisations to which information may need to be passed.** Where other bodies are providing services for or in conjunction with the NHS, those concerned must be aware of each others' information policies[10].

3.2 Subject to some important common elements (see paragraph 3.6), the precise arrangements for informing patients are for local decision, taking account of views expressed by community health councils, local patient groups, staff, and agencies with which the NHS body is in close contact. However, those concerned should bear in mind that:
  i as a general rule, patients should be told how information would be used before they are asked to provide it and must have the opportunity to discuss any aspects that are special to their treatment or circumstances;
  ii advice must be presented in a convenient form and be available both for general purposes and before a particular programme of care or treatment begins.

3.3 Methods of providing advice include:
  - leaflets enclosed with patients' appointment letters or provided when prescriptions are dispensed;
  - GP practice leaflets and/or notification on initial registration with a GP;
  - routinely providing patients with necessary information as a part of care planning;
  - identifying someone to provide further information if patients want it.

3.4 There must be arrangements for people whose first language is not English or who have restricted vision or reading skills.

---

[10] For example, general guidance for **local authority social services** was issued with LAC(88)17 HN(88)24 HN(FP)(88)22 and renewed by LASSL(92)9.

3.5 Notices in waiting areas, newsletters, and other publicity materials can help to reinforce the general approach, but are insufficient on their own.

3.6. **A model notice for patients is at _Annex A._** This may be adapted to local circumstances, though the core messages it contains are standard across the NHS and must **always** be identified. Patients registering with a GP should be made aware that certain basic personal information will be kept on a central register[11].

Patients' right of access to their own records

3.7 The _Patient's Charter_ identifies "the right to have access to your health records":

i subject to certain safeguards, patients may see their own manual health records made after 1 November 1991 and earlier records if they are necessary to understand the later ones (**Access to Health Records Act 1990**: see NHS Executive (1991) _Access to Health Records Act 1990: a guide for the NHS_). Patients do not have to give reasons for seeking access;

ii although there is no general statutory right to see manual records made before November 1991, access should be given whenever possible, subject to the judgment of the health professionals responsible for the patient's care and safeguards for other people who may have provided information about the patient;

iii there is specific guidance on access to records made at any time sought in connection with legal proceedings: see paragraph 5.5;

iv there are also rights of access under:

a the **Data Protection Act 1984** which, with some exemptions, entitles individuals to a copy of computerised information held about them;

b the **Access to Personal Files Act 1987** which concerns personal information held by local authority social services and may therefore be relevant in cases of joint care; and

c the **Access to Medical Reports Act 1988** in respect of reports for employers and insurance companies.

---

[11] The NHS Central Register for England and Wales (NHSCR) dates from 1951, having previously been part of the more general system of national registration begun during the Second World War. A computerised index now contains very basic personal details of all patients registered with a GP on or since 1 January 1991. **It does not contain clinical information**. The main functions of the NHSCR are to keep track of patients moving on and off registration lists and to control the issue of NHS numbers.

Chapter 4

Safeguarding information required for NHS and related purposes

Who has a duty of confidence?

4.1 The duty of confidence derives from the personal nature of the information recorded. It is unaffected by questions of who owns or holds particular records. Consequently, the following all have responsibilities for protecting information:

i **all NHS bodies and those carrying out functions on behalf of the NHS** have a common law duty of confidence to patients and a duty to support professional ethical standards of confidentiality;

ii **everyone working for or with the NHS** who records, handles, stores or otherwise comes across information has a personal common law duty of confidence to patients and to his or her employer[12]. This applies equally to those, such as students or trainees, on temporary placements;

iii **health professionals** have, by virtue of professional regulation, an ethical duty of confidence which, when considering whether information should be passed on, includes paying special regard to the health needs of the patient and to his or her wishes;

iv **other individuals and agencies** to whom information is passed legitimately may use it **only as authorised for specific purposes** and possibly subject to particular conditions.

Data Protection Act 1984

4.2 **All "personal data" (including patient information) relating to living individuals[13] that are held on a computer system are subject to the Data Protection Act 1984.** With the growth of information technology, this is increasingly the prime reference point for those using personal information: see _The Guidelines_ (3rd series, 1994) published by the Data Protection Registrar. The Act is underpinned by the **eight principles** at _Annex B._ NHS bodies that use computerised information must register with the DPR

---

[12] Non-NHS staff working in health care settings, such as hospital social workers or teachers in hospital schools, are subject to similar duties of confidence, as are social services staff and those of other caring agencies.

[13] In general the NHS should treat in confidence information about **deceased patients**, though the needs of relatives for certain information may require particular attention and sensitivity. Death certificates are not confidential. A deceased person's date and place of death are recorded on the NHS Central Index (see paragraph 3.6).

the purposes for which they hold personal information, sources and disclosures. It is a criminal offence to hold or disclose information in breach of the registration requirements of the Act.

Responsibility for passing on information

4.3 NHS bodies (and others performing NHS functions) are accountable for their decisions to pass on information. Such decisions should usually be taken by the health professional responsible for a patient's care and treatment or on the advice of a nominated senior professional within that body. Only the minimum identifiable information should be used: see paragraph 4.5.

4.4 If a patient wants information withheld from someone who might otherwise have received it in connection with his or her care or treatment, the patient should be informed of any health or social care implications or of other relevant factors (*eg* the importance for the patient of the long-term record held by the GP). The patient's wishes should be respected unless, as, for example, at paragraphs 5.2–7, there are overriding considerations to the contrary. The reason for not passing on information must be noted.

Non-identifiable information

Anonymised information

4.5 Where anonymised information[14] *would be sufficient for a particular purpose,* identifiable information should be omitted wherever possible. In that event, all reasonable steps must be taken to ensure that the recipient is unable to trace the patient's identity[15]. However, the fact that information has been anonymised **does not of itself remove the duty of confidence. It may still be passed on but only for a justifiable purpose.** The removal of personal details may in any case be insufficient to protect a patient's identity: for example, in some instances where the information relates to rare conditions, other characteristics or maybe to particular units or areas of the country.

Aggregated information

4.6 Making available aggregated information about performance and activity in the NHS is an important aspect

of accountability and a means of fostering public awareness of how taxpayers' money is spent and the range of services provided. Aggregated information is also vital for much research and development (see paragraph 4.20) and for certain pharmaceutical and other health-related purposes. However, aggregating selective information about a small number of patients may not always safeguard confidence adequately. Those with control of the information must make a judgement, taking into account clinical and other relevant considerations[16], as to the point at which aggregated material on its own cannot be regarded as personal and identifiable "patient information". In these circumstances, **provided that patients in general are made aware that personal information may be used to prepare statistics to support the sort of purposes at paragraph 1.2**, the aggregated information may be used or passed on for those purposes. *The Department of Health is giving further consideration to the use of aggregated or anonymised information.*

If confidence is breached

4.7 The unauthorised passing on of patient information by any member of staff or person in contract with the NHS is a serious matter, always warranting consideration of disciplinary action and possibly risking legal action by others. In addition health professionals may be subject to action by their regulatory bodies. **In their own interests and those of patients, all staff must be made aware of the possibly severe consequences of breaching patient confidence. NHS bodies are strongly advised to include a duty of confidence requirement in employment contracts or other documents setting out terms and conditions.** Staff should be assured that this is not intended to detract from the general climate of openness in the NHS and that, subject to their duty of confidence to patients, they have both rights and responsibilities to raise concerns about health care issues: see NHS Executive (1993) *Guidance for staff on relations with the public and the media.* Staff newly recruited, especially administrative staff who may need to see confidential information, should have their attention drawn to the NHS body's policies and procedures for protecting patient information.

4.8 Patients who feel that confidence has been breached may want to use the NHS complaints procedures,[17] which

---

[14] "Anonymised information" refers here to that from which a person's identity and other identifying details have been removed. "Aggregated information" (see paragraph 4.6), usually statistics, is compiled from personal information relating to a number of patients.

[15] There may be some circumstances (*eg* the surveillance of some rare conditions) in which, while it is necessary to be able to trace a patient, the removal or coding of his or her name or some other identifying features can provide an additional degree of confidentiality.

[16] Such as the type of information, size of the sample, degree of difficulty or means of identifying individuals, other relevant information to which recipients or a wider audience may have access, and economic, social or cultural factors.

[17] See interim guidance on new arrangements from 1 April 1996 in EL(95) 121.

will be published In March 1996, or those of professional bodies. They have a right under the *Patient's Charter* to be told how to complain or how to make comments or suggestions[18]. In the case of computerised information there is a statutory right to complain to the Data Protection Registrar (see DPR leaflet, *Your Complaint: What happens when you complain to the Data Protection Registrar*), as well as rights to take action for compensation if the individual has been damaged[19] and to have inaccurate personal information corrected or erased.

Patients unable to give consent

4.9 As the law stands[20], nobody is empowered to give consent on behalf of an adult. However, if a patient is unconscious or unable due to his or her mental or physical condition to give informed consent or to communicate a decision, decisions to pass on information will in practice usually be taken by the health professionals concerned, taking into account the patient's best interests and, as necessary, the views of relatives or carers. Such circumstances will usually arise when a patient has been unable to give informed consent to treatment. An earlier refusal to particular information being passed on, given while a patient had the capacity to decide, should, unless there are overriding considerations to the contrary, be regarded as decisive in circumstances similar to those envisaged by the patient.

Children and young people

4.10 **Young people aged 16 or 17** are regarded as adults for purposes of consent to treatment and are therefore entitled to the same duty of confidence as adults. **Children under 16** who have the capacity and understanding to take decisions about their own treatment are entitled also to decide whether personal information may be passed on and generally to have their confidence respected (*eg* they may be receiving treatment or counselling about which they do not wish their parents to know[21]). In other

instances, decisions to pass on personal information may be taken by a person with parental responsibility in consultation with the health professionals involved.

4.11 In **child protection** cases the overriding principle is to secure the best interests of the child. Therefore, if a health professional (or other member of staff) has knowledge of abuse or neglect it may be necessary to share this with others on a strictly controlled basis so that decisions relating to the child's welfare can be taken in the light of all relevant information[22].

Security measures

4.12 Ensuring the security and accuracy of patient information is a responsibility of management and staff at all levels: see NHS Executive (1992) *Information Systems Security: Top level policy for the NHS*. In particular:

i **arrangements for the storage and disposal of all patient information (both manually recorded and computer based) must protect confidentiality**;

ii **under the Data Protection Act security measures must be in place to protect computerised information.** Measures to protect information on the **NHS-wide networking system** are set out in EL(95) 108. The *NHS Security Reference Manual* (1996) contains further advice on computer security.

iii **care should be taken to ensure that unintentional breaches of confidence do not occur:** for example, by not leaving files, fax machines or computer terminals unattended, double-checking to avoid transmitting information to the wrong person, not allowing sensitive conversations to be overheard, and guarding against people seeking information by deception[23];

iv **where a non-NHS agency or individual is contracted to carry out NHS functions, the contract must draw attention to obligations on confidentiality** and require that patient information is:

a. treated and stored according to specified security standards; and

b. used only for purposes consistent with the terms of the contract.

Action in the event of confidence being breached (*eg* termination of contract) should be specified.

---

[18] The NHS complaints procedure should apply equally to services provided under contract to the NHS. Paragraph 4.12(iv) below emphasises that contracts with non-NHS agencies must include obligations on confidentiality.

[19] *i.e.* by inaccurate personal data or by loss or unauthorised destruction or disclosure of personal data: see DPR *Guideline* 5.

[20] Law Commission report 231 (1995) made proposals on decision-making for people who are mentally incapacitated. The Government announced in January 1996 that it did not intend to enact the Commission's draft Bill on mental incapacity as it stood but would issue a consultation document.

[21] In *Gillick* v *West Norfolk and Wisbech Health Authority [1986] AC 112* it was held that, where a child is under 16 but has sufficient understanding in relation to the proposed treatment to give (or withhold) consent, his or her consent (or refusal) should be respected. However, the child should be encouraged to involve parents or other legal guardians.

[22] See, *eg*, DH/BMA/Conference of Medical Royal Colleges (1994) *Child Protection: Medical Responsibilities*, section 4; UKCC, *Confidentiality: an elaboration of clause 9 of the second edition of the UKCC's Code of Professional Conduct for the Nurse, Midwife and Health Visitor*.

[23] Depending on the circumstances, such deception may well be a criminal and/or civil offence. Impersonating a medical practitioner is an offence under s.49 of the Medical Act 1983.

4.13 There are stipulated periods for which personal health records should be retained before being considered for destruction. A minimum of eight years is the general rule for hospital and community health services (see HC(89)20), but there are exceptions: maternity records should be retained for at least 25 years (HSG(94)11), those relating to patients under 18 at least until their 25th birthday (or 26th if a record was made when they were 17), and some mental health records for 20 years after care or treatment has ended[24]. EC guidance is that patient records used in connection with clinical trials should be kept for at least 15 years[25]. GP records should be retained for a minimum of 10 years (FHSL(34)30).

Coordinating care with social services and other agencies

4.14 In all areas of health and social care the various agencies involved, including the NHS, should be aiming to deliver a "seamless" service. In some instances particular agencies have a statutory obligation to assist each other or to work together[26]. Essential patient information must therefore be able to pass between the NHS, local authority social services and other services (such as housing, education, voluntary or independent bodies) where those agencies are contributing to or planning a programme of care, or where one may need to be initiated. The patient needs to be aware that some information sharing will be necessary and this can usually be discussed with him or her as part of the care planning process[27].

4.15 If the patient raises any objections, the possible consequences for a coordinated care programme should be explained and assurances given that other agencies would

---

[24] Records relating to patients who are mentally disordered within the meaning of the Mental Health Act 1983 should be retained for at least 20 years "from the date at which, in the opinion of the doctor concerned, the disorder has ceased or diminished to the point where no further care or treatment is considered necessary" (HC(89)20, paragraph 16 and Corrigenda).

[25] Note for Guidance: Good Clinical Practice for Trials on Medicinal Products in the European Community, section 3.17 (see *Pharmacology & Toxicology* 1990, **67**, 361–72).

[26] For example, the Children Act 1989, s.27 (local and health authorities), Education Act 1993, s.166 (education, health and local authorities), Mental Health Act 1983, s.117 (health and local authorities) and National Health Service Act 1977, s.22 (health, local and family health services authorities to cooperate to secure and advance the health and welfare of people in England and Wales).

[27] Complementary advice on handling patient information in cases of **severe mental illness** is given in Department of Health (1995) *Building Bridges*. The inclusion of a patient on a supervision register is of itself subject to the same considerations as patient information generally.

receive only information which they really need to know. However, as at paragraph 4.4, the patient's ultimate decision should be respected unless there are overriding considerations to the contrary: for example, in some cases involving a history of violence, or where an elderly frail person shows signs of non-accidental injury, it may be justifiable to pass information to another agency without his or her agreement (see paragraph 5.6).

4.16 When creating inter-agency registers or pooling information to assist joint commissioning of services, NHS (and other) bodies should ensure that patients know in general terms what is being done and to whom information may be passed: see paragraph 3.1.

Patients who are offenders

4.17 The Health Care Service for Prisoners, the probation service, police and other criminal justice agencies may be involved in the assessment and care (or continuing care following discharge from hospital or release from prison) of patients who have committed offences or have otherwise been involved with those agencies. This often applies to **mentally disordered offenders** and others with similar needs, including people seen by NHS or multi-agency assessment teams before or as a result of a court appearance. There should be agreed liaison arrangements which:

i as with links between health and social services, enable the passage of essential information between agencies that patients know are contributing to their care and support;

ii can handle sensitively the passing on of information that (as described in section 5) may be required by court order or can be justified to protect the public;

iii ensure that information passed on is used only for an authorised purpose;

Patients receiving social security benefits

4.18 HSG(94)8 asks hospital staff to notify local Benefit Agency offices when a patient receiving any social security benefit has been in hospital for four weeks. This is because benefit may need to be reduced after six weeks as an in-patient. The patient's consent must be obtained before such information is passed on.

Protecting public health

4.19 The surveillance of **communicable diseases** is essential to maintain high levels of disease prevention, to detect outbreaks and to inform and evaluate immunisation and other policies. This is dependent on the flow of information on a "need to know" basis between health professionals, microbiologists, Consultants in Communicable Disease Control (CCDCs), the Public Health Laboratory

Service and local authority Environmental Health Officers. Local authorities have particular responsibilities under the **Public Health (Control of Disease) Act 1984** and **Public Health (Infectious Diseases) Regulations 1988**, certain diseases being specifically "notifiable" by doctors to the "proper officer" of the authority, who is usually the CCDC. Staff must be reminded of these duties annually: see HSG(93)56[28]

Teaching and research

4.20 Advice to patients about the use of personal information must emphasise:

i the importance of teaching and research to the maintenance and improvement of care within the NHS, inter-agency care and public health generally;

ii that such information, anonymised or aggregated wherever possible, may sometimes be used for teaching and research (and that universities or other bodies carrying out approved research are required to treat it in confidence and must not use it for other purposes);

iii that any research proposals involving access to patient records require clearance by the relevant Local Research Ethics Committee[29], which must be satisfied in particular that:

  a arrangements to safeguard confidentiality are satisfactory;

  b any additional conditions relating to the use of information that the LREC thinks are necessary can be met;

  c any application to use *identifiable* patient information is fully justified: for example, because this is essential to a study of major importance to public health. If not, approval to proceed would not be given;

iv that their specific consent will be sought to any activity relating to teaching or research that would involve them personally;

v that any published research findings will not identify them without their specific agreement.

---

[28] See also paragraphs 5.2–3 and 5.6. Relevant responsibilities under the Public Health Act (Control of Diseases) Act 1984 outweigh the common law duty of confidence and are excluded from the provisions of the Data Protection Act.

[29] There are a few established exceptions to this practice, such as national morbidity surveys and post-marketing drug surveillance surveys using cohorts of at least 10,000 patients: see *Local Research Ethics Committees* (DH, 1991), paragraph 3.14 and Appendix A. LREC approval is not required for epidemiological surveys conducted for the purpose of communicable disease surveillance and control.

Particular restrictions on passing on information

4.21 NHS bodies or those carrying out NHS functions must not allow personal details of patients (most obviously names and addresses or the medical condition of named individuals) to be passed on or sold for fundraising or commercial marketing purposes.

4.22 There are some statutory restrictions on the disclosure of information relating to **HIV** and **AIDS**, other **sexually transmitted diseases, assisted conception** and **abortion**: see *Annex C*.[30]

Chapter 5

Passing on information for other purposes or as a legal requirement

Relatives, friends and carers

5.1 The *Patient's Charter* states that "if you agree, you can expect your relatives and friends to be kept up to date with the progress of your treatment". With the patient's consent, the significant role of carers may need to be recognised in the type of information provided: for example, on discharge from hospital and to make arrangements for continuing care.

Statutory requirements

5.2. In certain instances an NHS body or member of staff may have a statutory responsibility to pass on patient information. If so, prior consultation with the patient is not required. However, if the health professionals responsible for his or her care are not those required to pass on the information, the former should usually be consulted as to whether the clinical facts do indeed mean that disclosure is necessary. If in doubt, legal advice should be sought. The patient and relevant health professional should be informed as soon as possible that information has been passed on, and a note made in the patient's record.

5.3. The majority of statutory requirements concern forms of notification: for example, of births and deaths[31], communicable disease (see paragraph 4.18), abortion (Annex C),

---

[30] In the case of AIDS/HIV and other sexually transmitted diseases, these do not prevent the passage of essential information to Consultants in Communicable Disease Control.

[31] National Health Service Act 1977, s.124, and Regulations (1982 SI No 286).

substance misuse[32] and serious accidents[33]. There are also certain obligations to pass on information under the **Mental Health Act 1983**[34].

Litigation

5.4 The High Court has statutory powers to order:
  i the disclosure of documents before and during proceedings for personal injury or death;
  ii the production of information to an applicant and his or her legal, medical and professional advisers.

Such orders should specify clearly what information is required and by whom. If any aspect is unclear, clarification and/or legal advice should be sought without delay. The health professionals responsible for a patient's care and treatment should be consulted about the disclosure in case of a risk to the patient's (or someone else's) health. If there is a risk, legal advice should be sought on the possibility of seeking an amendment to the order. Where an order requires information about a patient who has not instigated a court action, that patient should be notified immediately in case he or she wishes to consider an appeal.

5.5 It is well-established practice that, at the patient's request, information relevant to legal proceedings may be released, usually to the patient's legal or medical adviser. The information should also be passed to lawyers acting for the NHS body concerned where the action involves the health authority, Trust or a member of staff. Where health care matters arise the relevant professional (if he or she is not the patient's medical adviser) should be informed and, if necessary, given the opportunity to comment. If the patient agrees, information may also be released to a third party involved in proceedings.

Release of information to protect the public

5.6 It may sometimes be justifiable to pass on patient information without consent or statutory authority. Disclosures for the "discovery of iniquity" are traditionally cited. Most commonly these involve the prevention of serious crime, but can extend to other dangers to the general public, such as a public health risk of violence, where, as already noted, essential information may need to be shared with other agencies[35].

5.7 Each case must be considered on its merits, the main criterion being whether the release of information to protect the public should prevail over the duty of confidence to the patient. The possible therapeutic consequences for the patient must be considered whatever the outcome. Decisions will sometimes be finely balanced and may concern matters on which NHS staff find it difficult to make a judgement. Therefore it may be necessary to seek legal or other specialist advice or to await or seek a court order. It is important not to equate "the public interest" with what may be "of interest" to the public[36].

Tackling serious crime

5.8 Passing on information to help tackle serious crime (see examples at *Annex D*) may be justified if the following conditions are satisfied:
  i without disclosure, the task of preventing, detecting or prosecuting the crime would be seriously prejudiced or delayed;
  ii information is limited to what is strictly relevant to a specific investigation;
  iii there are satisfactory undertakings that the information will not be passed on or used for any purpose other than the present investigation.

5.9 Requests for information relating to a number of patients in order to identify one or more is likely to be justified only if there is a very strong public interest.

Press and broadcasting

5.10 The maintenance of good relations with the press and broadcasting organisations is important. NHS bodies should ensure that someone with suitable experience and level of responsibility is available or contactable at all times to answer enquiries.

5.11 In law the same general rules apply to the passing of personal information to the media as in other circumstances. The patient's consent must therefore be obtained

---

[32] Misuse of Drugs Act 1971, s.10, and Regulations on the Notification of and Supply of Addicts (1973 SI No 799).

[33] In particular under the Health and Safety at Work etc Act 1974, Regulations on the Reporting of Injuries, Diseases and Dangerous Occurrences (1985 SI No 2023 and 1989 No 1457), and the Road Traffic Acts.

[34] S.13(2) (disclosures to and by approved social workers to enable them to assess patients) and provisions relating to relatives and "nearest relatives". S.117 requires health and local authorities to cooperate in the provision of after care services. See *Mental Health Act Code of Practice* (1993) (HSG(93)45).

[35] In practice, the sharing of information on a "need to know" basis to protect the public health can usually be regarded as an "NHS purpose" (as at paragraph 1.2).

[36] See, *eg, Eleventh Report of the Data Protection Registrar* (1995), Appendix 4

if he or she is *capable of taking a decision*. This applies whether or not the patient is a celebrity or public figure.

5.12 Where the patient is *unable to take a decision*, the provision of basic information may sometimes be judged to be in his or her best interests (*eg* by correcting misleading or damaging speculation). Where possible, relatives should be consulted, having regard, of course, to their own feelings and possible distress. For example, where the police have released the names and addresses of accident victims, the practice in most hospitals is to confirm the presence of a patient unless the patient or relatives have requested no publicity. In all such circumstances, **the NHS body must be prepared to justify a decision to release information**, which should usually be confined to a brief indication of progress in terms authorised by the relevant health professional.

5.13 If a patient or former patient has invited the media to report his or her treatment, the NHS body may comment in public, but should confine itself to factual information or the correction of any misleading assertions or published comment. The duty of confidence to the patient still applies. If in doubt, legal advice should be sought.

Department of Health
Health Promotion Division 4
March 1996

Annex A

Specimen notice for patients (see paragraph 3.6)

We *ask* you for information about yourself so that you can receive proper care and treatment.

We *keep* this information, together with details of your care, because it may be needed if we see you again.

We *may use* some of this information for other reasons: for example, to help us protect the health of the public generally and to see that the NHS runs efficiently, plans for the future, trains its staff, pays its bills and can account for its actions. Information may also be needed to help educate tomorrow's clinical staff and to carry out medical and other health research for the benefit of everyone.

Sometimes the law requires us to *pass on* information: for example, to notify a birth.

The NHS Central Register for England & Wales contains basic personal details of all patients registered with a general practitioner. The Register does not contain clinical information.

You have a right of access to your health records.

EVERYONE WORKING FOR THE NHS HAS A LEGAL DUTY TO KEEP INFORMATION ABOUT YOU CONFIDENTIAL.

You may be receiving care from other people as well as the NHS. So that we can all work together for your benefit we may need to share some information about you.

We only ever use or pass on information about you if people have a genuine need for it in your and everyone's interests. Whenever we can we shall remove details which identify you. The sharing of some types of very sensitive personal information is strictly controlled by law.

Anyone who receives information from us is also under a legal duty to keep it confidential.

The main reasons for which your information may be needed are:
- **giving you health care and treatment**
- **looking after the health of the general public**
- **managing and planning the NHS.** For example:
- making sure that our services can meet patient needs in the future
- paying your doctor, nurse, dentist, or other staff, and the hospital which treats you for the care they provide
- auditing accounts
- preparing statistics on NHS performance and activity (where steps will to be taken to ensure you cannot be identified)
- investigating complaints or legal claims
- **helping staff to review the care they provide to make sure it is of the highest standard**
- **training and educating staff** (but you can choose whether or not to be involved personally)
- **research** approved by the Local Research Ethics Committee. (If anything to do with the research would involve you personally, you will be contacted to see if you are willing to take part. You will not be identified in any published results without your agreement.)

If you agree your relatives, friends and carers will be kept up to date with the progress of your treatment.

If at any time you would like to know more about how we use your information you can speak to the person in charge of your care or to ....

Annex B

Data protection ACT 1984: the eight principles* (see paragraph 4.2)

1 The information to be contained in personal data shall be obtained, and personal data shall be processed, fairly and lawfully.
2 Personal data shall be held only for one or more specified lawful purposes.
3 Personal data held for any purpose or purposes shall not be used or disclosed in any manner incompatible with that purpose or purposes.
4 Personal data held for any purpose or purposes shall be adequate, relevant and not excessive in relation to that purpose or purposes.
5 Personal data shall be accurate and, where necessary, kept up to date.
6 Personal data held for any purpose or purposes shall not be kept longer than is necessary for that purpose or those purposes.
7 An individual shall be entitled:
   a at reasonable intervals and without undue delay or expense:
      i to be informed by any data user whether he holds personal data of which the individual is the subject; and
      ii to access to any such data held by a data user; and
   b where appropriate, to have such data corrected or erased.
8 Appropriate security measures shall be taken against unauthorised access to, or alteration, disclosure or destruction of, personal data and against accidental loss or destruction of personal data.

Annex C

Statutory restrictions on passing on information (see paragraph 4.21)

1 The **NHS (Venereal Diseases) Regulations 1974** and the **NHS Trusts (Venereal Diseases) Regulations 1991** prevent the disclosure of any identifying information about a patient with a sexually transmitted disease (including HIV and AIDS) other than to a medical practitioner (or to a person employed under the direction of a medical practitioner) in connection with and for the purpose of the treatment of the patient, or to prevent the spread of the disease. The regulations do **not** prevent the normal notification of other communicable diseases in such patients (as at paragraph 4.18 of the main guidance).
2 The **Human Fertilisation and Embryology Act 1990**, as amended by the **Human Fertilisation and Embryology (Disclosure of Information) Act 1992**, limits the circumstances in which information may be disclosed by centres licensed under the Act: see the Human Fertilisation and Embryology Authority's *Code of Practice* (HFEA, Paxton House, 30 Artillery Lane, London E1 7LS).
3 The **Abortion Regulations 1991**, made under the Abortion Act 1967, limit and define the circumstances in which information submitted under the Act to the Chief Medical Officer may be disclosed.

Annex D

Passing on information in connection with serious crime (see paragraph 5.8)

Passing on information to help prevent, detect or prosecute serious crime may sometimes be justified to protect the public. There is no absolute definition of "serious" crime, but section 116 of the Police and Criminal Evidence Act 1984 identifies some "serious arrestable offences". These include:

treason
murder
manslaughter
rape
kidnapping
certain sexual offences
causing an explosion
certain firearms offences
taking of hostages
hijacking
causing death by reckless driving
offences under prevention of terrorism legislation *(disclosures now covered by the Prevention of Terrorism Act 1989)*

*See Guideline 4 of *The Guidelines* issued by the Data Protection Registrar (3rd series, 1994), pp 51–69 *making a threat which if carried out would be likely to lead to:*

serious threat to the security of the state or to public order serious interference with the administration of justice or with the investigation of an offence death or serious injury substantial financial gain or serious financial loss to any person.

In other cases, it may be as well to seek legal advice before taking a decision to release information.

Produced by Department of Health
10021 HP 7k 1P Feb 97 SA (04)

54

The Caldicott Report on the review of patient-identifiable information – executive summary December 1997

The Caldicott Committee, Department of Health

Executive summary

i) In the light of the requirements in The Protection and Use of Patient Information and taking into account work undertaken by a joint Department of Health (DH) and British Medical Association (BMA) Working Group which has been considering NHS Information Management and Technology (IM&T) security and confidentiality, the Chief Medical Officer established the Caldicott Committee to review all patient-identifiable information which passes from National Health Service (NHS) organisations in England to other NHS or non-NHS bodies for purposes other than direct care, medical research, or where there is a statutory requirement for information.

ii) The purpose was to ensure that patient identifiable information is only transferred for justified purposes and that only the minimum necessary information is transferred in each case. Where appropriate, the Committee was asked to advise whether action to minimise risks of breach of confidentiality would be desirable.

iii) The work of the Committee was carried out in an open and consultative manner. Written submissions were sought from many organisations to identify existing concerns, and members of the Committee have met with representatives of a number of key bodies. Working groups containing a wide range of health professionals and managers were established to consider related groups of information flows and to take soundings on emerging findings.

iv) Some 86 flows of patient-identifiable information were mapped relating to a wide range of planning, operational or monitoring purposes. Some of these flows were exemplars, representing locally diverse information flows with broadly similar characteristics and purposes.

© The Caldicott Committee, Department of Health.

v) The Committee was greatly encouraged to discover that, within the context of current policy, all of the flows identified were for justifiable purposes. However, a number of the flows currently use more patient-identifiable information than is required to satisfy their purposes. Also many of the patient-identifiers currently used (eg name and address) could be omitted if a reliable, but suitably controlled, coded identifier could be used to support identification.

vi) It was recognised that some flows of information were likely to be missed and that flows commence, evolve or are discontinued with such frequency that specific recommendations could soon date. Although specific recommendations have been included where appropriate, in general the recommendations reflect this evolving picture by developing a direction of travel, outlining good practice principles and calling for regular reviews of activity within a clear framework of responsibility.

Summary of recommendations

Recommendation 1: Every dataflow, current or proposed, should be tested against basic principles of good practice. Continuing flows should be re-tested regularly.

Recommendation 2: A programme of work should be established to reinforce awareness of confidentiality and information security requirements amongst all staff within the NHS.

Recommendation 3: A senior person, preferably a health professional, should be nominated in each health organisation to act as a guardian, responsible for safeguarding the confidentiality of patient information.

Recommendation 4: Clear guidance should be provided for those individuals/bodies responsible for approving uses of patient-identifiable information.

Recommendation 5: Protocols should be developed to protect the exchange of patient-identifiable information between NHS and non-NHS bodies.

Recommendation 6: The identity of those responsible for monitoring the sharing and transfer of information within agreed local protocols should be clearly communicated.

Recommendation 7: An accreditation system which recognises those organisations following good practice with respect to confidentiality should be considered.

Recommendation 8: The NHS number should replace other identifiers wherever practicable, taking account of the consequences of errors and particular requirements for other specific identifiers.

Recommendation 9: Strict protocols should define who is authorised to gain access to patient identity where the NHS number or other coded identifier is used.

Recommendation 10: Where particularly sensitive information is transferred, privacy enhancing technologies (e.g. encrypting identifiers or "patient identifying information") must be explored.

Recommendation 11: Those involved in developing health information systems should ensure that best practice principles are incorporated during the design stage.

Recommendation 12: Where practicable, the internal structure and administration of databases holding patient-identifiable information should reflect the principles developed in this report.

Recommendation 13: The NHS number should replace the patient's name on Items of Service Claims made by General Practitioners as soon as practically possible.

Recommendation 14: The design of new systems for the transfer of prescription data should incorporate the principles developed in this report.

Recommendation 15: Future negotiations on pay and conditions for General Practitioners should, where possible, avoid systems of payment which require patient identifying details to be transmitted.

Recommendation 16: Consideration should be given to procedures for General Practice claims and payments which do not require patient-identifying information to be transferred, which can then be piloted.

Published by The Department of Health
© Crown Copyright 2001

Further information on Patient Confidentiality and Caldicott Guardians can be found on the following website:

http://www.doh.gov.uk/ipu/confiden/index.htm

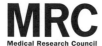
Personal information in medical research

Medical Research Council, 2000

Personal information in medical research

The MRC working group which prepared this guidance comprised:

Professor Andy Haines (Chair, Dept of Primary Care & Population Sciences, Royal Free & University College Medical School)
Dr Richard Ashcroft (University of Bristol / Imperial College School of Medicine)
Dr David Coggon (MRC Environmental Epidemiology Unit)
Dr Angela Coulter (The King's Fund/Picker Institute Europe)
Professor Len Doyal (Queen Mary & Westfield College)
Dr Elaine Gadd (Dept of Health)
Professor Charles Gillis (Dept of Public Health, University of Glasgow)
Dr Naomi Pfeffer (Consumers for Ethics in Research/ University of North London)
Professor Michael Wadsworth (MRC National Survey of Health & Development)
Mr Philip Walker (NHS Executive)
Mrs Madeleine Wang (Northern & Yorkshire Multi-Centre Research Ethics Committee)
Professor Simon Wessely (Dept of Psychological Medicine, Institute of Psychiatry)

Office staff
Dr Declan Mulkeen
Dr Imogen Evans
Dr Jenny Baverstock (2000)
Mr Stéphane Goldstein (1999)

Updates to this guidance are available on MRC's website: **www.mrc.ac.uk**
© 2000 Medical Research Council. October 2000.
Copies available from MRC External Communications **020 7636 5422**

Contents

Glossary

Personal information, as used in this guide, refers to all information about individuals, living or dead. This includes written and electronic records, opinions, images, recordings, and information obtained from samples. Although anonymised data is not, strictly speaking, personal information, its use is also covered in this guide.

Personal data, in the context of the 1998 Data Protection Act (Section 3.2, and Annex 3), comprise information about living people who can be identified from the data, or from combinations of the data and other information which the person in control of the data has, or is likely to have in future.

Anonymised data, are data prepared from personal information, but from which the person cannot be identified by the recipient of the information (see Sections 5.1–5.7). The term is used in the guide when referring to linked and unlinked anonymised data together.
  • **Linked Anonymised** data is anonymous to the people who receive and hold it (e.g. a research team), but contains information or codes that would allow others (e.g. those responsible for the individual's care) to identify people from it.
  • **Unlinked Anonymised data** contains no information that could reasonably be used, by anyone, to identify people.

Coded data is identifiable personal information in which the details that could identify people are concealed in a code, but which can be readily decoded by those using it. It is not "anonymised data" (see Section 5.2).

Confidential information is any information obtained by a person on the understanding that they will not disclose it to others, or obtained in circumstances where it is expected that they will not disclose it. The law assumes that whenever people give **personal information** to health professionals caring for them, it is confidential as long as it remains personally identifiable.

Sensitive information. The term "sensitive" is used in this guide to highlight the need for extra care in using information about mental health, sexuality and other areas where revealing confidential information is especially likely to cause embarrassment or discrimination. Note that "sensitive personal data" is defined in the 1998 Data Protection Act as including all information about physical or mental health or condition, or sexual life (Annex 3(B)).

1 Introduction

Much medical research revolves around information about people – their age, lifestyle, work, and health – drawn from medical records, scientific tests, surveys and interviews. Sometimes, the information also reveals facts about relatives and relationships. These types of information are sensitive and private for many people, although attitudes and expectations vary widely.

Respect for private life is a human right, and the ability to discuss information in confidence with others is rightly valued. Keeping control over facts about one's self can have an important role in a person's sense of security, freedom of action, and self respect. It can also protect against unfair discrimination.

The confidentiality of information patients give to doctors is central to the doctor-patient relationship, and to the public's trust in health care professions. There is little research evidence on how people view the use of this confidential information. The limited evidence available suggests that when asked, the vast majority are willing for information about them to be passed to others, under tight controls, if it will advance medical practice. But many people will not know how information about them might be used, and many others may not even know the sort of information that is contained in their medical records.

Although caution is therefore needed in using any personal medical information, this must be balanced against the potential for improving the quality of care by improving the flows of information within the health care system. At present, compared with what might be achieved:
  • information is fragmented, and too difficult to share. It is always difficult to build up a complete picture of the care and treatment people receive – from their GP and in hospital – in order to question whether this could be improved.

- information is often incomplete, and some activities are better documented than others. The results of hospital care tend to be well recorded, while the results of home care or preventive medicine are more difficult to measure and record.
- the information that is available is not analysed fully. Research into the effectiveness of the health services, and into factors affecting the health of people in the UK needs to be strengthened if we are to continue improving the health of the nation.

Medical Research Council staff and grantholders make widespread use of personal data in clinical research, in clinical trials, epidemiology, and other public health research. In 1972, the MRC set out its views on the conditions under which information about identifiable patients could be obtained and used in research. More detailed guidance was issued in 1985 and 1994. Since 1972, medical research based on records and surveys has led to many important advances in knowledge in the UK, including:

- recognition of new variant CJD and its relation to the BSE epidemic;
- improvements in the organisation and quality of cancer treatment;
- better understanding of suspected health hazards for example, Gulf War related illness and leukaemia in people living near to nuclear facilities;
- reliable evaluations of new preventive measures and treatments – for example, the benefits to people at risk of heart disease from aspirin, warfarin, cholesterol lowering drugs and vitamins;
- ways of reducing cot deaths;
- assessments of the health care needs of special groups in society, such as elderly people;
- identification of adverse drug reactions.

Over the same period, there have been no cases where doctors following these guidelines have been judged in law to have breached confidentiality. But some people involved in research do take exception to the way information about them is used, and many people have strong, general, concerns about the way public and private organisations use personal data.

From time to time, therefore, we have to ask whether the standards that researchers set reflect those society currently expects of us. Many people have a concern that modern information and communication technologies might lead to more casual, or frequent, infringements of privacy. And most people now expect the medical professions, and medical researchers, to be more open and accountable in their work, and to allow individuals more opportunity to be involved in decisions that affect them.

The last few years have also seen active discussion of the implications of the law on data protection for the use of confidential information in research. In 1998, the legal situation changed, with the passing of a new Data Protection Act, and a Human Rights Act guaranteeing respect for citizens' private lives.

Reflecting these changes, this booklet sets out the ethical and legal principles that should now guide the use of personal information in research, and provides a revised code of practice. It supersedes the guidance in the MRC ethics booklet *Responsibility in the use of Personal Medical Information for Research* (1994) and the relevant sections of the booklet *Responsibility in Investigations on Human Participants and Material and on Personal Information* (1992).

The NHS information strategy

At the time of writing, work is under way on an ambitious programme of changes in the NHS, including creating lifelong electronic health records for every person in the country, improved sharing and movement of information through an NHS information highway, and more effective use of information to inform NHS management. The strategy creates important opportunities to make some medical research easier and more effective, and to address some of the current concerns around the use of medical information in research. For example, it may become possible to widen the range of anonymised information that is available and useful for research. The strategy will also create new opportunities for health professionals and researchers to engage with members of the public to explain why information sharing is necessary. Researchers need to work with commitment and foresight to make the most of these long-term opportunities. At the same time, it has to be remembered that information systems designed to support routine health care cannot always be expected to provide the range or quality of information needed for original research.

The status of the guidance

This guidance is primarily for researchers supported by MRC, who are expected to follow it as a condition of funding. The guidance is prescriptive wherever this is appropriate, but like any code of practice, it cannot provide for every possible situation, and exceptions to the general rules will occasionally arise.

We hope that in addition the guidance will be informative and helpful to other researchers, to doctors and other health professionals whose patients' records may be involved in such research, to ethics committees, to others reviewing or supervising research, and to the public.

Scope

This guidance covers all uses of personal information whether or not it is "personal data" under the terms of the Data Protection Act, and whether or not it is confidential (see Glossary). Section 2 summarises the key principles that should guide ethical research, both in general situations, and in situations where research depends on using information without consent. Section 3 outlines the laws relating to confidentiality and personal information, how these relate to ethical principles, and discusses the areas where changes in practice may be needed. Section 4 analyses how the key principles should be applied in situations where consent can, and cannot be obtained. Sections 5, 6 and 7 give detailed advice on good practice, and are relevant to all research using personal information.

The guidance addresses the main uses of this information in medical research, including:

- collection of information as part of clinical trials or other patient-based research;
- use of information from general practice or hospital records to approach people to participate in studies;
- analysing patterns of disease and treatment outcomes from existing records;
- studying the health of people in a particular locality, or with a particular job or lifestyle.

The question of confidentiality often receives most attention in epidemiological or survey work when information is taken from medical records without the person's knowledge or consent, **but** researchers in every area of clinical and public health research need to respect confidentiality and protect the individual's interests by guarding against accidental or mischievous disclosures, and ensuring the information is not used in ways which could cause distress or harm.

Research use of tissue samples or DNA samples in conjunction with personal data raises special issues since:

- clinical samples, including stored blood, plasma and serum will often be used to answer questions unforeseen at the time they were collected;
- genetic analyses can reveal new information about an individual, their family members or raise concerns about insurance. Particular care needs to be taken when feeding back information and in the publication of material;
- this information raises special concerns when it is, or is seen as being, predictive of future health;
- some types of genetics research give rise to particular concern – for instance research relating to personality or cognitive function.

Samples, and the information obtained from them, cannot be treated in the same way as other data, and are the subject of separate MRC guidance *Collections of Human Tissue and Biological Samples for use in research.*

Disease registries often provide the starting points for research, and are an essential resource for improving the quality of health services. The NHS Plan[1] published in July 2000 recognises the importance of registries in improving disease management. The House of Commons Science and Technology Committee report "Cancer research – a fresh look"[2] underlined the importance of registries, and the impracticability of only using information in registries with express consent. Because registries are often established for purposes other than research, and because of their diversity, this guidance does not offer detailed advice on good practice. However, we would expect the general principles set out in Section 2 – such as the need to make people aware of how their information may be used – and much of the advice in Sections 5 through 7, to be applicable to research based on disease registries, and to registries maintained solely for research purposes.

Also, while we recognise that it is sometimes difficult to define clear boundaries between research and audit, this guide does not attempt to offer a code of practice for the wide range of activities and situations included in clinical audit. However, we hope that the advice will be helpful to some of those working in audit.

The guidance does not address in detail the question of consent to use information about children, or adults who are incapable of giving consent. Separate MRC ethics booklets give advice on research involving children (1991) and mentally incapacitated adults (1991). The ethical and legal issues in these areas have been actively discussed over the past ten years, and the Scottish Parliament has recently passed the Adults with Incapacity (Scotland) Act (2000), which creates a new framework for consent to research. New guidance will be prepared.

Updates and changes

MRC will keep this guidance under review. The law on confidentiality does not give specific direction on what can and cannot be done in various situations, but some points of law may be clarified in time. In some areas of work, the need for disclosures without consent should decrease with time.

This guide, and all other MRC ethics guides, are available on MRC's website – at **www.mrc.ac.uk** – and changes will be highlighted there as they arise.

---

[1] www.nhs.uk/nhsplan

[2] House of Commons Science and Technology Committee, Sixth report, Session 1999–2000.

2 Principles

2.1 General principles

The following principles should guide all MRC-funded research involving people or their information:

1 Personal information of any sort which is provided for health care, or obtained in medical research, must be regarded as confidential. Wherever possible people should know how information about them is used, and have a say in how it may be used. Research should therefore be designed to allow scope for consent, and normally researchers must ensure they have each person's explicit consent to obtain, hold, and use personal information. In most clinical research this is practicable.

2 All medical research using identifiable personal information, or using anonymised data from the NHS which is not already in the public domain, must be approved by a Research Ethics Committee.[3]

3 All personal information must be coded or anonymised as far as is possible and consistent with the needs of the study, and as early as possible in the data processing. Only personal identifiers that are essential should be held.

4 Each individual entrusted with patient information is personally responsible for their decisions about disclosing it. Health professionals disclosing information should, in particular, ensure they are familiar with the advice of the General Medical Council on disclosures for research. Health care organisations should be aware of the research conducted within the organisation, and should ensure research teams are accountable to them.

5 Researchers must ensure that personal information is handled only by health professionals or staff with an equivalent duty of confidentiality.

6 Principal investigators must take personal responsibility for ensuring (as far as is reasonably practical) that training, procedures, supervision, and data security arrangements are sufficient to prevent unauthorised breaches of confidentiality.

7 Researchers must also have procedures in place to minimise the risk of causing distress to the people they contact in the course of their research. Researchers must also be aware that, despite their best efforts, occasional untoward events may occur and plan for how to deal with these.

[3] Or, where appropriate, the Scottish Privacy Advisory Committee.

8 At the outset, researchers must decide what information about the results should be available to the people involved in the study once it is complete, and agree these plans with the Research Ethics Committee. However, researchers must also be prepared to reconsider if there are unforeseen findings from the study, and discuss the appropriate response with a research ethics committee.

2.2 Information disclosed without consent

2.2.1 Situations arise in which medical research questions can only be answered using personal medical information, but where it is not feasible for those responsible for the individual's care to contact all the relevant people to seek their consent. Based on the ethical and legal advice it has received (Section 3), the Medical Research Council considers that in some circumstances it is justifiable to use personal information, and disclose it to a limited number of other people, without consent.

2.2.2 The principles governing research using information without consent are:

1 Hospitals and practices involved in research must *develop* procedures for making patients aware that their information may sometimes be used for research, and explaining the reasons and safeguards. If patients object to their information being passed to others, patients should have the opportunity to discuss this with their doctor, and their objections must be respected.

2 When consent is impracticable confidential information can only be disclosed without consent only if:
   • the likely benefits to society outweigh the implications of the loss of confidentiality, so that it is clearly in the public interest for the research to be done;
   • there is no intention to feed information back to the individuals involved or take decisions that affect them, and;
   • there are no practicable alternatives of equal effectiveness.

Research must have been planned with confidentiality in mind: from the earliest stages of planning a study, researchers and/or those responsible for patient care should have given careful consideration to whether consent could be made practicable. The judgement that consent is impracticable is never that of the researcher alone: unless an ethics committee concurs, and health professionals agree to participate in the study on this basis, the research cannot take place.

3 The infringement of confidentiality must be kept to a minimum. Even where there is a strong justification for the study, the design must minimise the volume and

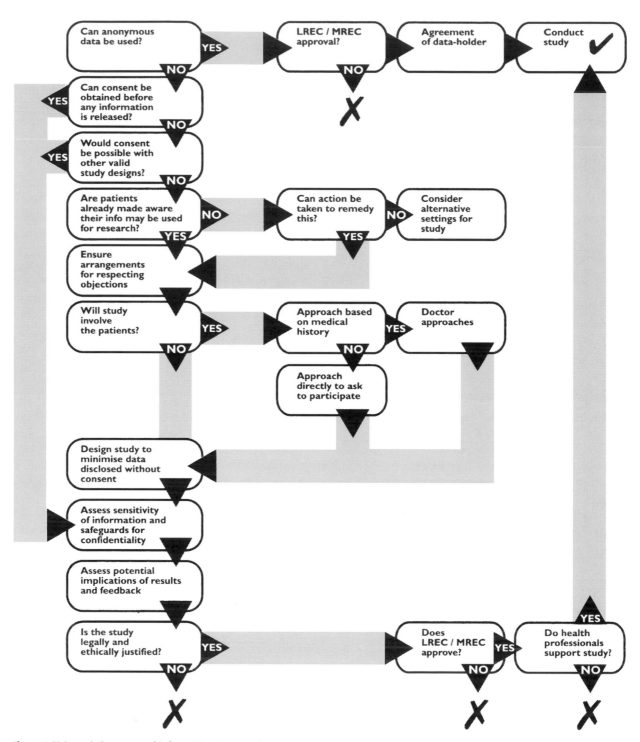

Figure 1 Using existing personal information in research
A simplified decision tree

sensitivity of the personal information that is disclosed, and the number of people who have access to it before it is coded or anonymised. If the disclosure made is to allow researchers to contact people, consent should be obtained then to gather the further information needed, and to hold and process their information.

2.2.3 The diversity of medical research makes it impossible to be prescriptive about the interpretation of these principles. Final decisions on the value *and* acceptability of a research protocol have to lie with the researchers, the health professionals, and the ethics committee involved, and the organisations which are responsible for supporting and overseeing the work.[4] When considering whether disclosures are justified, one useful aid to thinking might be to ask whether, if the proposed disclosure and the reasons for it became widely known, a reasonable person would see it as unacceptable. A second, narrower test might be to ask whether there are any grounds for supposing that, if consent could be sought effectively, people would be likely to refuse to allow their records to be used.

2.2.4 The conditions in which consent might be practical or impractical, ways of reducing the need for disclosures without consent, and the provision of advance information, are discussed further in sections 3 and 4.

3 The law as a guide to good practice

3.1 Confidentiality in law

3.1.1 In the UK, the confidentiality of personal information is addressed primarily in Common Law. The Data Protection Act 1998 superimposes on this a framework of rights and duties and principles governing the use of information in electronic form or structured paper records. These are discussed below, and Sections 3.3 to 3.6 consider how compliance with the law relates to ethical research practice.

3.1.2 In Common Law, anyone who receives information must respect its confidentiality (that is, not disclose it without consent or other strong justification) if they receive it on the understanding that it is confidential, or in circumstances where there is an implicit expectation that they will not reveal it to anyone else. But while Common Law establishes some core principles, it does not specify when confidential information may or may not be disclosed to others, in research or most other activities. Individuals and organisations using confidential information have to take

responsibility for deciding what is justified and acceptable on a case by case basis.

3.1.3 Common Law enshrines the principle that to disclose confidential information about a living person without consent is, generally speaking, to wrong an individual. In law, any information doctors have about their patients must be regarded as confidential, even addresses that might be publicly available elsewhere (for instance, in the electoral register), because the information is given in the expectation that it will not be passed on. Disclosing confidential personal information does not have to cause direct harm or distress for it to be unlawful – any unjustified use of confidential information that weakens trust in the doctor-patient relationship could also be seen as actionable.[5]

3.1.4 However, Common Law also recognises that it can be in the public interest for doctors to disclose confidential personal information, and that the nature and scale of the disclosure has to be balanced against the benefits to society. Interpretations of this balancing judgement vary, and there are few court rulings relevant to the sorts of limited disclosures involved in research. The legal advice to MRC is that the legality of using confidential information in research without consent, could only be judged on a case by case basis, taking into account:

- **necessity** – were there alternative, practicable, ways of conducting the study, which would have allowed consent to be obtained? Could anonymous data have been used?
- **sensitivity** – how much did the information reveal about the individual, and was it particularly likely to lead to worry or distress, or damage the doctorpatient relationship?
- **importance** – was the research well designed, and likely to make a significant contribution to knowledge in the area?
- **safeguards** – was the amount of information disclosed as small as possible? Were all reasonable steps taken to guard against unintended leaks of information and to maintain trust? Was the risk that the study or its findings might cause distress minimised?
- **independent review** – was the justification for the research reviewed by a Research Ethics Committee?
- **expectations** – if explicit consent was not possible, were there reasonable efforts to make people involved aware of how medical records were used, so they had an opportunity to raise any special concerns?

---

[4] Principally, the bodies employing researchers, such as MRC, Universities, NHS Trusts.

[5] That is, a person might have grounds for taking legal action against the person who disclosed it.

Since anonymised data derived from medical records is no longer information about identifiable people, disclosing it does not breach the duty of confidence to the patient, and these tests do not need to be applied.

3.1.5 Despite the fact that research projects may have been approved by a Research Ethics Committee, and authorised by a Health Authority or Trust, individual doctors remain accountable for their use of their patients' information. The same applies to those who receive confidential information: members of a research team must always be aware that they share a similar duty of confidence to doctors, and that revealing any personal information they hold without good reason – whether resulting from neglect, ignorance, or malice – is potentially actionable.

3.1.6 This is a controversial area of law, and MRC is aware that there are other interpretations of Common Law, some of which would argue for freer use of personal records, and some which hold that the public interest can only justify disclosing confidential information where there is an extraordinary threat to the health of the nation or individuals. MRC has sought to base its guidance on a position that can command broad support, and is consistent with the policies of the Department of Health[6] and General Medical Council.[7]

3.2 The Data Protection Act, the Human Rights Act and other statutory regulations

3.2.1 The UK's 1984 Data Protection Act, and the 1998 Data Protection Act, which replaces it, are both based on the concept of "fair processing". The main principles in the law are explained in Annex 3, but in brief, fair processing means that an individual should normally have the opportunity to know what organisations hold information about them, and why. When people give information, they should be told what it will be used for and to whom it will be passed. They will also be entitled to check records held about them and correct errors.

3.2.2 The Act covers only "personal data", which comprises information about living people who can be identified from the data, or identified from combinations of the data and other information which the person in control of the data is likely to have, either now, or at some future time. Data

which have previously been anonymised are outside the scope of the Act.

3.2.3 The law recognises that research needs special freedom to use information in ways not foreseen when it was first collected, and to archive and re-use data. Research work that is not used as a basis for decisions affecting the individuals involved, and which is unlikely to lead to substantial damage or distress, is given special exemptions in these areas (see Annex 3).

3.2.4 The law also sets conditions on when "sensitive personal data", such as information about health, religion, or ethnicity, can be processed. One condition is that the use of the data is necessary for medical purposes, (which are taken to include medical research and the management of healthcare services), *and* the processing is done by a health professional or a person with an equivalent duty of confidentiality. This condition is in addition to the need to conform to Common Law, and to other sections of the Data Protection Act.

3.2.5 Despite the exemptions mentioned above, the Act is important for research. Fair processing requires that when Health Authorities, hospitals, and doctors know patient information will probably be used for specific research projects, at the time it is collected, they must tell patients this. Health professionals and researchers must give careful thought to whether their use of information might cause substantial damage or distress. Information gathered primarily for research but which will also be used to inform clinical decisions, or which will result in individuals receiving significant new health information about themselves, must comply with every part of the Act.

3.2.6 The Human Rights Act (1998) (Annex 4) established the European Convention on Human Rights as part of UK law. This guarantees the right to respect for private and family life. The body of legal work on the interpretation of this right is still growing, but MRC's legal advice is that, like Common law, it provides for judgements on the balance between the rights of the individual and the legitimate needs of society.

3.2.7 Other relevant statutory regulations are listed and summarised at Annex 5.

Information about dead people, and historical records
3.2.8 The Data Protection Act does not apply to information about a person who is dead before the information is disclosed. Common Law on confidentiality, similarly, is not normally held to apply to information about dead people, although this is a grey area of the law. However, if the use of information about a dead person intruded on the privacy of their relatives – for example, because it revealed

---

[6] Health Service Guidance (96) 18 "The Protection and Use of Patient Information". Department of Health, March 1996.

[7] "Confidentiality: Protecting and Providing Information", GMC June 2000.

[8] See, for example, Canada's Tri-Council Policy Statement *Ethical Conduct for Research Involving Humans* (1998); New Zealand Health Information Privacy Code (1994).

Table 55.1. Controls on the use of information in medical research

	TYPE					
CONTROLS	**MEDICAL SOURCE**				**NON-MEDICAL SOURCE**	
	Information used in clinical care and research	**Information used in research only**				
		General personal information	Linked anonymised	Unlinked anonymised	Surveys and questionnaires	Research databases
Individual controls use of their information	Yes, if able to consent	Where possible	Where possible	No	Yes	No
Common Law on confidentiality	Yes	Yes	No	No	Yes	Yes
Data Protection Act applies in full	Yes	If results impact on individuals	If results impact on individuals	No	Yes	No
Data Protection Act applies with research exemptions	No	Yes, if no significant feedback	Assume yes, if no significant feedback	No	Yes	Yes
LREC / MREC approval	Yes	Yes	Yes	Yes	Expected*	Expected*

* MRC expects MREC or LREC approval or equivalent.

information about hereditary conditions or transmissible diseases – then the relatives might be able to take action under Human Rights legislation.

3.2.9 All NHS records are covered by the Public Records Act 1958: GPs' records become public records when they are forwarded to the appropriate local authorities after the death of the patient. While most public records are closed for 30 years, all NHS records relating to a person's physical or mental health are closed for 100 years. The few records kept for long term reference or research are fully open to the public after this point. The Public Records Office will sometimes allow bona fide social, historical or medical researchers access to records within this period, if confidentiality can be guaranteed.

3.3 Ethics and the law

3.3.1 The principles and arguments that underlie ethical reasoning about the use of personal information in research

are often broadly consistent with the legal principles discussed above. Interpretations of the law can vary widely, and some interpretations may permit uses of information that are unethical. Therefore, researchers and health professionals should ask first of all whether their actions will reflect ethical and professional codes, and secondly, whether their actions will be consistent with the law.

3.3.2 Over and above legal constraints, there is an ethical imperative not to engage in research which might harm an individual, whether by revealing personal information, or by leading to some intervention in a person's life – such as discovering new facts about their health – that might be against their interests, without their consent. As in all other areas, the presumption should be in favour of allowing individuals themselves to participate in any decision that might affect their interests. Research must not undermine trust in the confidentiality of the doctor-patient relationship, or respect for privacy and confidentiality. Even if it is apparent that a particular use of information cannot embarrass or harm an individual, researchers must ask whether their use of information goes against what a reasonable person might expect, and if so, whether it will, in the short or longer term, erode trust in health professionals or in medical research.

3.3.3 Despite the absence of legal protection, (see above) there is clearly an ethical obligation to continue to respect the confidentiality of medical information after death, and researchers should make sure that disclosures of information are fully justified. Many living people would be distressed by the thought that information about their private lives might be casually revealed after their deaths, especially in the years immediately after their death.

3.3.4 In dealing with disclosures without consent, many international and national ethical codes hold that research based only on records that will not directly affect the individual is one of the few areas where research without explicit consent can be justified. The consensus is that a balancing judgement is needed, setting the risks – often minimal – of harming the individual's interests or undermining respect for confidences more generally, against the likely long-term benefits of the research for society as a whole. However, there has been little emphasis on the need to ask first whether consent is practicable, or advice on how to weigh the different factors in reaching a balancing judgement.

3.3.5 The principles in Section 2, and the remainder of this guidance, draw on both ethical and legal advice.

3.4 Providing advance information about use of medical records

3.4.1 One of the most important steps that can be taken to address the ethical concerns, and to address the legal need for "fair data processing", is to ensure that all NHS patients, are made aware of how records are generally used in research. Explaining what is done, why, and what benefits might accrue, would protect the doctor-patient relationship, improve trust in research, and build realistic expectations of confidentiality. This was advocated by MRC in 1986, and became Department of Health policy in 1996[9], but is not yet widely practised in the Health Service.[10]

3.4.2 It is important, however, that this is not seen as consent to use medical records for any purpose, without either express permission, or proper consideration of the necessity, justification, and potential for harm.

3.4.3 We also have to bear in mind that it will take some time for information leaflets and notices to substantially change awareness of the uses of medical records. Other steps need to be taken, such as asking explicitly for agreement to the use of records in research at an appropriate time, which may be when new patients register with practices, or on first attendance at outpatients, or on admission to hospital.

3.4.4 Providing advance information also raises the question of how to respond when people object to their information being disclosed for research outside of the care team. A request for absolute confidentiality should be discussed with the patient, and has to be respected in all normal situations.[11] If a research study relevant to their health arose in future, their doctor would have to arrange to discuss the study with them and seek their explicit consent before passing on their name: in reality, time pressures would often mean that they would lose the opportunity to participate in the study.

3.4.5 Stated, general objections to disclosure without consent for unspecified studies should not prevent the inclusion of unlinked anonymised information about the patient in aggregated data or statistics (in contrast to the situation where a person declines to consent to a specific study).

3.5 Reducing the need to disclose confidential information

3.5.1 As previously mentioned, the long term development of the NHS Information Strategy will present opportunities to avoid disclosures of confidential information without consent. Better arrangements for data transfer, standardisation of diagnostic and treatment codes, and improvements in quality control, will gradually make anonymised data from IT systems more useful in research. Public awareness of how medical information is used will also increase.

3.5.2 In the medium term, improving the infrastructure for health services and public health research, especially in primary care, could reduce the need for disclosures, or their scale. Within the MRC's General Practice Research

---

[9] Health Service Guidance (96)18 *The Protection and Use of Patient Information.* Department of Health, March 1996.

[10] *Report on the Review of Patient-Identifiable Information.* The Caldicott Committee. Department of Health, 1997.

[11] Exceptions might occur if disclosure could prevent harm or death directly, or address other particularly serious and important problems.

Framework, the presence of research nurses in participating practices means that the preliminary work of selecting patients to receive invitations to participate in clinical trials or surveys can sometimes be done without any information leaving the primary care team until the patient has consented. Where patient details have to be checked centrally before invitations are sent, medical details can often be separated from names and addresses, and codes used to produce standard letters prepared without clerical staff seeing identifiable medical information.

3.5.3 Other primary care networks have, or are developing, similar arrangements and procedures. Researchers should always ask whether their questions can be answered by working only with practices that have the ability to handle information in this way.

3.6 Conclusions and implications for current practice

3.6.1 Clinical and public health research based on, or using, medical records and other personal information is essential if we are to continue to improve public health and health care – in which individuals, as citizens and members of society, have an obvious interest. On the basis of the advice summarised above, the Medical Research Council considers that it should be possible to undertake the full range of research needed in the UK, though some changes in practice are needed.

3.6.2 MRC's advice to health professionals providing information, and to researchers using information, is that they must remain aware that they can be held accountable for their decisions on the use of confidential information. On the question of consent, Common Law does not provide specific answers on when confidential information can and cannot be passed to others without consent, but the advice to MRC has been that use of personal information without explicit prior consent can be legally justified in certain circumstances. Health professionals and doctors must therefore ensure they are familiar with the advice from MRC, the Department of Health, the General Medical Council, and other bodies and should closely follow these guidelines to help ensure that their use of records is ethically and legally defensible, and to minimise the risk of any challenges.

3.6.3 Confidentiality remains a contentious area of law, and MRC cannot *guarantee* that researchers or doctors will *always* be safe from legal challenges by following the guidelines, or because their work has been approved by an Ethics Committee, even though ethics approval is very important. As the General Medical Council advises: "The decision of a research ethics committee would be taken into account by a court if a claim for breach of confidentiality were made, but the court's judgement would be based on its own assessment of whether the public interest was served."

3.6.4 Current practice varies across the country, but there are 4 areas in which change may be needed:
- patients must, as a matter of course, be given information about how their information may be used, and an opportunity to register and/or discuss their concerns throughout the health service. Where this is not the norm, researchers should press for change;[12]
- researchers have a duty to assess thoroughly, early in the design of a study, whether consent to use personal information is practicable, or could be made so, and to base research on explicit consent where practicable;
- researchers, health professionals and managers need to work together to develop the skills, information technology and infrastructure to facilitate records based research and reduce dependence on disclosures without consent;
- employers need to ensure that all staff using personal information in research have a duty of confidence that is well established through contracts, codes of conduct, and training.

Some of these changes in practice may mean higher research costs: MRC policy has always been to fund its research to the level reasonably needed for the work to be done well, safely, and ethically.

3.6.5 The research team's accountability to the NHS bodies responsible for the patients' care (assuming the researchers are not themselves NHS staff) can be an important safeguard. It is essential for those responsible for research in the NHS bodies involved to be aware of every study conducted, and to be able to call the research team to account if needed. Used as part of an effective research governance framework, honorary NHS contracts can play an important role in strengthening accountability. The Department of Health is currently (Autumn 2000) consulting on proposals for strengthening research governance in the NHS: MRC supports moves to strengthen governance frameworks, and to clarify roles and responsibilities.

---

[12] Model patient information leaflets or notices will be available from MRC's website in 2001, and a model is available in Health Service Guidance (96)18 *The Protection and Use of Patient Information*.

3.6.6 *The practicability of consent*

It is difficult to offer detailed advice on when consent is or is not practicable. The most common reasons why consent obtained through the team responsible for a person's healthcare may be impracticable are likely to be the sheer size of the group being surveyed, or the likelihood that many will be uncontactable. However, these obstacles have to be judged in the context of the structure of the relevant parts of the health service: what is impracticable in one setting is not necessarily impracticable everywhere. Other factors may include:

- before a person is asked to participate in a study, someone independent of their doctor, but with the doctor's permission, has to review their records, so that the decision to invite someone to participate is based on specific and uniform criteria;
- excluding people from whom consent cannot be obtained might bias a survey, so that people with a particular background, medical history, or attitude were disproportionately represented. For example, when studying apparent new health syndromes, or links between treatments and side effects, small or biased samples can give dangerously misleading results.

3.6.7 Very exceptionally, the nature of the research itself may be such that seeking consent, in itself, might cause harm or distress. As a hypothetical example, if a study aimed to examine correlations between parents' mental health and unexplained child deaths, it would be difficult to seek consent without risking causing serious distress. Similar dilemmas may occur in research using tissue samples to generate new information , and these situations are discussed in separate MRC guidance "Collections of Human Tissue and Biological Samples for use in research".

3.6.8 These rare situations call for careful consideration by researchers and ethics committees of where the balance of the patients' interests lies, and of:

- the scope to adopt special consent or counselling procedures that make informed consent achievable. It is important to bear in mind, however, that this standard of informed consent has to be reliably achieved throughout the study if it is to be acceptable.
- the public health importance of the question.
- the likely consequences of eventual publication of the results.

3.6.9 When the risks and the implications of not seeking consent have been fully assessed, the final decisions should be based on whether, despite these risks, it is in the public interest.

Scenarios

4 Using information with and without consent

Personal medical information is used in almost every type of clinical and public health research, and different research scenarios raise different ethical, practical and legal issues. Outlined below are some of the processes currently used in research. The scenarios are not intended as formulae for good practice, and do not cover every type of research, but are offered as examples for discussing how principles translate into practice, both when consent can be obtained and when it cannot. Whether a particular approach is ethical in a given case will depend on the circumstances of the project.

4.1 Approaching patients during medical care

> **Scenario A**
>
> Patients referred to a specialist centre in a teaching hospital are often involved in the centre's programmes of research on the causes and progression of a disease. Their participation is discussed with them by the consultant when they are first referred. A series of studies by a team of doctors, scientists and technicians draws together information on lifestyle, previous medical history, data from blood samples, X-rays, and CT scans, and information from hospital records about long-term outcomes.

> **Scenario B**
>
> A clinical trial of a new treatment is open to patients presenting in a general practice with defined symptoms. Their GP discusses their participation with them, before passing details to a trials office, to check eligibility and arrange entry in the trial.

4.1.1 In patient-based research involving direct contact with the individual, consent will always be possible, and, therefore, essential. There must be a written record of consent,[13] which includes written permission to use the

---

[13] In a few settings, signed consent is not appropriate, notably in self-administered, anonymous questionnaires – but the uses to which the information will be put must always be made clear to individuals before they fill in the form.

patient's information in the research, even if it seems a small issue alongside the patient's consent to participate in the research itself, and need not distract from this decision. Patients should also be aware that they have the right to opt out of a study at any time. The main ethical and practical questions, if any, about the use of personal information in these studies are likely to stem from:

- adequacy of data security and coding/anonymisation and, training and supervision of the group of people who will use the information;
- Longer term storage of the data, or re-use by other groups, or in other research areas.

These are generic questions that have to be addressed in every area, and are discussed in Section 5.

4.1.2 Consent will also be practicable and essential in most prospective studies – for instance, where a health professional takes details from patients knowing that the information will be used for research as well as for normal health care, consent must always be obtained. Researchers should also consider whether it is appropriate to seek permission to use the information again in other studies, and if so, what the patient needs to know about these studies.[14]

4.2.1 In each of these scenarios, the first question to ask is whether reasonable efforts have been made to make

4.2 Approaching patients from medical records

> **Scenario C**
>
> **Research based on linked anonymised data**
> To investigate the prevalence of asthma in a population, a study aims to research a cohort of new cases of asthma from a selection of patients from a network of General Practices. The GPs at the practices have already been part of a number of studies and each practice has the support of a part-time research nurse for studies of this kind. The nurse takes personal details of all the patients recorded as suffering from asthma or prescribed relevant medication, and replaces the names with a code before passing details to the research team. The research team identify a sub-set in each practice who should be invited to participate in more detailed studies, and the research nurse approaches them, using letters and information leaflets provided, to seek their consent.

[14] See Section 8.2.

> **Scenario D**
>
> **Disclosing names and addresses before consent is obtained**
> To study the health of an ageing population, a project aims to contact a large sample of the people aged 50–69 in several districts who are registered with local GPs, inviting them to complete a questionnaire and attend their practice for a check up and tests. The general practices consider that they cannot carry out the administrative work of making contact with each person and obtaining consent, even if paid, and instead, they provide the research team with names and addresses. A letter signed by the GP is then sent to each person, explaining the project and asking if they will participate. No other personal information is provided from the GP's records until a person has agreed to participate.

> **Scenario E**
>
> **Disclosing information about medical history**
> To test ways of maintaining the long-term health and quality of life of people with heart disease, a study needs to contact several tens of thousands of potential volunteers, with a history of angina, heart attacks, bypass surgery or other carefully defined conditions. A team of research nurses identifies people meeting these criteria from a range of different records at dozens of centres, and after checking with the GP, the trials office prepares letters to each individual, on behalf of their GP.

patients aware that their information may be used for research or other purposes not directly connected to their treatment (see Sections 2 and 3.4 above). This might seem unnecessary in Scenario C, which involves no disclosure of confidential information or personal data outside the General Practice, and is unlikely to raise legal or ethical issues other than those mentioned in 4.1.1 above. But even here, steps should be taken to make patients aware that personal information is used in research in the practice, and throughout the NHS, and that the care team includes research staff. In Scenarios D and E, making patients aware of how their information is used is not only ethically important, but would also help to minimise the risk of legal challenge to researchers and health professionals.

4.2.2 Scenarios D and E illustrate the situations that give rise to most ethical and legal uncertainty. Scenario D involves the disclosure of a limited amount of personal information given in confidence without consent, and the justification for this would need to be carefully considered by the health professionals and researchers involved, and by an ethics committee. If patients had previously been given general information about how their records might be used, and opportunity to raise objections, then this very limited disclosure would be unlikely to give rise to any serious objections. If patients had not been given information, then more caution would be needed: there would need to be a clear justification for conducting the research in this setting, and the potential benefits would have to outweigh the breach of confidence involved.

4.2.3 Scenario E involves disclosing information about medical history. While the number of people who have access to the information is strictly limited, the information is undoubtedly confidential and sensitive personal data, with potential to cause some embarrassment or perhaps even discrimination if disclosed. Many other types of medical information, such as information about mental health or sexuality, would be much more sensitive, and more likely to cause distress or embarrassment if disclosed.

4.2.4 If patients were aware of how their records might be used, the researchers, health professionals and ethics committee involved would need to satisfy themselves that the disclosure was necessary and justifiable, and that the information would be used properly (see 4.1.1). The detail of what patients were routinely told about their records, and the degree of sensitivity of the information, would be important factors in the decision. If patients were not aware that their information might be used in this way, this project would be unacceptable unless there were a strong justification, based on the absence of alternatives and clear potential to benefit health.

4.2.5 The reasons why consent cannot be obtained at the outset differ in Scenarios D and E. In D it is because of the practicality of GPs undertaking large amounts of additional administrative work, in writing letters, chasing and checking replies, and answering queries. In E direct access to medical records is needed to ensure the right people are identified using consistent and objective criteria, which requires appropriately trained and supervised researchers. In both scenarios, the disclosure of identifiable information might be reduced or even avoided if the study could be based in general practices with good facilities for doing research.

4.2.6 The second ethical issue that studies of this sort raise is how to contact people in a way that is unlikely to cause worry or embarrassment. The first approach to people identified from medical records should normally involve a letter signed by the health professional responsible for their care giving information about the research, or accompanied by a letter from the researcher which does so. As well as showing respect for the doctor-patient relationship, this is a vital step in checking that the information on which the researcher acts is up to date, and that those approached are not recently bereaved or likely to be distressed for any other reason. The advice of the person's doctor in this area must always be followed. The same principles apply to approaches based on data from disease registries.

4.2.7 It is acceptable for research teams to provide trained clerical support for the health professional, to prepare and distribute letters and related correspondence, if the clerical staff are bound by a duty of confidence, and the research cannot be in a setting where the care team has the capacity to do this themselves.

4.2.8 The initial letters sent to patients should normally cover all, or some of the following:

- why the research is being carried out, and how participation could help;
- how the patient has been selected;
- that the patient's doctor has considered, and fully supports, the study;
- that there is no obligation to participate, and that their decision will not affect their care;
- what will be involved i.e. in terms of time, interviews, treatment, examinations etc.;
- the benefits (if any) that participants can hope to gain from the research, and whether the study will involve any commitment of time, discomfort, or risk on their part;
- that confidentiality will be safeguarded;
- a contact point in the medical/research team for queries or information. If practical, this would be someone already known to the person;
- a reply form if the patient is willing to give permission without further discussion.

4.2.9 When it is proposed to visit a patient at home, advance notice should be given in the form of a letter from their doctor, explaining the purpose of the procedures, the reason, the name of the investigator, and how they will identify themselves. It must always be made clear that the patient is free to withdraw from the study at any stage. People should normally be given a simple response form with an SAE and adequate time to return it. Providing a Freephone number is also helpful. The care team or researchers should either confirm by telephone, or wait for positive written confirmation that the person is willing to meet them before calling in person. If the person has previously agreed to take part in the study, and knows a visit will be involved, then it is reasonable to assume that it is acceptable to call at the time suggested unless told otherwise.

4.2.10 Where the study relates to a well defined group, it is usually helpful to publicise the study through newsletters, support groups and similar channels, before, or at the same time as, making direct approaches to individuals. Information needs to be provided in a language that is easy to understand.

Contacting ward patients and patients attending clinics
4.2.11 If the people being contacted are in hospital, or attending a clinic, the patient should be asked first if they will see the researcher, or a member of the care team should introduce the patient to the researcher. Hospitals should also explain, in the information they give to patients, that they may be approached by researchers.

4.3 Research based on existing records and samples only

> **Scenario F**
>
> Stored tissue samples from former cancer patients are to be examined for biochemical markers that might hel predict how the disease will progress, and results will be related to data from medical records on the patient's condition, treatment and outcome. There will be no feedback to the patients, and there is no need to subsequently monitor the longer-term survival of the patients. Thus the data can be anonymised (unlinked) before the analysis, but names have to be used to identify patients and samples when the data are first gathered.

4.3.1 The fact that a study does not require contact with patients is not in itself a reason for not contacting people for consent, if consent is practicable. The justification for this study would need to be considered against the criteria in Section 2, in the same way as (D) and (E) above, though here, the minimal use of identifiable information would be a very important consideration. This type of research also raises the question of when it is right to create new biological information about an individual with or without consent, and these broader issues are dealt with in the MRC

ethics booklet "Collections of Human Tissue and Biological Samples for use in research".

> **Scenario G**
>
> Information from hospital records is to be analysed anonymously (unlinked) to identify risk factors predicting poor outcomes from surgery. As the hospital staff cannot be redeployed to extract and anonymise the information, a trained nurse or clerical officer from the research team is assigned to copy and anonymise the information.

4.3.2 Here too, although the justification for the study would still need to be considered by an Ethics Committee, the infringement of confidentiality is minimal, and there are unlikely to be significant ethical or legal objections to this aspect of the study.

4.4 Using information from non-medical sources to contact people

> **Scenario H**
>
> To address concerns about the safety of an industrial process, a research study aims to contact all those who lived in the vicinity of a plant, or who worked there, to survey their long-term health.

4.4.1 Direct approaches to members of the public identified from the electoral roll or other public sources do not require consent or agreement of the individual's doctor, but it is usually advisable to notify local General Practitioners before carrying out a study in an area. MRC expects medical studies of this sort to be reviewed by an LREC or MREC, even though it is not obligatory. Direct postal approaches are generally less likely to lead to distress or misunderstanding than "cold" telephone calls.

Selection by social or disability group
4.4.2 If the research focuses on the health of distinct socio-economic groups (e.g. homeless or disadvantaged people) or people of minority ethnic groups, researchers should consider whether community organisations or other bodies that might be able to represent their interests should be made aware of the study, and should have the opportunity of commenting on the research. When working in areas where there may be significant immigrant populations,

and when working with groups with sensory or learning disabilities, researchers should also check whether translators or some other help with communication is needed. It is also possible that some research participants may prefer interviewers of the same gender.

Selection by employment

4.4.3 Occupational surveys to assess risks from work activities, accidents, or from exposure to particular hazards or toxic substances are often based on employers' records. Prior to such a survey, discussions should take place with representatives of the staff involved, with management, the occupational health service, and where possible with the staff themselves. A normal approach would be through a letter confirming that the employer and Trade Union agreed to the study taking place. Publicity through newsletters etc. should also be considered, depending on the sensitivity of the issue being studied.

5 Safeguarding confidentiality

5.1 Anonymisation and coding

5.1.1 Information should be modified so that some, or all, of those who might see it are not aware of individual identities, as early as possible in data processing. Although anonymisation may introduce delays and increase risks of error, even a simple coding system provides a safeguard against accidental or mischievous release of confidential information.

5.1.2 It is important to distinguish between the different ways in which personal data can be modified to conceal identities. The definitions we have used in this guide are:

Coded information contains information which could readily identify people, but their identity is concealed by coding, the key to which is held by members of the research team using the information. This might be done, for example, to limit the number of people who had access to information about identifiable individuals, to reduce the risk of accidental disclosure, or when presenting results. This helps to meet legal and ethical obligations to protect personal information, but the research team still holds identifiable personal data, and the use of coded data falls within the scope of the Data Protection Act.

Linked Anonymised Data is anonymous to the research team that holds it, but contains coded information which could be used to identify people. The key to the code might,

for example, be held by those responsible for the individual's care, or by the custodians of a larger research database or register.

Unlinked Anonymised Data contains nothing that has reasonable potential to be used by anyone to identify individuals: the link to individuals has been irreversibly broken. As a minimum, unlinked anonymous data must not contain any of the following, or codes for the following:

* name, address, phone/fax. number, e-mail address, full postcode,
* NHS number, any other identifying reference number,
* photograph, or names of relatives.

5.1.3 With both linked and unlinked anonymised data, there is sometimes potential to deduce individuals' identities through combinations of information, either by the people handling research data, or by those who see the published results. The most important potential identifiers are:

* rare disease or treatment, especially if an easily noticed illness/disability is involved;
* partial post-code, or partial address;
* place of treatment or health professional responsible for care;
* rare occupation or place of work;
* combinations of birth date, ethnicity, place of birth, and date of death.

5.1.4 Researchers should always consider – when designing studies, before passing information to others, and before publishing information – whether data contain combinations of such information that might lead to identification of individuals or very small groups. Exactly how much of this potentially identifying information can be safely included in data that is assumed to be "unidentifiable" can only be judged on a case by case basis, taking into account the sample size, the ways in which results will be published and used, and all other circumstances of the study.

5.1.5 Both types of anonymisation *can help avoid the need to* disclose confidential medical information without consent. Linked data is typically used where it may be necessary to refer back to the original records for further information, or for verification, or if it is planned to provide feedback to patients or those responsible for their care. Unlinked data ensures absolute confidentiality, but by precluding follow-up, verification or feedback, may be incompatible with the research aims, or the interests of the participants and the health service.

5.1.6 **If it is practical and reliable**, the removal, or coding, of identifying information should be done within the team

---

[15] In the accepted information technology sense of the term, overcoming the accidental loss of some or all of the data stored on a system.

or organisation responsible for the individual's care. Where this is not possible, it is preferable for a member of the research team to help with the anonymisation rather than for identifiable information be used.

Anonymised data and ethical review

5.1.7 Research Ethics Committee approval is required for the use of coded and anonymised data from NHS medical records. The use of anonymous personal data is much easier to justify ethically and legally, but it must still only be used for bona fide research in the public interest. Removing all apparent personal identifiers will not always protect a patient's identity – for example in cases of rare disease – and anonymous data can still lead to new and disturbing information about groups or districts.

Data in Clinical Studies

5.1.8 In small scale clinical studies, which involve frequent reference by research and medical staff to current patients' conditions, encoding and decoding information can present a significant obstacle to effective team work, and increases the risk of an error that could affect the patient's care. Use of weaker codes (such as initials) in processing research data is acceptable where patients have already given consent to the use of their information in research as well as for their care, and when it can be guaranteed that only a small number of research staff will have access to the information.

5.2 The research team

Members of a research team who use personal medical information should be placed under a duty of confidentiality equivalent to that of a health professional. To reinforce this duty:

- Universities and other research organisations must ensure that all contracts and codes of conduct make clear that any breach of confidence is a grave disciplinary matter;
- team leaders must ensure all staff, students, visiting workers, and collaborators fully understand the standards expected, and the importance of confidentiality;
- team leaders and line managers should ensure that information and advice on principles and practice in this area is readily available.

5.2.1 The Medical Research Council's staff code already creates such an obligation, and it is reinforced by staff training and induction.

5.2.2 As discussed in section 3.6.5, MRC supports moves to clarify responsibilities for research governance in the NHS, and strengthen accountability of researchers to NHS bodies through ensuring better internal information systems and other means.

5.2.3 Access to personal information that is neither anonymised nor coded must be restricted to the smallest number that will allow the study to be done effectively. Access to encoded or anonymised data must also be under the control of the medical director or principal investigator, but the numbers with access can be larger.

5.3 Data security

Ensuring data are secure is a legal obligation under the Data Protection Act: the level of security, and the cost and effort involved, should reflect the nature of the information and the harm that might result from unauthorised disclosure or loss. Every research team must maintain written procedures for keeping electronic and written personal information secure, which must be enforced and reviewed at regular intervals. The measures needed to protect IT systems and data transfers, in particular, need frequent review and expert local advice should be sought. For this reason, the guidelines that follow should be viewed as a checklist, rather than as a comprehensive guide.

5.3.1 *Responsibilities*

There should be clearly assigned responsibilities for: overall management and control of research data; rapid response to breaches of security or leaks; management of the software; maintenance of backup regime and disaster recovery arrangements; ensuring duplicate files are kept to the minimum needed, controlling access rights, and changing access rights promptly when the team changes. The person or people responsible will normally report directly to the principal investigator on issues of data security.

5.3.2 Responsibilities for data security or disposal at the end of a project (see Section 7) must also be clear. If archived, data must be accorded the same level of security as when they were in active use. If destroyed, all copies of the data must be destroyed in a secure way. Records of destruction must be kept as these may be required for audit or other purposes later.

5.3.3 *Physical Environment*

- Rooms containing paper documents or computers should be accessible only to a limited number of authorised personnel;
- All relevant servers, routers, gateways and other critical equipment should be housed within a secure area;
- Workstations which are logged onto personal research data should not be left unattended;

- Data stored on laptop computers and other mobile machines are always at higher risk of loss or theft. Identifiable personal data should only be stored on these machines in special circumstances – for instance, when patients are interviewed and the data entered directly onto computer. Data thus stored on a laptop computer should then be transferred to a secure computer at the earliest opportunity and wiped from the portable's memory.

5.3.4 *Electronic Environment*

- Access rights to data and applications software should be clearly defined and staff authorised to access personal data should be formally notified in writing of the permissible scope of their access;
- For each application, system users should have a valid user system account name, i.e. a username ID, and a password known only to that user to prevent unauthorised use of systems. Users should be forced by systems to alter their passwords regularly – the frequency may vary according to the constraints of the system software but should be aimed at maintaining high levels of security. Passwords must not be written down or shared with other users under any circumstances. "Temporary" user accounts should not be used;
- A confidentiality warning message should be displayed on entering systems, informing the user that the system contains confidential information and is for authorised users only;
- Users should ensure that, at log-off, documents recently used and containing confidential information are cleared from applications on start up;
- Personal medical information should not normally be sent over the Internet via attached documents, FTP, or other systems. Where this has to be done, the data should be reliably encrypted. Databases transferred by mail should be sent by registered post.

6 Safeguarding other interests of the individual

6.1 Avoiding harm or distress

6.1.1 Apart from the possibility of allowing personal information to leak out by accident or through deliberate wrongdoing, researchers also need to be alert to the possibility of causing harm or distress through:

- approaching people or families who may be distressed, bereaved, or mentally ill;
- errors in the data used to contact people;
- feeding back findings to study participants and/or families (even where they have requested this);

- publishing findings which could be linked back to participants;
- publishing findings which lead to discrimination;
- allowing re-use of data for other purposes without proper ethical supervision.

6.1.2 The best safeguard against approaching the wrong people, or contacting people who may be distressed by the approach, is the role of the person's doctor in approving the approach, and, where possible, in making the initial approach. However, occasional errors are always possible, and research staff should be prepared to respond to mistakes sensitively and promptly.

6.1.3 The potential for harm to the interests of a defined group may be unavoidable where research has the potential to highlight that group as having, for example, poor health behaviour or being "at risk" from a particular local environmental hazard, or where the research may confirm stereotypes. Researchers must try to anticipate these issues before ethical review, and must consider whether any risk of harm is outweighed by longer term benefits to society, and/or to the group. Researchers must also consider consulting the groups involved, or their representatives, to explain their work, and listen to any concerns.

6.2 Feedback and publication

6.2.1 The question of when study participants should have access to new information specifically about them or their family that is generated in research is dealt with in the parallel MRC guide *Collections of Human Tissue and Biological Samples for use in research.*

6.2.2 The results of clinical trials, records-based research and epidemiological surveys can have substantial implications for individuals. People will be concerned about new risks, or potential side-effects of treatment, to which they may have been exposed, especially if they did not know about the research. Those who have a relevant illness will wonder whether this is as a result of the exposure or treatment. Researchers should liase with Health Authorities, Health Boards, General Practices, relevant consumer organisations or other bodies to ensure people have easy access to good information and advice, before publishing findings which are likely to be contentious or worrying.

6.2.3 The people who have participated in a study should, wherever feasible, be notified of the outcome of the study, and told of the general results. If researchers feel it is impossible or inappropriate to do this, the reasons should be discussed with the ethics committee when approval is sought.

6.2.4 Individuals and families must never be identified in publications without signed consent for that specific publication. Researchers must avoid publishing potential identifiers, such as date of birth or death, which might appear innocuous to the research team but which could reveal the patient's identity to close relatives or friends. Caution is also needed when publishing research about small groups of people, such as work on disease clusters, patient case series in a particular centre, and research on new treatments or rare adverse reactions, especially if the findings are likely to attract a lot of media attention. In these cases there is a particularly high risk that groups and cases may be identified by deduction.

7 Storage and re-use of research data

7.1 Storage

7.1.1 Research records need to be preserved for the longer-term for a number of reasons – other than for historical posterity. Firstly, records may be needed later on for scientific validation of research, or for future research and audit. Secondly, occasionally there is a need for access to records over the whole lifetime of patients, both by the patients themselves (who may have continuing long-term concerns about their own health) and their clinicians – for instance, where trials of novel treatments were involved.

7.1.2 MRC would expect that research records relating to clinical or public health studies should be maintained for twenty years, to allow adequate time for review, reappraisal, or further research, and to allow any concerns about the conduct or consequences of the work to be resolved. Beyond this date, full records may need to be retained for a few studies only, such as those which were of historical importance, where novel clinical interventions were first used, those which have proved controversial, or where research is ongoing. In the remaining clinical and public health studies, and all other studies for which consent was obtained, a subset of the original records, covering the protocol, the consent procedure, the people who consented to take part,[16] and any records of adverse effects should be retained until thirty years have elapsed.

7.1.3 MRC's expectation is that once a research team ceases to exist, when the team leader moves to another centre, or when the team stops working in a particular area, the responsibility for their information passes to the University, Hospital, or research centre. If records are to be stored in the long-term, a custodian must be designated for them, and the custodian's role must include ensuring that information is treated in confidence. If, in due course, the records are to be archived, this should be done in secure repositories. Areas where records may be consulted should be equally secure.

7.2 Re-use of data by third parties

7.2.1 Researchers obtaining information with consent should, wherever possible, anticipate likely needs to archive the data, and to share data sets with other researchers, and make this clear to the people involved. Consent to this should be distinct from consent to the primary use of the information. Existing data sets can be shared with other researchers provided this is not inconsistent with what participants were told about how the data would be used. For example, the use of clinical trial data for meta-analyses should not, in our opinion, require new consent.

7.2.2 In **any** case where research data are shared with another group for new studies:

- The custodian must ensure that the group accepts a duty of confidence and protects confidentiality through training procedures, etc, to the same standards as the custodian. Normally, only anonymised data should be passed on;
- The custodian must ensure that personal data are not passed to a country without legal protection for personal data equivalent to that in the UK, unless the custodian first assures themselves that the data will be adequately protected in practice. Under the terms of the Data Protection Act 1998, there are no special restrictions on transfers of identifiable data within the European Economic Area nations.[17] Outside of the EEA – e.g. for data sent to the USA, or any developing country – the custodian must either: remain able to control the use of the data transferred; anonymise the data; or obtain the individuals' explicit consent to send their data to another centre. Further details are available on the WebSite of the Office of the Data Protection Commissioner: www.dataprotection.gov.uk
- The third party must not pass on the data to any other group;
- Individuals may not be re-contacted except *via* their doctor, or, in the case of cohorts who have given consent, the original research group. Re-contacting individuals involved in past studies requires some sensitivity, as this

---

[16] Unless the study used anonymised and unlinked information.

[17] These are: Austria, Belgium, Denmark, Finland, France, Germany, Greece, Iceland, Ireland, Italy, Liechtenstein, Luxembourg, Netherlands, Norway, Portugal, Spain, Sweden and the UK.

may cause anxiety and – with the march of time – people may not wish to have a reminder from the past. Recontacting should therefore only be carried out if it is absolutely necessary, and only with LREC/MREC approval. It should be made clear in the information and consent documents that information from one study may be used in later studies;

- LREC/MREC approval is needed for any use of identifiable data, and for any unidentifiable data taken from NHS records not already in the public domain;
- LREC/MREC approval is not needed for re-use of unidentifiable data obtained directly from study participants, or for re-analysis, by any research group, of unidentifiable data from previous research;
- Where the research group that conducted the study no longer exists, the custodian of the data must ensure that the same standards are applied, and that LREC/MREC approval is obtained where necessary.

8 Information and consent forms

8.1 Patient leaflets and notices

8.1.1 The Department of Health guidelines *Protection and Use of Patient Information* (1996) provide advice on informing patients and a model notice that can be adapted to suit local needs. Centres active in research will normally wish to include some additional specific information about their research in patient leaflets. This could cover: the reasons for research; the fact that Universities (or other research organisations) work closely with the hospital or practice and regularly receive information; the main sources of funds for the research; that research is independently reviewed; and that all research staff have the same duty of confidence as the health professionals caring for them. Patients should also be told whom to contact if they have any concerns.

8.2 Consent procedures

8.2.1 Where patients are asked to participate in any clinical study, the patient information sheet must directly refer to the treatment of personal data, and explain:
- who will have access to their data;
- the confidentiality of the data (including reference to coding/anonymisation if necessary);
- what will happen to the data once the study is complete.

---

[18] Further advice information and consent forms can be found in the MREC Guidelines for Researchers on Patient Information Sheets.

8.2.2 Where information is being gathered for large scale or long-term studies, such as cohort studies, the information provided may need to include all or some of the following, depending on the nature of the study and the commitment the person is being asked to make:
- the types of studies the records or health data may be used for and the conditions that may be investigated;
- who will be responsible for custodianship of the information (normally this will be the person in charge of the study and/or the principal investigator) and to what organisation they belong;
- the arrangements for protecting the patient's confidentiality;
- who will have access to the data;
- the uses to which the data will be put;
- whether and how the individual or their doctor will be contacted again;
- the arrangements for actively feeding back information to participants, or providing access to research results;
- (if relevant) that anonymised and unlinked data may be passed on to other researchers;
- that they may ask to see the information held about them and withdraw from the study at any time (if the study design allows data linkage);
- who to contact if they have any concerns about the use of their data;
- what happens to the data once the study is complete;
- how they will find out about any change in the study's direction or custodianship.

8.2.3 If it is expected that data – apart from anonymised and unlinked data – may be used in other, secondary studies, the information may need to explain as well:
- any possible impact of secondary studies on their interests;
- how they can find out about secondary studies;
- what sorts of information might be passed to others, under what conditions;
- that secondary studies would have to be approved by an ethics committee.

Checklist for records-based research   Annex 1

Context

- Is the study based on a group of patients, or a data set, for which consent has already been obtained?
- Could the study (or parts of it) be done with consent?
- How well informed are patients in the hospitals/practices about how their information is used? What would they

reasonably expect? Have they had an opportunity to express any concerns?

Justification for the study

- How sensitive is the information involved? Are there any particular risks of harm or distress?
- What impact, if any, could the study findings have on the people involved?
- Do the benefits outweigh any foreseeable risks?
- If consent to the study is impracticable, do its potential benefits to people, as individuals or as members of society, outweigh the infringement of confidentiality, and any risks of harm or distress?

Conduct of the study

- If people are being approached, when are they being approached and why?
- If people are being approached, will they get adequate explanation of motives and safeguards, and of their right to opt out. Will it be clear to them that the doctor responsible for their care supports the approach?
- Will the information be anonymised (linked or unlinked) or encoded, and if so at which stage in the project?
- What people will have access to personal information during the study? Have they been made formally aware of their duty of confidence, and suitably trained?
- Do procedures for day to day work, electronic data security, and records storage offer adequate protection for personal information?
- What sorts of findings are likely, and what arrangements are there for these to be fed back to the people involved – if appropriate?
- What will happen to the data after the study is complete?

Responsibilities of a doctor providing personal information   Annex 2

A All health professionals have both a responsibility to protect their patients' confidentiality, and a responsibility for supporting high quality, ethical, research which is likely to benefit their patients as members of the UK public, in the longer term. Health professionals, and especially those involved in research, should ensure that patients are provided with effective information about how medical records are used, and why this is important. This should limit the occasions when responsibilities to patients and to research appear to conflict.

B Health professionals are personally responsible for assuring themselves that their use of confidential information is justified, that practical safeguards to protect confidentiality are in place, and, in particular, that Research Ethics Committee approval has been obtained. They should remember that the ultimate responsibility for protecting their patients' legal rights and *their employer's* interests lies with them, and should ensure they are familiar with guidance from the GMC and other bodies.

C Doctors should normally:
- write a letter to patients when they are first asked to participate in the study;
- ensure they know which patients will be involved, and provide researchers with any advice about patients' circumstances that will help them avoid causing worry or distress. Doctors may sometimes need to advise against approaching a particular individual, without necessarily giving any reason if the reason is itself confidential. This is especially important if the patients will be asked to consent to any physical examination or invasive procedures;
- ensure they are familiar with the design of the study and the safeguards, and able to answer patients' queries, even though the researchers may be the normal contact point for participants;
- when they can do so effectively, and it is consistent with the study design, doctors should anonymise *(linked or unlinked)* the information before passing it on to researchers.

The Data Protection Act 1998   Annex 3

Data protection principles

A The 1998 Act, like its predecessor, is based around a set of core principles.
1 Personal data shall be processed fairly and lawfully and, in particular, shall not be processed unless: (a) at least one of the conditions in Schedule 2 is met, and (b) in the case of sensitive personal data, at least one of the conditions in Schedule 3 is also met.
2 Personal data shall be obtained only for one or more specified and lawful purposes, and shall not be further processed in any manner incompatible with that purpose or those purposes.
3 Personal data shall be adequate, relevant and not excessive in relation to the purpose or purposes for which they are processed.
4 Personal data shall be accurate and, where necessary, kept up to date.

5 Personal data processed for any purpose or purposes shall not be kept for longer than is necessary for that purpose or those purposes.

6 Personal data shall be processed in accordance with the rights of data subjects under this Act.

7 Appropriate technical and organisational measures shall be taken against unauthorised or unlawful processing of personal data and against accidental loss or destruction of, or damage to, personal data.

8 Personal data shall not be transferred to a country or territory outside the European Economic Area unless that country or territory ensures an adequate level of protection for the rights and freedoms of data subject in relation to the processing of personal data.

Personal data means "data which relate to a living individual who can be identified (a) from those data), or, (b) from those data and other information which is in the possession of, or is likely to come into the possession of, the data controller."

The "data controller" is "a person who (either alone or jointly or in common with other persons) determines the purposes for which, and the manner in which any personal data are, or are to be, processed."

B The "sensitive data" referred to in the first principle includes all information relating to a person's physical or mental health or condition, sexual life, racial or ethnic origin, religious or *political beliefs*, trade union membership, or (alleged) crimes. The references to processing data "fairly and lawfully" draw in the concept of "fair processing" (such as ensuring people are not deceived as to the reasons why information is being collected from them) and also mean that anything which is unlawful under Common Law, cannot be acceptable under the Act.

C Ordinary personal data cannot be processed unless: (The conditions listed below are those most likely to be relevant).

Schedule 2

1 The data subject has given his consent to the processing. *(or)*

4 The processing is necessary in order to protect the vital interests of the data subject. *(or)*

5 The processing is necessary:
  (a) for the administration of justice [. . .]
  (d) for the exercise of any other functions of a public nature exercised in the public interest by any person. *(or)*

6 (1) The processing is necessary for the purposes of legitimate interests pursued by the data controller or by the third party or parties to whom the data are disclosed, except where the processing is unwarranted in any particular case by reason of prejudice to the rights and freedoms or legitimate interests of the data subject.

(2) The Secretary of Sate may by order specify particular circumstances in which this condition is, or is not, to be taken to be satisfied.

Schedule 3

In addition, sensitive data cannot be processed unless:

1 The data subject has given his explicit consent to the processing of the personal data. *(or)*

8 (1) The processing is necessary for medical purposes and is undertaken by:
  (a) a health professional, or
  (b) a personal who in the circumstances owes a duty of confidentiality which is equivalent to that which would arise if that person were a health professional.

(2) In this paragraph "medical purposes" includes the purposes of preventive medicine, medical diagnosis, medical research, the provision of care and treatment and the management of healthcare services.

D Use of data for medical research will normally be justifiable under Sections (1) or (6) of Schedule 2, and Sections (1) or (8) of Schedule 3. However, the fact that use of medical records is acceptable under these clauses of the Act does not necessarily mean it is lawful or fair: it also to be consistent with Common Law on confidentiality, and with general concepts of fairness.

E The Act recognises that research work and statistical work often require information to be processed in ways other than those for which it was collected, and that it is often unreasonable to expect members of the public to know about this processing, or to have the right to access the data. Research is given special exemptions in Section 33 of the Act.

Research, history and statistics

33(1) In this section, "research purposes" includes statistical or historical purposes; "the relevant conditions" in relation to any processing of personal data means the conditions:
  (a) that the data are not processed to support measures or decisions with respect to particular individuals, and
  (b) that the data are not processed in such a way that that substantial damage or substantial distress is, or is likely to be, caused to any data subject.

33(2) For the purposes of the second data protection principle, the further processing of personal data only for research purposes in compliance with the relevant conditions, is not to be regarded as incompatible with the purposes for which they are obtained.

33(3) Personal data which are processed only for research purposes are exempt may, notwithstanding the fifth data protection principle, be kept indefinitely.

33(4) Personal data which are processed only for research purposes are exempt from section 7 if –
(a) they are processed in compliance with the relevant conditions, and
(b) the published results of the research or any resulting statistics are not made available in a form which identifies data subjects or any of them.

(Note: Section 7 of the Act deals with individuals' right to access the data that organisations hold on them)

33(5) For the purposes of subsections (2) to (4) personal data are not to be treated as processed otherwise than for research purposes merely because the data are disclosed:
(a) to any person, for research purposes only
(b) to the data subject or a person acting on his behalf
(c) at the request, or with the consent, of the data subject or a person acting on his behalf
(d) in circumstances in which the person making the disclosure has reasonable grounds for believing that the disclosure falls within paragraph (a), (b), or (c).

The 1998 Human Rights Act   Annex 4

The 1998 Act incorporates the rights and freedoms set out in the 1950 European Convention on Human Rights into UK law. The Act gives UK courts the authority to rule that existing or new UK laws are incompatible with these rights and freedoms. The Act makes it unlawful for a public authority, by its acts or failures to act, to conduct itself in a manner incompatible with the Convention. Courts can hear cases brought by people affected by the actions or inaction of public bodies, and can order public bodies to make redress or pay damages.

The interpretation of the Act in the UK will take account of previous rulings by the European Court of Human Rights.

The Convention covers matters such as:
• protection of property
• the right to life
• prohibition of torture
• prohibition of slavery and forced labour
• right to liberty and security
• right to a fair trial
• prohibition of punishments without legal foundation
• right to respect for private and family life
• freedom of thought, conscience and religion
• freedom of expression
• freedom of assembly and association
• the right to marry

The Act sets out situations in which laws can restrict these rights, for example to prevent civil disturbance or protect public health, and possible justifications for public bodies infringing these rights. In relation to the right to respect for private and family life, the Act states:

1 Everyone has the right to respect for his private and family life, his home, and his correspondence.
2 There shall be no interference by a public authority with the exercise of this right except such as in accordance with the law and is necessary in a democratic society in the interests of national security, public safety or the economic well-being of the country, for the prevention of disorder or crime, for the protection of health or morals, or for the protection of the rights and freedoms of others.

The confidentiality of medical information about a person is seen as an integral part of respect for private and family life. Previous European cases dealing with disclosures of medical information in criminal cases and other areas have focussed on:
• whether the disclosure was in accordance with national law
• whether it was necessary
• whether it was proportionate (i.e. no greater than needed for the purpose).

Other statutory requirements   Annex 5

Aside from the Data Protection Act 1998, there are other statutes and regulations on the disclosure of information:
• The NHS (Venereal Diseases) Regulations 1974 and the NHS Trusts (Venereal Diseases) Directions 1991, prevent the disclosure of any identifying information about a patient examined or treated for a sexually transmitted disease (including HIV and AIDS) other than to a medical practitioner (or to a person employed under the direction of a medical practitioner) in connection with and for the purpose of either the treatment of the patient and/or the prevention of the spread of the disease.
• The Human Fertilisation and Embryology Act 1990, as amended by the Human Fertilisation and Embryology (Disclosure of Information) Act 1992, limits the circumstances in which information may be disclosed by centres licensed under the Act.

- The Abortion Regulations 1991 impose obligations on medical practitioners who carry out terminations of pregnancy to notify the Chief Medical Officer and to provide detailed information about the patient. The Chief Medical Officer may then only disclose that information in accordance with the provisions of the regulations.

Source: For the Record: managing records in NHS Trusts and Health Authorities', *Health Service Circular HSC 1999/053 (March 1999).*

Other publications in this series

The Ethical Conduct of Research on Children, December 1991 (reprinted 1993).

Responsibility in the use of Animals in Medical Research, July 1993.

Responsibility in the use of Personal Medical Information for Research – Principles and Guide to Practice, Prepared for Council's standing Committee on the Use of Medical Information for research, 1985. Reprinted with minor revisions as footnotes, September 1994. To be revised 2001.

Principles in the Assessment of Medical Research and Publicising results, January 1995.

MRC policy and procedure for inquiring into allegations of scientific misconduct, December 1997.

The Ethical Conduct of Research on the Mentally Incapacitated, December 1991Reprinted August 1993.

Collections of Human Tissue and Biological Samples for Use in Human Research. Available January 2001.

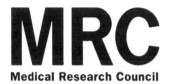

MRC

Medical Research Council

20 Park Crescent, London W1B 1AL
Telephone: 020 7636 5422   Facsimile: 020 7436 6179
Website: www.mrc.ac.uk

56

Use and disclosure of medical data
– guidance on the Application of the Data Protection Act, 1998
May 2002

The Information Commissioner

Table of contents

Information Commissioner's Foreword

The Data Protection Act 1998 presents a number of significant challenges to data controllers in the health sector. Over the course of the last year, I have seen a significant increase in the number of requests for assistance from

individuals. At the same time I have been asked to consider issues arising out the Department of Health electronic patient records project, issues in relation to cancer and other disease registries, and issues in relation to the use of patient data in research. Frequently these requests for advice have significant implications for the NHS as a whole and the Department of Health as well as for patients.

It seems to me that there are several reasons for the increase in requests for assistance and advice. Firstly there has been an extension of the scope of Data Protection from purely automated records to many classes of manual records. Whereas the 1984 Act only applied to computerised records, the 1998 Act applies fully to all patient records whether they are held on computer or in paper files, and whether they consist of hand written case notes or x-rays.

Secondly, it is clear that many practitioners are confused between the requirements of the Data Protection Act and those of the various regulatory and representative bodies within the sector including the GMC, MRC, and BMA. To some extent the advice issued by these different bodies may reflect their different roles. To some extent it may also reflect misunderstandings of the requirements of the Act. It is a common misconception, for instance, that the Act always requires the consent of data subjects to the processing of their data. At the same time, as private litigation increases throughout society, many health service bodies have adopted a more cautions approach towards the use and disclosure of patient data, fearing that uses and disclosures of data which previously seemed unexceptionable might attract action for a breach of confidence.

Thirdly, the demands that are placed on the health service are greater and more varied than ever before. Health Authorities, NHS Trusts and individual practitioners are increasingly involved in inter-agency initiatives, whether in the context of the Crime and Disorder Act or the joint delivery of health and social care with local authority social service departments. Meanwhile, the creation of a national system of electronic health records is likely to raise fresh questions about who is responsible for those records and who should be allowed access to them.

If steps are not taken to clarify the ground rules, then the uncertainty experienced by clinicians and NHS organisations may translate into concerns on the part of patients as to who has access to their records and on what basis their personal data are processed. In that context I welcome wholeheartedly statements by Department of Health Ministers that in the foreseeable future all processing of patient records should be on the basis of informed consent. I also welcome the decision of the NHS Executive to begin work on development of a Code of Practice that is aimed at producing coherent practical guidance for clinicians and health service bodies incorporating the different standards emanating from the different professional and representative bodies. The guidance that I have published is more limited in its ambition. My aim has been to clarify the minimum requirements of the Data Protection Act, providing answers to frequently asked questions such as:

• Is patient consent necessary for processing?
• If so, in what circumstances?
• If so, in what form?
• When is it necessary to anonymise data?
• When is it necessary to pseudonymise data?

Although as far as possible the Guidance attempts to provide practical examples of the steps that should be taken in order to achieve compliance with the requirements of the Act, the audience for the Guidance is not primarily practitioners but data protection officers, Caldicott Guardians and those charged with the development of the IT infrastructure of the NHS. It is, in other words a somewhat technical document that seeks to explain the enforceable requirements of the Data Protection Act rather than to describe "good practice".

The term "enforceable requirements" refers to the powers given to me by the Act to take action against data controllers whom I consider to be in breach of any of the eight Data Protection Principles in Schedule 1 of the Act. The Act does not, however, require that I take enforcement action on each occasion that I consider that there has been a breach. Before serving an enforcement notice I will not only measure the performance of the data controller against the standard set out in the guidance but also consider, as the Act requires, whether the actions of the data controller have caused damage or distress to any individual. I shall also have regard to the circumstances of different data controllers. For instances, as is explained in the section of the Guidance dealing with privacy enhancing technologies, in many cases it may be possible to process patient data, for instance for research or administrative purpose, without having access to the data which would identify particular patients. While I would not necessarily expect each GP practice to develop its own IT system capable of concealing the identities of patients from those who do not need to know them, I do expect those developing IT systems for use by GPs to build in such a capability and I would certainly consider action against a GP (or any other data controller) who did not make use of the features available on a system for maximising the privacy of patients.

Finally, I would like to thank all those who have contributed towards the development of this guidance. Some seventy responses were received to the initial consultation paper issued in May 2001. Since a number of these were received from representative bodies, the number of organisations who had input was actually much greater. I would also particularly like to thank those individuals and organisations who attended the consultative seminar which I held in October of last year. While there will inevitably be issues upon which I am asked to provide further clarification, I am certain that without the help of all those who contributed to the consultation I would have faced a far greater number of such requests.

Elizabeth France
May 2002

Chapter 1: Introduction

Scope of the Guidance

The Data Protection Act 1998 gives effect in UK law to EC Directive 95/46/EC, and introduces Eight Data Protection Principles that set out standards of information handling. These standards apply to all data controllers who process personal data. This guidance is concerned with the application of the Act with regards to the processing of information contained within 'health records'. The term, "Processing", includes the collection, use, and disclosure of personal data. The guidance is limited, in the main, to the requirements of the First Data Protection Principle and the Second Data Protection Principle. Further general advice regarding the other Principles, which cover such matters as data quality, rights of access, and security, can be found in *"The Data Protection Act 1998 – Legal Guidance"*, which is available on the Information Commissioner's website at **www.informationcommissioner.gov.uk**.

The term 'health record' is defined by Section 68 of the Act, and means any record which:

- consists of information relating to the physical or mental health or condition of an individual, and
- has been made by or on behalf of a health professional in connection with the care of that individual.

The term 'health professional' is also defined by the Act, and the definition is included in Appendix 2.

This Guidance will be of most value to individuals within organisations (including both the public and private sector) whose responsibilities include data protection, privacy and confidentiality issues. These may include data protection officers, Caldicott Guardians, or legal advisers. The Guidance sets out the requirements of the law and in some cases provides an indication of the issues that data controllers will need to consider when fulfilling their obligations under the Act. The Guidance also aims to provide an indication of the standard which the Information Commissioner will seek to enforce. It is not the intention of this Guidance to provide specific advice on all the possible uses and disclosures of patient information. Data controllers will need to apply the general advice provided here to their specific situations. Box 1 gives an indication of the areas upon which guidance is provided. These are treated more fully in Appendix 1.

Chapter 2: First Data Protection Principle

The First Data Protection Principle states:

"Personal data shall be processed fairly and lawfully and, in particular, shall not be processed unless –
a) at least one of the conditions in Schedule 2 is met, and
b) in the case of sensitive personal data, at least one of the conditions in Schedule 3 is also met"

The conditions is Schedules 2 and 3, referred to above, are listed in Appendix 2.

It is possible to identify a number of separate, albeit cumulative, requirements of this Principle:

- The requirement to satisfy a condition in Schedule 2 and Schedule 3;
- The requirement to collect personal data fairly;
- The requirement to process personal data lawfully.

The requirement to satisfy a condition in Schedule 2 and Schedule 3

In all cases data controllers must satisfy at least one of the conditions in Schedule 2 of the Act. In the context of health sector data controllers, the most relevant Schedule 2 conditions are likely to be:

Box 1

Examples of uses and disclosures of personal data

a) **Care & Treatment**
- Routine record keeping, consultation of records etc, in the course of the provision of care and treatment;
- Processing of records in the event of a medical emergency;
- Disclosures made by one health professional or organisation to another, e.g. where a GP refers a patient to a specialist;
- Clinical audit e.g. the monitoring of a patient care pathway against existing standards and benchmarks.

b) **Administration**
- Processing for administrative purposes, e.g. disclosure by a GP made in order to receive payment for treatment provided;
- Administrative audit, which may include studies designed to improve the efficiency of the NHS as an organisation, e.g. to support decisions about the allocation of resources.

c) **Research & Teaching**
- Statutory disclosures to disease registries and for epidemiological research;
- Non-statutory disclosures to disease registries and for epidemiological research;
- Clinical trials;
- Hospital-based teaching;
- University-based teaching.

d) **Use and disclosures for non-health purposes**
- Disclosures for Crime and Disorder Act 1998 purposes;
- Disclosures to the police;
- Disclosures to hospital chaplains;
- Disclosures to the media.

This list is not exhaustive. It is likely that data controllers will need to apply the requirements of the Act to uses and disclosures of health data that are not listed above.

- Processing with the consent of the data subject;
- Processing necessary to protect the vital interests of the data subject;
- Processing which is necessary for the exercise of functions of a public nature exercised in the public interest by any person;
- Processing which is necessary for the purposes of the legitimate interests pursued by the data controller or those of a third party to whom the data are disclosed, except where the processing is prejudicial to the rights and freedoms or legitimate interests of the data subject.

In practice, it is unlikely to be difficult to satisfy one of these conditions. The focus of this section of the Guidance is therefore on the Schedule 3 processing conditions, at least one of which must be satisfied when processing sensitive personal data. "Sensitive data" is defined in the Act and includes data that relates to the physical or mental health of data subjects. No distinction is drawn in the Act between, say, data relating to the mental health of patients and data relating to minor physical injuries: they are all sensitive.

The most relevant Schedule 3 conditions are likely to be:

- Processing with the explicit consent of the data subject;
- Processing necessary to protect the vital interests of the data subject or another person, where it is not possible to get consent;
- Processing necessary for the purpose of, or in connection with, legal proceedings (including prospective legal proceedings), obtaining legal advice, or is otherwise necessary for the purposes of establishing, exercising or defending legal rights;
- The processing is necessary for medical purposes and is undertaken by a health professional or a person owing a duty of confidentiality equivalent to that owed by a health professional.

The Act provides that included within the term 'medical purposes' are preventative medicine, medical diagnosis, medical research, the provision of care and treatment, and the management of healthcare services. This definition, with the exception of medical research, is taken from the Directive from which the Act is derived. The Commissioner considers that the term 'vital interests' refers to matters of life and death.

The Schedule 3 conditions have been supplemented by further conditions set out in the Data Protection (Processing of Sensitive Personal Data) Order 2000. The most likely conditions for the purposes of this Guidance are:

- Processing of medical data or data relating to ethnic origin for monitoring purposes;
- Processing in the substantial public interest, necessary for the purpose of research whose object is not to support decisions with respect to any particular data subject otherwise than with the explicit consent of the data subject and which is unlikely to cause substantial damage or substantial distress to the data subject or any other person.

The necessity test

Many of the conditions for processing set out in Schedule 2 and Schedule 3 specify that processing must be *necessary* for the purpose stated. In order to satisfy one of the conditions other than processing with consent, data controllers must be able to show that it would not be possible to achieve their purposes with a reasonable degree of ease without the processing of *personal* data. Where data controllers are able to achieve, with a reasonable degree of ease, a purpose using data from which the personal identifiers have been removed, this is the course of action that they must pursue. This may require the use of Privacy Enhancing Technologies (PETs) – Box below. What constitutes a 'reasonable degree of ease' is to be determined by taking into consideration issues including the technology available, and the form in which the personal data are held.

The Commissioner takes the view that when considering the issue of necessity, data controllers must consider objectively whether:

- Such purposes can be achieved only by the processing of personal data; and
- The processing is proportionate to the aim pursued.

This aspect of the First Principle is reinforced by the Third Data Protection Principle, which states that:

"Personal data shall be adequate, relevant and not excessive in relation to the purpose or purposes for which they are processed".

The disclosure of personal data where this is not actually necessary would be likely to contravene this Principle.

The requirement to collect personal data fairly

The Data Protection Principles are listed in Part 1 of Schedule 1 of the Act. Part 2 of Schedule 1 contains further statutory interpretation of the Act. Paragraph 2 of Part 2 sets out the obligation on data controllers to provide certain information to data subjects when collecting their personal data:

- The identity of the data controller;
- The identity of any representative nominated by the data controller for the purposes of the Act;

Box 2

Privacy Enhancing Technologies (PETs)

In a general sense, the term "PET" is used to refer to an IT design philosophy which seeks to deploy new technology in ways which enhance rather than undermine privacy. From this standpoint, the use of techniques such as encryption, password control and other measures designed to ensure that data are guarded with appropriate security can all be regarded as privacy enhancing technologies. Privacy, however, is not limited to security and confidentiality. A Privacy Enhancing approach to database design might allow the holding of patient preferences (e.g. consent to be contacted in connection with medical research), might prompt a clinician to check the personal details of a patient who has not visited a surgery for some years, and might force the periodic review of older records.

More specifically PETs have become associated with systems designed to protect the identity of patients by substituting true identifiers such as name, address or National Health Number with pseudonyms. The starting point is the implied requirement of Schedule 2 and 3 of the Act that, in the absence of consent, personal data should only be processed where it is necessary to do so. If it is never necessary to know the identity of the individuals to whom personal data relates, then the data should be anonymised by removing all personal identifiers. Anonymisation is a permanent process and once anonymised, it will never be possible to link the data to particular individuals.

However, permanent anonymisation may not always be acceptable. For instance a researcher may have no need to know the identity of the patients suffering from a particular condition. He or she may, however, need to know that the patient who was diagnosed with the condition on a particular date is the same patient who was diagnosed with a different condition on another date. Pseudonymisation, sometimes described as "reversible anonymisation" provides a solution. In effect a computer system is used to substitute true patient identifiers with pseudonyms. The true identities are not, however, discarded but retained in a secure part of the computer system allowing the original data to be reconstituted as and when this is required. Typically those making day-to-day uses of pseudonymised data would not have the "keys" allowing the data to be reconstituted.

Potentially there are many different applications for such PETs. For instance they might allow researchers to make more extensive use of medical records without increasing the risk of the misuse or accidental disclosure of patient details. They might prevent support staff from gaining access to information about the medical condition of patients while allowing access to the information necessary to perform administrative tasks.

The Commissioner expects that consideration will be given to the deployment of PETs in all significant new IT developments within the Health Service. She would also expect that data controllers within the Health Service make use of any privacy enhancing features of the software and hardware which they use.

- The purpose or purposes for which the data are to be processed; and
- Any further information which is necessary, having regard to the specific circumstances in which the data are or are to be processed, to enable the processing in respect of the data subject to be fair.

These details are often referred to as "fair processing information", "the fair processing code", or the "fair collection code". In this Guidance we refer to these details as "fair processing information".

The question of the nominated representative of the data controller is highly unlikely to arise in the context of health records, and is not therefore considered here. The other three requirements are considered separately, before discussing the timing and the level of detail to be provided.

Identity of the data controller

Care should be taken to ensure that the data subject knows the identity of the data controller(s) that will process his or her data. Information as to the identity of the data controller should be reasonably specific (e.g. a GPs practice, a NHS Trust etc). "The NHS" or "The Health Service" are not legal entities and therefore cannot be data controllers. Within a GP practice the assumption of data subjects is probably that the practice as a whole is the data controller and that other members of the practice may have access to their records. If there is any doubt, e.g. if a number of GP practices share the same premises, it is the duty of the GP practice to ensure that the patient knows the true position.

Data controllers must also be aware that with increased multi-agency working and initiatives (e.g. between a Trust and a social services department), it may not be immediately clear to data subjects as to who the data controller actually is. Indeed, there may be more than one data controller, in which case the identity of all data controllers should be communicated to data subjects.

Purpose or purposes of processing

When explaining the purpose or purposes for which information is to be processed, data controllers must strike a balance between providing an unnecessary amount of detail and providing information in too general terms. An explanation to the effect that personal data are to be processed for 'health care purposes' would be too general. On the other hand, an explanation that explained all the administrative systems in which patient data might be recorded, the use of data for diagnosis, for treatment etc would be excessive. (An explanation which is not sufficiently detailed is unlikely, in any event, to be sufficient to obtain the consent of the data subject to the processing of data should this be required. The question of consent is considered in more detail in Chapter 4).

Other information necessary to make the processing fair

The Act provides no guidance as to what further information should be provided to data subjects in order to make the processing of their data fair. Clearly this will vary from case to case and from patient to patient depending upon levels of understanding of how the NHS operates, command of English and the sensitivity of the data in question. However, among the information that it may be necessary to provide is the following:

- Information as to what data are to be or have been recorded, where this is in doubt. Patients are likely to expect that basic information will be recorded as to diagnosis and treatment. They may, however, be surprised to find that other information has been recorded whether this is an opinion of a doctor or the circumstances surrounding an injury. Unless patients have a reasonably clear idea of what is recorded about them, any consent to other uses or disclosures of their data may not be valid.
- Information as to specific disclosures. Given the sensitivity of medical data, data subjects should be informed of any non-routine disclosures of their data.
- Information as to whether any secondary uses or disclosures of data are optional. Where patients have a choice as to whether to provide information, to allow its disclosure to third parties or to object to certain uses or

disclosures, then the requirement of fairness suggests that these choices should be brought to their attention.

How much fair processing information should be provided?

Concern has been expressed that the fair processing rules may require the provision of very large amounts of information in which patients have no real interest. In the Commissioner's view this concern is misplaced. In effect the fair processing information provided should achieve two basic purposes:

- It should provide sufficient information to allow the patients to exercise their rights in relation to their data. Hence patients should be told who will process their data, including any disclosures of personal data (which will allow them to make subject access requests), whether it must be supplied (which will allow them to opt-out if they wish), and what information is contained in their record (which will allow them to give meaningful consent to its processing.)
- It should provide sufficient information to allow the individual to assess the risks to him or her in providing their data, in consenting to their wider use, in choosing not to object to their processing etc. This should have at least two consequences for data controllers. It should become clear that fair processing notices do not need to contain a large amount of detail about routine, administrative uses of data. It should also become clear that researchers engaged in open-ended studies are not prevented by the Act from soliciting patient data on the grounds that their fair processing notices cannot be sufficiently detailed. Fair processing notices in this case should simply need to make clear that the research in question is indeed open-ended, leaving the individual to assess the risk.

It may also be helpful to bear in mind that the fair processing rules do not mean that patients must be provided with information that they are known to already possess.

When should fair processing information be provided?

It is likely that there will be a number of standard purposes for which the personal data of all patients entering a hospital or registering with a GP will be processed, information about which can be provided to patients at the outset of the episode of care. In particular, patients may need to be told about typical flows of data between different NHS bodies. This information is relatively timeless and it is appropriate that patients are given it at an early opportunity. It would certainly be good practice to remind patients of this information from time to time, for instance by ensuring that leaflets containing the relevant information are available to patients.

Some patients may subsequently have their personal data processed for a number of additional purposes e.g. information about a cancer diagnosis may be passed to a cancer registry, or information may be passed to social services. Those patients who will have their personal data processed for these additional purposes will need to be provided with this further information, in order to satisfy the fair processing requirements. This type of information is specific to particular patients at particular times and should be given in context, at a time when individuals are able to make sense of it.

How should the fair processing information be given?

The provision of 'fair processing information' by means of a poster in the surgery or waiting room or by a notice in the local paper etc is unlikely to be sufficient to meet the requirements of the Act since not all patients will see or be able to understand such information. Such methods may, however, be used to supplement other forms of communication. Methods by which the fair processing information may be provided include a standard information leaflet, information provided face to face in the course of a consultation, information included with an appointment letter from a hospital or clinic, or a letter sent to a patient's home. The effort involved in providing this information may be minimised by integrating the process with existing procedures. Many GP practices, for instance, already provide leaflets to patients about how the practice operates. Such leaflets could easily incorporate the fair processing information. Doctors may be able to easily provide specific information to patients in the course of consultations. Only where such an opportunity does not present itself will it be necessary to contact patients separately, for instance, if they are to be invited to participate in a programme of research involving the disclosure of their medical records to a researcher who may wish to interview patients with particular medical conditions.

Obtaining data from a person other than the data subject

In many cases medical information will be obtained directly from the patient either because it has been supplied by the patient (e.g. a description of symptoms) or has been obtained by a medical examination conducted by the person creating the record (e.g. an observation of symptoms). In a significant proportion of cases, however, data will be obtained by other means, whether from a third party or generated by the person creating the record (e.g. a medical opinion based on symptoms presented).

The Act recognises that the provision of fair processing information when data are obtained other than from the data subject presents some difficulties. The following exceptions from the provision of the fair processing information may only be relied upon by data controllers where they have obtained personal data from someone other than the data subject. It should be stressed that the ability to rely on an exemption does not absolve the data controller from the overriding duty to process personal data fairly.

The exceptions are:
- Where providing the fair processing information would involve a disproportionate effort; or
- Where it is necessary for the data controller to record the information to be contained in the data, or to disclose the data, to comply with any legal obligation to which the data controller is subject, other than an obligation imposed by contract.

The term 'disproportionate effort' is not defined by the Act. In assessing what does or does not amount to disproportionate effort, the starting point must be that data controllers are **not** generally exempt from providing the fair processing information because they have not obtained data directly from the data subject. What does or does not amount to disproportionate effort is a question of fact to be determined in each and every case.

In deciding this, the Commissioner will take into account a number of factors, including the nature of the data, the length of time and the cost involved to the data controller in providing the information. The fact that the data controller has had to expend a substantial amount of effort and/or cost in providing the information does not necessarily mean that the Commissioner will reach the decision that the data controller can legitimately rely upon the disproportionate effort exception. In certain circumstances, the Commissioner would consider that such an effort could reasonably be expected. The above factors will always be balanced against the effect on the data subject and in this respect a relevant consideration would be the extent to which the data subject already knows about the processing of his or her personal data by the data controller.

Data controllers should note that the Data Protection (Conditions Under Paragraph 3 of Part II of Schedule 1) Order 2000 provides that any data controller claiming the benefit of the disapplication of the requirement to provide fair processing information must still provide this information to any individual who requests it. In addition a data controller who does not provide fair processing information because to do so would involve disproportionate effort must keep a record of the reasons why he believes the disapplication of the fair processing requirements is necessary.

In practice, the Commissioner thinks that it is increasingly unlikely that NHS data controllers will be able to rely successfully upon these provisions. While there will be many cases in which, say, a consultant, receives personal data from a person other than the data subject, for instance his or her GP, the GP will have obtained the data directly from the patient and will have therefore provided the necessary fair processing information. There is no need, in other words, for the consultant to rely upon the exception since the patient will already be in possession of the fair processing information.

One area, however, where the exception is likely to be of assistance is that of records created before the enactment of data protection legislation. The Commissioner would generally accept that it would involve disproportionate effort to write to all existing patients to provide the fair processing information. However, that information should be available to patients when they attend surgeries and clinics and would have to be given in the event of any non-routine uses or disclosures of personal data.

The exception may also be relevant for those carrying out records based research where records were created in the past without the intention of using them for research purposes. (This issue is considered in greater detail in the following chapter under the heading "The Research Exemption".)

Cases where the requirement to provide fair processing information does not apply

There are a number of circumstances in which the requirement to provide the fair processing information does not apply.

- Section 29 of the Act permits uses or disclosures of personal data for the purpose of the prevention of detection of crime or the prosecution or apprehension of offenders, even though the data subject was not informed of those uses or disclosures, if to inform the data subject might prejudice that purpose. This may be of relevance in the context of combating fraud and corruption, e.g. in circumstances where it may be alleged that a GP has sought payment from a Health Authority for treatment which was not given, or where it is alleged that a patient has claimed free treatment to which he or she is not entitled. The exemption may also justify the disclosure of medical information to the police investigating an alleged assault on a member of staff.

- Section 31(2)(a)(iii) of the Act may allow for the disclosure of personal data without a prior explanation having been given to the data subject if the disclosure is necessary for protecting members of the public against "dishonesty, malpractice or other seriously improper conduct by, or the unfitness or incompetence of, persons authorised to carry on any profession or activity". This would appear to allow disclosures, in certain cases, of patient data to bodies responsible for maintaining professional standards.

- Section 31(4)(iii) allows the disclosure of personal data to the Health Service Commissioners (the Ombudsman) if not to do so would prejudice the discharge of the functions of those bodies.

- Section 35 allows the disclosure of information without breach of, among other things, the First, Second and Third Principles where the disclosure is a requirement of law or for the purpose of establishing, exercising or defending legal rights.

Although the exemptions may be relevant in some cases, they are unlikely to be the basis for the routine or wholesale processing of data without the provision of the information specified in the fair processing information to the data subject. In many cases, even though an exemption is apparently available, it would be wrong to rely upon it since it would be unnecessary to do so.

An example would be a disclosure of personal data for medical research purposes made in accordance with an order under s.60 of the Health and Social Care Act 2001 (applicable only in England and Wales). An order might specify, for instance, that all clinicians making a diagnosis of cancer must make a report to a cancer registry. While superficially s.35 suggests that fair processing information need not be given to the patient since the disclosure is a requirement of the law, in fact it would not be proper to rely upon the exemption since to provide the fair processing information would not be inconsistent with the disclosure.

By contrast, a hospital might decide to disclose to the police relevant parts of the medical record of a patient who had assaulted a member of staff even though no fair processing information had been given, since in that case there would be prejudice to the s.29 purpose of the disclosure if the normal rules were followed.

The requirement to process personal data lawfully

In addition to the requirement to satisfy a condition in Schedule 2 and Schedule 3 of the Act, there is a general requirement that personal data are processed lawfully. While the Act does not provide any guidance on the meaning of the terms "lawful" or "unlawful", the natural meaning of unlawful has been broadly described by the Courts as "something which is contrary to some law or enactment or is done without lawful justification or excuse". In effect, the Principle means that a data controller must comply with all relevant rules of law whether derived from statute or common law, relating to the purpose and ways in which the data controller processes personal data. The following may be relevant when deciding whether personal data have been processed lawfully:

- Statutory prohibitions on use or disclosure: If the general law prevents a particular disclosure of personal data then there would also be a contravention of the lawful processing requirement of the Data Protection Act 1998 if a disclosure were made.
- The *ultra vires* rule and the rule relating to the excess of delegated powers, under which the data controller may only act within the limits of its legal powers: Public authorities such as the Department of Health or a NHS Trust might exceed their powers if, for instance, they were to make commercial use of patient data, e.g. by selling names and addresses to the manufacturers of medical equipment.
- Contractual restrictions on processing: this may be of particular relevance in the private health sector where the provision of treatment is on the basis of a contract between the patient and the clinician, clinic, hospital etc.
- Confidentiality arising from the relationship of the data controller with the data subject: this issue is considered separately in Chapter 4.
- Article 8 of the European Convention on Human Rights (the right to respect for private and family life, home and correspondence): the Human Rights Act 2000 underpins the Data Protection Act and other legislation. Public authorities are required to construe the legislation under which they operate in accordance with the European Convention on Human Rights and to ensure that their actions and those of their staff are consistent with it.

This list is by no means exhaustive. The various different considerations inevitably overlap. The key issue for the processing of health data is likely to be the common law duty of confidence. This is addressed in greater detail in Chapter 4. In brief, even though the Act does not explicitly require the consent of patients in order to process medical data, in many cases there is an implied requirement to obtain patient consent for the processing of data since to process without consent would involve a breach of a duty of confidence which, in turn, would involve a breach of the requirement in the Act to process personal data lawfully.

Chapter 3: The Second Data Protection Principle

The Second Data Protection Principle states:

"Personal data shall be obtained only for one or more specified and lawful purposes, and shall not be further processed in any manner incompatible with those purposes."

There are two means by which a data controller may specify the purpose or purposes for which the personal data are obtained:

- In a notice given by the data controller to the data subject in accordance with the fair processing requirements; or
- By notifying the purposes on a data controller's Data Protection Register entry, through the Notification procedures. (It should be noted that Notification to the Commissioner alone will not satisfy the fairness requirements of the First Principle).

These are cumulative and, except in cases where it is proposed to process personal data for purposes that were not envisaged at the time of collection, the information provided to the data subject will reflect the purposes notified to the Commissioner. The effect of the Principle is to reinforce the First Principle and also to limit the range of cases where data may be processed for purposes of which the data subject was not informed to ones which are *compatible* with those for which data were originally obtained.

The research exemption

The Act does envisage some exceptions to the Second Principle, notably where personal data are processed for the purposes of research (including statistical or historical purposes). These exceptions are set out in Section 33 of the Act, which is commonly known as 'the research exemption'. These exceptions can be applied where the processing (or further processing) is only for research purposes, and where the following conditions are met:

- The data are not processed to support measures or decisions relating to particular individuals; and
- The data are not processed in such a way that substantial damage or substantial distress is, or is likely to be, caused to any data subject.

Where the exemption applies:

- The further processing of personal data will not be considered incompatible with the purposes for which they were obtained. (It is important to note that the exemption does not excuse the data controller from complying with the part of the Second Principle that states that personal data shall be obtained only for one or more specified and lawful purposes);

• Personal data may be kept indefinitely (despite the Fifth Data Protection Principle which states that personal data should not be kept for longer than is necessary);
• Subject access does not have to be given provided that the results of the research or any resulting statistics are not made available in a form that identifies the data subject.

It is important to note that even where the exemption applies, the data controller is still required to comply with the rest of the Act, including the First and Second Principles. The data controller should ensure that at the time the data are collected, the data subject is made fully aware of what the data controller intends to do with the data. If the data controller subsequently decides to process the data in order to carry out further research of a kind that would not have been envisaged by the data subject at the time the data were collected, the data controller will need to comply with the fair processing requirements of the Act in respect of this processing.

The exemption cannot be used to justify the retention of records for longer than would normally be the case simply because the records might be used for research in the future. The exemption may only be used, in other words, if research is actually being carried out or there is a firm intention to use the records for that purpose.

The research exemption, combined with the special fair processing rules in relation to data obtained from someone other than the data subject, has implications for records based research. Two general cases may be distinguished. In the first case, it is proposed to conduct records based research by making use of current records or ones yet to be created. Patients should be informed, as part of the standard fair processing information, that their data may be used for research purposes designed to better understand and treat their conditions. The research exemption (insofar as compatibility with the Second Principle is concerned) is not relevant since these records will have been compiled both for the purpose of treatment and research.

In the second case, research is proposed using existing records of patients who are no longer being treated for their condition. Such records may be quite old. Those patients who may be contacted without involving disproportionate effort should be given fair processing information. Those patients who cannot be contacted without disproportionate effort need not be given the fair processing information although the researcher should record this fact. The research exemption permits the use of these data for research, providing that the conditions described above apply.

Chapter 4: Confidentiality

Chapter 2 considered, among other matters, the general requirement to process personal data lawfully. While there are potentially a large number of considerations which data controllers processing health data must take, in practice, the key issue in this context is likely to be the duty of confidence.

The duty of confidence is a common law concept rather than a statutory requirement. As such it derives from cases that have been considered by the Courts. Inevitably there are areas which have not been litigated, where it is impossible to state with any certainty whether a duty of confidence exists and, therefore, that the consent of patients is required for the processing of their data. Even where there is case law, it may be difficult to extrapolate general principles from the particular circumstances of the case. There is no certainty that a decision made many years ago by a court would be reflected in a decision made in the context of a modern NHS. In this chapter, we first provide a general introduction to the concept of confidentiality, its exceptions and the requirement to obtain the consent of patients for the processing of medical data. Then we attempt to describe the approach taken by the Commissioner in the area of health.

Confidentiality and exceptions to the duty of confidence

Personal data that are subject to a duty of confidence have a number of characteristics:
• The information is not in the public domain or readily available from another source;
• The information is of a certain degree of sensitivity, (more than "mere title tattle") such as medical data;
• The information has been provided with the expectation that it will only be used or disclosed for particular purposes. This expectation may arise because a specific undertaking has been given, because the confider places specific restrictions on the use of data which are agreed by the recipient, or because the relationship between the recipient and the data subject generally gives rise to an expectation of confidentiality, for instance as arises between a customer and a bank or a patient and a doctor.

The Courts have generally recognised three exceptions to the duty of confidence:
• Where there is a legal compulsion;
• Where there is an overriding duty to the public;
• Where the individual to whom the information relates has consented.

Certain disclosures of medical data have long been requirements of the law. Certain diseases are notifiable. More recently s.60 of the Health and Social Care Act 2001 creates a power for the Secretary of State to make orders (subject to various safeguards, and only applicable in England and Wales) requiring the disclosure of patient data that would otherwise be prevented by a duty of confidence. Courts may order the disclosure of patient data in particular cases.

Disclosures required by law are relatively easy to identify. Disclosures that may be justified as being in the public interest, by contrast, necessarily involve the exercise of judgment, balancing the rights of patients against the public good. For instance, a hospital *may* consider the disclosure of medical information to the police would be justified in the event of an assault on a member of staff but unjustified in the context of a minor theft. Because such decisions involve the exercise of judgment it is important that they are taken at an appropriate level and that sound procedures are developed for taking those decisions.

Consent

Most uses or disclosures of medical data will be justified by having obtained the consent of patients. There is no single definition of consent.

The EU Directive, for instance, defines consent as: *"… any freely given specific and informed indication of his wishes by which the data subject signifies his agreement to personal data relating to him being processed."* On one reading this definition suggests that the giving of consent may not legitimately be made a condition of receiving a service such as health care since to impose conditions might mean that consent had not been "freely given". Were a data controller to seek to rely upon consent as a condition of processing medical data (rather than one of the other possible conditions suggested in Chapter 2) such a strict reading of the definition in the Directive might invalidate the consent that had apparently been obtained.

In considering the common law duty of confidence, however, the courts have not generally found that consent is rendered invalid by having conditions attached, providing that those conditions are not unduly onerous. In considering the common law duty of confidence, it is this approach to consent that the Commissioner will follow, taking three key considerations.

Firstly, consent must be informed. The data subject must know, in other words, what are the proposed uses or disclosures of personal data. In effect a patient will be able to give informed consent if he or she has been supplied with the fair processing information discussed earlier. It

follows from this that a patient cannot be deemed to have consented to something of which he or she is ignorant.

Secondly, the person giving consent must have some degree of choice. "Consent" given under duress or coercion is not consent at all. By contrast consent which is entirely optional and may be withheld without any consequences is clearly valid. Between these two extremes is consent which is more or less conditional upon agreement to some other term or condition. It would not necessarily be unfair that a patient should be asked to consent to the disclosure of data by, for example, a GP to a Health Authority for administrative purposes as a condition of receiving treatment from that GP. By contrast it could be argued that a requirement to consent to the disclosure of data to a medical student as a condition of receipt of treatment in a NHS hospital was unfair.

Thirdly, there must be some indication that the data subject has given his or her consent. This may be express (i.e. explicit) or implied. Express consent is given by a patient agreeing actively, usually orally or in writing, to a particular use or disclosure of information. Implied consent is given when an individual takes some other action in the knowledge that in doing so he or she has incidentally agreed to a particular use or disclosure of information. For instance a patient who visits a GP for treatment may be taken to imply consent to the GP consulting his or her medical records to assist diagnosis. The Courts have not generally specified whether consent should be express or implied. It is clear, however, that for consent of any sort to be given, there must be some active communication between the parties. It would not be sufficient, for instance, to write to patients to advise them of a new use of their data and to assume that all who had not objected had consented to that new use. It is a mistake to assume that implied consent is a less valid form of consent than express. Both must be equally informed and both reflect the wishes of the patient. The advantage of express consent is that it is less likely to be ambiguous and may thus be preferred when the risk of misunderstanding is greater.

The Commissioner's approach to medical confidentiality

The Commissioner is not a general source of advice upon confidentiality. However, from time to time, for instance when asked to carry out an assessment of whether the processing of personal data seems likely to meet the requirements of the Act, she must necessarily take a view as to whether firstly, in her opinion, a duty of confidence has arisen and secondly, whether there has been a breach of that duty. Each case must be considered upon its merits. This section of the Guidance describes the general approach.

The Commissioner's general assumption is that the processing of health data (that is data relating to the physical or mental health of data subjects) by a health professional (see Appendix 2) is subject to a duty of confidence even though explicit consent for processing is not a requirement of Schedule 3 of the Act. This assumption is based upon case law, upon statements made by Ministers at the Department of Health, and upon the advice given by regulatory and representative bodies in the area. The Commissioner distinguishes between a number of broad categories.

As was noted earlier, in some cases, even though data may be subject to a duty of confidence, there may be a justification for disclosure or for secondary use. For instance, the disclosure of information relating to a notifiable disease or a disclosure on the basis of an Order made under s.60 of the Health and Social Care Act cannot be legitimately accused of involving breaches of confidence.

Some other uses and disclosures of data, for instance, routine record keeping, consultation of records etc, in the course of the provision of care and treatment or clinical audit are effectively conditions of receiving treatment. Providing that these uses and disclosures are, as a matter of fact, necessary in order to provide treatment in today's National Health Service, the Commissioner thinks that it is unlikely that a court would find that consent was invalid by virtue of being made a condition of treatment. Such uses and disclosures may be described as "mandatory" in the sense that acceptance of treatment by the patient will imply consent to these uses or disclosures. (Although it may be generally acceptable to make the giving of consent a condition of treatment, as is discussed in the next chapter, in individual cases where a particular use or disclosure of personal data might cause unwarranted damage or distress, there is a right to object. For instance consent for administrative staff to access medical data for legitimate administrative purposes might generally be a condition of treatment. However, in a particular case, a patient might object if the member of the administrative team was personally known to him or her.)

In most cases where consent is required in order to satisfy the common law duty of confidence, the Commissioner accepts that implied consent is valid. She does not accept that implied consent is a lesser form of consent. Providing that the fair collection information described in Chapter 2 has been provided at an appropriate time, including information as to whether data must be supplied or whether it is optional to do so, and the data subject accepts treatment and does not object to any uses or disclosures of data, then the Commissioner will consider that valid consent has been

given. There is an overlap, in other words, between the fair processing requirements of the Act and the consent requirements of the common law.

The Commissioner does, however, think that there are some occasions when express or explicit consent is required. These arise particularly where data have been collected previously without the relevant fair processing information having been provided. This might occur because data were collected before the Act came into force or because the purposes for which it is proposed that data are processed has changed since collection.

In deciding when express rather than implied consent should be obtained and when it is legitimate to make provision of treatment conditional upon agreement to certain uses or disclosures of personal data, the Commissioner will be influenced not only by any relevant case law but also by any Codes of Practice, advice or guidance issued by the Department of Health, NHS Executive, or any of the relevant representative or regulatory bodies. In individual cases she will also take into account any decision or advice given by Caldicott Guardians, or the Health Service Ombudsman.

Chapter 5: The right to object to processing

The Act does not create an overarching requirement that personal data, even sensitive personal data, may only be processed with the consent of data subjects. As was discussed in Chapter 4, however, in many cases it will only be permissible to process health data with the consent of patients not because this is an explicit requirement of the Data Protection Act but because it is a required by the common law duty of confidence and the Act requires that personal data are processed lawfully.

Although data controllers may not be under a duty to obtain patient consent, there are certainly cases where they should give patients the opportunity to object to the processing of their data. There are also cases where data subjects may legitimately object to the processing of their personal data. These issues are considered in this Chapter.

When should an opt-out be given?

The point was made in Chapter 2 that among the other information that should be provided to data subjects in order to make the processing of personal data fair may be information as to whether the proposed uses or disclosures of data are mandatory or optional. The failure to provide this information would be likely to result in personal data being unfairly collected.

In deciding whether to offer an opt-out, data controllers should attempt to distinguish between those uses and disclosures of data which are essential in order to treat patients within the health service and those which are not. By the term "essential" is meant those uses and disclosures without which treatment could not be given and those uses or disclosures which the law makes mandatory. Examples of essential uses and disclosures include:

- Routine record keeping, consultation of records etc, in the course of the provision of care and treatment;
- Processing of records in the event of a medical emergency;
- Clinical audit e.g. the monitoring of a patient care pathway against existing standards and benchmarks;
- Processing for administrative purposes, e.g. disclosure by a GP made in order to receive payment for treatment provided;
- Administrative audit, which may include studies designed to improve the efficiency of the NHS as an organisation, e.g. to support decisions about the allocation of resources;
- Statutory disclosures to disease registries or statutory disclosures for epidemiological research.

In effect these are necessary elements of the medical purpose for which it is proposed that patients' data are processed. Since it is unlikely to make good administrative sense to offer patients the opportunity to object to the processing of their data for any of the individual elements suggested, it would not make sense to provide an opt-out.

Examples of uses and disclosures that may not be essential include:

- Disclosures to social workers/social services departments;
- Teaching;
- Disclosures to hospital chaplains;
- Clinical trials;
- Disclosures to the media.

In effect these non-essential uses are either for secondary medical purposes, in particular teaching or research, or for non-medical purposes. (Please note: the lists are intended neither to be exhaustive nor to be authoritative. What may be an essential use or disclosure for one data controller may not be essential for another.)

Opt-outs as means of gaining consent

In many cases the requirement of the Data Protection Act to provide fair processing information overlaps with the requirement flowing from the common law duty of confidence to obtain consent for the use and disclosure of data.

For instance, patients register for the first time with, say, a cancer clinic. They are provided with standard fair processing information about uses and disclosures of personal data and are also advised that their records will be made available to researchers who may wish to contact them in the future. Any patients who do not object may be deemed to have consented to the disclosure and to being contacted by the researchers.

It is important to distinguish this case, where patients are registering for the first time and thus have not yet provided the clinic with any personal data, from that where the clinic would like to pass the records of former patients to a researcher. On the assumption that patient consent is required (i.e. there is no relevant order under s.60 of the Health and Social Care Act), and that the research exemption is not relevant (since in this case contact by the researcher might cause substantial distress) it would **not** be sufficient simply to write to former patients giving the opportunity to object. In that case it would be incorrect to infer either consent or an objection from a failure of a patient to respond. The patients would not, in other words, have been given the opportunity to signify consent to the processing of their data.

Where consent to the use or disclosure of personal data is sought after those data were collected, it will normally be necessary to obtain the express or explicit consent of patients.

The right to object to processing

An opt-out should be provided wherever patients have a real choice as to how their data are to be processed or wherever this is an appropriate means of gaining consent. In addition, data subjects also have rights to object to the processing of their data whether or not they have been given an opt-out.

Section 10 of the Act sets out the general right to object:

"... an individual is entitled at any time by notice in writing to a data controller to require the data controller at the end of such period as is reasonable in the circumstance to cease, or not to begin, processing or processing for a specified purpose or in a specified manner, any personal data of which he is the data subject, on the grounds that, for specified reasons –

(a) the processing of those data or their processing for that purpose or in that manner is causing or is likely to cause substantial damage or substantial distress to him or another, and
(b) that damage or distress is or would be unwarranted

Among the important points to note are that objections to processing under this section of the Act must be put in writing, and secondly that the grounds for objection are limited to cases where there is or is likely to be substantial and unwarranted damage or distress to the data subject or

Appendix 1

Examples of uses and disclosures

a) Care and treatment

Use or Disclosure	Schedule 2 Condition	Schedule 3 Condition	Fair Processing Information	Lawfulness	PETs	2DPP
Routine record-keeping; consultation of records etc	Condition 5 or 6	Condition 8	Ensure patient is aware of identity of data controller. Generally assumed patient is aware of these uses and disclosure.	Consent likely to be required to meet Common Law obligations but need not be 'explicit' in terms of DPA.	Data must be secure, but there is no general need to use a PET.	Not applicable.
Processing of records in the event of a medical emergency	Condition 5 or 6	Condition 3. Wrong to rely on this condition if patient has previously objected to this type of use.	General information should be provided, even though it could be assumed that patients would expect their data to be available in an emergency.	Consent likely to be required to meet Common Law obligations but need not be 'explicit' in terms of DPA. If patient was unable to consent, then the public interest may meet the Common Law requirements. Common Law would be breached if it was known that the patient objected to the disclosure.	Data must be secure, but there is no general need to use a PET.	Disclosure is compatible.
Disclosures made by one health professional or organisation to another	Condition 5 or 6	Condition 8. Only relevant information should be disclosed.	Any disclosures should be explained.	Consent likely to be required to meet Common Law obligations but need not be 'explicit' in terms of DPA.	Data must be secure, but there is no general need to use a PET.	Disclosure is compatible.
Clinical audit	Condition 5 or 6	Condition 8. Only relevant information should be disclosed.	Any disclosures should be explained.	Consent likely to be required to meet Common Law obligations but need not be 'explicit' in terms of DPA.	Strong argument for the use of PETs to protect the identity of patients.	Satisfied by a notice given to patients. Where this was not possible, it may be possible to rely on S33.

b) Administration

Processing for administrative purposes	Condition 5 or 6	Condition 8. Only relevant information should be disclosed.	Purposes should be explained in general terms.	Consent likely to be required to meet Common Law obligations but need not be 'explicit' in terms of DPA.	Only disclose patient ID if it is intended to contact the patient. Use of PETs is encouraged.	Disclosure is compatible.
Administrative audit	Condition 5 or 6	Condition 8. Only relevant information should be disclosed.	Uses and disclosures should be explained.	Consent likely to be required to meet Common Law obligations but need not be 'explicit' in terms of DPA.	Strong argument for the use of PETs to protect the identity of patients.	Satisfied by a notice given to patients. If not given, it may be possible to rely on S33.

c) Research and teaching

Statutory disclosures to disease registries or statutory disclosures for epidemiological research	Condition 5 or 6	Condition 8. Only relevant information should be disclosed.	Uses and disclosures should be explained.	Common Law obligations met if there is a statutory requirement to disclose e.g. notifiable diseases, or s60 of Health & Social Care Act 2001 (England and Wales only).	Strong argument for the use of PETs to protect the identity of patients.	Satisfied by a notice given to patients. If not given, it may be possible to rely on S33.
Non-statutory disclosures to disease registries or non-statutory disclosures for epidemiological research	Condition 5 or 6	Condition 8. Only relevant information should be disclosed.	Uses and disclosures should be explained, including that this use of personal data is optional.	Consent likely be required to meet Common Law obligations, but need not be 'explicit' in terms of DPA. Patients have the right to object.	Strong argument for the use of PETs to protect the identity of patients.	Satisfied by a notice given to patients. If not given, it may be possible to rely on S33.
Clinical trials	Condition 1, 5 or 6	Condition 1 or 8. Only relevant information should be disclosed.	Uses and disclosures should be explained, including that this use of personal data is optional.	Consent required to meet Common Law obligations, and is likely to be 'explicit' in terms of DPA.	Strong argument for the use of PETs to protect the identity of patients.	Satisfied by a notice given to patients. S33 is unlikely to be appropriate.
Teaching	Condition 1, 5 or 6	Condition 1, or 8. Only relevant information should be disclosed.	Uses and disclosures should be explained, including that this use of personal data is optional, and whether it is hospital or university based teaching.	Consent likely to be required to meet Common Law obligations, but need not be 'explicit' in terms of DPA. Patients have the right to object.	Strong argument for the use of PETs to protect the identity of patients.	Satisfied by a notice given to patients. S33 is unlikely to be appropriate.

(cont.)

d) Uses and disclosures for non-health purposes

Use or Disclosure	Schedule 2 Condition	Schedule 3 Condition	Fair Processing Information	Lawfulness	PETs	2DPP
Disclosures for Crime and Disorder Act purposes	Condition 5 or 6	Condition 1 or 7. Only relevant information should be disclosed.	Uses and disclosures should be explained, unless prejudicial to S29.	Consent likely to be required to meet Common Law obligations (unless another exception to the duty of confidence applies), but need not be 'explicit' in terms of DPA.	Data must be secure, and anonymised data should be used where possible.	Satisfied by a notice given to patients. If S29 applies, a notice may not be required.
Disclosures to the police	Condition 5 or 6	Condition 7	Uses and disclosures should be explained, unless prejudicial to S29.	Consent not required if disclosure is in the public interest, or if required by law (e.g. court order).	Data must be secure, but there is no general need to use a PET.	Satisfied by a notice given to patients. If S29 applies, a notice may not be required.
Disclosures of religious affiliation to Chaplains	Condition 1. Condition 4 may apply in very limited circumstances.	Condition 1. Condition 3 may apply in very limited circumstances.	Uses and disclosures should be explained.	Consent required, unless individual unable to give consent.	Data must be secure, but there is no general need to use a PET.	Satisfied by obtaining consent of patient.
Disclosures to the media	Condition 1 or 6	Condition 1	Uses and disclosures should be explained.	Consent likely to be required to meet Common Law obligations.	Data must be secure, but there is no general need to use a PET.	Satisfied by obtaining consent of patient.

another person. (There will be many cases where it is good practice to act upon an objection made by means other than writing. It would also be good practice to respect an individual's wishes even if they could not demonstrate that the damage or distress caused to them was *substantial.*)

A data controller in receipt of a written objection to processing must, within 21 days, inform the person making the objection in writing whether it has complied or intends to comply with the request or must state its grounds for refusing to do so.

The Act gives no comprehensive guidance as to the valid grounds for objecting to the processing of health data, although it makes clear that the interests of the data controller will outweigh those of the person objecting to the processing of data if the processing of data is on the basis of any of the following four Schedule 2 conditions:

• The data subject has given his consent (this condition will be relevant where the person objecting to the processing is a person other than the data subject);

• The processing is necessary for the performance of a contract or for entering into a contract at the request of the data subject;

• The processing is necessary for compliance with legal obligations (for instance a disclosure made on a statutory basis);

• The processing is necessary to protect the vital interests of the data subject (this condition will also only be relevant where the person objecting to the processing is a person other than the data subject).

In the absence of any clearer guidance in the Act, data controllers must judge each objection to processing which is received on its merits. For instance, two individuals may object to their GP to the processing of their data for administrative purposes. In the case of the first, no grounds for the objection are advanced and the GP may be justified in continuing to process the patient's data for administrative purposes despite the objection (on the assumption that the patient continues to accept treatment). In the second case, a patient objects to the use of data for administrative purposes because a member of the administrative staff in the practice is known to the patient personally and he or she does not wish the details of their medical condition to be disclosed to that person. In this case it is far easier to see that substantial damage or distress might be caused to the patient and it is likely that the GP will decide to make separate administrative arrangements for this patient.

In addition to the general right to object to processing which is, as we have seen, a qualified right, there is an absolute right to object to the use of personal data for direct marketing purposes.

Appendix 1: Practical application

In this section we seek to apply the analysis of the Principles as discussed in the preceding chapters. Here, the application is limited to those examples listed in the Introduction, but should be sufficiently informative to allow a similar application of the Act to other uses and disclosures of health data.

The tables should not be read in isolation, but in the context of the discussion found in the preceding chapters. Please refer to Chapter 1 for a full description of the use and disclosure headings.

The tables on the preceding pages are broken down into 4 broad areas:

a) Care and treatment;
b) Administration;
c) Research and teaching;
d) Uses and disclosures for non-health purposes.

Appendix 2: Glossary of terms

Data controller: A person who (either jointly or in common with other persons) determines the purposes for which and the manner in which personal data are, or are to be, processed.

Data subject: An individual who is the subject of personal data.

Health professional: Means any of the following:

a) a registered medical practitioner (a "registered medical practitioner" includes any person who is provisionally registered under section 15 or 21 of the Medical Act 1983 and is engaged in such employment as is mentioned in subsection (3) of that section.)

b) a registered dentist as defined by section 53(1) of the Dentists Act 1984,

c) a registered optician as defined by section 36(1) of the Opticians Act 1989,

d) a registered pharmaceutical chemist as defined by section 24(1) of the Pharmacy Act 1954 or a registered person as defined by Article 2(2) of the Pharmacy (Northern Ireland) Order 1976,

e) a registered nurse, midwife or health visitor,

f) a registered osteopath as defined by section 41 of the Osteopaths Act 1993,

g) a registered chiropractor as defined by section 43 of the Chiropractors Act 1994,

h) any person who is registered as a member of a profession to which the Professions Supplementary to Medicine Act 1960 for the time being extends,

i) a clinical psychologist, child psychotherapist or speech therapist,

j) a music therapist employed by a health service body, and

k) a scientist employed by such a body as head of department.

Health record: Any record which consists of information relating to the physical or mental health or condition of an individual, and has been made by or on behalf of a health professional in connection with the care of that individual.

Personal data: Data which relate to a living individual who can be identified from those data, or from those data and other information which is in the possession of, or is likely to come into the possession of, the data controller and includes any expression of opinion about the individual and any indication of the intentions of the data controller or any other person in respect of the individual.

Processing: In relation to information or data, processing means obtaining, recording or holding the information or data, or carrying out any operation or set of operations on the information or data.

Appendix 3: Schedule 2 and schedule 3 conditions

Schedule 2:

1 The data subject has given their consent to the processing.

2 The processing is necessary –
   a) for the performance of a contract to which the data subject is a party, or
   b) for the taking of steps at the request of the data subject with a view to entering into a contract.

3 The processing is necessary to comply with any legal obligation to which the data controller is subject, other than an obligation imposed by contract.

4 The processing is necessary in order to protect the vital interests of the data subject.

5 The processing is necessary –
   a) for the administration of justice,
   b) for the exercise of any functions conferred by or under any enactment,
   c) for the exercise of any functions of the Crown, a Minister of the Crown or a government department, or
   d) for the exercise of any other functions of a public nature exercised in the public interest.

6 The processing is necessary for the purposes of legitimate interests pursued by the data controller or by the third party or parties to whom the data are disclosed, except where the processing is unwarranted in any particular case because of prejudice to the rights and freedoms or legitimate interests of the data subject. The Secretary of State may by order specify particular circumstances in which this condition is, or is not, to be taken to be satisfied.

Schedule 3:

1 The data subject has given their explicit consent to the processing of the personal data.

2 The processing is necessary for the purposes of exercising or performing any right or obligation which is conferred or imposed by law on the data controller in connection with employment. The Secretary of State may by order specify cases where this condition is either excluded altogether or only satisfied upon the satisfaction of further conditions.

3 The processing is necessary –
   a) in order to protect the vital interests of the data subject or another person, in a case where –
      i. consent cannot be given by or on behalf of the data subject, or
      ii. the data controller cannot reasonably be expected to obtain the consent of the data subject, or
   b) in order to protect the vital interests of another person, in a case where consent by or on behalf of the data subject has been unreasonably withheld.

4 The processing –
   a) is carried out in the course of its legitimate activities by any body or association which exists for political, philosophical, religious or trade-union purposes and which is not established or conducted for profit,
   b) is carried out with appropriate safeguards for the rights and freedoms of data subjects,
   c) relates only to individuals who are either members of the body or association or who have regular contact with it in connection with its purposes, and
   d) d) does not involve disclosure of the personal data to a third party without the consent of the data subject.

5 The information contained in the personal data has been made public as a result of steps deliberately taken by the data subject.

6 The processing –
   a) is necessary for the purpose of, or in connection with, any legal proceedings (including prospective legal proceedings),

b) is necessary for the purpose of obtaining legal advice, or

c) is otherwise necessary for the purposes of establishing, exercising or defending legal rights.

7 The processing is necessary –
   a) for the administration of justice,
   b) for the exercise of any functions conferred by or under any enactment, or
   c) for the exercise of any functions of the Crown, a Minister of the Crown or a government department.

   The Secretary of State may by order specify cases where this condition is either excluded altogether or only satisfied upon the satisfaction of further conditions.

8 The processing is *necessary* for medical purposes (including the purposes of preventative medicine, medical diagnosis, medical research, the provision of care and treatment and the management of healthcare services) and is undertaken by –
   a) a health professional (as defined in the Act), or
   b) a person who owes a duty of confidentiality which is equivalent to that which would arise if that person were a health profes- sional.

9 The processing –
   a) is of sensitive personal data consisting of information as to racial or ethnic origin,
   b) is necessary for the purpose of identifying or keeping under review the existence or absence of equality of opportunity or treatment between persons of different racial or ethnic origins, with a view to enabling such equality to be promoted or maintained, and
   c) is carried out with appropriate safeguards for the rights and freedoms of data subjects. The Secretary of State may by order specify circumstances in which such processing is, or is not, to be taken to be carried out with appropriate safeguards for the rights and freedoms of data subjects.

10 The personal data are processed in circumstances specified in an order made by the Secretary of State.

Data Protection (Processing of Sensitive Personal Data) Order 2000:

Relevant conditions –

7 Processing of medical data or data relating to ethnic origin for monitoring purposes.

9 Processing in the substantial public interest, necessary for the purpose of research whose object is not to support decisions with respect to any particular data subject otherwise than with the explicit consent of the data subject and which is unlikely to cause substantial damage or substantial distress to the data subject or any other person.

(B) Vulnerable participants

57

Guidelines for the ethical conduct of medical research involving children

Royal College of Paediatrics and Child Health:
Ethics Advisory Committee

These guidelines are written for everyone involved in the planning, review, and conduct of research with children. The Royal College of Paediatrics and Child Health's first guidelines (then the British Paediatric Association) were published in 1980. Since then, there has been significant progress in the understanding of children's interests, in legal requirements, and in the proper regulation of research. The revised guidelines take account of such developments. General guidelines relating to all medical research provide an essential background to this document on research with children.[1-9] These guidelines are based on six principles:

(1) Research involving children is important for the benefit of all children and should be supported, encouraged and conducted in an ethical manner

(2) Children are not small adults; they have an additional, unique set of interests

(3) Research should only be done on children if comparable research on adults could not answer the same question

(4) A research procedure which is not intended directly to benefit the child subject is not necessarily either unethical or illegal

(5) All proposals involving medical research on children should be submitted to a research ethics committee

(6) Legally valid consent should be obtained from the child, parent or guardian as appropriate. When parental consent is obtained, the agreement of school age children who take part in research should also be requested by researchers.

Correspondence to: Professor Neil McIntosh, Department of Child Life and Health, 20 Sylvan Place, Edinburgh EH9 1UW, UK.

These guidelines were produced initially by the Ethics Advisory Committee of the British Paediatric Association in 1992* and have been modified and updated by the Royal College of Paediatrics and Child Health Ethics Advisory Committee in 1999†.

* Chairman, Professor C Normand; Members, Dr P Alderson, Miss G Brykczynska, Professor R Cooke, Professor The Rev G Dunstan CBE, Professor Dame J Lloyd DBE, Mr J Montgomery, Dr R Nicholson, Professor M Pembrey.

† Chairman, Professor N McIntosh; Members, Mr P Bates, Miss G Brykczynska, Professor The Rev G Dunstan CBE, Dr A Goldman, Professor D Harvey, Dr V Larcher, Dr D Mc Crae, Dr A McKinnon, Dr M Patton, Dr J Saunders, Mrs P Shelley.

[1] Royal College of Physicians. *Research on healthy volunteers.* London: The College, 1988.

[2] Royal College of Physicians. *Research involving patients.* London: The College, 1990.

[3] Royal College of Physicians. *Guidelines on the practice of ethics committees involved in medical research involving human subjects.* 3rd ed. London: The College, 1996.

Arch. Dis. Child. 2000; 82(2): 1777–182 Permission granted by BMJ Publishing Group.

[4] NHS Management Executive. *Guidelines on local research ethics committees.* London: NHS Management Executive, 1991.

[5] World Medical Association. *The declaration of Helsinki.* Ferney-Voltaire, France: The Association, 1996; revised in 1975, 1983 and 1989.

[6] United Kingdom Central Council on Nursing, Midwifery and Health Visiting. *Exercising accountability: A framework to assist nurses, midwives, and health visitors to consider ethical aspects of professional practice.* London: The Council, 1989.

[7] Nicholson R, ed. *Medical research with children: ethics, law and practice.* Oxford: Oxford University Press, 1986.

[8] National Commission for the Protection of Human Subjects of Biomedical and Behavioral Research. *Research involving children: report and recommendations.* Washington DC: Department of Health, Education and Welfare, 1977.

[9] Alderson P. *Choosing for children: parents' consent to surgery.* Oxford: Oxford University Press, 1990.

The special implications of fetal research are considered by the *Polkinghorne Report.*[10]

Value of ethical research with children

Medical research involving children is an important means of promoting child health and wellbeing. Such research includes systematic investigation into normal childhood development and the aetiology of disease, as well as careful scrutiny of the means of promoting health and of diagnosing, assessing, and treating disease. It is also important to validate in children the beneficial results of research conducted in adults.

Research with children is worthwhile if each project:
* has an identifiable prospect of benefit to children
* is well designed and well conducted
* does not simply duplicate earlier work
* is not undertaken primarily for financial or professional advantage
* involves a statistically appropriate number of subjects
* eventually is to be properly reported.

Comprehensive registers such as the National Perinatal Epidemiology Unit's register of perinatal research and the National Research Register help to promote high standards. They publicise worthwhile projects and good practice; they help to prevent unnecessary duplication; and by recording unpublished work they provide valuable information.

Children's interests

Children are unique as a research group for many reasons. They are the only people, in British law, on whose behalf other individuals may consent to medical procedures. Many children are vulnerable, easily bewildered and frightened, and unable to express their needs or defend their interests. Potentially with many decades ahead of them, they are likely to experience, in their development and education, the most lasting benefits or harms from research.

To facilitate both the child's health care and longer term research, general practitioners should be notified of all research on their paediatric patients. Long term follow up of research interventions may be of particular benefit to child subjects. Yet this means still more intrusion into their lives, as records are shared and computerised. Children may be less able than adults to challenge records about themselves. There is therefore a duty on researchers to respect

---

[10] *Review of the guidance on the research use of fetuses and fetal material (The Polkinghorne Report).* London: Her Majesty's Stationery Office, 1989 Cm762.

confidentiality, and keep up to date with data protection and legislation on access to health records.

More needs to be known about how children are affected by their experiences as patients and research subjects, and what support they need. It is desirable to encourage psychosocial research conducted independently and in conjunction with physiological research. Research will then further the task of caring for the whole child within the family.

Research shares this task when it is more than research *on* children, and is research *with* them, learning from their responses and attending to their interests as perceived by the child and parents. ("Parents" in these guidelines refers to parents, guardians, or adults legally entitled to give consent on the child's behalf.) This partnership should accord with the *Declaration of Helsinki* in that concern for the interests of the subject must always prevail over those of science and society.

Must the research involve children?

In principle, the informed and willing consent of human research subjects should be sought whenever possible. Yet there are complications in obtaining the consent of minors. Research and innovative treatment on humans should only be undertaken after adequate basic research. Research with children should be undertaken only if work with adults is clearly not feasible. When a choice of age groups is possible, older children should be involved in preference to younger ones, although much valuable research can only be done with younger children and babies.

Some treatments, such as organ transplantation, may involve a range of procedures. Each separate new procedure should be tested with informed willing adults when possible, with time to assess at least the medium term effects, before the procedure is attempted with children. The urgent desire to offer babies and children the potential benefits of medical innovation is laudable. Yet childhood is a vulnerable, formative time, when harms can have serious impact as well as being potentially long lasting. Potential harms should therefore be assessed carefully before children are put at risk.

Increasingly, research experience is regarded as an essential qualification for promotion in medicine. Research work can offer valuable training that may improve the quality of doctors' clinical practice. An inquiring mind disciplined to test hypotheses by the approved canons of research while sensitive to the vulnerability of child patients should be seen as a valued professional asset in a paediatrician.

However, great care should be exercised by supervisory senior staff over the choice of research projects. The criteria for worthwhile research, listed above, must govern the selection of projects whether primarily undertaken as part of medical training or for the advancement of knowledge.

Potential benefits, harm, and cost

There are no general statutory provisions covering research on human beings. In the absence of relevant case law, earlier cautions against research on minors that offer no direct benefit to the child subject[11] have been replaced by qualified support.[5,12] This has not been challenged in the courts. The attempt to protect children absolutely from the potential harms of research denies any of them the potential benefits. We therefore support the premise that research that is of no intended benefit to the child subject is not necessarily unethical or illegal. Such research includes observing and measuring normal development, assessing diagnostic methods, the use of "healthy volunteers" and of placebos in controlled trials.

The importance of evaluating potential benefits, harms, and costs in research on human beings, and ways of doing so,[7] have been discussed repeatedly. A summary of discussion points is included in these guidelines to illustrate how complex such evaluations can be. Our aim, rather than to provide answers, is to list questions for researchers and ethics committees to consider.

Assessment of potential benefit includes reviewing estimates of:

Magnitude

- How is the knowledge gained likely to be used?
- In research into treatment how severe is the problem which the research aims to alleviate?
- How common is the problem?

Probability

- How likely is the research to achieve its aims?

Beneficiaries

- Is the research intended to benefit the child subjects, and/or other children?

[11] Medical Research Council. Responsibility in investigations on human subjects: In: *Report of the Medical Research Council for the year 1962–63: 21–5*. London: Her Majesty's Stationery Office, 1964.

[12] Dworkin G. Legality of consent to non-therapeutic medical research on infants and young children. *Arch Dis Child* 1978; **51**:443–6.

Resources

- Will potential benefits be limited because they are very expensive, or require unusually highly trained professionals?

Assessment of potential harm included estimates of:

Types of intervention

- How invasive or intrusive is the research? (psychosocial research should be assessed as carefully as physical research)

Magnitude

- How severe may the harms associated with research procedures be?

Probability

- How likely are the harms to occur?

Timing

- Might adverse effects be brief or long lasting, immediate or not evident until years later?

Equity

- Are a few children drawn into too many projects simply because they are available?
- Are researchers relying unduly on children who already have many problems?

Interim finding

- If evidence of harm in giving or withholding certain treatment emerges during the trial, how will possible conflict between the interests of the child subjects and of valid research be managed?

Assessment of potential harm also includes reviewing personal estimates

Children's responses are varied, often unpredictable, and alter as children develop, so that generalisations about risk tend to be controversial. A procedure that does not bother one child arouses severe distress in another. Researchers sometimes underestimate high risk of pain if the effects are brief, whereas the child or parents may consider the severe transient pain is not justified by the hoped for benefit. There is evidence that tolerance of pain increases with age and maturity when the child no longer perceives medical interventions as punitive.[13–15]

Some potential harms may not be obvious without careful consideration of their consequences. For example, with research into serious genetic disorders that present in adult life, presymptomatic diagnosis in a child, while it may be beneficial, may also have very harmful effects, and may affect the child's opportunities and freedom of choice.[16]

Risks may be estimated as minimal, low or high

Minimal (the least possible) risk describes procedures such as questioning, observing, and measuring children, provided that procedures are carried out in a sensitive way, and that consent has been given. Procedures with minimal risk include collecting a single urine sample (but not by aspiration), or using blood from a sample that has been taken as part of treatment.

Low risk describes procedures that cause brief pain or tenderness, and small bruises or scars. Many children fear needles and for them low rather than minimal risks are often incurred by injections and venepuncture.

High risk procedures such as lung or liver biopsy, arterial puncture, and cardiac catheterisation are not justified for research purposes alone. They should be carried out only when research is combined with diagnosis or treatment intended to benefit the child concerned.

We believe that research in which children are submitted to more than minimal risk with only slight, uncertain or no benefit to themselves deserves serious ethical consideration. The most common example of such research involves blood sampling. Where children are unable to give consent, by reason of insufficient maturity or understanding, their parents or guardians may consent to the taking of blood for non-therapeutic purposes, provided that they have been given and understand a full explanation of the reasons for blood sampling and have balanced its risk to their child. Many children fear needles, but with careful explanation of the reason for venepuncture and an understanding of the

effectiveness of local anaesthetic cream, they often show altruism and allow a blood sample to be taken. We believe that this has to be the child's decision. We believe that it is completely inappropriate to insist on the taking of blood for non-therapeutic reasons if a child indicates either significant unwillingness before the start or significant stress during the procedure.

Despite careful selection, children in clinical trials have social and emotional problems that are mainly unpredictable.[17] Provision for necessary, continuing, emotional support should be built into the research design.

Assessment of potential cost includes reviewing:

Resources

• How much medical, nursing and other professional time is required for informing and supporting families, and for collecting data?

• Are sufficient staff available without prejudicing the care of patients?

• Are the costs of reducing and preventing harms included in the protocol (such as information material for staff and families, local anaesthetic cream (for example, EMLA), autolet)

• How much family time is required for collecting data, or attending clinics?

• How will their extra expenses be paid?

• Are reasonable costs allowed for collecting, collating, and analysing data, for writing and disseminating the reports, and for informing research subjects of the results?

Statistics

• Are enough children involved to make a statistically valid sample, and to allow for withdrawals during longer studies?

• Is the planned number of subjects unnecessarily high?

Inconvenience

• How much inconvenience to families is justified (such as extra visits to clinics)?

• All medical research, whether or not associated with therapy, requires careful evaluation, as well as the safeguards described in the next two sections.

[13] Haslam D. Age of perception of pain. *Psychological Science* 1969; **15**:86–7.

[14] Petrillo D, Danger P. *Emotional care of hospitalised children.* New York: Lippincott, 1980.

[15] Jacox A, ed. *Pain: a sourcebook for nurses and other health professionals.* Boston: Little Brown, 1977.

[16] British Paediatric Association Ethics Advisory Committee. *Testing children for late onset genetic disorders.* London: BPA Statement, 1996.

[17] Kinmonth A, Lindsay M, Baum J. Social and emotional complications in a clinical trial among adolescents with diabetes mellitus. *BMJ* 1983; **286**:952–4.

Research ethics committees

As assessment of benefit and harm is complex, children are best protected if projects are reviewed at many levels, by researchers, funding and scientific bodies, research ethics committees, the research assistants and nurses working with child subjects, the children, and their parents. Everyone concerned (except young children) has some responsibility.

Ethics is about good practice, and each research ethics committee considering a project involving children should be advised by people with a close, practical knowledge of babies and children, such as a registered sick children's nurse. They may be research ethics committee members, persons co-opted, or members of a subcommittee.

Given that valuable research can range from the descriptive using qualitative methods to that requiring statistical analysis, research ethics committees need to have or to co-opt members with a breadth of experience adequate to assess such research.

Multicentre research ethics committees (MRECs) have the task of reviewing all research taking place in five or more centres, and protocols approved by the MREC cannot be amended by a local research ethics committee (LREC). It is therefore particularly important that multicentre studies in children are always assessed after such advice and that LRECs are advised accordingly. LRECs considering multicentre protocols should ensure that there are no local objections to the study (for example, over researched groups, ethnic factors, research facilities, local investigators).

The duties of LRECs have been clearly described.[3,4] Those of MRECs have also been outlined.[18] It is important that committees are satisfied that each project:
- sets out to answer a useful question or questions
- is designed in the best possible way to answer the questions
- will work in practice (such as in the safety of drugs and techniques, age appropriate interventions, and prevention of too many studies being carried out in one ward).

Both MRECs and LRECs may also wish to know how researchers plan to monitor and respond to any signs of distress in child subjects. This may involve helping children to withdraw from the study. LRECs have the additional responsibility of monitoring the progress of studies.[19]

---

[18] NHS Executive. *Ethics committee review of multi-centre research.* HSG(97)23. London: Department of Health, 1997.

[19] International Conference on Harmonisation of Technical Requirements for Registration of Pharmaceuticals for Human Use (ICH Harmonised Tripartite Guidelines). *Guideline for good clinical practice.* Geneva: IFPMA, 1997.

Research ethics committees are faced with the paradox of trying to be both stringent assessors and an approachable forum for helping researchers to resolve problems. They have to compromise between aiming for the perfect protocol in advance and encouraging researchers to respond to families' unpredictable responses, which may require changes in the research design later on.

Consent and assent

"Consent", in this section, describes the positive agreement of a person; "assent" refers to acquiescence. The law relating to research on children (children defined by law as those under 18 years) has never been clearly established. The application of general principles indicates that, where children have "sufficient understanding and intelligence to understand what is proposed", it is they and not their parents whose consent is required by law.[20] A reasoned refusal by a child to participate in research is likely to be taken as evidence of such understanding, and it would be unwise to rely on parental consent in such circumstances. If the child is insufficiently mature to consent, then valid parental consent must be obtained.

The physical integrity of children, as of all other people, is protected by law. Unless they, or their parents or guardians acting on their behalf, agree to it, nothing can be done lawfully that involves touching them. Research with children must normally be carried out only with the consent of parent, guardian or child. Some research based on observation, collating information from notes and tests already performed for therapeutic purposes may, however, be permissible without consent because it does not involve touching the child.

A general exception to the requirement for consent is the provision of medical care in an emergency. If emergency medical, surgical, and neonatal care are to be improved, research is necessary. On many, but not all, such occasions, it may be impracticable, or meaningless, to attempt immediately to obtain informed consent for the proposed research procedures from parents or guardians. To require such an attempt always to be made could also inhibit much potentially valuable research.

Provided, therefore, that the specific approval of a research ethics committee has been obtained for the project overall, it would be ethical to carry out research on children on such occasions of extreme urgency without obtaining consent. It is possible, however, that it would still be unlawful if the research were not expected to benefit the

---

[20] Gillick -v- West Norfolk AHA. 3 All Er 402, at 423–4.

child in question, although legal action would be unlikely. The parents or guardians and, where appropriate, the child must be informed about the research as soon as possible afterwards: a requirement in ethics as in courtesy.

Parental consent will probably not be valid if it is given against the child's interests. This means that parents can consent to research procedures that are intended directly to benefit the child, but that research that does not come into this category can only be validly consented to if the risks are sufficiently small to mean that the research can be reasonably said not to go against the child's interests.[21] Even when it is not legally required, researchers should obtain the assent or agreement of school age children to their involvement in the research, and should always ensure that the child does not object.

Legally valid consent is both freely given and informed. For consent to be freely given researchers must:
• offer families no financial inducement, although expenses should be paid
• exert no pressure on families
• give them as much time as possible (some days for a major study) to consider whether to take part in the project
• encourage families to discuss the project with – for example, their relatives, or primary health carers
• tell them that they may refuse to take part, or may withdraw at any time, even if they have signed a consent form
• say that they need not give a reason for withdrawing, although their reason may help the researchers and other children in the study
• assure them that the child patient's treatment will not be prejudiced by withdrawal from the research
• encourage parents to stay with their child during procedures
• respond to families' questions, anxiety or distress throughout the study.

Consent is not a single response; it involves willing commitment that may falter during a long, difficult project. Families may need to be supported and informed frequently. Children's ability to consent develops as they learn to make increasingly complex and serious decisions. Ability may relate to experience rather than to age, and even very young children appear to understand complex issues. They should therefore be informed as fully as possible about the research in terms they can understand.

For consent to be informed, researchers must discuss with families:
• the purpose of the research
• whether the child stands to benefit directly and, if so, how; the difference between research and treatment

[21] S -v- S. 3 All ER 107, at 111.

• the meaning of relevant research terms (such as placebos)
• the nature of each procedure, how often or for how long each may occur
• the potential benefits and harms (both immediate and long term)
• the name of a researcher whom they can contact with inquiries
• the name of the doctor directly responsible for the child
• how children can withdraw from the project. Researchers will also:
• willingly explain and answer questions throughout the project
• ensure that other staff caring for child subjects know about the research, and can also explain it if necessary
• give clearly written leaflets for families to keep
• should report the results of research to the families involved.

When explaining relevant terms, researchers need to discuss with families the consent implications. For example, consenting to a double blind randomised trial means not minding which of a choice of treatments the child will have, and that neither the family nor their doctor will know which treatment has been given until the trial has been completed.

These guidelines are designed to benefit children who take part in research, children who may be helped by the research findings, and medical research itself. Researchers who observe high standards will continue to enjoy public support and cooperation.

Commentary

The Ethics Committee of the British Paediatric Association (BPA), now the Royal College of Paediatrics and Child Health (RCPCH), has prepared guidelines on the planning, conduct, and review of research on children. Two of their basic principles are that "research involving children is important for the benefit of all children" and that "a research procedure not intended directly to benefit the child subject is not necessarily either unethical or illegal". Research is necessary to ensure that children receive fully informed care.

Analysis of blood is an essential part of many research programmes – for example, the determination of nutritional status and the evaluation of therapeutic drugs. Taking blood is often painful, it sometimes leaves a worrying bruise, and the experience can be distressing. Debate both in and out of the Councils of the BPA/RCPCH has centred on whether taking blood from children poses a minimal or a low risk. Procedures that have a low risk are usually inappropriate if the child involved is unlikely to benefit from the experience.

Blood taken by a skilled person poses only a minimal risk of physical harm, except possibly the taking of a separate sample of blood from a very immature infant. It is the pain and distress and the memory of it that might cause more than minimal harm.

Taking blood from children can be a positive experience. Children, like adults, are capable of being generous and doing something worthwhile even if it means they experience discomfort. Parents when they are fully informed usually consent to their babies experiencing the brief pain of blood taking if the investigation might be to the benefit of other infants. It seems to me that for blood taking to be a minimal risk, it is important that all concerned know what is happening, that the moment when the blood is taken is appropriate, that the procedure is skilfully performed, and that all steps are taken to reduce the amount of pain the child experiences – for example, by using local anaesthetic creams.

Some children, however, like some adults are frightened of needles and the sight of blood. The guidance originally stated that "Many children fear needles and to them low rather than minimal risks are often incurred by injection and venepuncture". It now says "Many children fear needles, but with careful explanation of the reason for the venepuncture and an understanding of the effectiveness of anaesthetic cream, they often show altruism, and allow a blood sample to be taken". I welcome the move to a more positive position. It is in the common interest of children. But it makes it more, rather than less, necessary for research workers to be able to *recognise* when a child is very upset whether by the thought of the procedure or at the time of the procedure and to *accept* this distress as genuine dissent from being involved. The child's feelings are not to be sacrificed.

I hope that the number of children who get very upset at the thought of needles or the sight of blood will fall as accident and emergency departments strive to ensure that when children attend for treatment, the experience enhances rather than undermines their confidence in modern clinical care.

Professor Sir David Hull
Emeritus Professor

58

Clinical investigation of medicinal products in the paediatric population
ICH Harmonised tripartite guideline

International Conference on Harmonisation of Technical Requirements for Registration of Pharmaceuticals for Human Use

Recommended for Adoption at Step 4 of the ICH Process on 20 July 2000 by the ICH Steering Committee

This Guideline has been developed by the appropriate ICH Expert Working Group and has been subject to consultation by the regulatory parties, in accordance with the ICH Process. At Step 4 of the Process the final draft is recommended for adoption to the regulatory bodies of the European Union, Japan and USA.

Clinical investigation of medicinal products in the pediatric population

ICH Harmonised Tripartite Guideline

Having reached *Step 4* of the ICH Process at the ICH Steering Committee meeting on 19 July 2000, this guideline is recommended for adoption to the three regulatory parties to ICH

Table of contents

Clinical investigation of medicinal products in the pediatric population

1 Introduction

1.1 Objectives of the guidance

The number of medicinal products currently labeled for pediatric use is limited. It is the goal of this guidance to encourage and facilitate timely pediatric medicinal product development internationally. The guidance provides an outline of critical issues in pediatric drug development and approaches to the safe, efficient, and ethical study of medicinal products in the pediatric population.

1.2 Background

Other ICH documents with relevant information impacting on pediatric studies include:

E2: Clinical Safety Data Management
E3: Structure and Content of Clinical Study Reports
E4: Dose-Response Information to Support Drug Registration
E5: Ethnic Factors in the Acceptability of Foreign Clinical Data
E6: Good Clinical Practice: Consolidated Guideline
E8: General Considerations for Clinical Trials
E9: Statistical Principles for Clinical Trials
E10: Choice of Control Group in Clinical Trials
M3: Nonclinical Safety Studies for the Conduct of Human Clinical Trials for Pharmaceuticals
Q1: Stability Testing
Q2: Validation of Analytical Procedures
Q3: Impurity Testing

1.3 Scope of the guidance

Specific clinical study issues addressed include: (1) considerations when initiating a pediatric program for a medicinal product; (2) timing of initiation of pediatric studies during medicinal product development; (3) types of studies (pharmacokinetic, pharmacokinetic/pharmacodynamic (PK/PD), efficacy, safety); (4) age categories; and (5) ethics of pediatric clinical investigation. This guidance is not intended to be comprehensive; other ICH guidances, as well as documents from regional regulatory authorities and pediatric societies, provide additional detail.

1.4 General principles

Pediatric patients should be given medicines that have been appropriately evaluated for their use. Safe and effective pharmacotherapy in pediatric patients requires the timely development of information on the proper use of medicinal products in pediatric patients of various ages and, often, the development of pediatric formulations of those products. Advances in formulation chemistry and in pediatric study design will help facilitate the development of medicinal products for pediatric use. Drug development programs should usually include the pediatric patient

population when a product is being developed for a disease or condition in adults and it is anticipated the product will be used in the pediatric population. Obtaining knowledge of the effects of medicinal products in pediatric patients is an important goal. However, this should be done without compromising the well-being of pediatric patients participating in clinical studies. This responsibility is shared by companies, regulatory authorities, health professionals, and society as a whole.

2 Guidance

2.1 Issues when initiating a pediatric medicinal product development program

Data on the appropriate use of medicinal products in the pediatric population should be generated unless the use of a specific medicinal product in pediatric patients is clearly inappropriate. The timing of initiation of clinical studies in relation to studies conducted in adults, which may be influenced by regional public health and medical needs, is discussed in section 2.3. Justification for the timing and the approach to the clinical program needs to be clearly addressed with regulatory authorities at an early stage and then periodically during the medicinal product development process. The pediatric development program should not delay completion of adult studies and availability of a medicinal product for adults.

The decision to proceed with a pediatric development program for a medicinal product, and the nature of that program, involve consideration of many factors, including:

- The prevalence of the condition to be treated in the pediatric population
- The seriousness of the condition to be treated
- The availability and suitability of alternative treatments for the condition in the pediatric population, including the efficacy and the adverse event profile (including any unique pediatric safety issues) of those treatments
- Whether the medicinal product is novel or one of a class of compounds with known properties
- Whether there are unique pediatric indications for the medicinal product
- The need for the development of pediatric-specific endpoints
- The age ranges of pediatric patients likely to be treated with the medicinal product
- Unique pediatric (developmental) safety concerns with the medicinal product, including any nonclinical safety issues
- Potential need for pediatric formulation development

Of these factors, the most important is the presence of a serious or life-threatening disease for which the medicinal product represents a potentially important advance in therapy. This situation suggests relatively urgent and early initiation of pediatric studies.

Information from nonclinical safety studies to support a pediatric clinical program is discussed in ICH M3, section 11. It should be noted that the most relevant safety data for pediatric studies ordinarily come from adult human exposure. Repeated dose toxicity studies, reproduction toxicity studies and genotoxicity tests would generally be available. The need for juvenile animal studies should be considered on a case-by-case basis and be based on developmental toxicology concerns.

2.2 Pediatric formulations

There is a need for pediatric formulations that permit accurate dosing and enhance patient compliance. For oral administration, different types of formulations, flavors and colors may be more acceptable in one region than another. Several formulations, such as liquids, suspensions, and chewable tablets, may be needed or desirable for pediatric patients of different ages. Different drug concentrations in these various formulations may also be needed. Consideration should also be given to the development of alternative delivery systems.

For injectable formulations, appropriate drug concentrations should be developed to allow accurate and safe administration of the dose. For medicinal products supplied as single-use vials, consideration should be given to dose-appropriate single-dose packaging.

The toxicity of some excipients may vary across pediatric age groups and between pediatric and adult populations, e.g., benzyl alcohol is toxic in the preterm newborn. Depending on the active substance and excipients, appropriate use of the medicinal product in the newborn may require a new formulation or appropriate information about dilution of an existing formulation. International harmonization on the acceptability of formulation excipients and of validation procedures would help ensure that appropriate formulations are available for the pediatric population everywhere.

2.3 Timing of studies

During clinical development, the timing of pediatric studies will depend on the medicinal product, the type of disease being treated, safety considerations, and the efficacy and safety of alternative treatments. Since development of pediatric formulations can be difficult and time consuming, it is important to consider the development of these formulations early in medicinal product development.

2.3.1 Medicinal products for diseases predominantly or exclusively affecting pediatric patients

In this case, the entire development program will be conducted in the pediatric population except for initial safety and tolerability data, which will usually be obtained in adults. Some products may reasonably be studied only in the pediatric population even in the initial phases, e.g., when studies in adults would yield little useful information or expose them to inappropriate risk. Examples include surfactant for respiratory distress syndrome in preterm infants and therapies targeted at metabolic or genetic diseases unique to the pediatric population.

2.3.2 Medicinal products intended to treat serious or life-threatening diseases, occurring in both adults and pediatric patients, for which there are currently no or limited therapeutic options

The presence of a serious or life-threatening disease for which the product represents a potentially important advance in therapy suggests the need for relatively urgent and early initiation of pediatric studies. In this case, medicinal product development should begin early in the pediatric population, following assessment of initial safety data and reasonable evidence of potential benefit. Pediatric study results should be part of the marketing application database. In circumstances where this has not been possible, lack of data should be justified in detail.

2.3.3 Medicinal products intended to treat other diseases and conditions

In this case, although the medicinal product will be used in pediatric patients, there is less urgency than in the previous cases and studies would usually begin at later phases of clinical development or, if a safety concern exists, even after substantial postmarketing experience in adults. Companies should have a clear plan for pediatric studies and reasons for their timing. Testing of these medicinal products in the pediatric population would usually not begin until Phase 2 or 3. In most cases, only limited pediatric data would be available at the time of submission of the application, but more would be expected after marketing. The development of many new chemical entities is discontinued during or following Phase 1 and 2 studies in adults for lack of efficacy or an unacceptable side effect profile. Therefore, very early initiation of testing in pediatric patients might needlessly expose these patients to a compound that will be of no benefit. Even for a nonserious disease, if the medicinal product represents a major therapeutic advance for the pediatric population, studies should begin early in development, and the submission of pediatric data would be expected in the application. Lack of data should be justified in detail. Thus, it is important to carefully weigh benefit/risk and therapeutic need in deciding when to start pediatric studies.

2.4 Types of studies

The principles outlined in ICH E4, E5, E6, and E10 apply to pediatric studies. Several pediatric-specific issues are worth noting. When a medicinal product is studied in pediatric patients in one region, the intrinsic (e.g., pharmacogenetic) and extrinsic (e.g., diet) factors[1] that could impact on the extrapolation of data to other regions should be considered.

When a medicinal product is to be used in the pediatric population for the same indication(s) as those studied and approved in adults, the disease process is similar in adults and pediatric patients, and the outcome of therapy is likely to be comparable, extrapolation from adult efficacy data may be appropriate. In such cases, pharmacokinetic studies in all the age ranges of pediatric patients likely to receive the medicinal product, together with safety studies, may provide adequate information for use by allowing selection of pediatric doses that will produce blood levels similar to those observed in adults. If this approach is taken, adult pharmacokinetic data should be available to plan the pediatric studies.

When a medicinal product is to be used in younger pediatric patients for the same indication(s) as those studied in older pediatric patients, the disease process is similar, and the outcome of therapy is likely to be comparable, extrapolation of efficacy from older to younger pediatric patients may be possible. In such cases, pharmacokinetic studies in the relevant age groups of pediatric patients likely to receive the medicinal product, together with safety studies, may be sufficient to provide adequate information for pediatric use.

An approach based on pharmacokinetics is likely to be insufficient for medicinal products where blood levels are known or expected not to correspond with efficacy or where there is concern that the concentration-response relationship may differ between the adult and pediatric

populations. In such cases, studies of the clinical or the pharmacological effect of the medicinal product would usually be expected.

Where the comparability of the disease course or outcome of therapy in pediatric patients is expected to be similar to adults, but the appropriate blood levels are not clear, it may be possible to use measurements of a pharmacodynamic effect related to clinical effectiveness to confirm the expectations of effectiveness and to define the dose and concentration needed to attain that pharmacodynamic effect. Such studies could provide increased confidence that achieving a given exposure to the medicinal product in pediatric patients would result in the desired therapeutic outcomes. Thus, a PK/PD approach combined with safety and other relevant studies could avoid the need for clinical efficacy studies.

In other situations where a pharmacokinetic approach is not applicable, such as for topically active products, extrapolation of efficacy from one patient population to another may be based on studies that include pharmacodynamic endpoints and/or appropriate alternative assessments. Local tolerability studies may be needed. It may be important to determine blood levels and systemic effects to assess safety.

When novel indications are being sought for the medicinal product in pediatric patients, or when the disease course and outcome of therapy are likely to be different in adults and pediatric patients, clinical efficacy studies in the pediatric population would be needed.

2.4.1 Pharmacokinetics

Pharmacokinetic studies generally should be performed to support formulation development and determine pharmacokinetic parameters in different age groups to support dosing recommendations. Relative bioavailability comparisons of pediatric formulations with the adult oral formulation typically should be done in adults. Definitive pharmacokinetic studies for dose selection across the age ranges of pediatric patients in whom the medicinal product is likely to be used should be conducted in the pediatric population.

Pharmacokinetic studies in the pediatric population are generally conducted in patients with the disease. This may lead to higher intersubject variability than studies in normal volunteers, but the data better reflect clinical use.

For medicinal products that exhibit linear pharmacokinetics in adults, single-dose pharmacokinetic studies in the pediatric population may provide sufficient information for dosage selection. This can be corroborated, if indicated, by sparse sampling in multidose clinical studies. Any nonlinearity in absorption, distribution, and elimination in adults and any difference in duration of effect

---

[1] In the ICH E5 guideline on Ethnic Factors in the Acceptance of Foreign Data, factors which may result in different drug responses to a drug in different populations are categorized as intrinsic ethnic factors or extrinsic ethnic factors. In this document, these categories are referred to as intrinsic factors and extrinsic factors, respectively.

between single and repeated dosing in adults would suggest the need for steady state studies in the pediatric population. All these approaches are facilitated by knowledge of adult pharmacokinetic parameters. Knowing the pathways of clearance (renal and metabolic) of the medicinal product and understanding the age-related changes of those processes will often be helpful in planning pediatric studies.

Dosing recommendations for most medicinal products used in the pediatric population are usually based on milligram (mg)/kilogram (kg) body weight up to a maximum adult dose. While dosing based on mg/square meter body surface area might be preferred, clinical experience indicates that errors in measuring height or length (particularly in smaller children and infants) and calculation errors of body surface area from weight and height are common. For some medications (e.g., medications with a narrow therapeutic index, such as those used in oncology), surface-area-guided dosing may be necessary, but extra care should be taken to ensure proper dose calculation.

Practical considerations to facilitate pharmacokinetic studies

The volume of blood withdrawn should be minimized in pediatric studies. Blood volumes should be justified in protocols. Institutional Review Boards/Independent Ethics Committees (IRB's/IEC's) review and may define the maximum amount of blood (usually on a milliliters (mL)/kg or percentage of total blood volume basis) that may be taken for investigational purposes. Several approaches can be used to minimize the amount of blood drawn and/or the number of venipunctures.

• Use of sensitive assays for parent drugs and metabolites to decrease the volume of blood required per sample
• Use of laboratories experienced in handling small volumes of blood for pharmacokinetic analyses and for laboratory safety studies (blood counts, clinical chemistry)
• Collection of routine, clinical blood samples wherever possible at the same time as samples are obtained for pharmacokinetic analysis
• The use of indwelling catheters, etc., to minimize distress as discussed in section 2.6.5.
• Use of population pharmacokinetics and sparse sampling based on optimal sampling theory to minimize the number of samples obtained from each patient. Techniques include:
  - Sparse sampling approaches where each patient contributes as few as 2 to 4 observations at predetermined times to an overall "population area-under-the-curve"

  - Population pharmacokinetic analysis using the most useful sampling time points derived from modeling of adult data

2.4.2 Efficacy

The principles in study design, statistical considerations and choice of control groups detailed in ICH E6, E9, and E10 generally apply to pediatric efficacy studies. There are, however, certain features unique to pediatric studies. The potential for extrapolation of efficacy from studies in adults to pediatric patients or from older to younger pediatric patients is discussed in section 2.4. Where efficacy studies are needed, it may be necessary to develop, validate, and employ different endpoints for specific age and developmental subgroups. Measurement of subjective symptoms such as pain requires different assessment instruments for patients of different ages. In pediatric patients with chronic diseases, the response to a medicinal product may vary among patients not only because of the duration of the disease and its chronic effects but also because of the developmental stage of the patient. Many diseases in the preterm and term newborn infant are unique or have unique manifestations precluding extrapolation of efficacy from older pediatric patients and call for novel methods of outcome assessment.

2.4.3 Safety

ICH guidances on E2 topics and ICH E6, which describe adverse event reporting, apply to pediatric studies. Age-appropriate, normal laboratory values and clinical measurements should be used in adverse event reporting. Unintended exposures to medicinal products (accidental ingestions, etc.) may provide the opportunity to obtain safety and pharmacokinetic information and to maximize understanding of dose-related side effects.

Medicinal products may affect physical and cognitive growth and development, and the adverse event profile may differ in pediatric patients. Because developing systems may respond differently from matured adult organs, some adverse events and drug interactions that occur in pediatric patients may not be identified in adult studies. In addition, the dynamic processes of growth and development may not manifest an adverse event acutely, but at a later stage of growth and maturation. Long-term studies or surveillance data, either while patients are on chronic therapy or during the posttherapy period, may be needed to determine possible effects on skeletal, behavioral, cognitive, sexual, and immune maturation and development.

2.4.4 Postmarketing information

Normally the pediatric database is limited at the time of approval. Therefore, postmarketing surveillance is particularly important. In some cases, long-term follow-up studies may be important to determine effects of certain medications on growth and development of pediatric patients. Postmarketing surveillance and/or long-term follow-up studies may provide safety and/or efficacy information for subgroups within the pediatric population or additional information for the entire pediatric population.

2.5 Age classification of pediatric patients

Any classification of the pediatric population into age categories is to some extent arbitrary, but a classification such as the one below provides a basis for thinking about study design in pediatric patients. Decisions on how to stratify studies and data by age need to take into consideration developmental biology and pharmacology. Thus, a flexible approach is necessary to ensure that studies reflect current knowledge of pediatric pharmacology. The identification of which ages to study should be medicinal product-specific and justified.

If the clearance pathways of a medicinal product are well established and the ontogeny of the pathways understood, age categories for pharmacokinetic evaluation might be chosen based on any "break point" where clearance is likely to change significantly. Sometimes, it may be more appropriate to collect data over broad age ranges and examine the effect of age as a continuous covariant. For efficacy, different endpoints may be established for pediatric patients of different ages, and the age groups might not correspond to the categories presented below. Dividing the pediatric population into many age groups might needlessly increase the number of patients required. In longer term studies, pediatric patients may move from one age category to another; the study design and statistical plans should prospectively take into account changing numbers of patients within a given age category.

The following is one possible categorization. There is, however, considerable overlap in developmental (e.g., physical, cognitive, and psychosocial) issues across the age categories. Ages are defined in completed days, months, or years.

- Preterm newborn infants
- Term newborn infants (0 to 27 days)
- Infants and toddlers (28 days to 23 months)
- Children (2 to 11 years)
- Adolescents (12 to 16–18 years (dependent on region))

2.5.1 Preterm newborn infants
The study of medicinal products in preterm newborn infants presents special challenges because of the

unique pathophysiology and responses to therapy in this population. The complexity of and ethical considerations involved in studying preterm newborn infants suggest the need for careful protocol development with expert input from neonatologists and neonatal pharmacologists. Only rarely will it be possible to extrapolate efficacy from studies in adults or even in older pediatric patients to the preterm newborn infant.

The category of preterm newborn infants is not a homogeneous group of patients. A 25-week gestation, 500-gram (g) newborn is very different from a 30-week gestation newborn weighing 1,500 g. A distinction should also be made for lowbirth-weight babies as to whether they are immature or growth retarded. Important features that should be considered for these patients include: (1) gestational age at birth and age after birth (adjusted age); (2) immaturity of renal and hepatic clearance mechanisms; (3) protein binding and displacement issues (particularly bilirubin); (4) penetration of medicinal products into the central nervous system (CNS); (5) unique neonatal disease states (e.g., respiratory distress syndrome of the newborn, patent ductus arteriosus, primary pulmonary hypertension); (6) unique susceptibilities of the preterm newborn (e.g., necrotizing enterocolitis, intraventricular hemorrhage, retinopathy of prematurity); (7) rapid and variable maturation of all physiologic and pharmacologic processes leading to different dosing regimens with chronic exposure; and (8) transdermal absorption of medicinal products and other chemicals. Study design issues that should be considered include: (1) weight and age (gestational and postnatal) stratification; (2) small blood volumes (a 500-g infant has 40 mL of blood); (3) small numbers of patients at a given center and differences in care among centers; and (4) difficulties in assessing outcomes.

2.5.2 Term newborn infants (0 to 27 days)
While term newborn infants are developmentally more mature than preterm newborn infants, many of the physiologic and pharmacologic principles discussed above also apply to term infants. Volumes of distribution of medicinal products may be different from those in older pediatric patients because of different body water and fat content and high body-surface-area-to-weight ratio. The blood-brain barrier is still not fully mature and medicinal products and endogenous substances (e.g., bilirubin) may gain access to the CNS with resultant toxicity. Oral absorption of medicinal products may be less predictable than in older pediatric patients. Hepatic and renal clearance mechanisms are immature and rapidly changing; doses may need to be adjusted over the first weeks of life. Many examples of increased susceptibility to toxic effects of medicinal

products result from limited clearance in these patients (e.g., chloramphenicol grey baby syndrome). On the other hand, term newborn infants may be less susceptible to some types of adverse effects (e.g., aminoglycoside nephrotoxicity) than are patients in older age groups.

2.5.3 Infants and toddlers (28 days to 23 months)

This is a period of rapid CNS maturation, immune system development and total body growth. Oral absorption becomes more reliable. Hepatic and renal clearance pathways continue to mature rapidly. By 1 to 2 years of age, clearance of many drugs on a mg/kg basis may exceed adult values. The developmental pattern of maturation is dependent on specific pathways of clearance. There is often considerable inter-individual variability in maturation.

2.5.4 Children (2 to 11 years)

Most pathways of drug clearance (hepatic and renal) are mature, with clearance often exceeding adult values. Changes in clearance of a drug may be dependent on maturation of specific metabolic pathways.

Specific strategies should be addressed in protocols to ascertain any effects of the medicinal product on growth and development. Children achieve several important milestones of psychomotor development that could be adversely affected by CNS-active drugs. Entry into school and increased cognitive and motor skills may affect a child's ability to participate in some types of efficacy studies. Factors useful in measuring the effects of a medicinal product on children include skeletal growth, weight gain, school attendance, and school performance. Recruitment of patients should ensure adequate representation across the age range in this category, as it is important to ensure a sufficient number of younger patients for evaluation. Stratification by age within this category is often unnecessary, but it may be appropriate to stratify patients based on pharmacokinetic and/or efficacy endpoint considerations.

The onset of puberty is highly variable and occurs earlier in girls, in whom normal onset of puberty may occur as early as 9 years of age. Puberty can affect the apparent activity of enzymes that metabolize drugs, and dose requirements for some medicinal products on a mg/kg basis may decrease dramatically (e.g., theophylline). In some cases, it may be appropriate to specifically assess the effect of puberty on a medicinal product by studying pre- and postpubertal pediatric patients. In other cases, it may be appropriate to record Tanner stages of pubertal development or obtain biological markers of puberty and examine data for any potential influence of pubertal changes.

2.5.5 Adolescents (12 to 16–18 years (dependent on region))

This is a period of sexual maturation; medicinal products may interfere with the actions of sex hormones and impede development. In certain studies, pregnancy testing and review of sexual activity and contraceptive use may be appropriate.

This is also a period of rapid growth and continued neurocognitive development. Medicinal products and illnesses that delay or accelerate the onset of puberty can have a profound effect on the pubertal growth spurt and, by changing the pattern of growth, may affect final height. Evolving cognitive and emotional changes could potentially influence the outcome of clinical studies.

Many diseases are also influenced by the hormonal changes around puberty (e.g., increases in insulin resistance in diabetes mellitus, recurrence of seizures around menarche, changes in the frequency and severity of migraine attacks and asthma exacerbations). Hormonal changes may thus influence the results of clinical studies.

Within this age group, adolescents are assuming responsibility for their own health and medication. Noncompliance is a special problem, particularly when medicinal products (for example, steroids) affect appearance. In clinical studies compliance checks are important. Recreational use of unprescribed drugs, alcohol and tobacco should be specifically considered.

The upper age limit varies among regions. It may be possible to include older adolescents in adult studies, although issues of compliance may present problems. Given some of the unique challenges of adolescence, it may be appropriate to consider studying adolescent patients (whether they are to be included in adult or separate protocols) in centers knowledgeable and skilled in the care of this special population.

2.6 Ethical issues in pediatric studies

The pediatric population represents a vulnerable subgroup. Therefore, special measures are needed to protect the rights of pediatric study participants and to shield them from undue risk. The purpose of this section is to provide a framework to ensure that pediatric studies are conducted ethically.

To be of benefit to those participating in a clinical study, as well as to the rest of the pediatric population, a clinical study must be properly designed to ensure the quality and interpretability of the data obtained. In addition, participants in clinical studies are expected to benefit from the clinical study except under the special circumstances discussed in ICH E6, section 4.8.14.

2.6.1 Institutional Review Board/Independent Ethics Committee (IRB/IEC)

The roles and responsibilities of IRB's/IEC's as detailed in ICH E6 are critical to the protection of study participants. When protocols involving the pediatric population are reviewed, there should be IRB/IEC members or experts consulted by the IRB/IEC who are knowledgeable in pediatric ethical, clinical, and psychosocial issues.

2.6.2 Recruitment

Recruitment of study participants should occur in a manner free from inappropriate inducements either to the parent(s)/legal guardian or the study participant. Reimbursement and subsistence costs may be covered in the context of a pediatric clinical study. Any compensation should be reviewed by the IRB/IEC.

When studies are conducted in the pediatric population, an attempt should be made to include individuals representing the demographics of the region and the disease being studied, unless there is a valid reason for restricting enrollment.

2.6.3 Consent and assent

As a rule, a pediatric subject is legally unable to provide informed consent. Therefore pediatric study participants are dependent on their parent(s)/legal guardian to assume responsibility for their participation in clinical studies. Fully informed consent should be obtained from the legal guardian in accordance with regional laws or regulations. All participants should be informed to the fullest extent possible about the study in language and terms they are able to understand. Where appropriate, participants should assent to enroll in a study (age of assent to be determined by IRB's/IEC's or be consistent with local legal requirements). Participants of appropriate intellectual maturity should personally sign and date either a separately designed, written assent form or the written informed consent. In all cases, participants should be made aware of their rights to decline to participate or to withdraw from the study at any time. Attention should be paid to signs of undue distress in patients who are unable to clearly articulate their distress. Although a participant's wish to withdraw from a study must be respected, there may be circumstances in therapeutic studies for serious or lifethreatening diseases in which, in the opinion of the investigator and parent(s)/legal guardian, the welfare of a pediatric patient would be jeopardized by his or her failing to participate in the study. In this situation, continued parental (legal guardian) consent should be sufficient to allow participation in the study. Emancipated or mature minors (defined by local laws) may be capable of giving autonomous consent.

Information that can be obtained in a less vulnerable, consenting population should not be obtained in a more vulnerable population or one in which the patients are unable to provide individual consent. Studies in handicapped or institutionalised pediatric populations should be limited to diseases or conditions found principally or exclusively in these populations, or situations in which the disease or condition in these pediatric patients would be expected to alter the disposition or pharmacodynamic effects of a medicinal product.

2.6.4 Minimizing risk

However important a study may be to prove or disprove the value of a treatment, participants may suffer injury as a result of inclusion in the study, even if the whole community benefits. Every effort should be made to anticipate and reduce known hazards. Investigators should be fully aware before the start of a clinical study of all relevant preclinical and clinical toxicity of the medicinal product. To minimize risk in pediatric clinical studies, those conducting the study should be properly trained and experienced in studying the pediatric population, including the evaluation and management of potential pediatric adverse events.

In designing studies, every attempt should be made to minimize the number of participants and of procedures, consistent with good study design. Mechanisms should be in place to ensure that a study can be rapidly terminated should an unexpected hazard be noted.

2.6.5 Minimizing distress

Repeated invasive procedures may be painful or frightening. Discomfort can be minimized if studies are designed and conducted by investigators experienced in the treatment of pediatric patients.

Protocols and investigations should be designed specifically for the pediatric population (not simply re-worked from adult protocols) and approved by an IRB/IEC as described in section 2.6.1.

Practical considerations to ensure that participants' experiences in clinical studies are positive and to minimize discomfort and distress include the following:

- Personnel knowledgeable and skilled in dealing with the pediatric population and its age-appropriate needs, including skill in performing pediatric procedures
- A physical setting with furniture, play equipment, activities, and food appropriate for age
- The conduct of studies in a familiar environment such as the hospital or clinic where participants normally receive their care

- Approaches to minimize discomfort of procedures, such as:
  - Topical anesthesia to place IV catheters
  - Indwelling catheters rather than repeated venipunctures for blood sampling
  - Collection of some protocol-specified blood samples when routine clinical samples are obtained

IRB's/IEC's should consider how many venipunctures are acceptable in an attempt to obtain blood samples for a protocol and ensure a clear understanding of procedures if an indwelling catheter fails to function over time. The participant's right to refuse further investigational procedures must be respected except as noted in section 2.6.3.

59

Guidelines for researchers and for ethics committees on psychiatric research involving human participants – executive summary

Royal College of Psychiatrists
July 2001

1   The responsibility for the ethical conduct of research rests firmly on the principal investigator.

2.1   In considering whether a procedure is research or not, LRECs and researchers are referred to the Royal College of Physicians (1996) guidelines, paragraph 6.4.

"The distinction between medical research and innovative medical practice derives from the *intent*. In medical *practice* the predominant intent is to benefit the *individual patient* consulting the clinician, not to gain knowledge of general benefit, though such knowledge may emerge from the clinical experience gained. In medical *research* the primary intention is to advance knowledge so that *patients in general* may benefit: the individual patient may or may not benefit directly."

2.2   It is in the interests of everyone that high quality research should be fostered and supported. Ethics Committees (throughout the report, "Ethics Committees" refers to "Research Ethics Committees dealing with human participants") need to check that the research they approve is of adequate quality. Because of the immense value of research, it is unacceptable that individuals from any segments of the population be disallowed by virtue of their being members of that group from participation in research that is necessary to improve the understanding of disorders from which they are particularly likely to suffer. The difficulties that must be faced in this connection with groups whose capacity to consent is limited are considered further below in paragraph 5. Nevertheless, it is a basic ethical principle that psychiatric patients, like all other patients, must be able to benefit from the fruits of research and, hence, they must have the opportunity to participate freely in sound research.

2.3   Ethics Committees should be required to assess the levels of risk in all research that they review and they should not approve projects in which the risk is regarded as excessive when considered in the light of all the circumstances, and of the potential benefits. With research regarded by the Ethics Committee as within an acceptable risk level, there is the additional requirement that all participants should be adequately informed about the nature of research, its possible risks and potential benefits, so that they can make up their own minds, on an informed basis, with respect to whether or not they are willing to take part in the study.

2.4   Ethics Committees should refuse to approve research where the funding body is of a kind that raises serious doubts about its track record on abuses of research findings.

2.5   Ethics Committees should require applicants to state whether the Funding Body (or any other interested party) places any constraints on publication. If any such constraints exist, the Ethics Committee must satisfy itself that they are reasonable in type and degree, that they are explicit and time-limited, and that they do not involve risk of censorship or distortion of findings or prevention of publication.

3.1   All research that involves human subjects directly or indirectly, and that is undertaken by the staff of any discipline (paid or honorary or emeritus) of an institution, comes within the remit of its relevant Ethics Committee, irrespective of whether or not the participants are its patients, and irrespective of where the research is undertaken. Similarly, irrespective of who undertakes the research, all research that involves the institution's patients, clients, students or staff as participants in the research falls within the Ethics Committee remit.

3.2   Routine clinical audit based solely on perusal of records must be conducted in an ethical manner and it is the responsibility of Ethics Committees to ensure that this is the case. This will require their obtaining written details of the procedures to be followed. It is up to the committee to decide whether to delegate this responsibility to someone acting on their behalf (such as the Clinical Director), or to consider the procedures in committee. Either way, however, the ultimate responsibility lies with the Ethics Committee and it is their duty to ensure that the necessary ethical needs have been met. Patient information sheets and consent forms should not be required for such case note audit and, once a set of procedures has been agreed, it should not be necessary to reconsider the procedures until it is proposed to change them.

Research into audit that involves any form of new information from patients or staff (such as by questionnaire or interview), or any form of intrusion into routine procedures (such as by video- or audio-tape recording or observation by researchers), or any form of participation in a comparison of procedures (whether or not by random allocation) should be subject to the same form of individual application required for other research applications to the Ethics Committee. Patient information and consent forms should ordinarily be required.

3.3 As with any other type of research involving human subjects, approval of research using records and archived samples must be sought from the appropriate Ethics Committee which will need to consider the usual ethical issues with respect to purposes, reputability of researchers, lack of inappropriate constraints on publication, source of funding and the other matters outlined in this document. In addition, as also recommended by the Royal College of Physicians (1999), the Ethics Committee should have specifically agreed to exempt the research from the general requirement for individual consent from each research subject. In that respect, our recommendation on research using records and archived samples follows the same principles as those that apply to clinical audit.

3.3a Individual consent should not be necessary for group analyses of anonymised data but the Ethics Committee should ensure that the required anonymisation has been achieved before the data are made available. Custodians of pooled data sets should have their own Ethics Committees to review applications for use of those sets.

3.3b Individual consent should not be necessary for analyses of personalized records provided that no contact with participants is envisaged, that access to records is controlled by a custodian (who must not be the investigator) who has the responsibility for checking the details of what is proposed, and that no data will be published that could directly or indirectly identify individuals.

3.3c Archived data may be used without individual consent to trace individual patients or volunteers in order to ask if they are willing to participate in a study. However, the planned study must have received ethical approval and all the usual expectations of individual informed consent apply to participation in any aspect of the research required for individual contact or new information/samples from individuals.

3.3d The use of personal records for tracing, when the records are not themselves the basis for identification of potential participants in research, should be dealt with in the same way as the use of archived records for tracing. For this to be generally possible, the legal acceptability of this procedure under Data Protection rules will have to be made explicit. Ethics Committees should ensure that the method of tracing to be used is discrete (see paragraph 4.13).

3.4 LRECs and researchers should be aware of the continued ethical and legal relevance of the therapeutic vs. nontherapeutic distinction as embodied in a number of current guidelines. However, rather than relying on the distinction as made, they should assess each research project on its merits according to the general principles outlined above, having regard in particular to the risks & benefits to potential participants. We recommend that steps should be taken to remove the distinction between therapeutic and nontherapeutic research.

3.5 Each research proposal should be assessed on an individual basis with respect to its individual merits and risks. The details of all procedures should be considered with regard to their possible intrusiveness, invasiveness, or distress-provoking properties in relation to the target group of participants. Researchers should be expected to have taken appropriate steps to keep all of these potentially negative features to a minimum.

3.6 All pilot studies, at all stages and of all kinds, fall within the remit of the Ethics Committees. It is acceptable, however, for the early stages of pilot work to proceed without formal application provided that a second opinion (by someone approved by the Committee to act on its behalf) is obtained and that the view is taken that the risks are trivial (as likely to be viewed by participants), that the study is being ethically undertaken, and that satisfactory informed consent is being obtained from all participants.

3.7 Ethics Committees should be prepared dispassionately to investigate any complaints over possibly unethical practice in relation to any research falling within their area of responsibility.

3.8 It is the responsibility of Ethics Committees to ensure that appropriate mechanisms for dealing with concerns over possible fraud are available and are operated in a fair and efficient manner.

4.1 Ethics Committees must consider the scientific quality of the study they are asked to approve, and the adequate provision of expert advice within the research team on the handling of risk situations. The degree of scientific scrutiny should be proportionate to the risks involved. Untoward incidents arising during the course of a study should be reported to the Ethics Committees, as a matter of routine.

4.2 A person's clinical care should not be affected by their unwillingness to take part in a study, or their withdrawal from the study during its course. No reason for nonparticipation or withdrawal need be given. The Ethics Committee needs to determine that, in these circumstances, it is practical for normal care to be provided. Participation in a study, similarly, should not result in a person receiving a worse standard of care than ordinarily expectable; the Ethics Committee should determine that the research design will not have that adverse effect.

4.2a Comparison groups are an essential part of research designs to evaluate the efficacy of treatment. When a treatment known to be effective is ordinarily available, this treatment should usually be chosen as the comparison for the new treatment being investigated; this is both scientifically and ethically appropriate. Placebo controls may, however, be justified and ethically acceptable if the science require it and their use is not against the best interests of the individual.

4.2b Therapeutic trials must be undertaken with attention to the necessary steps required to provide adequate assessment of risks and benefits. Trials must be terminated when findings show either that a treatment is ineffective or that it is associated with an unacceptable risk of harm. For the latter to be apparent, there must be systematic monitoring of untoward effects; these must be reported to the Ethics Committee.

4.3 It is reasonable that participants in research should be reimbursed for their time, expenses and inconvenience. Ethics Committees, however, need to ensure that the payments are not at such a high level that they constitute an inducement to participate.

4.4 The guideline on payment to researchers is the same as that on payment to participants.

4.5 Participants should not be included without their knowledge or agreement in a study involving personal contact (see paragraphs 3.3 re the exceptions with respect to group analyses of archived data). Ordinarily, participants must also be informed about the purposes of the research in which they are being asked to participate. There are occasional cases in which the essence of the scientific design requires a degree of deception. Such research needs to be carefully considered with regard to its ethical acceptability, but it may be acceptable if scientifically essential and if there is appropriate debriefing at the conclusion of the experiment.

4.6 All personal medical information belongs to the patient who has the right to refuse for this information (either with respect to participation in a study or to findings from the research) to be passed on to his/her medical carer unless the safety of others is in jeopardy (see paragraph 4.8). If such refusal constitutes a sufficient danger to the participant (because of other treatments given in ignorance of the research intervention), it would be unethical to put the patient at risk by inclusion in the study.

4.7 Acceptable research governance requires that research teams have agreed procedures for minimizing the risks to staff involved in the research.

4.8 Research findings, like clinical findings, should in all ordinary circumstances be regarded as confidential and should not be passed on to others without the participant's explicit permission. There are, however, rare circumstances in which the law (and/or good clinical and ethical practice) requires that confidentiality be breached. The criteria for when this rare occurrence can be considered to arise are the same in research as in clinical practice. When the nature of the research means that it is likely that findings could have implications for other family members, this contingency should be discussed at the point of obtaining informed consent, with the aim of obtaining agreement for disclosure.

4.9 All researchers working directly with children should have a police check for crimes relating to children before starting such work.

4.10 Researchers should be strongly encouraged to provide feedback to participants on the general findings and implications of research in which they have participated.

4.11 When research involves clinically valid assessments relevant for individual diagnosis, it should be expected that participants will be informed on all findings that have substantial medical significance for them as individuals. This must be done by someone who understands the clinical implications of the findings and the information must be given in a clinically sensitive manner. However, when the findings are of unknown significance or when they have meaning only at a group level, feedback should not be expected. For studies from which the findings are likely to be of this kind, the information sheet should be explicit that individual feedback will not be provided.

4.12   Research data should be subject to the same safeguards on security and confidentiality as clinical data. The custodianship of the data should be the responsibility of the named lead researcher for the study that collected the data initially but, given appropriate safeguards, the data may be shared with collaborating researchers under the concept of extended confidentiality.

4.13   Researchers need to be aware that letters and telephone calls to potential participants, especially when using addresses and telephone numbers that may no longer be applicable, may be intercepted by third parties. This possibility requires attention to the need to avoid initial communications that, implicitly or explicitly, include personal information that could inadvertently provide a breach of confidentiality.

4.14   Informed consent must be obtained if it is envisaged that a portion of a biological sample obtained for a clinical purpose may also be used for research.

4.15   Ethics Committees should emphasize to their organizations and to the applicants asking for ethical approval of studies the need to avoid undue overload on research participants.

4.16   It is good research (and ethics) practice to consult members of the community to be studied when planning studies. As appropriate to the individual study, such consultation might involve consumers, professionals, community members or ethnic/religious groups.

5.1   Ordinarily, it is necessary that potential participants actively opt in to a study. Opt-out procedures with respect to parents consenting on behalf of children may be ethically acceptable, however, for large scale studies involving routine type procedures carrying no significant risk so long as certain safeguards are provided and the details of what is proposed have been approved by the appropriate Ethics Committee. It will always be necessary for the children to be given appropriate information, for them to give or withhold their consent, and their refusal should be accepted.

5.2   Participants should ordinarily have the right to decide for themselves whether or not they wish to participate in a study, and professionals should not have the right to

refuse access when the potential participant is known to the researcher through some other route. An exception arises when the patient is currently under active treatment and the carer considers that the research could jeopardize the care being provided.

5.3   Researchers have a responsibility to ensure that all respondents have a clearly written, readily understandable, information sheet that is explicit on the purpose of the study, the procedures involved, what is required of the participants, details of the lead researcher and contact person, any significant risks, and the right to decline to take part (or to withdraw during the study) without giving a reason and without detriment to normal treatment.

5.4   Ordinarily, a written consent should be obtained; this should specify that the information sheet has been given, read and understood, and that what is involved has been explained to the satisfaction of the participant.

5.5   Scrupulous care must be taken by researchers to avoid undue influence on potential participants to agree to take part in research. Attention is particularly necessary with respect to payments to participants, the dangers of pressure implicit in hierarchical relationships, and the pressures (and opportunities) that may be perceived by detained persons.

5.6   The capacity to give consent is task- and time-specific, it constitutes a graded dimension of understanding, and it is something that can be influenced to some degree. Researchers should seek to help respondents achieve the capacity needed for the specific decision needed. Although, legally, a categorical decision on whether a person is competent to give consent is required, individuals whose capacity falls below that level should be helped to understand what is involved and to participate in decision-making. Ethics Committees should satisfy themselves that the materials and process used to facilitate understanding are adequate.

5.6a   It is good research practice to engage children in the decision-making process even when they lack the capacity to give consent. The issues with respect to assessing capacity outlined in paragraph 5.6 apply to children. Parents should be able to authorize children's participation in research provided it presents no more than minimal risks. If the research involves risks that are greater than minimal, it could be ethically acceptable if the scientific need is sufficiently great, specifically applies to children, and could not be met with research on competent adults. A strong case would need to be made in this circumstance and, in addition to parental assent, it would be essential for there to be unambiguous support from an independent professional with respect to both scientific needs and ethical acceptability. With procedures that are more intrusive than required for ordinary clinical care, a child's refusal should be accepted as a sufficient reason not to proceed, irrespective of parental consent.

5.6b No individuals should be disqualified by virtue of their group membership from participating in research (as a result of incompetence to give consent or other reason) that could be of benefit in relation to the disease, disorder, or disability from which they suffer. It is ethically acceptable to proceed without personal informed consent provided that a specified set of conditions has been met. These include the relevance of the research, the fact that the research cannot be undertaken with validity in less vulnerable groups with the same disorder, the assent of the individual's closest relative or cohabiting partner, the support of both the person's professional carer and an independent clinician, minimal risks, and approval by the appropriate Ethics Committee. However, as with children, the patient's refusal should be accepted as sufficient reason not to proceed irrespective of other consents.

5.6c It is ethical to waive consent in the study of emergency treatments for life-threatening situations affecting individuals who are incompetent to give consent, provided the principles outlined in paragraph 5.6b have been followed. The specifics in such emergency situations differ, however, in two respects. It is acceptable to proceed without the assent of a relative if that cannot be obtained in time (but not ethical to proceed in the face of a relative's objection); and the risk-benefits should be judged in relation to those associated with existing treatments or outcomes (rather than minimal risks in an absolute sense). In planning research that deals with these circumstances, there should be appropriate consultation with the relevant user groups (see paragraph 4.16).

5.6d Active steps should be taken to help individuals with learning difficulties to achieve sufficient understanding for them to give informed consent. Even when this is not possible, the individuals should be helped to be involved in the decision-making process. When the competence to give consent is lacking, research may be ethically acceptable if it is relevant to learning difficulties, it is not against the individuals best interests, it does not intrude unreasonably on the person's privacy or freedom of action, appropriate assent has been obtained from a close relative, the procedures have been approved by an independent professional, the study has the support of relevant user group representatives

and the study as a whole has been approved by the relevant Ethics Committee.

5.6e There are risks of perceived covert coercion if staff and students who are in a hierarchical relationship with the researcher are approached to volunteer to participate in research. It is usually desirable to avoid the use of such groups in research and, if their use is needed, there must be a reasoned case included in the Ethics Committee application; this must specify how the coercion concern will be dealt with.

5.6f For detained patients the general principles of 5.6 apply, but especial care is needed to ensure that there is no possibility of perceived coercion and that an independent professional opinion has been obtained. For research on detained patients to be ethically acceptable, the focus of the research must be relevant for their disorders, it must not be possible for the research to be undertaken in a valid and generalizable fashion with less vulnerable groups, it must not be against their individual best interests, and particular care must be taken to ensure that the informed consent is real. Ordinarily, too, it should be expected that the research procedures should be noninvasive. Invasive research may be ethically acceptable but particularly strong justification with respect to risk benefits would be essential (see paragraph 5.6a).

5.6g For prisoners, the same general principles as those outlined for detained patients apply with respect to possibly perceived coercion but in most cases there is not the same issue with respect to competence. In the few instances where that is relevant, a comparable set of procedures should be followed at the individual level. When competence is not in doubt, the main concern is to ensure that the research, and the procedures of obtaining consent, provide adequate protection to the individual. Ethics Committees should consider whether, given the nature of a particular study, independent advice should be sought regarding the ethical acceptability of the study.

6.1 Uniformity should be sought on expectations regarding which studies need to be submitted to Ethics Committees. The legal implications of disregarding Ethics Committee decisions should also be clarified.

6.2 Committee membership should reflect the range of research and clinical skills relevant to the applications that they consider, the range of disciplines involved in the case of patients with disorders in the field covered, and should include both lay members and people who reflect the interests of patients and their families. It is highly desirable that the Chair or Vice Chair be a lay person. Sufficient experts in clinical and research aspects of mental health should be included in the membership of Committees to cover the range of research topics they are likely to have to deal with.

6.3   Ethics Committees should have a properly resourced professional administration.

6.4   Attention should be paid to the design of application forms to ensure that all necessary details of the study and ethical issues are provided in a standard way.

6.5   Ethical review of studies must include an appropriate degree of scientific scrutiny and continuation of ethical approval should be made contingent on the researchers providing information on any changes in design, funding, or personnel involved.

6.6   Studies of nonpatient samples or samples of patients obtained from registers separate from local centres should ordinarily be considered by the appropriate local ethics committee, rather than being passed on to a multicentre ethics committee. When research involves several centres (but below the number requiring referral to a multicentre committee), the relevant local Ethics Committees should decide on which one should take the lead, with the expectation that the other committees would accept their decision unless there were some special additional considerations to be taken into account.

6.7   Formal declaration of potential conflicts of interest should be expected of all members of Ethics Committees and, if these create a possible problem in relation to individual applications, affected members should withdraw during their discussion.

Reproduced by permission of the Royal College of Psychiatrists.

The full text is available from
Publications Department
Royal College of Psychiatrists
17 Belgrave Square
London SW1X 8PG

Tel: 020 7235 2351
Fax: 020 7245 1231

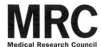

The ethical conduct of research on the mentally incapacitated

Medical Research Council

Working Party on Research on the Mentally Incapacitated
Published December 1991 – (Reprinted August 1993)

The Working Party submitted its report to the Council in July 1991. The Council endorsed its recommendations and agreed that its report should be published.

Introduction

The Working Party on Research on the Mentally Incapacitated was established by the Medical Research Council (MRC) in July 1988.[1] The Council proposed the following terms of reference:

(i) to consider the adequacy or otherwise of existing MRC statements and the published guidance from other bodies about the conduct of non-therapeutic research investigations in the special circumstances of research on the mentally incapacitated;

(ii) to consider whether, in the light of (i), the Council should formulate new guidance, and if so prepare advice on the ethical conduct of research on the mentally incapacitated taking account of the existing guidance and supplementing, extending and modifying it where necessary;

(iii) to make recommendations to the Council.

The Working Party membership was as follows:

Mrs Renee Short (Chairman)
Dr J L T Birley
Mr I C Dodds-Smith
Professor R E Kendell
Mr W H Wells
Professor J K Wing

This is no longer applicable in Scotland following the introduction of the Adults with Incapacity (Scotland) Act in 2000.
© Medical Research Council.

1 Background

1.1 The Council's general stance on ethical matters is set out in the Statement first published in the Council's Annual Report for 1962–63 (Cmnd 2382) and subsequently reprinted as a booklet 'Responsibility in Investigations on Human Subjects'.

1.2 In the years which followed publication of the Council's Statement, other bodies have taken an interest in the ethical conduct of medical research In 1984 the Council formally consulted the Royal College of Physicians of London (RCP), the then Department of Health and Social Security (DHSS) and Sir Douglas Black (as an independent adviser) and reached the view that the leadership in ethical matters had now passed, rightly and properly, to the profession. Specifically, the RCP's 1984 booklet 'Guidelines on the Practice of Ethics Committees in Medical Research' (subsequently revised in 1990) could be regarded as an up-to-date and practical expression of the principles first promulgated by the Council in its 1962–63 Statement The Council saw no pressing need to consider revising the 1962–63 Statement at that stage.

1.3 In the course of a wide ranging discussion of ethical issues in 1987, Council again endorsed the general principles contained in the 1962–63 Statement but agreed that a succession of recent events had made it timely to consider whether to say more on some of the difficult issues facing those engaged in clinical research, in particular research on children and on the mentally incapacitated. Council therefore agreed to establish two Working Parties to advise on research on each of these groups. Explicit in the decision to seek this advice was the realisation that the guidance on such research given in the Council's 1962–63 Statement was now out of line with that given by other reputable bodies, and with accepted good practice in clinical research.

1.4 One important development since the Council's 1962–63 Statement has been the establishment of Local Research Ethics Committees (LRECs) Advice on the constitution and role of such Committees was published in 1973 by the RCP and subsequently updated in 1984 and 1990 (see paragraph 1 2) In 1975 the then DHSS issued a circular (HSC(15)153) urging all health authorities to ensure that research conducted under their auspices was subject to ethical review It is now accepted that any medical research project involving human subjects must be submitted for approval to the appropriate LREC, the Council's own rules governing programme and project grants have for some years required all such applications to have prior LREC approval (and that of all relevant LRECs in the case of multicentre studies). There are similar requirements in respect of directly supported research. In 1991 the Department of Health intends to issue a further circular on LRECs to Health Authorities (now published). This includes guidance on the issue of consent to research in general, and in the special circumstances of research involving mentally incapacitated people. The content of these and other relevant guidelines is discussed in section 5 below.

2 Method of working

2.1 We met on 5 occasions; at our first meeting we agreed that as the question of consent (see 3.2.1) was central to our task, our advice might be more helpful to the Council if our proposed terms of reference were broadened to include all forms of research. We therefore deleted the term 'non-therapeutic'.

2.2 In accordance with our terms of reference we took written and oral evidence from a number of organisations and from various individuals, both in their own right and as representatives of professional bodies. We are grateful to the then President of the RCP for an early sight of drafts of the College's 1990 report on 'Research Involving Patients' and of their 1990 'Guidelines on the Practice of Ethics Committees in Medical Research Involving Human Subjects'. We regard both as providing valuable and up-to-date advice. We did not consider it appropriate to go over all the ground covered in these and other recent documents discussing the general ethical issues surrounding medical research, our report and recommendations should be read in the context of the advice offered by the RCP and other authoritative bodies. We recommend that the Council should continue to review its stance on ethical matters both generally and in relation to specific issues at regular intervals to ensure that it takes appropriate account of contemporary public and professional opinion.

2.3 The issues we considered had much in common with those being considered by the Council's Working Party on Research on Children. One of our members was also a member of that Working Party and was therefore able to keep each group informed of the other's progress. Communication between the working Parties was further enhanced by the exchange of minutes and draft reports, and by discussions between the legal experts We were from the outset fully aware of the legal problems associated with research in this area; we chose to concentrate in the first instance on defining the ethical issues and only then considered the legal position. This was somewhat clarified but by no means resolved by a recent judgement by the House of Lords (see 7.2.1 below).

3 Definitions

3.1 Mental incapacity

3.1.1 We agreed that for our purposes mental incapacity should be defined as incompetence to give consent. Various categories of person are included in this definition; we are primarily concerned with the mentally ill, the mentally handicapped, the demented and the unconscious. Some of these persons will never have the capacity to give consent, some will lose it irrevocably and in some it will be present at times but not at others.

3.2 Consent

3.2.1 Seeking the consent of an individual to participation in research reflects the right of that individual to self-determination and also his fundamental right to be free from bodily interference whether physical or psychological. These are ethical principles recognised by English law as legal rights. We identified three elements to consent in its broadest sense – the information given, the capacity to understand it and the voluntariness of any decision taken.

3.2.2 At the most basic level, failure to supply information about the nature and purpose of what is proposed may lead to a claim that the interference with the research subject's body constitutes a trespass to person. Thus it should be made clear to the subject that he is being invited to participate in research even if what is proposed is part of normal treatment. If a person then freely consents that consent is real provided there has been no misrepresentation of the facts. However, additional information, for instance, on possible risks and alternatives is required in a suitable form before it can properly be said that the researcher has fully discharged his general duty to put the subject in a position to make a rational judgement about whether to participate.

3.2.3 Whether a person has the capacity to understand the information depends on the ability to comprehend the nature and purpose of any course of action and the short and long-term risks and benefits of what is proposed. An individual may be in a position to consent to take part in some studies but not others: capacity to consent will depend not only on the nature of the research itself but also on the nature of the explanation.

3.2.4 Consent must also be voluntarily given and therefore must not be obtained through either implicit or explicit coercion.

3.3 Therapeutic and non-therapeutic research*

*Note: therapeutic research is here used as an umbrella term to cover research not only on the treatment of disease but also on its prevention (eg, by vaccination) and on diagnostic procedures.

3.3.1 The primary intention of all medical research is to acquire knowledge that will be of benefit to humanity as a whole – to all who are or may become ill. Although a number of our expert witnesses used terms such as 'unproblematic and problematic' research or 'single and dual intention' research we have preferred to retain the more usual usage of therapeutic and non-therapeutic research. Therapeutic research is directly concerned with treatment and thus offers the possibility of immediate benefit to participants. Direct benefit to participants in non-therapeutic research is either unlikely or long delayed.

3.3.2 As the Council's 1962–63 Statement recognised, it may initially be difficult to make a clear distinction between innovative therapeutic procedures and research. Nevertheless, at some stage such procedures must be subjected to disciplined investigation.

4 The position set out in the council's 1962–63 statement

4.1 As part of our terms of reference we considered it necessary to offer some comments on the guidance contained in the Council's 1962–63 Statement on consent, these we have appended to this report.

4.2 The Council's 1962–63 Statement does not use the term 'mental incapacity' but includes reference to the 'mentally subnormal' and the 'mentally disordered'. Nor does it use the terms 'therapeutic' and 'non-therapeutic' research, it does, however, make a distinction between 'procedures contributing to the benefit of the individual' and 'procedures not of direct benefit to the individual, These two categories correspond broadly to those we have defined as therapeutic and non-therapeutic research.

4.3 In relation to procedures contributing to the benefit of the individual (ie, therapeutic research) the Statement does not explicitly address the question of adults unable to consent.

4.4 The Statement is clear about the requirements for the inclusion of those unable to consent in procedures which are not of direct benefit to them (ie, non-therapeutic research). Any person taking part in such procedures must volunteer 'in the full sense of the word'. The Statement reads:

"It should be clearly understood that the possibility or probability that a particular investigation will be of benefit to humanity or to posterity would afford no defence in the event of legal proceedings. The individual has rights that the law protects and nobody can infringe those rights for the public good In investigations of this type it is, therefore, always necessary to ensure that the true consent of the subject is explicitly obtained."

"When true consent cannot be obtained, procedures which are of no direct benefit and which might carry a risk of harm to the subject should not be undertaken."

5 Other guidance on research on mentally incapacitated people

5.1 The Declaration of Helsinki, drawn up by the World Medical Association in 1964 and revised by the World Medical Assembly in 1975 and 1983, states that freely given informed consent should be obtained from those participating in any medical research but that "where physical or mental incapacity makes it impossible to obtain informed consent ... permission from the responsible relative replaces that of the subject in accordance with national legislation". This statement is not of much assistance to researchers in the UK where the law does not recognise as effective the proxy consent of a relative other than in the case of consent on behalf of a minor by a parent or a legally appointed guardian, or by some other person having a care, custody or residence order.

5.2 In 1990 the Committee of Ministers of the Council of Europe issued a Recommendation (No.R(90)3) to Governments of member states to adopt legislation or measures to ensure implementation of a set of principles concerning medical research on human beings. Principle 3 includes the statement that "No medical research may be carried out without informed, free, express and specific consent of the person undergoing it." Principles 4 and 5 state:

Principle 4

A legally incapacitated person may only undergo medical research where authorised by Principle 5 and if his legal representative, or an authority or an individual authorised or designated under his national law, consents. If the legally incapacitated person is capable of understanding, his consent is also required and no research may be undertaken if he does not give his consent.

Principle 5

1. A legally incapacitated person may not undergo medical research unless it is expected to produce a direct and significant benefit to his health.

2. However, by way of exception, national law may authorise research involving a legally incapacitated person which is not of direct benefit to his health when that person offers no objection, provided that the research is to the benefit of persons in the same category and that the same scientific results cannot be obtained by research on persons who do not belong to this category."

5.3 In July 1990 the European Commission issued guidelines, prepared by the Committee for Proprietary Medicinal Products, on Good Clinical Practice for Trials on Medicinal Products in the European Community. These guidelines do not yet have statutory force in the UK, but it is proposed to require all member states to make them part of national law and it appears likely that they will represent national law by 1992. The guidelines cover a number of issues from ethics committees to consent in trials of medicinal products.

Paragraph 1.13 states:

"If the subject is incapable of giving personal consent (eg, unconsciousness or severe mental illness or disability), the inclusion of such patients may be acceptable if the ethics committee is, in principle, in agreement and if the investigator is of the opinion that participation will promote the welfare and interest of the subject. The

agreement of a legally valid representative that participation will promote the welfare interest of the subject should also be recorded by a dated signature. If neither signed informed consent nor witnessed signed verbal consent are possible, this fact must be documented with reasons by the investigator".

Paragraph 1.14 states:

"Consent must always be given by the signature of the subject in a non-therapeutic study, ie, when there is no direct clinical benefit to the subject."

5.4 The RCP's 1990 report 'Research involving Patients' also emphasises that, with some exceptions such as observational research which carries no risk and is not intrusive, patients should know that they are taking part in research and that research should only be carried out with their consent.

5.5 The RCP report emphasises that many mentally handicapped and mentally ill patients will be able to give consent. It continues:

"A strong ethical case can be made out for non-therapeutic research (involving only minimal risk) in mentally handicapped patients because only through better understanding of their condition can care for such patients be improved. We think that the best guidance under these circumstances might be that there should be agreement by the close relatives or guardians and that the mentally handicapped individual seems to agree to the procedure.'

5.6 This report, together with the RCP's 1990 'Guidelines on the Practice of Ethics Committees in Medical Research Involving Human Subjects'*, recommends that the considerations quoted above in relation to mentally handicapped adults are relevant to therapeutic and non-therapeutic research involving mentally ill patients who cannot give consent or whose consent is in doubt. The RCP's reports emphasise, however, that no patient who refuses or resists should be included in research.

5.7 The Royal College of Psychiatrists' (RCPsych) 1990 'Guidelines for Ethics of Research Committees on Psychiatric Research involving Human Subjects' puts the case for psychiatric research as follows:

"Research is as essential in psychiatry as in any other branch of medicine. While there are ethical problems in carrying out research, it is unethical for the profession to fail to do research because this deprives present and future patients of the possibility of more informed and better treatment as well as the (more distant) prospect of prevention of psychiatric disorder."

5.8 The RCPsych Guidelines emphasise that "The majority of psychiatric patients are as capable of giving consent as are other patients". On the question of 'incompetent' patients, they point out that many suffer from conditions, such as mental handicap and dementia, in which advances are most needed and which cannot be obtained by studying other patients. The Guidelines recommend a 'common sense' approach to research in such circumstances. They do not distinguish explicitly between therapeutic and non-therapeutic research but emphasise that the LREC should decide in the usual way whether the research is acceptable in terms of the balance of benefits, discomfort and risks, and suggest that in most cases the research worker should discuss the research with one or more close relatives. If there is no relative, or the patient expresses the wish that his relatives should not be consulted (confidentiality may be an important issue in this and other contexts), they recommend consulting an independent person approved by the LREC who knows the patient well and will protect his interests. Whatever the views of third parties, the Guidelines state that no research should proceed if the patient refuses, or appears to refuse, either in words or actions.

5.9 We have had the opportunity to see in draft form the Department of Health's 1991 Circular on Local Research Ethics Committees (now published) which states at para 3.9:

"Some research proposals will draw their subjects from groups of people who may find it difficult or impossible to give their consent, for example the OnCOn scious, the very elderly, the mentally disordered or some other vulnerable group In considering these proposals the LREC should seek appropriate specialist advice and they will' need to examine the proposal with particular care to satisfy themselves that proceeding without valid consent is ethically acceptable."

In relation to research on mentally disordered people, the Circular refers LRECs and researchers to the RCPsych's guidelines, and states at para 4.11:

"Proposals for research where capacity to consent is impaired will need particularly careful consideration by the LREC, with regard to its acceptability in terms of the balance of benefits, discomforts and risks for the individual patient and the need to advance knowledge so that people with mental disorder may benefit."

6 The ethical case for including mentally incapacitated people in research

General

6.1.1 Many people with mental impairment or disorder will be capable of giving or withholding consent to their inclusion in research and should be free to do so. We have given some thought to who should decide whether an individual has the capacity to consent to a particular project. When that individual is a patient in the care of a physician other than the research worker, this physician should be approached for an informed and independent judgement. When the individual concerned is not in the direct care of a physician, or that physician is the research worker, the view of a relative, friend or other person acceptable to the LREC should be sought. When there is any doubt about an individual's mental capacity to consent, an independent person should be present when consent is sought and should sign a document stating that they were present when the project was discussed.

6.1.2 It is clear from the material discussed in section 5 above that there is a consensus, with which we concur, that a principled case can be made on ethical grounds for research involving people who cannot consent. There are a number of situations in which knowledge that is badly needed for the sake of those suffering from various forms of mental handicap or mental illness can only be acquired by research on people who are themselves suffering from these conditions and as a consequence lack the mental capacity to consent.

6.1.3 At the same time, there is agreement on the need for strict safeguards for such research. In particular:
- those unable to consent should take part in research only if it relates to their condition and if the relevant knowledge could not be gained by research in persons able to consent
- all projects must be approved by the appropriate LREC(s)
- the inclusion of an individual unable to consent should be subject to the agreement of an informed, independent person acceptable to the LREC that that individual's welfare and interests have been properly safeguarded
- those included in the research do not object or appear to object in either words or action

6.1.4 We are not seeking to argue that the need to seek consent for research can be waived for the mentally incapacitated or any other class of person. Rather, we believe that it is now widely accepted by authoritative individuals and bodies that there are circumstances in which it is ethically acceptable for another person to review the balance of risk and benefit (if any) associated with participation in a project and to give or withhold their agreement that the welfare and interests of a subject who is unable to consent have been properly safeguarded. The precise role of this person will depend upon the nature of the proposed research and is discussed separately below for therapeutic and non-therapeutic research. In all cases, everything possible should be done to explain the nature of, and reasons for, research procedures to mentally incapacitated people who have some measure of understanding.

6.2 Therapeutic research

6.2.1 We believe that subject to the safeguards listed at 6.1.3 above there is a strong ethical case for including those who cannot consent in therapeutic research; indeed we would argue that. in circumstances where participation is in their best interests, their exclusion would be unethical.

6.2.2 The inclusion in therapeutic research of an individual who cannot consent must be subject to the agreement of a relative, friend or person acceptable to the LREC and not directly involved in the research that, weighing the likely benefits and the possible risks of harm to the individual concerned, that individual's welfare has been properly safeguarded and participation in the research is in his best interests.

6.3 Non-therapeutic research

6.3.1 Because it might infringe the rights of a group which society should take particular care to protect, the participation of people who cannot consent in non-therapeutic research raises more complex ethical issues. We do not seek to argue that a mentally incapacitated person's participation in non-therapeutic research is directly in his interests. But we recognise that there are circumstances in which it is important to gain knowledge which may be of benefit to mentally incapacitated people in general and which can only be acquired as a result of research which involves those who are unable to consent.

6.3.2 We therefore believe that there is a strong case for including those unable to consent in such research, but it is essential that the safeguards listed at 6.1.3 are observed, and that those included are placed at no more than negligible risk of harm.

6.3.3 The degree of risk involved in a project should be given particularly careful scrutiny by the LREC when mentally incapacitated people are to be included. There have been various attempts to describe and define degrees of risk. We use the term negligible risk to mean that the risks of harm anticipated in the proposed research are not greater, considering the probability and magnitude of physiological or psychological harm or discomfort, than those ordinarily encountered in daily life or during the performance of routine physical or psychological examination or tests. Examples of procedures involving negligible risk would include the observation of behaviour, non-invasive physiological monitoring, physical examinations, changes in diet and obtaining blood and urine specimens. We discuss risk in non-therapeutic research in the context of the law in para 7.3.4 below.

6.3.4 We are clear that participation in such research of an individual unable to consent can only be ethical if a relative, friend or person acceptable to the LREC and not directly involved in the research agrees that participation would place that individual at no more than negligible risk of harm and is therefore not against that individual's interests.

7 The legal position

7.1 General

7.1.1 Our primary task was to advise on ethical issues; however we have considered it proper to comment on the legal position, partly because the Council's stance set out in the 1962/63 Statement derives from it and partly because it raises a number of complex issues. As was the case when the Council developed the 1962/63 Statement, one is dealing not with statute law but with common law principles as developed by judges in case law. The applicable case law focuses upon conventional medical treatment rather than treatment in the context of research or non-therapeutic research. Nevertheless, the decisions help to indicate the likely attitude of the courts.

England, Wales and Northern Ireland

7.1.2 The Mental Health Act 1983 for England and Wales and the Mental Health (Northern Ireland) Order 1986 for Northern Ireland include certain provisions relating to consent procedures relevant to the administration of particular types of treatment to mentally disordered patients for their disorder but in principle detention under these statutes does not bear upon the ability of a person to give a valid consent. The legislation does not address the question of research. However, the Department of Health and Welsh Office have issued a Code of Practice which includes guidance on the treatment of patients suffering from mental disorder.

7.1.3 Under common law principles, research involving adults who cannot consent faces two important legal obstacles. The first is that since one has a right to determine what is done with one's body it is an unlawful act (trespass to person) for anyone, regardless of his intention, to touch or otherwise interfere with the bodily integrity of an adult without his consent. The second is that there is no provision in English law for anyone to give consent on behalf of another adult. Thus while in respect of minors (under 18) unable to consent, parents may consent to treatment on behalf of their children, or the court may exercise its wardship jurisdiction, no-one – not even the next of kin – has the power to consent on behalf of an adult unable to consent himself through mental disability. Moreover, it is now established that no court has any jurisdiction with respect to such a person to consent on his behalf. Judges have suggested that this is an area suitable for parliamentary intervention, but in the meantime, rather than purport to give a proxy consent on behalf of the person concerned, the courts have been prepared to make binding declarations as to whether the actions of those involved in the particular proposed procedure are legal.

7.2 Therapeutic research

England, Wales and Northern Ireland

7.2.1 Case law in the past has established the legality of bodily interference without consent in certain circumstances, such as the physical contact of every day social activity and emergency treatment to protect life. Most recently, in a landmark decision (in Re F 1989), the House of Lords established that a doctor in England, Wales and Northern Ireland can lawfully give any treatment to an adult patient who is incapable of consenting through mental incapacity provided such treatment is performed in accordance with a responsible body of relevant professional opinion and in the best interests of the patient ie, it is carried out in order either to save life or to ensure improvement or prevent deterioration in his physical or mental health. The court also endorsed as good practice consultation with relatives and others concerned with the care of the patient. The particular case involved the sterilisation of a mentally handicapped woman: the court declared that in cases of this type involving major treatment of an irreversible nature, the public interest additionally required the express approval of the court. It has not, however, been suggested that standard curative or prophylactic treatment of the mentally incapacitated normally requires court approval (see in Re E, 1991).

7.2.2 While the judgement in Re F concerned conventional medical treatment and not research, we agree with the conclusion of the RCP 1990 Report 'Research Involving Patients', that the principle enunciated should equally apply when the treatment in question is still in the research phase. An experimental medicinal procedure may be the only appropriate therapy and provided the relevant health professional acts with proper skill and care and in the best interests of the patient, neither liability for trespass nor negligence should arise.

7.2.3 The Code of Practice issued under the Mental Health Act 1983 emphasises that patients should be informed of the nature, purpose and likely effects of the treatment proposed in a suitable manner even if they lack capacity to consent to the treatment.

7.2.4 We are clear that, provided the necessary safeguards are in place, the ethical grounds for including mentally incapacitated people in therapeutic research (and indeed for not denying them the opportunity to participate in research that offers the prospect of improving their health) are so great, that it would be contrary to accepted good practice to be deterred by the comparative lack of clarity surrounding the legal position. However, it may be prudent for doctors contemplating special categories of treatment of a serious and irreversible nature in a research context to consider whether it is appropriate to seek endorsement of their actions by the court, no doubt in consultation with the relevant ethics committee.

7.3 Non-therapeutic research

England, Wales and Northern Ireland

7.3.1 In the main, the legal arguments to which the Council referred in its 1962/63 Statement (see paragraph 4.4) are still pertinent with respect to procedures involving bodily interventions or which place an individual at risk of harm. We have, however, argued on ethical grounds that a mentally incapacitated person should not be excluded from the opportunity to contribute to the welfare of other mentally incapacitated people, and possibly to his own welfare, provided no more than minimal risk of harm is involved.

7.3.2 That this is widely accepted is illustrated by the fact that the Council and other reputable funding bodies have not been paralysed by lack of clarity in the law, but have supported work of this type for some time.

7.3.3 As a legal matter, any interference with a person's body will only be lawful if it is justified on the basis of some legally recognised principle. It has been noted above that the courts in England and Wales and Northern Ireland now accept that it is in the public interest to ensure that those unable to consent should not be deprived of appropriate medical treatment but it must be stressed that the courts have not yet considered whether there is any public interest basis for allowing any form of non-therapeutic intervention in a person who, through mental incapacity, is unable to consent. In recent cases concerning issues of consent, the Courts have emphasised the need to establish what is in the best interests of the individual. This may suggest that health professionals will be exposed to legal action if they are responsible for allowing such a person, who has no prospect of immediate personal benefit, to be exposed to any risk purely in the interest of advancing knowledge. If this is correct, researchers should be clear that, although appropriate on ethical grounds, the approval of an ethics committee or a relative or some other independent person is unlikely to be recognised by the law as an adequate substitute for the consent of the research subject.

7.3.4 However, it seems to us that a case can be made out that it is not in the public interest for persons suffering from mental incapacity to be excluded from socially responsible behaviour purely through lack of consent competence. Where the risk attending participation in non-therapeutic research into mental disorder is minimal and a reasonable person with that disorder but able to consent is likely to accept that risk when told that such research might lead to advances in treatment, it would be strange if a person unable to consent because of that disorder should be imputed with a wholly different attitude to the welfare of the class of persons of which he is a member. It seems to us that provided the welfare of the individual in the broadest sense is properly considered by the ethics committee and, in addition, by an informed person independent of the researcher, and participation is not found to be against his best interests because the risk of harm is minimal, the subject's participation may be viewed by the courts as in the public interest and lawful. For these purposes it is difficult to define minimal risk in all the contexts that may arise but it would seem unlikely that the courts would countenance exposing a mentally incapacitated person to a risk (having regard to probability and magnitude of physical or psychological harm or discomfort) beyond what is normally encountered in daily life or in the routine medical or psychological examination of a normal person.

7.3.5 The Law Commission has undertaken a review of a variety of matters concerning the mentally incapacitated including issues of consent competence and has recently published a Consultation Paper In due course, this may lead to legislation but not in the immediate future. In the meantime, in view of the legal uncertainty, the only sure legal protection for researchers concerned about their position would be for them to seek a declaration from the court that the proposed research procedures are legal.

8 Summary and recommendations

8.1 Many people with mental impairment or disorder are able to consent to their inclusion in research provided care is taken to explain it to them. When there is doubt about an individual's mental capacity, we recommend that a judgement on his ability to consent should be sought from the physician responsible. When the individual is not under the care of a physician, or the physician is involved in the proposed research, a view should be sought from a relative, friend or other person acceptable to the LREC.

8.2 There is a strong case for allowing those unable to consent to participate in medical research provided safeguards are observed. We recommend that an individual unable to consent should be included in research only if it relates to his condition and the relevant knowledge could not be gained by research in persons able to consent and

it is approved by the appropriate LREC(s)

he does not object or appear to object in either words or action

an informed, independent person acceptable to the LREC agrees that the individual's welfare and interests have been properly safeguarded and in the case of therapeutic research, weighing the likely benefits and the possible risk of harm to the individual concerned, participation is in that individual's best interests

in the case of non-therapeutic research, that participation would place the individual at no more than negligible risk of harm and is not against that individual's interests.

8.3 We recommend that the Council should revise its guidance on research on mentally incapacitated people so as not to exclude research satisfying these conditions.

The ethical conduct of reseach on the mentally incapacitated

Appendix

The council's 1962–63 statement: consent

The Council's Statement* has played an important role in the development of the discussion of the ethics of medical research. The position set out in it with respect to consent is, however, now seriously out of line with contemporary thinking. The root of the problem lies in the general statement which reads:

"In the case of procedures directly connected with the management of the condition in the particular individual, the relationship is essentially that between doctor and patient. Implicit in this relationship is the willingness on the

---

* The Council has agreed that its 1962–63 Statement should be withdrawn and a revised version should be issued.

part of the subject to be guided by the judgement of his medical attendant. Provided, therefore, that the medical attendant is satisfied that there are reasonable grounds for believing that a particular new procedure will contribute to the benefit of that particular patient, either by treatment, prevention or increased understanding of his case, he may assume the patient's consent to the same extent as he would were the procedure entirely established practice."

While we would readily accept that trust between doctor and patient continues to be central to good clinical practice, we would suggest that it can no longer be assumed that the patient will or indeed should be guided solely by the judgement of his medical attendant, or that there are any circumstances (other than some emergencies) where the doctor can assume consent.

It is now generally accepted that the doctor has a duty to explain to his patient the pros and cons of the various courses of action open to him in offering treatment or measures intended to prevent or ameliorate a given condition. If this is so for treatment, it must hold even more strongly for research. There is unanimity among those we consulted that for most classes of research the patient must understand that he is taking part in research and give his consent to his participation in that research (examples cited by the Royal College of Physicians of London of studies for which patients' consent need not be sought include the examination of anonymised specimens collected in the course of ordinary medical practice, and observational research involving no contact with or risk to patients).

This guidance is no longer applicable in Scotland following the introduction of the Adults with Incapacity (Scotland) Act 2000

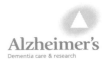
Alzheimer's
Dementia care & research

Volunteering for research into dementia
November 2000

Alzheimer's Society

A great deal of research is currently being carried out into the causes of dementia, diagnosis and treatments. The progress that is being made is only possible because people with dementia and their carers are willing to participate in research.

Range of research

There are many different ways in which people with dementia can take part in research. They may, for example, be asked to give a sample of their blood for use in genetic research or may be asked to take part in a drug trial.

While it is important that research is carried out, it is also important that the rights of the person with dementia are respected and their dignity maintained.

Types of research

- Therapeutic research refers to research that may be of benefit to the person with dementia, either during the project itself or once it has been concluded.
- Non-therapeutic research will not directly benefit those who are participating, but will add to the general body of knowledge about dementia. The findings may benefit people with dementia in the future.

If the research is non-therapeutic this must be made clear to the person with dementia before they decide whether or not to take part.

Consent

Consent must be obtained from the person with dementia before any research is carried out, even if it is simply a

question of an extra blood sample. The carer's agreement is not sufficient.

Consent must be adequately informed and voluntary. The person with dementia must be aware of the purpose of the research and what is involved.

No pressure should be exerted on the person with dementia to take part in research if they are unwilling to do so, even if the carer is in favour.

The person with dementia should be given plenty of time to consider whether to participate. They may first wish to consult their family or GP. It should be made clear that even if they do agree to participate they are free to change their mind and withdraw at any point.

The person with dementia should also be reassured that any support or services they receive will not be affected by whether or not they agree to take part in research.

The person with dementia should, in most cases, be given an information sheet giving details of the research and the name, address and telephone number of the researcher and their supervisor. If they do agree to take part in the research they will usually be asked to sign a consent form.

Unable to consent?

Occasionally a person with dementia will be included in a therapeutic research project even though they are not able to give their informed consent. This can only happen if the doctor concerned believes that the research will be of direct benefit to the person with dementia.

There are a few rare occasions when the person with dementia will be included in non-therapeutic research, despite not being able to give their informed consent. This can only happen if:

• It can be shown that important information that may benefit people with dementia in the future cannot be gained in any other way and

• There is almost no risk for the person concerned.

Although the actual decision to include someone with dementia in research without obtaining their consent can only be made by the doctor, relatives should, of course, be consulted.

Research ethics committees

All research undertaken by doctors and other health professionals which involves human subjects must be approved by a research ethics committee.

Research ethics committees have been set up to ensure that:

• The research undertaken is morally justifiable

• The highest standards of practice are maintained

• The likely benefits of any research outweigh any possible risks, and

• Participants' rights are properly safeguarded.

Although not all kinds of research involving people with dementia will go through a research ethics committee, all researchers should make every effort to preserve high standards.

Randomised controlled trials

If someone with dementia is invited to participate in research on a new drug, you may hear the phrase 'randomised controlled trial' mentioned.

A randomised control trial is a procedure in which a group of people receiving a new treatment is compared with a 'control group' of similar people who may be receiving a different treatment, a placebo treatment (that is a dummy treatment or sugar pill) or no treatment at all.

The effects of the new treatment would be very difficult to measure without such comparisons. Participants are randomly allocated to the treatment or control group by means of a mathematical formula or a computerised system to safeguard against any bias.

You may also hear the terms 'blind' and 'double blind' used to describe a trial.

• 'Blind' means that the person participating is not aware of whether they are receiving the new treatment or are one of the control group.

• 'Double blind' means that those carrying out the research do not know which participants are receiving the treatment and which are controls. Because of this their observations are less likely to be biased.

People with dementia should be told that if they agree to participate in randomised trials they may be given the new treatment, or an existing treatment, or a placebo.

It should be made clear that if someone with dementia receives a drug during a trial which appears to be of benefit, this does not mean that they can automatically continue with the drug once the trial is over.

Checklist of questions

Before taking part in any research, the person with dementia and their carer should consider the following points:

General

• What is the purpose of the research?

• What does the research involve for the person with dementia and will they benefit from participating?

• Will the carer be involved and if so how?

• Where will the research take place, how many sessions will there be and over what period of time?

• How will confidentiality be maintained?

• Who will have access to questionnaires and will this information be destroyed once the research is complete?

• If transport is needed, will this be arranged and if there are expenses will these be met?

• Are there plans to tell people about the results of the research and if so how and when?

Health-related research

In addition you may need to ask:

• Has the research been approved by a research ethics committee?

• Is the research likely to cause any discomfort or distress?

• If the research involves treatment what are the risks and likely side-effects?

• If the research involves treatment which appears to benefit the person with dementia can they continue with the treatment once the research is completed?

Complaints

If you have any worries or complaints about the research first take it up with the person in charge. If you are still not satisfied seek advice from the Alzheimer's Society or your local advice agency.

For further information call the Alzheimer's Helpline 0845 300 0336

Alzheimer's Society, Gordon House, 10 Greencoat Place, London SW1P 1PH. Telephone 020 7306 0606. Fax 020 7306 0808. Email info@alzheimers.org.uk. Website www.alzheimers.org.uk. Registered Charity No. 296645. Company Limited by Guarantee Registered in England No. 2115499

62

Knowledge to care: research and development in hospice and specialist palliative care – executive summary

National Council for Hospice and Specialist Palliative Care Services

1 This report in Council's series of Occasional Papers aims to promote high quality research in hospice and specialist palliative care, and to encourage all those working in this field to improve the quality of care through the application of research findings.

2 Involvement in research is one of the elements defining a specialist palliative care service and the implementation of evidence-based practice is a key aspect of service quality. All professions should develop evidence-based practice as an important tool in the continuous improvement of care.

3 Research is defined as the systematic pursuit of knowledge through observation, experiment and analysis. Research in health care can involve any discipline and includes:

- clinical research
- health services research
- sociological and health psychology research
- epidemiological research
- economic evaluation

4 The principles of medical ethics should be considered in all research situations. This involves balancing the fundamental principles of autonomy, beneficence (doing good), non-maleficence (doing no harm) and justice. Research design must be approached with ethical principles in mind whether or not any clinical intervention is involved, and participation should be on the basis of free and informed consent. It is essential for each research proposal involving patients or their carers to be approved by a research ethics committee.

5 Any research project should begin with specific "research questions" to be answered, and build on

previous knowledge in the field which should (if necessary) be collected together through a careful literature search. The appropriate research methods have to be chosen in the light of these research questions. Expert advice on methods, especially the advice of a statistician for quantitative studies, should be obtained at the earliest possible stage in the project.

6 There are particular risks and difficulties to be aware of in palliative care research, around:

- the use of quality of life, symptom or functional ability questionnaires
- adequate sample size, recruitment and attrition
- the attribution of outcomes (cause and effect)
- access to patients, and the use of substitutes or "proxies"

7 Each hospice/specialist palliative care service should appoint, either on its own or jointly with other services in the district:

- a senior clinician, or non-clinical academic, to have overall responsibility for research and development
- a senior clinician, who may be the same person as above, to oversee the use of evidence-based guidelines
- a Research Committee to formulate and prioritise an overall research strategy and ensure the quality of project

8 There are strong arguments for research in hospice and specialist palliative care to be undertaken on a multi-centre basis, and every specialist palliative care service should have some involvement in a local or regional research network, which may include links to an academic department of palliative care.

9 There should be formal arrangements for the supervision of staff undertaking research, informal opportunities for support, and access to appropriate educational facilities.

Those working towards a higher degree or other recognised qualification will usually need a supervisor who holds an appointment in an academic institution.

Occasional Paper 16. Glickman, M., October 1999

Reproduced by permission of the National Council for Hospice and Specialist Palliative Care Services

The full report can be found on
http://www.hospice-spc-council.org.uk

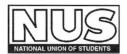

63

NUS guidelines for student participation in medical experiments and guidance for students considering participation in medical drug trials

National Union of Students

NUS produced these Guidelines in consultation with the Independent Clinical Research Contractors and the Association of the British Pharmaceutical Industry following the deaths of two students in the 1980s.

1 Student participation must be on a truly voluntary basis free from academic or financial pressure.

2 To ensure the above, no student should undertake experiments for ANY academic or researcher who tutors or lectures that student or who is involved in their academic assessment.

3 To ensure the above, payments for participation in experiment should be standardised, in both NHS and private research at rates of payments which compensate the student for expenses and inconvenience. There should be no financial incentive to participate.

4 A national computerised register of those participating in all experiments should be kept which records incidents

of side effect or ill health but which can also be used to identify individuals submitting themselves to a large number of experiments.

5 College authorities must monitor their own students' participation and tackle the unhealthy concentration of experiment participation among students involved in medical faculties and the associated natural sciences.

6 At any time a student should be able to free themselves from a previously agreed series of experiments.

7 Students should not sign documents which indemnify researchers against legal action. The NHS and private research companies should make their own insurance arrangements.

8 The scientific and medical authorities should indicate clearly the degree of risk involved. Obvious differences can be highlighted between the testing of totally new drugs and those which are already on the market but simply up for certification in the UK.

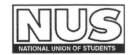

Guidance for students considering participation in medical drug trials

A drug is any substance administered to human being for experimental purposes. If you are considering participation in a drug trial please reject any action which is in contravention of these basic requirements.

1 For all students taking part the study must involve no more than minimal risk.
2 No financial inducement or coercion should colour your judgement and payment must never be offered for risk.
3 There must be close qualified medical supervision for the whole period of the trial and not just when the drugs are administered.
4 Full resuscitation equipment and facilities must be on hand, with trained staff to use them.
5 Confidentiality must be maintained throughout and beyond the trial.
6 The organisation should hold full insurance and compensate without regard to negligence.
7 You must authorise, and they must request, your permission to access your past medical history from your general practitioner. Full records must be maintained by the organisation and by your GP.

8 Only sign a consent form that you have read in full, and that gives you the right of withdrawal from the study at any time without having to give a reason.
9 You should be healthy at the time of the trial and undergo a full medical examination.
10 Do not withhold any information regarding any food you may have eaten or drugs you may have taken (this includes common non-prescription medicines, prescription medicines and alcohol).
11 You should report immediately any unusual sensations you may experience during the trial, and subsequently to your GP.
12 Leave at least 12 weeks between any trials you participate in, and inform the company of any previous trials.
13 Before participating, ask the organisation for proof of membership of the Association of Independent Clinical Research Contractors.
14 Always remember that whether the drug is 'tried and tested' or new on the market, you may individually suffer adverse reaction.

If you are ever approached by, or hear of any company carrying out drug trials which do not conform to the above standards you should refuse to participate and immediately inform your student union welfare officer or the National Union of Students.

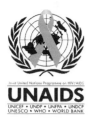

64

Ethical considerations in HIV preventive vaccine research
UNAIDS guidance document May 2000

Joint United Nations Programme on HIV/AIDS (UNAIDS)

UNAIDS/00.07E (English original) May 2000

UNAIDS, 20 avenue Appia, 1211 Geneva 27, Switzerland
Tel. (+41 22) 791 46 51 – Fax (+41 22) 791 41 87
E-mail: unaids@unaids.org – Internet:
http://www.unaids.org

Contents

Introduction

As we enter the third decade of the AIDS pandemic, there still remains no effective HIV preventive vaccine. As the numbers of those infected by HIV and dying from AIDS increase dramatically, the need for such a vaccine becomes ever more urgent. Several HIV candidate vaccines are at various stages of development. However, the successful development of effective HIV preventive vaccines is likely to require that many different candidate vaccines be studied simultaneously in different populations around the world. This in turn will require a large international cooperative effort drawing on partners from various health sectors, intergovernmental organizations, government, research institutions, industry, and affected populations. It will also require that these partners be able and willing to address the difficult ethical concerns that arise during the development of HIV vaccines.

In an effort to elucidate these ethical concerns, and to create forums where they could be discussed in full by those presently involved in, or considering, HIV vaccine development activities, the UNAIDS Secretariat convened meetings in Geneva (twice), Brazil, Thailand, Uganda and

Washington during 1997–1999. These meetings included lawyers, activists, social scientists, ethicists, vaccine scientists, epidemiologists, representatives of NGOs, people living with HIV/AIDS, and people working in health policy. In the regional meetings, efforts were made to include people from a number of countries from that particular region. The entire process involved people from a total of 33 countries.[1] The goals were to: (1) identify and discuss ethical elements specific to development of HIV preventive vaccines; (2) reach consensus when possible, and elucidate different positions, when not; (3) progress in ability to address these matters during pending or proposed HIV vaccine research.

In the present document, UNAIDS seeks to offer guidance emanating from this process. This document does not purport to capture the extensive discussion, debate, consensus, and disagreement which occurred at these meetings. Rather it highlights, from UNAIDS' perspective, some of the critical elements that must be considered in HIV vaccine development activities. Where these are adequately addressed, in UNAIDS' view, by other existing texts, there is no attempt to duplicate or replace these texts, which should be consulted extensively throughout HIV vaccine development activities. Such texts include: the Nuremberg Code (1947); the Declaration of Helsinki, first adopted by the World Medical Association in 1964 and subsequently amended in 1975, 1983, 1989 and 1996; the Belmont Report – Ethical Principles and Guidelines for the Protection of Human Subjects of Research, issued in 1979 by the US National Commission for the Protection of Human Subjects of Biomedical and Behavioral Research; the International Ethical Guidelines for Biomedical Research Involving Human Subjects, issued by the Council for International Organizations of Medical Sciences (CIOMS) in 1993 (and developed in close cooperation with WHO); the World Health Organization's Good Clinical Practice (WHO GCP) Guideline (1995); and the International Conference on Harmonisation's Good Clinical Practice (ICH GCP) Guideline (1996).

It is hoped that this document will be of use to potential research participants, investigators, community members, government representatives, pharmaceutical companies, and ethical and scientific review committees involved in HIV preventive vaccine development. It suggests standards,

as well as processes for arriving at standards, and can be used as a frame of reference from which to conduct further discussion at the international, national, and local levels.

Context

The HIV/AIDS pandemic is characterized by unique biological, social and geographical factors that, among other things, affect the balance of risks and benefits for individuals and communities who participate in HIV vaccine development activities. These factors may require that additional efforts are made to address the needs of participating individuals and communities, including their urgent need for a HIV vaccine, their need to have their rights protected and their welfare promoted in the context of HIV vaccine development activities, and their need to be able to be full and equal participants. These factors include the following:

• The global burden of disease and death related to HIV is increasing at a rate unmatched by any other pathogen. For many countries, it is already the leading cause of death. Currently available treatments are inadequate because they do not lead to cure, but at best slow the progression of disease. The most effective treatment for slowing HIV-related disease progression, antiretroviral medication, is complicated to administer, requires close medical monitoring, is extremely costly, and can cause significant adverse effects. Because of this, antiretroviral medication is not readily available to the vast majority of people affected by HIV/AIDS. These are people living in developing countries and in marginalized communities in developed countries. There is therefore an ethical imperative to seek, as urgently as possible, a globally effective and accessible vaccine, to complement other prevention strategies. Furthermore, this ethical imperative demands that HIV preventive vaccines be developed to address the situation of those people and populations most vulnerable to infection.

• Genetically distinct subtypes of HIV have been described, and different HIV subtypes are predominant in different regions and countries. Yet the relevance of these subtypes to potential vaccine-induced protection is not clearly understood. Thus, it is not known whether a vaccine targeted at one subtype will protect against infection from another subtype; and it is likely that a vaccine directed at a particular subtype will need to be tested in a population in which that subtype is prevalent. Therefore, developing a vaccine that is effective in the populations with the greatest incidence of HIV is likely to require experimental vaccines be tested in those populations, even though these populations may for a variety of reasons be relatively vulnerable

[1] For a full description of the process and participants, see "Final Report, UNAIDS-Sponsored Regional Workshops to discuss Ethical Issues in Preventive HIV Vaccine Trials", available from UNAIDS. See also Guenter, Esparza, and Macklin: Ethical considerations in international HIV vaccine trials: summary of a consultative process conducted by the Joint United Nations Programme on HIV/AIDS (UNAIDS). *Journal of Medical Ethics* (February 2000), vol. 26, No. 1: 37–43.

to exploitation and harm in the context of HIV vaccine development. Additional efforts may need to be made to overcome this vulnerability.

• Some candidate vaccines may be conceived and manufactured in laboratories of one country (sponsor country or countries), usually in the developed world, and tested in human populations in another country (host country or countries), often in the developing world.

[The term 'sponsor' has usually referred to the individual or institution who either owns the candidate vaccine or provides the material resources necessary to carry out the vaccine development programme. Traditionally, the sponsor has been thought of as a single corporate entity, such as a pharmaceutical company. In modern vaccine development programmes there are commonly multiple sponsors including one or more corporations, one or more national governments and one or more international agencies.] The potential imbalance of such a situation demands particular attention to factors that will address the differing perspectives, interests and capacities of sponsors and hosts with the goal of encouraging the urgent development of effective vaccines, in ethically acceptable manners, and their early distribution to populations most in need. In this regard, potential host countries and communities should be encouraged and given the capacity to make decisions for themselves regarding their participation in HIV vaccine development, based on their own health and human development priorities, in a context of equal collaboration with sponsors.

• HIV/AIDS is a condition that is both highly feared and stigmatized. This is in large part because it is associated with blood, death, sex, and activities which are often not legally sanctioned, such as commercial sex, men having sex with men, and substance abuse. These are issues which are difficult to address openly – at a societal and individual level. As a result, people affected by HIV/AIDS can experience stigma, discrimination, and even violence; and governments and communities continue to deny the existence and prevalence of HIV/AIDS. Furthermore, vulnerability to HIV infection and to the impact of AIDS is greater where people are marginalized due to their social, economic and legal status. These factors increase the risk of social and psychological harm for people participating in HIV vaccine research. Additional efforts must be made to address these increased risks, and to ensure that the risks participants take are justified by the benefits they receive by virtue of their participation in the research. A key means by which to protect participants and the communities from which they come is to ensure that the community in which the research is carried out is meaningfully involved in the design, implementation,

and distribution of results of vaccine research, including the involvement of representatives from marginalized communities from which participants are drawn, where possible and appropriate.

Suggested guidance

Given the global nature of the epidemic, the devastation being wreaked in some countries by it, the fact that vaccine(s) may be the best longterm solution by which to control the epidemic, especially in developing countries, and the potentially universal benefits of effective HIV vaccines, there is an ethical imperative for global support to the effort to develop these vaccines. This effort will require intense international collaboration and coordination over time, including among countries with scientific expertise and resources, and among countries where candidate vaccines could be tested but whose infrastructure, resource base, and scientific and ethical capacities could be insufficient at present. Though HIV vaccines should benefit

---

Guidance Point I: HIV vaccines development

Given the severity of the HIV/AIDS pandemic in human, public health, social, and economic terms, sufficient capacity and incentives should be developed to foster the early and ethical development of effective vaccines, both from the point of view of countries where HIV vaccine trials may be held, and from the point of view of sponsors of HIV vaccine trials. Donor countries and relevant international organizations should join with these stakeholders to promote such vaccine development.

---

all those in need, it is imperative that they benefit the populations at greatest risk of infection. Thus, HIV vaccine development should ensure that the vaccines are appropriate for use among such populations, among which it will be necessary to conduct trials; and, when developed, they should be made available and affordable to such populations.

Because HIV vaccine development activities take time, are complex, and require infrastructure, resources and international collaboration,

• potential sponsor countries and host countries should immediately include HIV vaccine development in their regional and national AIDS prevention and control plans.

• potential host countries should assess how they can and should participate in HIV vaccine development activities either nationally or on a regional basis, including identifying resources, establishing partnerships, conducting national information campaigns, strengthening their scientific and ethical sectors, and including a vaccine research component to complement other prevention interventions.

- potential donors and international agencies should make early and sustained commitments to allocate sufficient funds to make a vaccine a reality, including funds to strengthen ethical and scientific capacity in countries where multiple trials will have to be conducted and to purchase and distribute future vaccines.
- potential sponsors should establish partnerships with potential host countries, and begin discussions regarding community consultations, strengthening necessary scientific and ethical components, and eventual plans for equitable distribution of the benefits of research.

Although making a safe and effective vaccine reasonably available to the population where it was tested is a basic ethical requirement, some have argued that it could be a disincentive for industry to conduct studies in countries with large populations, or that it could constitute an undue inducement for a resource-poor country or community to "cooperate". Given the severity of the epidemic, it is imperative that sufficient incentives exist, both through financial rewards in the marketplace and through public subsidies, to foster development of effective vaccines while also ensuring that vaccines are produced and distributed in a fashion that actually makes them available to the populations at greatest risk.

Guidance Point 2: Vaccine availability

Any HIV preventive vaccine demonstrated to be safe and effective, as well as other knowledge and benefits resulting from HIV vaccine research, should be made available as soon as possible to all participants in the trials in which it was tested, as well as to other populations at high risk of HIV infection. Plans should be developed at the initial stages of HIV vaccine development to ensure such availability.

As health and research communities build HIV preventive vaccine research programmes, attention needs to be given immediately to how a successful vaccine, and other benefits resulting from the research, will be made readily and affordably available to the communities and countries where such a vaccine is tested, as well as to other communities and countries at high risk for HIV infection. This

process of discussion and negotiation should start as soon as possible and should be carried on through the course of the research.

At a minimum, the parties directly concerned should begin this discussion before the trials commence. This discussion should include representatives from relevant stakeholders in the host country, such as representatives from the executive branch, health ministry, local health authorities, and relevant scientific and ethical groups. It should also include representatives from the communities from which participants are drawn, people living with HIV/AIDS, and NGOs representing affected communities. The discussions should include decisions regarding payments, royalties, subsidies, technology and intellectual property, as well as distribution costs, channels and modalities, including vaccination strategies, target populations, and number of doses.

Furthermore, the discussion concerning availability and distribution of an effective HIV vaccine should engage international organizations, donor governments and bilateral agencies, representatives from wider affected communities, international and regional NGOs and the private sector. These should not only consider financial assistance regarding making vaccines available, but should also help to build the capacity of host governments and communities to negotiate for and implement distribution plans.

Potential host countries and communities have the right, and the responsibility, to take decisions regarding the nature of their participation in HIV vaccine research. Yet disparities in economic wealth, scientific experience, and technical capacity among countries and communities can lead to undue influence over and possible exploitation of host countries and communities. The development of an HIV vaccine will require international cooperative research, which should transcend, in an ethical manner, such disparities. Real or perceived disparities should be resolved in a way that ensures equality in decision-making and action. The desired relationship is one of collaboration among equals. Factors that may increase vulnerability to exploitation of host countries and communities may include, but are not limited to, the following:

- level of the proposed community's economic capacity, such as is reflected in the Human Development Index of the UNDP
- community/cultural experience with, and/or understanding of, scientific research
- local political awareness of the importance and process of vaccine research
- local infrastructure, personnel, and technical capacity for providing HIV health care and treatment options

---

Guidance Point 3: Capacity building

Strategies should be implemented to build capacity in host countries and communities so that they can practise meaningful self-determination in vaccine development, can ensure the scientific and ethical conduct of vaccine development, and can function as equal partners with sponsors and others in a collaborative process.

- ability of individuals in the community to provide informed consent, including the effect of class, gender, and other social factors on the potential for freely given consent
- level of experience and capacity for conducting ethical and scientific review, and
- local infrastructure, personnel, and technical capacity for conducting the proposed research.

Strategies to overcome these disparities could involve:

- scientific exchange, and knowledge and skills transfer between sponsor countries and institutions, and host countries and communities
- capacity-building programmes in the science and ethics of vaccine development by relevant scientific institutions and international organizations
- support to development of national and local ethical review capacity (see *Guidance Point 6*)
- support to affected communities and communities from which participants are drawn regarding information, education, and capacity and consensus-building on vaccine development, and
- early involvement of affected communities in the design and implementation of vaccine development plans and protocols (see *Guidance Point 5*).

In order to be ethical, clinical trials of vaccines should be based on scientifically valid research protocols, and the scientific questions posed should be rigorously formulated in a research protocol that is capable of providing reliable responses. Valid scientific questions relevant to HIV vaccine development are those that seek:

- to gain scientific information on the safety, immunogenicity (ability to induce immune responses against HIV) and efficacy (degree of protection) of candidate vaccines
- to determine immunological correlates or surrogates in order to identify the protective mechanisms and how they can be elicited
- to compare different candidate vaccines; and
- to test whether vaccines effective in one population are effective in other populations.

Guidance Point 4: Research protocols and study populations

In order to conduct HIV vaccine research in an ethically acceptable manner, the research protocol should be scientifically appropriate, and the desired outcome of the proposed research should potentially benefit the population from which research participants are drawn.

Furthermore, the selection of the research population should be based on the fact that its characteristics are relevant to the scientific issues raised; and the results of the research will potentially benefit the selected population. In this sense, the research protocol should:

- justify the selection of the research population from a scientific point of view
- outline how the risks undertaken by the participants of that population are balanced by the potential benefits to that population
- address particular needs of the proposed research population
- demonstrate how the candidate vaccine being tested is expected to be beneficial to the population in which testing occurs, and
- establish safeguards for the protection of research participants from potential harm arising from the research.

These general principles will be further elaborated below.

Involvement of community representatives should not be seen as a single encounter, nor as one-directional. The orientation of community involvement should be one of partnership – towards mutual education and consensus-building regarding all aspects of the vaccine development programme. There should be established a continuing forum for communication and problem-solving on all aspects of the vaccine development programme from phase I through phase III and beyond, to the distribution of a safe, effective, licensed vaccine. All participating parties should define the nature of this ongoing relationship. It

---

Guidance Point 5: Community participation

To ensure the ethical and scientific quality of proposed research, its relevance to the affected community, and its acceptance by the affected community, community representatives should be involved in an early and sustained manner in the design, development, implementation, and distribution of results of HIV vaccine research.

should include appropriate representation of the community on committees charged with the review, approval, and monitoring of the HIV vaccine research. Like investigators and sponsors, communities should assume appropriate responsibility for assuring the successful completion of the trial and of the programme.

Appropriate community representatives should be determined through a process of broad consultation. Members of the community who may contribute to a vaccine development process include representatives of the research population eligible to serve as research participants, other members of the community who would be among the intended beneficiaries of the developed vaccine, relevant nongovernmental organizations, persons living with HIV/AIDS, community leaders, public health officials, and those who provide health care and other services to people living with and affected by HIV.

Participation of the community in the planning and implementation of a vaccine development strategy can provide the following benefits:

- information regarding the health beliefs and understanding of the study population
- input into the design of the protocol
- input into an appropriate informed consent process
- insight into the design of risk reduction interventions
- effective methods for disseminating information about the trial and its outcomes
- information to the community-at-large on the proposed research
- trust between the community and researchers
- equity in choice of participants
- equity in decisions regarding level of standard of care and treatment and its duration, and
- equity in plans for applying results and vaccine distribution.

Guidance Point 6: Scientific and ethical review

HIV preventive vaccine trials should only be carried out in countries and communities that have the capacity to conduct appropriate independent and competent scientific and ethical review.

Proposed HIV vaccine research protocols should be reviewed by scientific and ethical review committees that are located in, and include membership from, the country and community where the research is proposed to take place. This process ensures that the proposed research is analysed from the scientific and ethical viewpoints by individuals who are familiar with the conditions prevailing in the potential research population.

Some countries do not currently have the capacity to conduct independent, competent and meaningful scientific and ethical review. If the country's capacity for scientific and ethical review is inadequate, the sponsor should be responsible for ensuring that adequate structures are developed in the host country for scientific and ethical review prior to the start of the research. Care should be taken to minimize the potential for conflicts of interest, while providing assistance in capacity-building for scientific and ethical review. Capacity-building for scientific and ethical review may also be developed in collaboration with international agencies, organizations within the host country, and other relevant parties.

Guidance Point 7: Vulnerable populations

Where relevant, the research protocol should describe the social contexts of a proposed research population (country or community) that create conditions for possible exploitation or increased vulnerability among potential research participants, as well as the steps that will be taken to overcome these and protect the dignity, safety, and welfare of the participants.

Some countries or communities, often described as "developing", have been perceived as inappropriate participants for some phases of clinical research, due to a real or perceived increased level of vulnerability to exploitation or harm. The usefulness of the " developing/developed" terminology for assessing risk of harm and exploitation, however, is limited. It refers primarily to economic considerations, which are not the only relevant factors in HIV vaccine research. It also establishes two fixed categories, whereas in reality, countries and communities are distributed along a spectrum, characterized by a variety of different factors that affect risk. It is more useful to identify the *particular* aspects of a social context that create conditions for exploitation or increased vulnerability for the pool of participants that has been selected. These aspects should be described in the protocol, as should the measures that will be taken to overcome them. In some potential research populations (countries or communities), conditions affecting potential vulnerability or exploitation may be so severe that ensuring adequate safeguards is not possible. In such populations, HIV preventive vaccine research should not be conducted.

Some factors to be considered are those listed in ***Guidance Point 3*** which influence the disparity in real or perceived power as between sponsors and host countries, as well as the factors listed below that can also increase the nature and level of risk of harm to participants:

- governmental, institutional or social stigmatization or discrimination on the basis of HIV status
- inadequate ability to protect HIV-related human rights, and to prevent HIV-related discrimination and stigma, including those arising from participation in an HIV vaccine trial
- social and legal marginalization of groups from which participants might be drawn, e.g. women, injecting drug users, men having sex with men, sex workers
- limited availability, accessibility and sustainability of health care and treatment options
- limited ability of individuals or groups in the community to understand the research process
- limited ability of individuals to understand the informed consent process
- limited ability of individuals to be able to give freely their informed consent in the light of prevailing class, gender, and other social and legal factors, and
- lack of meaningful national/local scientific and ethical review.

Initial stages in a vaccine development programme entail research in laboratories and among animals. The transition from this preclinical phase to a phase I clinical trial, in which testing involves the administration of the candidate vaccine to human subjects to assess safety and immunogenicity, is a time when risks may not be yet well defined. Furthermore, specific infrastructures are often required in order to ensure the safety and care of the research participants at these stages. For these reasons, the first administration of a candidate HIV vaccine in humans should generally be conducted in less vulnerable research populations, usually in the country of the sponsor.

There may be situations, however, where developing countries choose to conduct phases I/II and/or III (large-scale trials to assess efficacy) among their populations that are relatively vulnerable to risk and exploitation. For instance, this could occur where an experimental HIV vaccine is directed primarily towards a viral strain that does not exist in the sponsor country but does exist in the potential host country. Conducting phase I/II trials in the country where the strain exists may be the only way to determine whether safety and immunogenicity are acceptable in that particular population, prior to conducting a phase III trial. A country may also decide that, due to the high level of HIV risk to its population and the gravity of HIV/AIDS already in country, it is willing to test a vaccine concept that is not being tested in another country. Such a decision may result in obvious benefits to the country in question if an effective vaccine is found. It may also provide an important capacity-building experience, if phase I or phase II trials are

---

Guidance Point 8: Clinical trial phases

As phases I, II, and III in the clinical development of a preventive vaccine all have their own particular scientific requirements and specific ethical challenges, the choice of study populations for each trial phase should be justified in advance in scientific and ethical terms in all cases, regardless of where the study population is found. Generally, early clinical phases of HIV vaccine research should be conducted in communities that are less vulnerable to harm or exploitation, usually within the sponsor country. However, countries may choose, for valid scientific and public health reasons, to conduct any phase within their populations, if they are able to ensure sufficient scientific infrastructure and sufficient ethical safeguards.

---

conducted in a host country prior to a phase III trial being initiated there.

Establishing a vaccine development programme that entails the conduct of some, most, or all of its clinical trial components in a country or community that is relatively vulnerable to harm or exploitation is ethically justified if:

- the vaccine is anticipated to be effective against a strain of HIV that is an important public health problem in the country
- the country and the community either have, or with assistance can develop or be provided with, adequate scientific and ethical capability and administrative and health infrastructure for the successful conduct of the proposed research
- community members, policy makers, ethicists and investigators in the country have determined that their residents will be adequately protected from harm or exploitation, and that the vaccine development programme is necessary for and responsive to the health needs and priorities in their country; and
- all other conditions for ethical justification as set forth in this document are satisfied.

In cases in which it is decided to carry out phase I or phase II trials first in a country other than the sponsor country, due consideration should be given to conducting them simultaneously in the country of the sponsor, where this is practical and ethical. Also, when the host country or community is not familiar with conducting biomedical research in human subjects, phase I/II trials that have been performed in the country of the sponsor should ordinarily be repeated in the community in which the phase III trials are to be conducted.

Participation in HIV preventive vaccine research may involve physiological, psychological and social risks. With regard to the physiological risks, the purpose of an HIV preventive vaccine is to induce an immunological response in the human body to counteract the HIV virus if it enters the body, or to prevent it from entering at all. Vaccines currently being considered for human trials are not capable of causing infection, i.e. they do not include replicating HIV.[2] Several candidate HIV vaccines have been tested in laboratories, and some have been tested in human subjects. Not all of these candidate vaccines are the same, and not all candidate vaccines carry the same risks for harm. Thus far, however, significant adverse biological effects have not been observed. Nevertheless, some of the more likely physiological risks of participating in vaccine research include the following:

Guidance Point 9: Potential harms

The nature, magnitude, and probability of all potential harms resulting from participation in an HIV preventive vaccine trial should be specified in the research protocol as fully as can be reasonably done, as well as the modalities by which to address these, including provision for the highest level of care to participants who experience adverse reactions to the vaccine, compensation for injury related to the research, and referral to psychosocial and legal support, as necessary.

- A person who has received a candidate vaccine and is then exposed to HIV may have a greater risk of developing established infection, or of progressing more rapidly once infected, than if the vaccine had not been administered. This potential harm has not been observed in trials thus far.
- An HIV vaccine may require that several injections be given over months or years, resulting in pain, occasional skin reactions, and possibly other biological adverse events, such as fever and malaise.
- Injuries may be sustained due to research-related activities during the course of the trial.

The potential for adverse reactions to the candidate vaccine, as well as possible injuries related to HIV vaccine

research, should be described, as far as possible, in the research protocol and fully explained in the informed consent process. Both the protocol and the consent process should also describe the nature of medical treatment to be provided for injuries, as well as compensation for harm incurred due to research-related activities, including the process by which it is decided whether an injury will be compensated. HIV infection acquired during participation in an HIV preventive vaccine trial should not be considered an injury subject to compensation unless it is directly attributable to the vaccine itself, or to direct contamination through research-related activities. In addition to compensation for biological/medical injuries, appropriate consideration should be given to compensation for social or economic harms, e.g. job loss as a result of testing positive following vaccine administration.

With regard to psychosocial risks, participation in a complicated, lengthy trial involving intensely intimate matters, involving repeated HIV testing, and involving exposure to culturally different scientific and medical concepts may cause anxiety, stress, depression, as well as stress between partners in a relationship. Participation, if it becomes publicly known, may also cause stigma and discrimination against the participant if s/he is perceived to be HIV-infected. Finally, some people may develop a positive HIV test after receiving a candidate HIV vaccine, even though they are not truly infected with HIV, i.e. a 'false positive' HIV test. This may result in the same negative social consequences that exist for those actually HIV-infected. The protocol should describe these, as well as ensure that the research occurs in communities where confidentiality can be maintained and where participants will have access to, and can be referred to, ongoing psychosocial services, including counselling, social support groups, and legal support. Consideration should also be given to setting up an ombudsperson who can intervene with outside parties, if necessary and requested, on behalf of participants, as well as to providing documentation to participants that they can use to show that their "false positive" is due to their participation in research.[3]

Some of the activities related to the conduct of HIV vaccine trials should benefit those who participate. At a minimum, participants should:
- have regular and supportive contact with health care workers and counsellors throughout the course of the trial
- receive comprehensive information regarding HIV transmission and how it can be prevented

---

[2] Some of the most effective viral vaccines are based on live-attenuated viruses and some investigators have proposed a similar approach for HIV vaccines. Any decision regarding testing a live-attenuated HIV vaccine in humans would have to be carefully assessed in view of the significant safety concerns associated with such a vaccine approach.

[3] When a vaccine is tested, laboratory techniques should be available to differentiate HIV-positivity due to vaccination from that due to actual HIV infection.

- receive access to HIV prevention methods, including male and female condoms, and clean injecting equipment, where legal
- have access to a pre-agreed care and treatment package for HIV/AIDS if they become HIV-infected while enrolled in the trial (see **Guidance Point 16**)
- receive compensation for time, travel and inconvenience for participation in the trials, and
- if the vaccine is effective, develop protective immunity to HIV.

A vaccine with proven efficacy in preventing infection or disease from HIV does not currently exist. Therefore, the use of a placebo control arm is ethically acceptable in appropriately designed protocols.

Participants in the control arm of a future phase III HIV preventive vaccine trial should receive an HIV vaccine known to be safe and effective when such is available, unless there are compelling scientific reasons which justify the use of a placebo. Compelling scientific reasons to use a placebo rather than a known effective HIV vaccine in the research population include the following:
- The effective HIV vaccine is not believed to be effective against the virus that is prevalent in the research population.
- There are convincing reasons to believe that the biological conditions that prevailed during the initial trial demonstrating efficacy were so different from the conditions in the proposed research population that the results of the initial trial cannot be directly applied to the research population under consideration.

In an effort to address the concern of lack of benefit to those randomly placed in a placebo control arm, apart from the benefits described in **Guidance Point 10**, it is recommended that the provision to these persons of another vaccine, such as for hepatitis B or tetanus, be considered. The appropriateness of such a step should be analysed in terms of the scientific requirements of the trial, the health needs of the population of participants, and the balance of benefits and risks to the active versus control arms of the trial.

A process of consultation between community representatives, researchers, sponsor(s) and regulatory bodies should be used to design an effective informed consent strategy and process. Issues such as illiteracy, language and cultural barriers, and diminished personal autonomy should be addressed in this consultative process. In some communities, special efforts may be required to achieve adequate understanding of 'cause and effect', 'contagion', 'placebo', 'double blind', and other concepts involved in the scientific design of the research.

HIV preventive vaccine trials require informed consent at a number of stages. The first stage consists of screening candidates for eligibility for participation in the trial, which will involve, among other things, an assessment of the individual's risk-taking behaviour and a test for HIV status. Informed consent should be obtained during this screening process after the candidate has received all material information regarding the screening procedures, as well as an outline of the vaccine trial in which he will be invited to enrol, if found eligible. Fully informed consent should also be given for the test for HIV status, which should also be accompanied by pre-and post-test counselling, and referral to clinical and social support services, if found positive.

The second stage at which informed consent is required occurs once a person is judged eligible for enrolment.

That individual should then be given full information concerning the nature and length of participation in the trial, including the risks and benefits posed by participation, so that s/he is able to give informed consent to participate.

Once enrolled, efforts should then be made throughout the trial to obtain assurance that the participation continues to be on a basis of free consent and understanding of what is happening. Informed consent, with pre- and post-test counselling, should also be given for any repeated tests for HIV status. Throughout all stages of the trial and consent process, there should be assurance by the investigator that the information is understood before consent is given.

In some communities, it is customary to require the authorization of a third party, such as a community elder, in order for investigators to enter the community to invite individual members to participate in research. Other situations which make individual informed consent difficult include those in which an individual requires approval of another person or group in order to make decisions, where there is coercion, and where there is a cultural tradition of sharing risks and responsibilities, e.g. in some cultures where men hold the prerogative in marital relationships, where there is parental control of women, and/or where there are strong influences by community and/or religion or hierarchy (see *Guidance Point 13*). Such authorization or influence must not be used as a substitute for individual informed consent. Nor should trials be conducted where truly individual and free consent cannot be obtained. Authorization by a third party in place of individual informed consent is permissible only in the case of some minors who have not attained the legal age of consent to participate in a trial. In cases where it is proposed that minors will be enrolled as research participants, specific and full justification for their enrolment must be given, and their own consent must be obtained in light of their evolving capacities (see *Guidance Point 18*).

In addition to the standard content of informed consent, prior to participation in an HIV vaccine trial, each prospective participant must be informed, using appropriate language and technique, of the following specific details:

- Prospective participants of phase II and III trials of HIV preventive vaccines should be informed that they have been chosen as prospective participants because they are at relatively high risk of HIV infection.
- Prospective participants for phase I, II and III trials should be informed that they will receive counselling and access to the means of risk reduction (in particular, male and female condoms, and clean injecting equipment, where legal) concerning how to reduce their risk of infection; and that in spite of these risk reduction efforts, some of the participants may become infected, particularly in the

case of phase III trials where large numbers of participants at high risk are participating.

- They should be informed that it is not known whether the experimental vaccine will prevent HIV infection or disease, and further, that some of the participants will receive a placebo instead of the candidate HIV vaccine, when such is the case.
- They should be informed of the specific risks for physical harm, as well as for psychological and social harm, and of the types of treatment and compensation that are available for harm, and of services to which they may be referred should harm occur.
- All prospective participants of phase I, II or III trials should be informed of the nature and duration of care and treatment that is available, and how it can be accessed, if they become infected with HIV during the course of the trial (see *Guidance Point 16*).

Guidance Point 13: Informed consent – special measures

Special measures should be taken to protect persons who are, or may be, limited in their ability to provide informed consent due to their social or legal status.

There are several categories of persons who are legally competent to consent to participate in a trial, and who have sufficient cognitive capacity to consent, but who may have limitations in their freedom to make independent choices. Those who plan, review, and conduct vaccine trials should be alert to the problems presented by the involvement of such persons, and either exclude such persons, if their vulnerability cannot be addressed, or take appropriate steps to ensure meaningful and independent ongoing informed consent, respect their rights, foster their well-being, and protect them from harm. The following are individuals or groups who should be given extra consideration with regard to their ability to provide informed consent in HIV preventive vaccine trials:

- Persons who are junior or subordinate members of hierarchical structures may be vulnerable to undue influence or coercion in that they may fear retaliation if they refuse cooperation with authorities. Such persons include members of the armed forces, students, government employees, prisoners, and refugees.
- Persons who engage in illegal or socially stigmatized activities are vulnerable to undue influence and threats presented by possible breaches of confidentiality and action by legal forces. Such persons include sex workers, intravenous drug users, and men who have sex with men.

- Persons who are impoverished or dependent on welfare programmes are vulnerable to being unduly influenced by offers of what others may consider modest material or health inducements.
- Women living in cultures where their autonomy as individuals is not sufficiently recognized are vulnerable to influence and coercion from male partners, family, or community members.

Steps that might be taken to ensure that ongoing free and informed consent is given by participants from these groups include:

- appointment of an independent ombudsperson and/or group to monitor these issues
- expansion of the responsibilities of the clinical trial monitor to include adherence to the informed consent and counselling process, or appointment of an independent counselling monitor
- training of the counsellors on these issues, and
- group counselling and/or interaction with local NGOs representing the groups from which such participants are drawn.

Reducing the risk of HIV infection throughout the trial among participants is an essential ethical component of HIV preventive vaccine trials. All trial participants should receive comprehensive counselling concerning methods of decreasing the risk of transmission of HIV. This should include the basic principles of safe sexual practice and safe use of injection equipment, as well as education concerning general health and treatment of sexually transmitted infections (STIs). Investigators should provide trial participants appropriate access to condoms, sterile injecting equipment (where legal) and treatment for other STIs. All trial participants should also be counselled prior to enrolling in a clinical trial regarding the potential benefits and risks of post-exposure prophylaxis with antiretroviral medication, and how it can be accessed in the community.

Guidance Point 14: Risk-reduction interventions

Appropriate risk-reduction counselling and access to prevention methods should be provided to all vaccine trial participants, with new methods being added as they are discovered and validated.

The technique and frequency of counselling should be agreed upon by the community-host government-investigator-sponsor partnership, and should be based upon reliable information about the prevailing social and behavioural characteristics of the study population. Consideration should be given to providing counselling

through an agency or organisation that is independent of the investigators in order to prevent any real or perceived conflict of interest. Local capacity should be developed to employ such means in a culturally suitable and sustainable fashion, guided by the best scientific data.

The provision of counselling to reduce risk should be monitored to ensure quality and to minimize the potential conflict of interest between the risk-reduction goals and the vaccine trial's scientific goals. As new methods of prevention are discovered and validated, these must be added to the preventive methods being offered to trial participants.

The value of informed consent depends primarily on the ongoing quality of the process by which it is conducted, and

---

Guidance Point 15: Monitoring informed consent and interventions

A plan for monitoring the initial and continuing adequacy of the informed consent process and risk-reduction interventions, including counselling and access to prevention methods, should be agreed upon before the trial commences.

---

not solely on the structure and content of the informed consent document. The informed consent process should be designed to empower participants to allow them to make appropriate decisions. Similarly, there are many ways in which risk reduction (counselling and access to means of prevention) can be conducted, with some methods being more effective than others in conveying the relevant information and in reducing risk behaviour.

A method for monitoring the adequacy of these processes should be designed and agreed upon by the community-host-government-investigator-sponsor partnership. Consideration should be given to the expansion of the responsibilities of the clinical trial monitor to include adherence to the informed consent and counselling process, and/or the appointment of an independent counselling monitor, as suggested in *Guidance Point 13*. The appropriateness of such plans should be determined by the scientific and ethical review committees that are responsible for providing prior and continuing review of the trial. This recommendation supplements the usual guidelines for the monitoring of vaccine trials for safety and compliance with scientific and ethical standards and regulatory requirements.

Sponsors need to ensure care and treatment for participants who become HIV-infected during the course of the trial. At present, there is no universal consensus regarding the level of care and treatment that should be provided. This was evidenced at the UNAIDS-sponsored regional workshops to discuss ethical issues in preventive HIV vaccine trials at which the following three different conclusions were reached. Care and treatment for those who become infected should be provided:

Guidance Point 16: Care and treatment

Care and treatment for HIV/AIDS and its associated complications should be provided to participants in HIV preventive vaccine trials, with the ideal being to provide the best proven therapy, and the minimum to provide the highest level of care attainable in the host country in light of the circumstances listed below. A comprehensive care package should be agreed upon through a host/community/ sponsor dialogue which reaches consensus prior to initiation of a trial, taking into consideration the following:
- level of care and treatment available in the sponsor country
- highest level of care available in the host country
- highest level of treatment available in the host country, including the availablity of antiretroviral therapy outside the research context in the host country
- availability of infrastructure to provide care and treatment in the context of research
- potential duration and sustainability of care and treatment for the trial participant.

- at the level of that offered in the sponsor country, and should include preventive risk behaviour counselling, general HIV care and treatment, post-exposure prophylaxis and antiretroviral therapy, according to the best scientific evidence for effectiveness available at the time of the trial; and should last at least for the duration for the trial, and longer, if so negotiated
- at a level decided upon by the host country, e.g. it might include immunological monitoring, physician visits, prevention and treatment of opportunistic infections, and palliative care, but not necessarily antiretroviral therapy; and should be made reasonably available for the lifetime of the participants
- at a level consistent with that available in the host country; there is no imperative to provide a level of care consistent with that in the sponsoring country, or with the highest available in the world.

Competing considerations that have led to disagreement about the standard of care and treatment include:
- the need to achieve equity in care and treatment for all participants in HIV vaccine trials globally; in particular, to achieve equity between potential participants from sponsor countries and host countries
- an ethical obligation of sponsors to provide care and treatment according to their resources
- concern that a high level of care and treatment will constitute undue incentives and inducements for countries and communities to participate
- concern that governments might abdicate on their responsibility to provide care and treatment if sponsors fill this role
- governments' desire to be able to attract research into their countries in order to address the critical need of their populations for an HIV preventive vaccine
- the right and responsibility of sovereign nations and communities to determine for themselves the balance of risks and benefits they are willing to accept.

In the light of these competing concerns, it is recommended that:
- A consensus on the standard/level of care and treatment, its duration, and who will bear the costs should be reached prior to a decision to host HIV vaccine development.
- This consensus should emerge from an extensive dialogue involving the above-mentioned competing concerns among sponsors, and representatives from the potential host country and communities from which potential trial participants would be drawn, e.g. government officials, national scientific and ethical communities, affected populations, relevant NGOs, local religious and community leaders.
- Such a consensus should aim for achieving, as closely as possible, the ideal of provision of the best proven therapy for trial participants, in the light of relevant conditions and concerns.
- Sponsors should seek, at a minimum, to ensure access to a level of care and treatment that approaches the best proven care and treatment that are attainable in the potential host country.
- Those participating in the planning of vaccine development programmes should seek to provide a comprehensive care and treatment package based, at a minimum, on standards of care developed by the community, but also taking into account the additional resources and higher standards brought by the sponsor into the research setting.
- Sponsors should contribute to the building up of both the research capacity and the health care delivery capacity of the community where the research is to be carried out, in such a way that they become integrated into the infrastructure of the community.

Such a care and treatment package should include, but not be limited to, some or all of the following items, depending on the type of research, the setting, and the consensus reached by all interested parties before the trials begin:

- counselling
- preventive methods and means
- treatment for other STIs
- tuberculosis prevention and treatment
- prevention/treatment of opportunistic infections
- nutrition
- palliative care, including pain control and spiritual care
- referral to social and community support
- family planning
- home-based care
- antiretroviral therapy

Women, including pregnant women, potentially pregnant women and breast-feeding women, should be eligible for enrolment in HIV preventive vaccine trials, both as a matter of equity and because in many communities throughout the world women are at high risk of HIV infection. Therefore, the safety, immunogenicity, and efficacy of candidate vaccines should be established for women, and for their fetus and breast-fed child, where applicable. In these situations, the clinical trials should be designed with the intent of establishing the effects of the candidate vaccine on the health of the woman and the fetus and/or breast-fed infant, where applicable.

Guidance Point 17: Women

As women, including those who are potentially pregnant, pregnant, or breast-feeding, should be recipients of future HIV preventive vaccines, women should be included in clinical trials in order to verify safety, immunogenicity, and efficacy from their standpoint. During such research, women should receive adequate information to make informed choices about risks to themselves, as well as to their fetus or breast-fed infant, where applicable.

Although the enrolment of pregnant, potentially pregnant, or breast-feeding women complicates the analysis of risks and benefits, because both the women and the fetus or infant could be benefited or harmed, such women should be viewed as autonomous decision-makers, capable of making an informed choice for themselves and for their fetus or child. As with all research participants, steps should be taken to ensure that pregnant or breast-feeding women who are enrolled in vaccine trials are capable of giving informed consent, as indicated in *Guidance Points 12* and *13*. Furthermore, in order for (pregnant) women to be able to make an informed choice for their fetus/breast-fed infant,

they should be duly informed about any potential for teratogenesis and other risks to the fetus, and/or the breast-fed infant. If there are risks related to breast-feeding, they should be informed of the availability of nutritional substitutes and other supportive services.

Children[4], including infants and adolescents, should be eligible for enrolment in HIV preventive vaccine trials, both as a matter of equity and as a function of the fact that in many communities throughout the world children are at high risk of HIV infection. Infants born to HIV-infected mothers are at risk of becoming infected during birth and during the post-partum period through breast-feeding. Many adolescents are also at high risk of infection due to sexual activity, lack of access to HIV prevention education and means, and engagement in injecting drug use.

Guidance Point 18: Children

As children should be recipients of future HIV preventive vaccines, children should be included in clinical trials in order to verify safety, immunogenicity, and efficacy from their standpoint. Efforts should be taken to design vaccine development programmes that address the particular ethical and legal considerations relevant for children, and safeguard their rights and welfare during participation.

Therefore, vaccine development programmes should consider the needs of children for an effective HIV vaccine; should explore the legal, ethical and health considerations relevant to their participation in vaccine research; and should enrol children in clinical trials designed to establish safety, immunogencity, and efficacy for their age groups, once they can be so enrolled in terms of meeting the health needs and ethical considerations relevant to their situation. Those designing vaccine development programmes that might include children should do so in consultation with groups dedicated to the protection and promotion of the rights and welfare of children, both at international and national levels.

Unless exceptions are authorized by national legislation in the host country, consent to participate in an HIV vaccine trial must be secured from the parent or guardian of a child who is a minor before the enrolment of the child as a participant in a vaccine trial. The consent of one parent is

---

[4] As defined by the Convention on the Rights of the Child, Article 1: "...a child means every human being below the age of eighteen years unless, under the law applicable to the child, majority is attained earlier."

generally sufficient, unless national law requires the consent of both. Every effort should be made to obtain consent to participate in the trial also from the child according to the evolving capacities of the child.

In some jurisdictions, individuals who are below the age of consent are authorized to receive, without the consent or awareness of their parents or guardians, such medical services as abortion, contraception, treatment for drug or alcohol abuse, treatment of sexually transmitted diseases, etc. In some of these jurisdictions, such minors are also authorized to consent to serve as participants in research in the same categories without the agreement or the awareness of their parents or guardians provided the research presents no more than "minimal risk". However, such authorization does not justify the enrolment of minors as participants in vaccine trials without the consent of their parents or guardians.

In some jurisdictions, some individuals who are below the general age of consent are regarded as "emancipated" or "mature" minors and are authorized to consent without the agreement or even the awareness of their parents or guardians. These may include those who are married, parents, pregnant or living independently. When authorized by national legislation, minors in these categories may

consent to participation in vaccine trials without the permission of their parents or guardians.

The Joint United Nations Programme on HIV/AIDS (UNAIDS) is the leading advocate for global action on HIV/AIDS. It brings together seven UN agencies in a common effort to fight the epidemic: the United Nations Children's Fund (UNICEF), the United Nations Development Programme (UNDP), the United Nations Population Fund (UNFPA), the United Nations International Drug Control Programme (UNDCP), the United Nations Educational, Scientific and Cultural Organization (UNESCO), the World Health Organization (WHO) and the World Bank.

UNAIDS both mobilizes the responses to the epidemic of its seven cosponsoring organizations and supplements these efforts with special initiatives. Its purpose is to lead and assist an expansion of the international response to HIV on all fronts: medical, public health, social, economic, cultural, political and human rights. UNAIDS works with a broad range of partners – governmental and NGO, business, scientific and lay – to share knowledge, skills and best practice across boundaries.

Produced with environment friendly materials

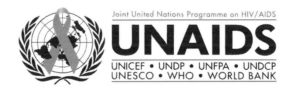

Joint United Nations Programme on HIV/AIDS (UNAIDS)
UNAIDS - 20 avenue Appia - 1211 Geneva 27 - Switzerland
Telephone: (+41 22) 791 46 51 - Fax: (+41 22) 791 41 87
E-mail: unaids@unaids.org - Internet: http://www.unaids.org

International research

65

2002 international ethical guidelines for biomedical research involving human subjects

Council for International Organisations of Medical Sciences (CIOMS)

See the CIOMS website for the complete text of the publication. http://www.cioms.ch/

Guideline 1: Ethical justification and scientific validity of biomedical research involving human beings

The ethical justification of biomedical research involving human subjects is the prospect of discovering new ways of benefiting people's health. Such research can be ethically justifiable only if it is carried out in ways that respect and protect, and are fair to, the subjects of that research and are morally acceptable within the communities in which the research is carried out. Moreover, because scientifically invalid research is unethical in that it exposes research subjects to risks without possible benefit, investigators and sponsors must ensure that proposed studies involving human subjects conform to generally accepted scientific principles and are based on adequate knowledge of the pertinent scientific literature.

Commentary on Guideline 1

Among the essential features of ethically justified research involving human subjects, including research with identifiable human tissue or data, are that the research offers a means of developing information not otherwise obtainable, that the design of the research is scientifically sound, and that the investigators and other research personnel are competent. The methods to be used should be appropriate to the objectives of the research and the field of study. Investigators and sponsors must also ensure that all who participate in the conduct of the research are qualified by virtue of their education and experience to perform competently in their roles. These considerations should be

adequately reflected in the research protocol submitted for review and clearance to scientific and ethical review committees (Appendix I).

Scientific review is discussed further in the Commentaries to Guidelines 2 and 3: *Ethical review committees* and *Ethical review of externally sponsored research*. Other ethical aspects of research are discussed in the remaining guidelines and their commentaries. The protocol designed for submission for review and clearance to scientific and ethical review committees should include, when relevant, the items specified in Appendix I, and should be carefully followed in conducting the research.

Guideline 2: Ethical review committees

All proposals to conduct research involving human subjects must be submitted for review of their scientific merit and ethical acceptability to one or more scientific review and ethical review committees. The review committees must be independent of the research team, and any direct financial or other material benefit they may derive from the research should not be contingent on the outcome of their review. The investigator must obtain their approval or clearance before undertaking the research. The ethical review committee should conduct further reviews as necessary in the course of the research, including monitoring of the progress of the study.

Commentary on Guideline 2

Ethical review committees may function at the institutional, local, regional, or national level, and in some cases at the international level. The regulatory or other governmental authorities concerned should promote uniform standards across committees within a country, and, under all systems, sponsors of research and institutions in which the investigators are employed should allocate sufficient resources to the review process. Ethical review committees may receive money for the activity of reviewing protocols, but under no circumstances may payment be offered or accepted for a review committee's approval or clearance of a protocol.

Scientific review   According to the Declaration of Helsinki (*Paragraph 11*), medical research involving humans must conform to generally accepted scientific principles, and be based on a thorough knowledge of the scientific literature, other relevant sources of information, and adequate laboratory and, where indicated, animal experimentation. Scientific review must consider, inter alia, the study design, including the provisions for avoiding or minimizing risk and for monitoring safety. Committees competent to review and approve scientific aspects of research proposals must be multidisciplinary.

Ethical review   The ethical review committee is responsible for safeguarding the rights, safety, and well-being of the research subjects. Scientific review and ethical review cannot be separated: scientifically unsound research involving humans as subjects is ipso facto unethical in that it may expose them to risk or inconvenience to no purpose; even if there is no risk of injury, wasting of subjects' and researchers' time in unproductive activities represents loss of a valuable resource. Normally, therefore, an ethical review committee considers both the scientific and the ethical aspects of proposed research. It must either carry out a proper scientific review or verify that a competent expert body has determined that the research is scientifically sound. Also, it considers provisions for monitoring of data and safety.

If the ethical review committee finds a research proposal scientifically sound, or verifies that a competent expert body has found it so, it should then consider whether any known or possible risks to the subjects are justified by the expected benefits, direct or indirect, and whether the proposed research methods will minimize harm and maximize benefit. (See Guideline 8: *Benefits and risks of study participation*.) If the proposal is sound and the balance of risks to anticipated benefits is reasonable, the committee should then determine whether the procedures proposed for obtaining informed consent are satisfactory and those proposed for the selection of subjects are equitable.

Ethical review of emergency compassionate use of an investigational therapy   In some countries, drug regulatory authorities require that the so-called compassionate or humanitarian use of an investigational treatment be reviewed by an ethical review committee as though it were research. Exceptionally, a physician may undertake the compassionate use of an investigational therapy before obtaining the approval or clearance of an ethical review committee, provided three criteria are met: a patient needs emergency treatment, there is some evidence of possible effectiveness of the investigational treatment, and there is no other treatment available that is known to be equally effective or superior. Informed consent should be obtained according to the legal requirements and cultural standards of the community in which the intervention is carried out. Within one week the physician must report to the ethical review committee the details of the case and the action taken, and an independent health-care professional must confirm in writing to the ethical review committee the treating physician's judgment that the use of the investigational intervention was justified according to the three specified criteria. (See also Guideline 13 Commentary section: *Other vulnerable groups*.)

National (centralized) or local review   Ethical review committees may be created under the aegis of national or local health administrations, national (or centralized) medical research councils or other nationally representative bodies. In a highly centralized administration a national, or centralized, review committee may be constituted for both the scientific and the ethical review of research protocols. In countries where medical research is not centrally administered, ethical review is more effectively and conveniently undertaken at a local or regional level. The authority of a local ethical review committee may be confined to a single institution or may extend to all institutions in which biomedical research is carried out within a defined geographical area. The basic responsibilities of ethical review committees are:

– to determine that all proposed interventions, particularly the administration of drugs and vaccines or the use of medical devices or procedures under development, are acceptably safe to be undertaken in humans or to verify that another competent expert body has done so;
– to determine that the proposed research is scientifically sound or to verify that another competent expert body has done so;
– to ensure that all other ethical concerns arising from a protocol are satisfactorily resolved both in principle and in practice;
– to consider the qualifications of the investigators, including education in the principles of research practice, and the conditions of the research site with a view to ensuring the safe conduct of the trial; and

– to keep records of decisions and to take measures to follow up on the conduct of ongoing research projects.

Committee membership National or local ethical review committees should be so composed as to be able to provide complete and adequate review of the research proposals submitted to them. It is generally presumed that their membership should include physicians, scientists and other professionals such as nurses, lawyers, ethicists and clergy, as well as lay persons qualified to represent the cultural and moral values of the community and to ensure that the rights of the research subjects will be respected. They should include both men and women. When uneducated or illiterate persons form the focus of a study they should also be considered for membership or invited to be represented and have their views expressed.

A number of members should be replaced periodically with the aim of blending the advantages of experience with those of fresh perspectives.

A national or local ethical review committee responsible for reviewing and approving proposals for externally sponsored research should have among its members or consultants persons who are thoroughly familiar with the customs and traditions of the population or community concerned and sensitive to issues of human dignity.

Committees that often review research proposals directed at specific diseases or impairments, such as HIV/AIDS or paraplegia, should invite or hear the views of individuals or bodies representing patients with such diseases or impairments. Similarly, for research involving such subjects as children, students, elderly persons or employees, committees should invite or hear the views of their representatives or advocates.

To maintain the review committee's independence from the investigators and sponsors and to avoid conflict of interest, any member with a special or particular, direct or indirect, interest in a proposal should not take part in its assessment if that interest could subvert the member's objective judgment. Members of ethical review committees should be held to the same standard of disclosure as scientific and medical research staff with regard to financial or other interests that could be construed as conflicts of interest. A practical way of avoiding such conflict of interest is for the committee to insist on a declaration of possible conflict of interest by any of its members. A member who makes such a declaration should then withdraw, if to do so is clearly the appropriate action to take, either at the member's own discretion or at the request of the other members. Before withdrawing, the member should be permitted to offer comments on the protocol or to respond to questions of other members.

Multi-centre research Some research projects are designed to be conducted in a number of centres in different communities or countries. Generally, to ensure that the results will be valid, the study must be conducted in an identical way at each centre. Such studies include clinical trials, research designed for the evaluation of health service programmes, and various kinds of epidemiological research. For such studies, local ethical or scientific review committees are not normally authorized to change doses of drugs, to change inclusion or exclusion criteria, or to make other similar modifications. They should be fully empowered to prevent a study that they believe to be unethical. Moreover, changes that local review committees believe are necessary to protect the research subjects should be documented and reported to the research institution or sponsor responsible for the whole research programme for consideration and due action, to ensure that all other subjects can be protected and that the research will be valid across sites.

To ensure the validity of multi-centre research, any change in the protocol should be made at every collaborating centre or institution, or, failing this, explicit inter-centre comparability procedures must be introduced; changes made at some but not all will defeat the purpose of multi-centre research. For some multi-centre studies, scientific and ethical review may be facilitated by agreement among centres to accept the conclusions of a single review committee; its members could include a representative of the ethical review committee at each of the centres at which the research is to be conducted, as well as individuals competent to conduct scientific review. In other circumstances, a centralized review may be complemented by local review relating to the local participating investigators and institutions. The central committee could review the study from a scientific and ethical standpoint, and the local committees could verify the practicability of the study in their communities, including the infrastructures, the state of training, and ethical considerations of local significance.

In a large multi-centre trial, individual investigators will not have authority to act independently, with regard to data analysis or to preparation and publication of manuscripts, for instance. Such a trial usually has a set of committees which operate under the direction of a steering committee and are responsible for such functions and decisions. The function of the ethical review committee in such cases is to review the relevant plans with the aim of avoiding abuses.

Sanctions Ethical review committees generally have no authority to impose sanctions on researchers who violate ethical standards in the conduct of research involving humans. They may, however, withdraw ethical approval of a research project if judged necessary. They should be required to monitor the implementation of an approved protocol and its progression, and to report to institutional or governmental authorities any serious or continuing non-compliance with ethical standards as they are reflected in protocols that they have approved or in the conduct of the studies. Failure to submit a protocol to the committee should be considered a clear and serious violation of ethical standards.

Sanctions imposed by governmental, institutional, professional or other authorities possessing disciplinary power should be employed as a last resort. Preferred methods of control include cultivation of an atmosphere of mutual trust, and education and support to promote in researchers and in sponsors the capacity for ethical conduct of research.

Should sanctions become necessary, they should be directed at the non-compliant researchers or sponsors. They may include fines or suspension of eligibility to receive research funding, to use investigational interventions, or to practise medicine. Unless there are persuasive reasons to do otherwise, editors should refuse to publish the results of research conducted unethically, and retract any articles that are subsequently found to contain falsified or fabricated data or to have been based on unethical research. Drug regulatory authorities should consider refusal to accept unethically obtained data submitted in support of an application for authorization to market a product. Such sanctions, however, may deprive of benefit not only the errant researcher or sponsor but also that segment of society intended to benefit from the research; such possible consequences merit careful consideration.

Potential conflicts of interest related to project support Increasingly, biomedical studies receive funding from commercial firms. Such sponsors have good reasons to support research methods that are ethically and scientifically acceptable, but cases have arisen in which the conditions of funding could have introduced bias. It may happen that investigators have little or no input into trial design, limited access to the raw data, or limited participation in data interpretation, or that the results of a clinical trial may not be published if they are unfavourable to the sponsor's product. This risk of bias may also be associated with other sources of support, such as government or foundations. As the persons directly responsible for their work, investigators should not enter into agreements that interfere unduly with their access to the data or their ability to analyse the data independently, to prepare manuscripts, or to publish them. Investigators must also disclose potential or apparent conflicts of interest on their part to the ethical review committee or to other institutional committees designed to evaluate and manage such conflicts. Ethical review

committees should therefore ensure that these conditions are met. See also *Multi-centre research*, above.

Guideline 3: Ethical review of externally sponsored research

An external sponsoring organization and individual investigators should submit the research protocol to ethical and scientific review in the country of the sponsoring organization, and the ethical standards applied should be no less stringent than they would be for research carried out in that country. The health authorities of the host country, as well as a national or local ethical review committee, should ensure that the proposed research is responsive to the health needs and priorities of the host country and meets the requisite ethical standards.

Commentary on Guideline 3

Definition The term *externally sponsored research* refers to research undertaken in a host country but sponsored, financed, and sometimes wholly or partly carried out by an external international or national organization or pharmaceutical company with the collaboration or agreement of the appropriate authorities, institutions and personnel of the host country.

Ethical and scientific review Committees in both the country of the sponsor and the host country have responsibility for conducting both scientific and ethical review, as well as the authority to withhold approval of research proposals that fail to meet their scientific or ethical standards. As far as possible, there must be assurance that the review is independent and that there is no conflict of interest that might affect the judgement of members of the review committees in relation to any aspect of the research. When the external sponsor is an international organization, its review of the research protocol must be in accordance with its own independent ethical-review procedures and standards.

Committees in the external sponsoring country or international organization have a special responsibility to determine whether the scientific methods are sound and suitable to the aims of the research; whether the drugs, vaccines, devices or procedures to be studied meet adequate standards of safety; whether there is sound justification for conducting the research in the host country rather than in the country of the external sponsor or in another country; and whether the proposed research is in compliance with the ethical standards of the external sponsoring country or international organization.

Committees in the host country have a special responsibility to determine whether the objectives of the research are responsive to the health needs and priorities of that country. The ability to judge the ethical acceptability of various aspects of a research proposal requires a thorough understanding of a community's customs and traditions. The ethical review committee in the host country, therefore, must have as either members or consultants persons with such understanding; it will then be in a favourable position to determine the acceptability of the proposed means of obtaining informed consent and otherwise respecting the rights of prospective subjects as well as of the means proposed to protect the welfare of the research subjects. Such persons should be able, for example, to indicate suitable members of the community to serve as intermediaries between investigators and subjects, and to advise on whether material benefits or inducements may be regarded as appropriate in the light of a community's gift-exchange and other customs and traditions.

When a sponsor or investigator in one country proposes to carry out research in another, the ethical review committees in the two countries may, by agreement, undertake to review different aspects of the research protocol. In short, in respect of host countries either with developed capacity for independent ethical review or in which external sponsors and investigators are contributing substantially to such capacity, ethical review in the external, sponsoring country may be limited to ensuring compliance with broadly stated ethical standards. The ethical review committee in the host country can be expected to have greater competence for reviewing the detailed plans for compliance, in view of its better understanding of the cultural and moral values of the population in which it is proposed to conduct the research; it is also likely to be in a better position to monitor compliance in the course of a study. However, in respect of research in host countries with inadequate capacity for independent ethical review, full review by the ethical review committee in the external sponsoring country or international agency is necessary.

Guideline 4: Individual informed consent

For all biomedical research involving humans the investigator must obtain the voluntary informed consent of the prospective subject or, in the case of an individual who is not capable of giving informed consent, the permission of a legally authorized representative in accordance with applicable law. Waiver of informed consent is to be regarded as uncommon and exceptional, and must in all cases be approved by an ethical review committee.

Commentary on Guideline 4

General considerations Informed consent is a decision to participate in research, taken by a competent individual who has received the necessary information; who has adequately understood the information; and who, after considering the information, has arrived at a decision without having been subjected to coercion, undue influence or inducement, or intimidation.

Informed consent is based on the principle that competent individuals are entitled to choose freely whether to participate in research. Informed consent protects the individual's freedom of choice and respects the individual's autonomy. As an additional safeguard, it must always be complemented by independent ethical review of research proposals. This safeguard of independent review is particularly important as many individuals are limited in their capacity to give adequate informed consent; they include young children, adults with severe mental or behavioural disorders, and persons who are unfamiliar with medical concepts and technology (see Guidelines 13, 14, 15).

Process Obtaining informed consent is a process that is begun when initial contact is made with a prospective subject and continues throughout the course of the study. By informing the prospective subjects, by repetition and explanation, by answering their questions as they arise, and by ensuring that each individual understands each procedure, investigators elicit their informed consent and in so doing manifest respect for their dignity and autonomy. Each individual must be given as much time as is needed to reach a decision, including time for consultation with family members or others. Adequate time and resources should be set aside for informed-consent procedures.

Language Informing the individual subject must not be simply a ritual recitation of the contents of a written document. Rather, the investigator must convey the information, whether orally or in writing, in language that suits the individual's level of understanding. The investigator must bear in mind that the prospective subject's ability to understand the information necessary to give informed consent depends on that individual's maturity, intelligence, education and belief system. It depends also on the investigator's ability and willingness to communicate with patience and sensitivity.

Comprehension The investigator must then ensure that the prospective subject has adequately understood the information. The investigator should give each one full opportunity to ask questions and should answer them honestly, promptly and completely. In some instances the investigator may administer an oral or a written test or otherwise determine whether the information has been adequately understood.

Documentation of consent   Consent may be indicated in a number of ways. The subject may imply consent by voluntary actions, express consent orally, or sign a consent form. As a general rule, the subject should sign a consent form, or, in the case of incompetence, a legal guardian or other duly authorized representative should do so. The ethical review committee may approve waiver of the requirement of a signed consent form if the research carries no more than minimal risk – that is, risk that is no more likely and not greater than that attached to routine medical or psychological examination – and if the procedures to be used are only those for which signed consent forms are not customarily required outside the research context. Such waivers may also be approved when existence of a signed consent form would be an unjustified threat to the subject's confidentiality. In some cases, particularly when the information is complicated, it is advisable to give subjects information sheets to retain; these may resemble consent forms in all respects except that subjects are not required to sign them. Their wording should be cleared by the ethical review committee. When consent has been obtained orally, investigators are responsible for providing documentation or proof of consent.

Waiver of the consent requirement   Investigators should never initiate research involving human subjects without obtaining each subject's informed consent, unless they have received explicit approval to do so from an ethical review committee. However, when the research design involves no more than minimal risk and a requirement of individual informed consent would make the conduct of the research impracticable (for example, where the research involves only excerpting data from subjects' records), the ethical review committee may waive some or all of the elements of informed consent.

Renewing consent   When material changes occur in the conditions or the procedures of a study, and also periodically in long-term studies, the investigator should once again seek informed consent from the subjects. For example, new information may have come to light, either from the study or from other sources, about the risks or benefits of products being tested or about alternatives to them. Subjects should be given such information promptly. In many clinical trials, results are not disclosed to subjects and investigators until the study is concluded. This is ethically

acceptable if an ethical review committee has approved their non-disclosure.

Cultural considerations   In some cultures an investigator may enter a community to conduct research or approach prospective subjects for their individual consent only after obtaining permission from a community leader, a council of elders, or another designated authority. Such customs must be respected. In no case, however, may the permission of a community leader or other authority substitute for individual informed consent. In some populations the use of a number of local languages may complicate the communication of information to potential subjects and the ability of an investigator to ensure that they truly understand it. Many people in all cultures are unfamiliar with, or do not readily understand, scientific concepts such as those of placebo or randomization. Sponsors and investigators should develop culturally appropriate ways to communicate information that is necessary for adherence to the standard required in the informed consent process. Also, they should describe and justify in the research protocol the procedure they plan to use in communicating information to subjects. For collaborative research in developing countries the research project should, if the necessary, include the provision of resources to ensure that informed consent can indeed be obtained legitimately within different linguistic and cultural settings.

Consent to use for research purposes biological materials (including genetic material) from subjects in clinical trials   Consent forms for the research protocol should include a separate section for clinical-trial subjects who are requested to provide their consent for the use of their biological specimens for research. Separate consent may be appropriate in some cases (e.g., if investigators are requesting permission to conduct basic research which is not a necessary part of the clinical trial), but not in others (e.g., the clinical trial requires the use of subjects' biological materials).

Use of medical records and biological specimens   Medical records and biological specimens taken in the course of clinical care may be used for research without the consent of the patients/subjects only if an ethical review committee has determined that the research poses minimal risk, that the rights or interests of the patients will not be violated, that their privacy and confidentiality or anonymity are assured, and that the research is designed to answer an important question and would be impracticable if the requirement for informed consent were to be imposed. Patients have a right to know that their records or specimens may be used for research. Refusal or reluctance of individuals to agree to participate would not be evidence of impracticability sufficient to warrant waiving informed consent. Records and specimens of individuals who have specifically rejected such uses in the past may be used only in the case of public health emergencies. (See Guideline 18 Commentary, *Confidentiality between physician and patient*.)

Secondary use of research records or biological specimens
Investigators may want to use records or biological specimens that another investigator has used or collected for use, in another institution in the same or another country. This raises the issue of whether the records or specimens contain personal identifiers, or can be linked to such identifiers, and by whom. (See also Guideline 18: *Safeguarding confidentiality*) If informed consent or permission was required to authorize the original collection or use of such records or specimens for research purposes, secondary uses are generally constrained by the conditions specified in the original consent. Consequently, it is essential that the original consent process anticipate, to the extent that this is feasible, any foreseeable plans for future use of the records or specimens for research. Thus, in the original process of seeking informed consent a member of the research team should discuss with, and, when indicated, request the permission of, prospective subjects as to: i) whether there will or could be any secondary use and, if so, whether such secondary use will be limited with regard to the type of study that may be performed on such material; ii) the conditions under which investigators will be required to contact the research subjects for additional authorization for secondary use; iii) the investigators' plans, if any, to destroy or to strip of personal identifiers the records or specimens; and iv) the rights of subjects to request destruction or anonymization of biological specimens or of records or parts of records that they might consider particularly sensitive, such as photographs, videotapes or audiotapes.

(See also Guidelines 5: *Obtaining informed consent: Essential information for prospective research subjects*; 6: *Obtaining informed consent: Obligations of sponsors and investigators*; and 7: *Inducement to participate*.)

Guideline 5: Obtaining informed consent: Essential information for prospective research subjects

Before requesting and individual's consent to participate in research, the investigator must provide the following information, in language or another form of communication that the individual can understand:

1) that the individual is invited to participate in research, the reasons for considering the individual suitable for the research, and that participation is voluntary;

2) that the individual is free to refuse to participate and will be free to withdraw from the research at any time without penalty or loss of benefits to which he or she would otherwise be entitled;

3) the purpose of the research, the procedures to be carried out by the investigator and the subject, and an explanation of how the research differs from routine medical care;

4) for controlled trials, an explanation of features of the research design (e.g., randomization, double-blinding), and that the subject will not be told of the assigned treatment until the study has been completed and the blind has been broken;

5) the expected duration of the individual's participation (including number and duration of visits to the research centre and the total time involved) and the possibility of early termination of the trial or of the individual's participation in it;

6) whether money or other forms of material goods will be provided in return for the individual's participation and, if so, the kind and amount;

7) that, after the completion of the study, subjects will be informed of the findings of the research in general, and individual subjects will be informed of any finding that relates to their particular health status;

8) that subjects have the right of access to their data on demand, even if these data lack immediate clinical utility (unless the ethical review committee has approved temporary or permanent non-disclosure of data, in which case the subject should be informed of, and given, the reasons for such non-disclosure);

9) any foreseeable risks, pain or discomfort, or inconvenience to the individual (or others) associated with participation in the research, including risks to the health or well-being of a subject's spouse or partner;

10) the direct benefits, if any, expected to result to subjects from participating in the research;

11) the expected benefits of the research to the community or to society at large, or contributions to scientific knowledge;

12) whether, when and how any products or interventions proven by the research to be safe and effective will be made available to subjects after they have completed their participation in the research, and whether they will be expected to pay for them;

13) any currently available alternative interventions or courses of treatment;

14) the provisions that will be made to ensure respect for the privacy of subjects and for the confidentiality of records in which subjects are identified;

15) the limits, legal or other, to the investigators' ability to safeguard confidentiality, and the possible consequences of breaches of confidentiality;

16) policy with regard to the use of results of genetic tests and familial genetic information, and the precautions in place to prevent disclosure of the results of a subject's genetic tests to immediate family relatives or to others (e.g., insurance companies or employers) without the consent of the subject;

17) the sponsors of the research, the institutional affiliation of the investigators, and the nature and sources of funding for the research;

18) the possible research uses, direct or secondary, of the subject's medical records and of biological specimens taken in the course of clinical care (see also Guidelines 4 and 18 Commentaries);

19) whether it is planned that biological specimens collected in the research will be destroyed at its conclusion, and, if not, details about their storage (where, how, for how long, and final disposition) and possible future use, and that subjects have the right to decide about such future use, to refuse storage, and to have the material destroyed (see Guideline 4 Commentary);

20) whether commercial products may be developed from biological specimens, and whether the participant will receive monetary or other benefits from the development of such products;

21) whether the investigator is serving only as an investigator or as both investigator and the subject's physician;

22) the extent of the investigator's responsibility to provide medical services to the participant;

23) that treatment will be provided free of charge for specified types of research-related injury or for complications associated with the research, the nature and duration of such care, the name of the organization or individual that will provide the treatment, and whether there is any uncertainty regarding funding of such treatment;

24) in what way, and by what organization, the subject or the subject's family or dependants will be compensated for disability or death resulting from such injury (or, when indicated, that there are no plans to provide such compensation);

25) whether or not, in the country in which the prospective subject is invited to participate in research, the right to compensation is legally guaranteed;

26) that an ethical review committee has approved or cleared the research protocol.

Guideline 6: Obtaining informed consent: obligations of sponsors and investigators

Sponsors and investigators have a duty to:

– refrain from unjustified deception, undue influence, or intimidation;

– seek consent only after ascertaining that the prospective subject has adequate understanding of the relevant facts and of the consequences of participation and has had sufficient opportunity to consider whether to participate;

– as a general rule, obtain from each prospective subject a signed form as evidence of informed consent – investigators should justify any exceptions to this general rule and obtain the approval of the ethical review committee (see Guideline 4 Commentary, *Documentation of consent*);

– renew the informed consent of each subject if there are significant changes in the conditions or procedures of the research or if new information becomes available that could affect the willingness of subjects to continue to participate; and

– renew the informed consent of each subject in long-term studies at pre-determined intervals, even if there are no changes in the design or objectives of the research.

Commentary on Guideline 6

The investigator is responsible for ensuring the adequacy of informed consent from each subject. The person obtaining informed consent should be knowledgeable about the research and capable of answering questions from prospective subjects. Investigators in charge of the study must make themselves available to answer questions at the request of subjects. Any restrictions on the subject's opportunity to ask questions and receive answers before or during the research undermines the validity of the informed consent.

In some types of research, potential subjects should receive counselling about risks of acquiring a disease unless they take precautions. This is especially true of HIV/AIDS vaccine research (see *Guidance Points in the UNAIDS Guidance Document on Ethical Considerations in HIV Preventive Vaccine Research, Guidance Point 14*, pp. 38–39).

Withholding information and deception   Sometimes, to ensure the validity of research, investigators withhold certain information in the consent process. In biomedical research, this typically takes the form of withholding information about the purpose of specific procedures. For example, subjects in clinical trials are often not told the purpose of tests performed to monitor their compliance with the protocol, since if they knew their compliance was being monitored they might modify their behaviour and hence invalidate results. In most such cases, the prospective subjects are asked to consent to remain uninformed of the purpose of some procedures until the research is completed; after the conclusion of the study they are given the omitted information. In other cases, because a request for permission to withhold some information would jeopardize the validity of the research, subjects are not told that some information has been withheld until the research has been completed. Any such procedure must receive the explicit approval of the ethical review committee.

Active deception of subjects is considerably more controversial than simply withholding certain information. Lying to subjects is a tactic not commonly employed in biomedical research. Social and behavioural scientists, however, sometimes deliberately misinform subjects to study their attitudes and behaviour. For example, scientists have pretended to be patients to study the behaviour of health-care professionals and patients in their natural settings.

Some people maintain that active deception is never permissible. Others would permit it in certain circumstances. Deception is not permissible, however, in cases in which the deception itself would disguise the possibility of the subject being exposed to more than minimal risk. When deception is deemed indispensable to the methods of a study the investigators must demonstrate to an ethical review committee that no other research method would suffice; that significant advances could result from the research; and that nothing has been withheld that, if divulged, would cause a reasonable person to refuse to participate. The ethical review committee should determine the consequences for the subject of being deceived, and whether and how deceived subjects should be informed of the deception upon completion of the research. Such informing, commonly called "debriefing", ordinarily entails explaining the reasons for the deception. A subject who disapproves of having been deceived should be offered an opportunity to refuse to allow the investigator to use information thus obtained. Investigators and ethical review committees should be aware that deceiving research subjects may wrong them as well as harm them; subjects may resent not having been informed when they learn that they have participated in a study under false pretences. In some studies there may be justification for deceiving persons other than the subjects by either withholding or disguising elements of information. Such tactics are often proposed, for example, for studies of the abuse of spouses or children. An ethical review committee must review and approve all proposals to deceive persons other than the subjects. Subjects are entitled to prompt and honest answers to their questions; the ethical review committee must determine for each study whether others who are to be deceived are similarly entitled.

Intimidation and undue influence Intimidation in any form invalidates informed consent. Prospective subjects who are patients often depend for medical care upon the physician/investigator, who consequently has a certain credibility in their eyes, and whose influence over them may be considerable, particularly if the study protocol has a therapeutic component. They may fear, for example, that refusal to participate would damage the therapeutic relationship or result in the withholding of health services. The physician/investigator must assure them that their decision on whether to participate will not affect the therapeutic relationship or other benefits to which they are entitled. In this situation the ethical review committee should consider whether a neutral third party should seek informed consent.

The prospective subject must not be exposed to undue influence. The borderline between justifiable persuasion and undue influence is imprecise, however. The researcher should give no unjustifiable assurances about the benefits, risks or inconveniences of the research, for example, or induce a close relative or a community leader to influence a prospective subject's decision. See also Guideline 4: *Individual informed consent.*

Risks Investigators should be completely objective in discussing the details of the experimental intervention, the pain and discomfort that it may entail, and known risks and possible hazards. In complex research projects it may be neither feasible nor desirable to inform prospective participants fully about every possible risk. They must, however, be informed of all risks that a 'reasonable person' would consider material to making a decision about whether to participate, including risks to a spouse or partner associated with trials of, for example, psychotropic or genital-tract medicaments. (See also Guideline 8 Commentary, *Risks to groups of persons.*)

Exception to the requirement for informed consent in studies of emergency situations in which the researcher anticipates that many subjects will be unable to consent Research protocols are sometimes designed to address conditions occurring suddenly and rendering the patients/subjects incapable of giving informed consent. Examples are head trauma, cardiopulmonary arrest and stroke. The investigation cannot be done with patients who can give informed consent in time and there may not be time to locate a person having the authority to give permission. In such circumstances it is often necessary to proceed with the research interventions very soon after the onset of the condition in order to evaluate an investigational treatment or develop the desired knowledge. As this class of emergency exception can be anticipated, the researcher must secure the review and approval of an ethical review committee before initiating the study. If possible, an attempt should be made to identify a population that is likely to develop the condition to be studied. This can be done readily, for example, if the condition is one that recurs periodically in individuals; examples include grand mal seizures and alcohol binges. In such cases, prospective subjects should be contacted while fully capable of informed consent, and invited to consent to their involvement as research subjects during future periods of incapacitation. If they are patients of an independent physician who is also the physician-researcher, the physician should likewise seek their consent while they are fully capable of informed consent. In all cases in which approved research has begun without prior consent of patients/subjects incapable of giving informed consent because of suddenly occurring conditions, they should be given all relevant information as soon as they are in a state to receive it, and their consent to continued participation should be obtained as soon as is reasonably possible.

Before proceeding without prior informed consent, the investigator must make reasonable efforts to locate an individual who has the authority to give permission on behalf of an incapacitated patient. If such a person can be located and refuses to give permission, the patient may not be enrolled as a subject. The risks of all interventions and procedures will be justified as required by Guideline 9. (*Special limitations on risks when research involves individuals who are not capable of giving consent.*) The researcher and the ethical review committee should agree to a maximum time of involvement of an individual without obtaining either the individual's informed consent or authorization according to the applicable legal system if the person is not able to give consent. If by that time the researcher has not obtained either consent or permission – owing either to a failure to contact a representative or a refusal of either the patient or the person or body authorized to give permission – the participation of the patient as a subject must be discontinued. The patient or the person or body providing authorization should be offered an opportunity to forbid the use of data derived from participation of the patient as a subject without consent or permission.

Where appropriate, plans to conduct emergency research without prior consent of the subjects should be publicized within the community in which it will be carried out. In the design and conduct of the research, the ethical review committee, the investigators and the sponsors should be responsive to the concerns of the community. If there is cause for concern about the acceptability of the research in the community, there should be a formal consultation with representatives designated by the community. The research should not be carried out if it does not have substantial support in the community concerned. (See Guideline 8 Commentary, *Risks to groups of persons.*)

Exception to the requirement of informed consent for inclusion in clinical trials of persons rendered incapable of informed consent by an acute condition   Certain patients with an acute condition that renders them incapable of giving informed consent may be eligible for inclusion in a clinical trial in which the majority of prospective subjects will be capable of informed consent. Such a trial would relate to a new treatment for an acute condition such as sepsis, stroke or myocardial infarction. The investigational treatment would hold out the prospect of direct benefit and would be justified accordingly, though the investigation might involve certain procedures or interventions that were not of direct benefit but carried no more than minimal risk; an example would be the process of randomization or the collection of additional blood for research purposes. For such cases the initial protocol submitted for approval to the ethical review committee should anticipate that some patients may be incapable of consent, and should propose for such patients a form of proxy consent, such as permission of the responsible relative. When the ethical review committee has approved or cleared such a protocol, an investigator may seek the permission of the responsible relative and enrol such a patient.

Guideline 7: Inducement to participate

Subjects may be reimbursed for lost earnings, travel costs and other expenses incurred in taking part in a study; they may also receive free medical services. Subjects, particularly those who receive no direct benefit from research, may also be paid or otherwise compensated for inconvenience and time spent. The payments should not be so large, however, or the medical services so extensive as to induce prospective subjects to consent to participate in the research against their better judgment ("undue inducement"). All payments, reimbursements and medical services provided to research subjects must have been approved by an ethical review committee.

Commentary on Guideline 7

Acceptable recompense   Research subjects may be reimbursed for their transport and other expenses, including lost earnings, associated with their participation in research. Those who receive no direct benefit from the research may also receive a small sum of money for inconvenience due to their participation in the research. All subjects may receive medical services unrelated to the research and have procedures and tests performed free of charge.

Unacceptable recompense Payments in money or in kind to research subjects should not be so large as to persuade them to take undue risks or volunteer against their better judgment. Payments or rewards that undermine a person's capacity to exercise free choice invalidate consent. It may be difficult to distinguish between suitable recompense and undue influence to participate in research. An unemployed person or a student may view promised recompense differently from an employed person. Someone without access to medical care may or may not be unduly influenced to participate in research simply to receive such care. A prospective subject may be induced to participate in order to obtain a better diagnosis or access to a drug not otherwise available; local ethical review committees may find such inducements acceptable. Monetary and in-kind recompense must, therefore, be evaluated in the light of the traditions of the particular culture and population in which they are offered, to determine whether they constitute undue influence. The ethical review committee will ordinarily be the best judge of what constitutes reasonable material recompense in particular circumstances. When research interventions or procedures that do not hold out the prospect of direct benefit present more than minimal risk, all parties involved in the research – sponsors, investigators and ethical review committees – in both funding and host countries should be careful to avoid undue material inducement.

Incompetent persons Incompetent persons may be vulnerable to exploitation for financial gain by guardians. A guardian asked to give permission on behalf of an incompetent person should be offered no recompense other than a refund of travel and related expenses.

Withdrawal from a study A subject who withdraws from research for reasons related to the study, such as unacceptable side-effects of a study drug, or who is withdrawn on health grounds, should be paid or recompensed as if full participation had taken place. A subject who withdraws for any other reason should be paid in proportion to the amount of participation. An investigator who must remove a subject from the study for wilful noncompliance is entitled to withhold part or all of the payment.

Guideline 8: Benefits and risks of study participation

For all biomedical research involving human subjects, the investigator must ensure that potential benefits and risks are reasonably balanced and risks are minimized.

- Interventions or procedures that hold out the prospect of direct diagnostic, therapeutic or preventive benefit for the individual subject must be justified by the expectation that they will be at least as advantageous to the individual subject, in the light of foreseeable risks and benefits, as any available alternative. Risks of such 'beneficial' interventions or procedures must be justified in relation to expected benefits to the individual subject.
- Risks of interventions that do not hold out the prospect of direct diagnostic, therapeutic or preventive benefit for the individual must be justified in relation to the expected benefits to society (generalizable knowledge). The risks presented by such interventions must be reasonable in relation to the importance of the knowledge to be gained.

Commentary on Guideline 8

The Declaration of Helsinki in several paragraphs deals with the well-being of research subjects and the avoidance of risk. Thus, considerations related to the well-being of the human subject should take precedence over the interests of science and society (*Paragraph 5*); clinical testing must be preceded by adequate laboratory or animal experimentation to demonstrate a reasonable probability of success without undue risk (*Paragraph 11*); every project should be preceded by careful assessment of predictable risks and burdens in comparison with foreseeable benefits to the subject or to others (*Paragraph 16*); physician-researchers must be confident that the risks involved have been adequately assessed and can be satisfactorily managed (*Paragraph 17*); and the risks and burdens to the subject must be minimized, and reasonable in relation to the importance of the objective or the knowledge to be gained (*Paragraph 18*).

Biomedical research often employs a variety of interventions of which some hold out the prospect of direct therapeutic benefit (beneficial interventions) and others are administered solely to answer the research question (non-beneficial interventions). Beneficial interventions are justified as they are in medical practice by the expectation that they will be at least as advantageous to the individuals concerned, in the light of both risks and benefits, as any available alternative. Non-beneficial interventions are assessed differently; they may be justified only by appeal to the knowledge to be gained. In assessing the risks and benefits that a protocol presents to a population, it is appropriate to consider the harm that could result from forgoing the research.

Paragraphs 5 and 18 of the Declaration of Helsinki do not preclude well-informed volunteers, capable of fully appreciating risks and benefits of an investigation, from participating in research for altruistic reasons or for modest remuneration.

Minimizing risk associated with participation in a randomized controlled trial   In randomized controlled trials subjects risk being allocated to receive the treatment that proves inferior. They are allocated by chance to one of two or more intervention arms and followed to a predetermined end-point. (Interventions are understood to include new or established therapies, diagnostic tests and preventive measures.) An intervention is evaluated by comparing it with another intervention (a control), which is ordinarily the best current method, selected from the safe and effective treatments available globally, unless some other control intervention such as placebo can be justified ethically (See Guideline 11).

To minimize risk when the intervention to be tested in a randomized controlled trial is designed to prevent or postpone a lethal or disabling outcome, the investigator must not, for purposes of conducting the trial, withhold therapy that is known to be superior to the intervention being tested, unless the withholding can be justified by the standards set forth in Guideline 11. Also, the investigator must provide in the research protocol for the monitoring of research data by an independent board (Data and Safety Monitoring Board); one function of such a board is to protect the research subjects from previously unknown adverse reactions or unnecessarily prolonged exposure to an inferior therapy. Normally at the outset of a randomized controlled trial, criteria are established for its premature termination (stopping rules or guidelines).

Risks to groups of persons   Research in certain fields, such as epidemiology, genetics or sociology, may present risks to the interests of communities, societies, or racially or ethnically defined groups. Information might be published that could stigmatize a group or expose its members to discrimination. Such information, for example, could indicate, rightly or wrongly, that the group has a higher than average prevalence of alcoholism, mental illness or sexually transmitted disease, or is particularly susceptible to certain genetic disorders. Plans to conduct such research should be sensitive to such considerations, to the need to maintain confidentiality during and after the study, and to the need to publish the resulting data in a manner that is respectful of the interests of all concerned, or in certain circumstances not to publish them. The ethical review committee should ensure that the interests of all concerned are given due consideration; often it will be advisable to have individual consent supplemented by community consultation.

[The ethical basis for the justification of risk is elaborated further in Guideline 9]

Guideline 9: Special limitations on risk when research involves individuals who are not capable of giving informed consent

When there is ethical and scientific justification to conduct research with individuals incapable of giving informed consent, the risk from research interventions that do not hold out the prospect of direct benefit for the individual subject should be no more likely and not greater than the risk attached to routine medical or psychological examination of such persons. Slight or minor increases above such risk may be permitted when there is an overriding scientific or medical rationale for such increases and when an ethical review committee has approved them.

Commentary on Guideline 9

The low-risk standard: Certain individuals or groups may have limited capacity to give informed consent either because, as in the case of prisoners, their autonomy is limited, or because they have limited cognitive capacity. For research involving persons who are unable to consent, or whose capacity to make an informed choice may not fully meet the standard of informed consent, ethical review committees must distinguish between intervention risks that do not exceed those associated with routine medical or psychological examination of such persons and risks in excess of those.

When the risks of such interventions do not exceed those associated with routine medical or psychological examination of such persons, there is no requirement for special substantive or procedural protective measures apart from those generally required for all research involving members of the particular class of persons. When the risks are in excess of those, the ethical review committee must find: 1) that the research is designed to be responsive to the disease affecting the prospective subjects or to conditions to which they are particularly susceptible; 2) that the risks of the research interventions are only slightly greater than those associated with routine medical or psychological examination of such persons for the condition or set of clinical circumstances under investigation; 3) that the objective of the research is sufficiently important to justify exposure of the subjects to the increased risk; and 4) that the interventions are reasonably commensurate with the clinical interventions that the subjects have experienced or may be expected to experience in relation to the condition under investigation.

If such research subjects, including children, become capable of giving independent informed consent during the research, their consent to continued participation should be obtained.

There is no internationally agreed, precise definition of a "slight or minor increase" above the risks associated with routine medical or psychological examination of such persons. Its meaning is inferred from what various ethical review committees have reported as having met the standard. Examples include additional lumbar punctures or bone-marrow aspirations in children with conditions for which such examinations are regularly indicated in clinical practice. The requirement that the objective of the research be relevant to the disease or condition affecting the prospective subjects rules out the use of such interventions in healthy children.

The requirement that the research interventions be reasonably commensurate with clinical interventions that subjects may have experienced or are likely to experience for the condition under investigation is intended to enable them to draw on personal experience as they decide whether to accept or reject additional procedures for research purposes. Their choices will, therefore, be more informed even though they may not fully meet the standard of informed consent.

(See also Guidelines 4: *Individual informed consent*; 13: *Research involving vulnerable persons*; 14: *Research involving children*; and 15: *Research involving individuals who by reason of mental or behavioural disorders are not capable of giving adequately informed consent.*)

Guideline 10: Research in populations and communities with limited resources

Before undertaking research in a population or community with limited resources, the sponsor and the investigator must make every effort to ensure that:

– the research is responsive to the health needs and the priorities of the population or community in which it is to be carried out; and

– any intervention or product developed, or knowledge generated, will be made reasonably available for the benefit of that population or community.

Commentary on Guideline 10

This guideline is concerned with countries or communities in which resources are limited to the extent that they are, or may be, vulnerable to exploitation by sponsors and investigators from the relatively wealthy countries and communities.

Responsiveness of research to health needs and priorities
The ethical requirement that research be responsive to the health needs of the population or community in which it is carried out calls for decisions on what is needed to fulfil the requirement. It is not sufficient simply to determine that a disease is prevalent in the population and that new or further research is needed: the ethical requirement of "responsiveness" can be fulfilled only if successful interventions or other kinds of health benefit are made available to the population. This is applicable especially to research conducted in countries where governments lack the resources to make such products or benefits widely available. Even when a product to be tested in a particular country is much cheaper than the standard treatment in some other countries, the government or individuals in that country may still be unable to afford it. If the knowledge gained from the research in such a country is used primarily for the benefit of populations that can afford the tested product, the research may rightly be characterized as exploitative and, therefore, unethical.

When an investigational intervention has important potential for health care in the host country, the negotiation that the sponsor should undertake to determine the practical implications of "responsiveness", as well as "reasonable availability", should include representatives of stakeholders in the host country; these include the national government, the health ministry, local health authorities, and concerned scientific and ethics groups, as well as representatives of the communities from which subjects are drawn and nongovernmental organizations such as health advocacy groups. The negotiation should cover the health-care infrastructure required for safe and rational use of the intervention, the likelihood of authorization for distribution, and decisions regarding payments, royalties, subsidies, technology and intellectual property, as well as distribution costs, when this economic information is not proprietary. In some cases, satisfactory discussion of the availability and distribution of successful products will necessarily engage international organizations, donor governments and bilateral agencies, international nongovernmental organizations, and the private sector. The development of a health-care infrastructure should be facilitated at the onset so that it can be of use during and beyond the conduct of the research.

Additionally, if an investigational drug has been shown to be beneficial, the sponsor should continue to provide it to the subjects after the conclusion of the study, and pending its approval by a drug regulatory authority. The sponsor is unlikely to be in a position to make a beneficial investigational intervention generally available to the community or population until some time after the conclusion of the study, as it may be in short supply and in any case cannot be made generally available before a drug regulatory authority has approved it.

For minor research studies and when the outcome is scientific knowledge rather than a commercial product, such complex planning or negotiation is rarely, if ever, needed. There must be assurance, however, that the scientific knowledge developed will be used for the benefit of the population.

Reasonable availability   The issue of "reasonable availability" is complex and will need to be determined on a case-by-case basis. Relevant considerations include the length of time for which the intervention or product developed, or other agreed benefit, will be made available to research subjects, or to the community or population concerned; the severity of a subject's medical condition; the effect of withdrawing the study drug (e.g., death of a subject); the cost to the subject or health service; and the question of undue inducement if an intervention is provided free of charge.

In general, if there is good reason to believe that a product developed or knowledge generated by research is unlikely to be reasonably available to, or applied to the benefit of, the population of a proposed host country or community after the conclusion of the research, it is unethical to conduct the research in that country or community. This should not be construed as precluding studies designed to evaluate novel therapeutic concepts. As a rare exception, for example, research may be designed to obtain preliminary evidence that a drug or a class of drugs has a beneficial effect in the treatment of a disease that occurs only in regions with extremely limited resources, and it could not be carried out reasonably well in more developed communities. Such research may be justified ethically even if there is no plan in place to make a product available to the population of the host country or community at the conclusion of the preliminary phase of its development. If the concept is found to be valid, subsequent phases of the research could result in a product that could be made reasonably available at its conclusion.

(See also Guidelines 3: *Ethical review of externally sponsored research*; 12: *Equitable distribution of burdens and benefits*; 20: *Strengthening capacity for ethical and scientific review and biomedical research*; and 21: *Ethical obligation of external sponsors to provide health-care services*.)

Note on Guideline 11

'Best current intervention' is the term most commonly used to describe the active comparator that is ethically preferred in controlled clinical trials. For many indications, however, there is more than one established 'current' intervention and expert clinicians do not agree on which is superior. In other circumstances in which there are several established 'current' interventions, some expert clinicians recognize one as superior to the rest; some commonly prescribe another because the superior intervention may be locally unavailable, for example, or prohibitively expensive or unsuited to the capability of particular patients to adhere to a complex and rigorous regimen. 'Established effective intervention' is the term used in this Guideline to refer to all such interventions, including the best and the various alternatives to the best. In some cases an ethical review committee may determine that it is ethically acceptable to use an established effective intervention as a comparator, even in cases where such an intervention is not considered the best current intervention.

Guideline 11: Choice of control in clinical trials

As a general rule, research subjects in the control group of a trial of a diagnostic, therapeutic, or preventive intervention should receive an established effective intervention. In some circumstances it may be ethically acceptable to use an alternative comparator, such as placebo or "no treatment".

Placebo may be used:
– when there is no established effective intervention;
– when withholding an established effective intervention would expose subjects to, at most, temporary discomfort or delay in relief of symptoms;
– when use of an established effective intervention as comparator would not yield scientifically reliable results and use of placebo would not add any risk of serious or irreversible harm to the subjects.

Commentary on Guideline 11

General considerations for controlled clinical trials   The design of trials of investigational diagnostic, therapeutic or preventive interventions raises interrelated scientific and ethical issues for sponsors, investigators and ethical review committees. To obtain reliable results, investigators must compare the effects of an investigational intervention on subjects assigned to the investigational arm (or arms) of a trial with the effects that a control intervention produces in subjects drawn from the same population and assigned to its control arm. Randomization is the preferred method for assigning subjects to the various arms of the clinical trial unless another method, such as historical or literature controls, can be justified scientifically and ethically. Assignment to treatment arms by randomization, in addition to its usual scientific superiority, offers the advantage of tending to render equivalent to all subjects the foreseeable benefits and risks of participation in a trial.

A clinical trial cannot be justified ethically unless it is capable of producing scientifically reliable results. When the objective is to establish the effectiveness and safety of an investigational intervention, the use of a placebo control is often much more likely than that of an active control to produce a scientifically reliable result. In many cases the ability of a trial to distinguish effective from ineffective interventions (its assay sensitivity) cannot be assured unless the control is a placebo. If, however, an effect of using a placebo would be to deprive subjects in the control arm of an established effective intervention, and thereby to expose them to serious harm, particularly if it is irreversible, it would obviously be unethical to use a placebo.

Placebo control in the absence of a current effective alternative The use of placebo in the control arm of a clinical trial is ethically acceptable when, as stated in the Declaration of Helsinki (Paragraph 29), "no proven prophylactic, diagnostic or therapeutic method exists." Usually, in this case, a placebo is scientifically preferable to no intervention. In certain circumstances, however, an alternative design may be both scientifically and ethically acceptable, and preferable; an example would be a clinical trial of a surgical intervention, because, for many surgical interventions, either it is not possible or it is ethically unacceptable to devise a suitable placebo; for another example, in certain vaccine trials an investigator might choose to provide for those in the 'control' arm a vaccine that is unrelated to the investigational vaccine.

Placebo-controlled trials that entail only minor risks A placebo-controlled design may be ethically acceptable, and preferable on scientific grounds, when the condition for which patients/subjects are randomly assigned to placebo or active treatment is only a small deviation in physiological measurements, such as slightly raised blood pressure or a modest increase in serum cholesterol; and if delaying or omitting available treatment may cause only temporary discomfort (e.g., common headache) and no serious

adverse consequences. The ethical review committee must be fully satisfied that the risks of withholding an established effective intervention are truly minor and short-lived.

Placebo control when active control would not yield reliable results A related but distinct rationale for using a placebo control rather than an established effective intervention is that the documented experience with the established effective intervention is not sufficient to provide a scientifically reliable comparison with the intervention being investigated; it is then difficult, or even impossible, without using a placebo, to design a scientifically reliable study. This is not always, however, an ethically acceptable basis for depriving control subjects of an established effective intervention in clinical trials; only when doing so would not add any risk of serious harm, particularly irreversible harm, to the subjects would it be ethically acceptable to do so. In some cases, the condition at which the intervention is aimed (for example, cancer or HIV/AIDS) will be too serious to deprive control subjects of an established effective intervention.

This latter rationale (*when active control would not yield reliable results*) differs from the former (*trials that entail only minor risks*) in emphasis. In trials that entail only minor risks the investigative interventions are aimed at relatively trivial conditions, such as the common cold or hair loss; forgoing an established effective intervention for the duration of a trail deprives control subjects of only minor benefits. It is for this reason that it is not unethical to use a placebo-control design. Even if it were possible to design a so-called "non-inferiority", or "equivalency", trial using an active control, it would still not be unethical in these circumstances to use a placebo-control design. In any event, the researcher must satisfy the ethical review committee that the safety and human rights of the subjects will be fully protected, that prospective subjects will be fully informed about alternative treatments, and that the purpose and design of the study are scientifically sound. The ethical acceptability of such placebo-controlled studies increases as the period of placebo use is decreased, and when the study design permits change to active treatment ("escape treatment") if intolerable symptoms occur (*WHO Good Clinical Practice Guidelines, 1995*).

Exceptional use of a comparator other than an established effective intervention An exception to the general rule is applicable in some studies designed to develop a therapeutic, preventive or diagnostic intervention for use in a country or community in which an established effective intervention is not available and unlikely in the foreseeable future to become available, usually for economic or logistic reasons. The purpose of such a study is to make available to the population of the country or community an effective alternative to an established effective intervention that is locally unavailable. Accordingly, the proposed investigational intervention must be responsive to the health needs of the population from which the research subjects are recruited and there must be assurance that, if it proves to be safe and effective, it will be made reasonably available to that population. Also, the scientific and ethical review committees must be satisfied that the established effective intervention cannot be used as comparator because its use would not yield scientifically reliable results that would be relevant to the health needs of the study population. In these circumstances an ethical review committee can approve a clinical trial in which the comparator is other than an established effective intervention, such as placebo or no treatment or a local remedy.

However, some people strongly object to the exceptional use of a comparator other than an established effective intervention because it could result in exploitation of poor and disadvantaged populations. The objection rests on three arguments:

• Placebo control could expose research subjects to risk of serious or irreversible harm when the use of an established effective intervention as comparator could avoid the risk.
• Not all scientific experts agree about conditions under which an established effective intervention used as a comparator would not yield scientifically reliable results.
• An economic reason for the unavailability of an established effective intervention cannot justify a placebo-controlled study in a country of limited resources when it would be unethical to conduct a study with the same design in a population with general access to the effective intervention outside the study.

Placebo control when an established effective intervention is not available in the host country   The question addressed here is: when should an exception be allowed to the general rule that subjects in the control arm of a clinical trial should receive an established effective intervention?

The usual reason for proposing the exception is that, for economic or logistic reasons, an established effective intervention is not in general use or available in the country in which the study will be conducted, whereas the investigational intervention could be made available, given the finances and infrastructure of the country.

Another reason that may be advanced for proposing a placebo-controlled trial is that using an established effective intervention as the control would not produce scientifically reliable data relevant to the country in which the

trial is to be conducted. Existing data about the effectiveness and safety of the established effective intervention may have been accumulated under circumstances unlike those of the population in which it is proposed to conduct the trial; this, it may be argued, could make their use in the trial unreliable. One reason could be that the disease or condition manifests itself differently in different populations, or other uncontrolled factors could invalidate the use of existing data for comparative purposes.

The use of pacebo control in these circumstances is ethically controversial, for the following reasons:

1. Sponsors of research might use poor countries or communities as testing grounds for research that would be difficult or impossible in countries where there is general access to an established effective intervention, and the investigational intervention, if proven safe and effective, is likely to be marketed in countries in which an established effective intervention is already available and it is not likely to be marketed in the host country.
2. The research subjects, both active-arm and control-arm, are patients who may have a serious, possibly life-threatening, illness. They do not normally have access to an established effective intervention currently available to similar patients in many other countries. According to the requirements of a scientifically reliable trial, investigators, who may be their attending physicians, would be expected to enrol some of those patients/subjects in the placebo-control arm. This would appear to be a violation of the physician's fiduciary duty of undivided loyalty to the patient, particularly in cases in which known effective therapy could be made available to the patients.

An argument for exceptional use of placebo control may be that a health authority in a country where an established effective intervention is not generally available or affordable, and unlikely to become available or affordable in the foreseeable future, seeks to develop an affordable intervention specifically for a health problem affecting its population. There may then be less reason for concern that a placebo design is exploitative, and therefore unethical, as the health authority has responsibility for the population's health, and there are valid health grounds for testing an apparently beneficial intervention. In such circumstances an ethical review committee may determine that the proposed trial is ethically acceptable, provided that the rights and safety of subjects are safeguarded.

Ethical review committees will need to engage in careful analysis of the circumstances to determine whether the use of placebo rather than an established effective intervention is ethically acceptable. They will need to be satisfied that an established effective intervention is truly unlikely to become available and implementable in that country.

This may be difficult to determine, however, as it is clear that, with sufficient persistence and ingenuity, ways may be found of accessing previously unattainable medicinal products, and thus avoiding the ethical issue raised by the use of placebo control.

When the rationale of proposing a placebo-controlled trial is that the use of an established effective intervention as the control would not yield scientifically reliable data relevant to the proposed host country, the ethical review committee in that country has the option of seeking expert opinion as to whether use of an established effective intervention in the control arm would invalidate the results of the research.

An "equivalency trial" as an alternative to a placebo-controlled trial An alternative to a placebo-control design in these circumstances would be an "equivalency trial", which would compare an investigational intervention with an established effective intervention and produce scientifically reliable data. An equivalency trial in a country in which no established effective intervention is available is not designed to determine whether the investigational intervention is superior to an established effective intervention currently used somewhere in the world; its purpose is, rather, to determine whether the investigational intervention is, in effectiveness and safety, equivalent to, or almost equivalent to, the established effective intervention. It would be hazardous to conclude, however, that an intervention demonstrated to be equivalent, or almost equivalent, to an established effective intervention is better than nothing or superior to whatever intervention is available in the country; there may be substantial differences between the results of superficially identical clinical trials carried out in different countries. If there are such differences, it would be scientifically acceptable and ethically preferable to conduct such 'equivalency' trials in countries in which an established effective intervention is already available.

If there are substantial grounds for the ethical review committee to conclude that an established effective intervention will not become available and implementable, the committee should obtain assurances from the parties concerned that plans have been agreed for making the investigational intervention reasonably available in the host country or community once its effectiveness and safety have been established. Moreover, when the study has external sponsorship, approval should usually be dependent on the sponsors and the health authorities of the host country having engaged in a process of negotiation and planning, including justifying the study in regard to local health-care needs.

Means of minimizing harm to placebo-control subjects Even when placebo controls are justified on one of the bases set forth in the guideline, there are means of minimizing the possibly harmful effect of being in the control arm.

First, a placebo-control group need not be untreated. An add-on design may be employed when the investigational therapy and a standard treatment have different mechanisms of action. The treatment to be tested and placebo are each added to a standard treatment. Such studies have a particular place when a standard treatment is known to decrease mortality or irreversible morbidity but a trial with standard treatment as the active control cannot be carried out or would be difficult to interpret [*International Conference on Harmonisation (ICH) Guideline: Choice of Control Group and Related Issues in Clinical Trials, 2000*]. In testing for improved treatment of life-threatening diseases such as cancer, HIV/AIDS, or heart failure, add-on designs are a particularly useful means of finding improvements in interventions that are not fully effective or may cause intolerable side-effects. They have a place also in respect of treatment for epilepsy, rheumatism and osteoporosis, for example, because withholding of established effective therapy could result in progressive disability, unacceptable discomfort or both.

Second, as indicated in Guideline 8 Commentary, when the intervention to be tested in a randomized controlled trial is designed to prevent or postpone a lethal or disabling outcome, the investigator minimizes harmful effects of placebo-control studies by providing in the research protocol for the monitoring of research data by an independent Data and Safety Monitoring Board (DSMB). One function of such a board is to protect the research subjects from previously unknown adverse reactions; another is to avoid unnecessarily prolonged exposure to an inferior therapy. The board fulfils the latter function by means of interim analyses of the data pertaining to efficacy to ensure that the trial does not continue beyond the point at which an investigational therapy is demonstrated to be effective. Normally, at the outset of a randomized controlled trial, criteria are established for its premature termination (stopping rules or guidelines).

In some cases the DSMB is called upon to perform "conditional power calculations", designed to determine the probability that a particular clinical trial could ever show that the investigational therapy is effective. If that probability is very small, the DSMB is expected to recommend termination of the clinical trial, because it would be unethical to continue it beyond that point.

In most cases of research involving human subjects, it is unnecessary to appoint a DSMB. To ensure that research is carefully monitored for the early detection of adverse events, the sponsor or the principal investigator appoints an individual to be responsible for advising on the need to consider changing the system of monitoring for adverse events or the process of informed consent, or even to consider terminating the study.

Guideline 12: Equitable distribution of burdens and benefits in the selection of groups of subjects in research

Groups or communities to be invited to be subjects of research should be selected in such a way that the burdens and benefits of the research will be equitably distributed. The exclusion of groups or communities that might benefit from study participation must be justified.

Commentary on Guideline 12

General considerations   Equity requires that no group or class of persons should bear more than its fair share of the burdens of participation in research. Similarly, no group should be deprived of its fair share of the benefits of research, short-term or long-term; such benefits include the direct benefits of participation as well as the benefits of the new knowledge that the research is designed to yield. When burdens or benefits of research are to be apportioned unequally among individuals or groups of persons, the criteria for unequal distribution should be morally justifiable and not arbitrary. In other words, unequal allocation must not be inequitable. Subjects should be drawn from the qualifying population in the general geographic area of the trial without regard to race, ethnicity, economic status or gender unless there is a sound scientific reason to do otherwise.

In the past, groups of persons were excluded from participation in research for what were then considered good reasons. As a consequence of such exclusions, information about the diagnosis, prevention and treatment of diseases in such groups of persons is limited. This has resulted in a serious class injustice. If information about the management of diseases is considered a benefit that is distributed within a society, it is unjust to deprive groups of persons of that benefit. Such documents as the *Declaration of Helsinki* and *Guidance Points in the UNAIDS Guidance Document on Ethical Considerations in HIV Preventive Vaccine Research*, and the policies of many national governments and professional societies, recognize the need to redress these injustices by encouraging the participation of previously excluded groups in basic and applied biomedical research.

Members of vulnerable groups also have the same entitlement to access to the benefits of investigational interventions that show promise of therapeutic benefit as persons not considered vulnerable, particularly when no superior or equivalent approaches to therapy are available.

There has been a perception, sometimes correct and sometimes incorrect, that certain groups of persons have been overused as research subjects. In some cases such overuse has been based on the administrative availability of the populations. Research hospitals are often located in places where members of the lowest socioeconomic classes reside, and this has resulted in an apparent overuse of such persons. Other groups that may have been overused because they were conveniently available to researchers include students in investigators' classes, residents of long-term care facilities and subordinate members of hierarchical institutions. Impoverished groups have been overused because of their willingness to serve as subjects in exchange for relatively small stipends. Prisoners have been considered ideal subjects for Phase I drug studies because of their highly regimented lives and, in many cases, their conditions of economic deprivation.

Overuse of certain groups, such as the poor or the administratively available, is unjust for several reasons. It is unjust to selectively recruit impoverished people to serve as research subjects simply because they can be more easily induced to participate in exchange for small payments. In most cases, these people would be called upon to bear the burdens of research so that others who are better off could enjoy the benefits. However, although the burdens of research should not fall disproportionately on socioeconomically disadvantaged groups, neither should such groups be categorically excluded from research protocols. It would not be unjust to selectively recruit poor people to serve as subjects in research designed to address problems that are prevalent in their group – malnutrition, for example. Similar considerations apply to institutionalized groups or those whose availability to the investigators is for other reasons administratively convenient.

Not only may certain groups within a society be inappropriately over-used as research subjects, but also entire communities or societies may be over-used. This has been particularly likely to occur in countries or communities with insufficiently well-developed systems for the protection of the rights and welfare of human research subjects. Such over-use is especially questionable when the populations or communities concerned bear the burdens of participation in research but are extremely unlikely ever to enjoy the benefits of new knowledge and products developed as a result of the research. (See Guideline 10: *Research in populations and communities with limited resources.*)

Guideline 13: Research involving vulnerable persons

Special justification is required for inviting vulnerable individuals to serve as research subjects and, if they are selected, the means of protecting their rights and welfare must be strictly applied.

Commentary on Guideline 13

Vulnerable persons are those who are relatively (or absolutely) incapable of protecting their own interests. More formally, they may have insufficient power, intelligence, education, resources, strength, or other needed attributes to protect their own interests.

General considerations   The central problem presented by plans to involve vulnerable persons as research subjects is that such plans may entail an inequitable distribution of the burdens and benefits of research participation. Classes of individuals conventionally considered vulnerable are those with limited capacity or freedom to consent or to decline to consent. They are the subject of specific guidelines in this document (Guidelines 14, 15) and include children, and persons who because of mental or behavioural disorders are incapable of giving informed consent. Ethical justification of their involvement usually requires that investigators satisfy ethical review committees that:

– the research could not be carried out equally well with less vulnerable subjects;
– the research is intended to obtain knowledge that will lead to improved diagnosis, prevention or treatment of diseases or other health problems characteristic of, or unique to, the vulnerable class – either the actual subjects or other similarly situated members of the vulnerable class;
– research subjects and other members of the vulnerable class from which subjects are recruited will ordinarily be assured reasonable access to any diagnostic, preventive or therapeutic products that will become available as a consequence of the research;
– the risks attached to interventions or procedures that do not hold out the prospect of direct health-related benefit will not exceed those associated with routine medical or psychological examination of such persons unless an ethical review committee authorizes a slight increase over this level of risk (Guideline 9); and,
– when the prospective subjects are either incompetent or otherwise substantially unable to give informed consent, their agreement will be supplemented by the permission of their legal guardians or other appropriate representatives.

Other vulnerable groups   The quality of the consent of prospective subjects who are junior or subordinate members of a hierarchical group requires careful consideration, as their agreement to volunteer may be unduly influenced, whether justified or not, by the expectation of preferential treatment if they agree or by fear of disapproval or retaliation if they refuse. Examples of such groups are medical and nursing students, subordinate hospital and laboratory personnel, employees of pharmaceutical companies, and members of the armed forces or police. Because they work in close proximity to investigators, they tend to be called upon more often than others to serve as research subjects, and this could result in inequitable distribution of the burdens and benefits of research.

Elderly persons are commonly regarded as vulnerable. With advancing age, people are increasingly likely to acquire attributes that define them as vulnerable. They may, for example, be institutionalized or develop varying degrees of dementia. If and when they acquire such vulnerability-defining attributes, and not before, it is appropriate to consider them vulnerable and to treat them accordingly.

Other groups or classes may also be considered vulnerable. They include residents of nursing homes, people receiving welfare benefits or social assistance and other poor people and the unemployed, patients in emergency rooms, some ethnic and racial minority groups, homeless persons, nomads, refugees or displaced persons, prisoners, patients with incurable disease, individuals who are politically powerless, and members or communities unfamiliar with modern medical concepts. To the extent that these and other classes of people have attributes resembling those of classes identified as vulnerable, the need for special protection of their rights and welfare should be reviewed and applied, where relevant.

Persons who have serious, potentially disabling or life-threatening diseases are highly vulnerable. Physicians sometimes treat such patients with drugs or other therapies not yet licensed for general availability because studies designed to establish their safety and efficacy have not been completed. This is compatible with the Declaration of Helsinki, which states in Paragraph 32: *"In the treatment of a patient, where proven . . . therapeutic methods do not exist or have been ineffective, the physician, with informed consent from the patient, must be free to use unproven or new . . . therapeutic measures, if in the physician's judgement it offers hope of saving life, re-establishing health or alleviating suffering"*. Such treatment, commonly called 'compassionate use', is not properly regarded as research, but it can contribute to ongoing research into the safety and efficacy of the interventions used.

Although, on the whole, investigators must study less vulnerable groups before involving more vulnerable groups, some exceptions are justified. In general, children are not suitable for Phase I drug trials or for Phase I or II vaccine trials, but such trials may be permissible after studies in adults have shown some therapeutic or preventive effect. For example, a Phase II vaccine trial seeking evidence of immunogenicity in infants may be justified when a vaccine has shown evidence of preventing or slowing progression of an infectious disease in adults, or Phase I research with children may be appropriate because the disease to be treated does not occur in adults or is manifested differently in children.

Guideline 14: Research involving children

Before undertaking research involving children, the investigator must ensure that:
– the research might not equally well be carried out with adults;
– the purpose of the research is to obtain knowledge relevant to the health needs of children;
– a parent or legal representative of each child has given permission;
– the agreement (assent) of each child has been obtained to the extent of the child's capabilities; and,
– a child's refusal to participate or continue in the research will be respected.

Commentary on Guideline 14

Justification of the involvement of children in biomedical research The participation of children is indispensable for research into diseases of childhood and conditions to which children are particularly susceptible (cf. vaccine trials), as well as for clinical trials of drugs that are designed for children as well as adults. In the past, many new products were not tested for children though they were directed towards diseases also occurring in childhood; thus children either did not benefit from these new drugs or were exposed to them though little was known about their specific effects or safety in children. Now it is widely agreed that, as a general rule, the sponsor of any new therapeutic, diagnostic or preventive product that is likely to be indicated for use in children is obliged to evaluate its safety and efficacy for children before it is released for general distribution.

Assent of the child The willing cooperation of the child should be sought, after the child has been informed to the extent that the child's maturity and intelligence permit. The age at which a child becomes legally competent to give consent differs substantially from one jurisdiction to another; in some countries the "age of consent" established in their different provinces, states or other political subdivisions varies considerably. Often children who have not yet reached the legally established age of consent can understand the implications of informed consent and go through the necessary procedures; they can therefore knowingly agree to serve as research subjects. Such knowing agreement, sometimes referred to as assent, is insufficient to permit participation in research unless it is supplemented by the permission of a parent, a legal guardian or other duly authorized representative.

Some children who are too immature to be able to give knowing agreement, or assent, may be able to register a 'deliberate objection', an expression of disapproval or refusal of a proposed procedure. The deliberate objection of an older child, for example, is to be distinguished from the behaviour of an infant, who is likely to cry or withdraw in response to almost any stimulus. Older children, who are more capable of giving assent, should be selected before younger children or infants, unless there are valid scientific reasons related to age for involving younger children first.

A deliberate objection by a child to taking part in research should always be respected even if the parents have given permission, unless the child needs treatment that is not available outside the context of research, the investigational intervention shows promise of therapeutic benefit, and there is no acceptable alternative therapy. In such a case, particularly if the child is very young or immature, a parent or guardian may override the child's objections. If the child is older and more nearly capable of independent informed consent, the investigator should seek the specific approval or clearance of the scientific and ethical review committees for initiating or continuing with the investigational treatment. If child subjects become capable of independent informed consent during the research, their informed consent to continued participation should be sought and their decision respected.

A child with a likely fatal illness may object or refuse assent to continuation of a burdensome or distressing intervention. In such circumstances parents may press an investigator to persist with an investigational intervention against the child's wishes. The investigator may agree to do so if the intervention shows promise of preserving or prolonging life and there is no acceptable alternative treatment. In such cases, the investigator should seek the specific approval or clearance of the ethical review committee before agreeing to override the wishes of the child.

Permission of a parent or guardian The investigator must obtain the permission of a parent or guardian in accordance with local laws or established procedures. It may be assumed that children over the age of 12 or 13 years are usually capable of understanding what is necessary to give adequately informed consent, but their consent (assent) should normally be complemented by the permission of a parent or guardian, even when local law does not require such permission. Even when the law requires parental permission, however, the assent of the child must be obtained.

In some jurisdictions, some individuals who are below the general age of consent are regarded as "emancipated" or "mature" minors and are authorized to consent without the agreement or even the awareness of their parents or guardians. They may be married or pregnant or be already parents or living independently. Some studies involve investigation of adolescents' beliefs and behaviour regarding sexuality or use of recreational drugs; other research addresses domestic violence or child abuse. For studies on these topics, ethical review committees may waive parental permission if, for example, parental knowledge of the subject matter may place the adolescents at some risk of questioning or even intimidation by their parents.

Because of the issues inherent in obtaining assent from children in institutions, such children should only exceptionally be subjects of research. In the case of institutionalized children without parents, or whose parents are not legally authorized to grant permission, the ethical review committee may require sponsors or investigators to provide it with the opinion of an independent, concerned, expert advocate for institutionalized children as to the propriety of undertaking the research with such children.

Observation of research by a parent or guardian A parent or guardian who gives permission for a child to participate in research should be given the opportunity, to a reasonable extent, to observe the research as it proceeds, so as to be able to withdraw the child if the parent or guardian decides it is in the child's best interests to do so.

Psychological and medical support Research involving children should be conducted in settings in which the child and the parent can obtain adequate medical and psychological support. As an additional protection for children, an investigator may, when possible, obtain the advice of a child's family physician, paediatrician or other health-care provider on matters concerning the child's participation in the research.

(See also Guideline 8: *Benefits and risks of study participation*; Guideline 9: *Special limitations on risks when* *subjects are not capable of giving consent*; and Guideline 13: *Research involving vulnerable persons.*)

Guideline 15: Research involving individuals who by reason of mental or behavioural disorders are not capable of giving adequately informed consent

Before undertaking research involving individuals who by reason of mental or behavioural disorders are not capable of giving adequately informed consent, the investigator must ensure that:

– such persons will not be subjects of research that might equally well be carried out on persons whose capacity to give adequately informed consent is not impaired;
– the purpose of the research is to obtain knowledge relevant to the particular health needs of persons with mental or behavioural disorders;
– the consent of each subject has been obtained to the extent of that person's capabilities, and a prospective subject's refusal to participate in research is always respected, unless, in exceptional circumstances, there is no reasonable medical alternative and local law permits overriding the objection; and,
– in cases where prospective subjects lack capacity to consent, permission is obtained from a responsible family member or a legally authorized representative in accordance with applicable law.

Commentary on Guideline 15

General considerations Most individuals with mental or behavioural disorders are capable of giving informed consent; this Guideline is concerned only with those who are not capable or who because their condition deteriorates become temporarily incapable. They should never be subjects of research that might equally well be carried out on persons in full possession of their mental faculties, but they are clearly the only subjects suitable for a large part of research into the origins and treatment of certain severe mental or behavioural disorders.

Consent of the individual The investigator must obtain the approval of an ethical review committee to include in research persons who by reason of mental or behavioural disorders are not capable of giving informed consent. The willing cooperation of such persons should be sought to the extent that their mental state permits, and any objection on their part to taking part in any study that has no components designed to benefit them directly should always be respected. The objection of such an individual to an investigational intervention intended to be of therapeutic benefit should be respected unless there is no reasonable medical alternative and local law permits overriding the objection. The agreement of an immediate family member or other person with a close personal relationship with the individual should be sought, but it should be recognized that these proxies may have their own interests that may call their permission into question. Some relatives may not be primarily concerned with protecting the rights and welfare of the patients. Moreover, a close family member or friend may wish to take advantage of a research study in the hope that it will succeed in "curing" the condition. Some jurisdictions do not permit third-party permission for subjects lacking capacity to consent. Legal authorization may be necessary to involve in research an individual who has been committed to an institution by a court order.

Serious illness in persons who because of mental or behavioural disorders are unable to give adequately informed consent   Persons who because of mental or behavioural disorders are unable to give adequately informed consent and who have, or are at risk of, serious illnesses such as HIV infection, cancer or hepatitis should not be deprived of the possible benefits of investigational drugs, vaccines or devices that show promise of therapeutic or preventive benefit, particularly when no superior or equivalent therapy or prevention is available. Their entitlement to access to such therapy or prevention is justified ethically on the same grounds as is such entitlement for other vulnerable groups.

Persons who are unable to give adequately informed consent by reason of mental or behavioural disorders are, in general, not suitable for participation in formal clinical trials except those trials that are designed to be responsive to their particular health needs and can be carried out only with them.

(See also Guidelines 8: *Benefits and risks of study participation*; 9: *Special limitations on risks when subjects are not capable of giving consent*; and 13: *Research involving vulnerable persons*.)

Guideline 16: Women as research participants

Investigators, sponsors or ethical review committees should not exclude women of reproductive age from biomedical research. The potential for becoming pregnant during a study should not, in itself, be used as a reason for precluding or limiting participation. However, a thorough discussion of risks to the pregnant woman and to her fetus is a prerequisite for the woman's ability to make a rational decision to enrol in a clinical study. In this discussion, if participation in the research might be hazardous to a fetus or a woman if she becomes pregnant, the sponsors/investigators should guarantee the prospective subject a pregnancy test and access to effective contraceptive methods before the research commences. Where such access is not possible, for legal or religious reasons, investigators should not recruit for such possibly hazardous research women who might become pregnant.

Commentary on Guideline 16

Women in most societies have been discriminated against with regard to their involvement in research. Women who are biologically capable of becoming pregnant have been customarily excluded from formal clinical trials of drugs, vaccines and medical devices owing to concern about undetermined risks to the fetus. Consequently, relatively little is known about the safety and efficacy of most drugs, vaccines or devices for such women, and this lack of knowledge can be dangerous.

A general policy of excluding from such clinical trials women biologically capable of becoming pregnant is unjust in that it deprives women as a class of persons of the benefits of the new knowledge derived from the trials. Further, it is an affront to their right of self-determination. Nevertheless, although women of child-bearing age should be given the opportunity to participate in research, they should be helped to understand that the research could include risks to the fetus if they become pregnant during the research.

Although this general presumption favours the inclusion of women in research, it must be acknowledged that in some parts of the world women are vulnerable to neglect or harm in research because of their social conditioning to submit to authority, to ask no questions, and to tolerate pain and suffering. When women in such situations are potential subjects in research, investigators need to exercise special care in the informed consent process to ensure that they have adequate time and a proper environment in which to take decisions on the basis of clearly given information.

Individual consent of women In research involving women of reproductive age, whether pregnant or non-pregnant, only the informed consent of the woman herself is required for her participation. In no case should the permission of a spouse or partner replace the requirement of individual informed consent. If women wish to consult with their husbands or partners or seek voluntarily to obtain their permission before deciding to enrol in research, that is not only ethically permissible but in some contexts highly desirable. A strict requirement of authorization of spouse or partner, however, violates the substantive principle of respect for persons.

A thorough discussion of risks to the pregnant women and to her fetus is a prerequisite for the woman's ability to make a rational decision to enrol in a clinical study. For women who are not pregnant at the outset of a study but who might become pregnant while they are still subjects, the consent discussion should include information about the alternative of voluntarily withdrawing from the study and, where legally permissible, terminating the pregnancy. Also, if the pregnancy is not terminated, they should be guaranteed a medical follow-up.

(See also Guideline 17: *Pregnant women as research participants.*)

Guideline 17: Pregnant women as research participants

Pregnant women should be presumed to be eligible for participation in biomedical research. Investigators and ethical review committees should ensure that prospective subjects who are pregnant are adequately informed about the risks and benefits to themselves, their pregnancies, the fetus and their subsequent offspring, and to their fertility.

Research in this population should be performed only if it is relevant to the particular health needs of a pregnant woman or her fetus, or to the health needs of pregnant women in general, and, when appropriate, if it is supported by reliable evidence from animal experiments, particularly as to risks of teratogenicity and mutagenicity.

Commentary on Guideline 17

The justification of research involving pregnant women is complicated by the fact that it may present risks and potential benefits to two beings – the woman and the fetus – as well as to the person the fetus is destined to become. Though the decision about acceptability of risk should be made by the mother as part of the informed consent process, it is desirable in research directed at the health of the fetus to obtain the father's opinion also, when possible. Even when evidence concerning risks is unknown or ambiguous, the decision about acceptability of risk to the fetus should be made by the woman as part of the informed consent process.

Especially in communities or societies in which cultural beliefs accord more importance to the fetus than to the woman's life or health, women may feel constrained to participate, or not to participate, in research. Special safeguards should be established to prevent undue inducement to pregnant women to participate in research in which interventions hold out the prospect of direct benefit to the fetus. Where fetal abnormality is not recognized as an indication for abortion, pregnant women should not be recruited for research in which there is a realistic basis for concern that fetal abnormality may occur as a consequence of participation as a subject in research.

Investigators should include in protocols on research on pregnant women a plan for monitoring the outcome of the pregnancy with regard to both the health of the woman and the short-term and long-term health of the child.

Guideline 18: Safeguarding confidentiality

The investigator must establish secure safeguards of the confidentiality of subjects' research data. Subjects should be told the limits, legal or other, to the investigators' ability to safeguard confidentiality and the possible consequences of breaches of confidentiality.

Commentary on Guideline 18

Confidentiality between investigator and subject Research relating to individuals and groups may involve the collection and storage of information that, if disclosed to third parties, could cause harm or distress. Investigators should arrange to protect the confidentiality of such information by, for example, omitting information that might lead to the identification of individual subjects, limiting access to the information, anonymizing data, or other means. During the process of obtaining informed consent the investigator should inform the prospective subjects about the precautions that will be taken to protect confidentiality.

Prospective subjects should be informed of limits to the ability of investigators to ensure strict confidentiality and of the foreseeable adverse social consequences of breaches of confidentiality. Some jurisdictions require the reporting to appropriate agencies of, for instance, certain communicable diseases or evidence of child abuse or neglect. Drug regulatory authorities have the right to inspect clinical-trial records, and a sponsor's clinical-compliance audit staff may require and obtain access to confidential data. These and similar limits to the ability to maintain confidentiality should be anticipated and disclosed to prospective subjects.

Participation in HIV/AIDS drug and vaccine trials may impose upon the research subjects significant associated risks of social discrimination or harm; such risks merit consideration equal to that given to adverse medical consequences of the drugs and vaccines. Efforts must be made to reduce their likelihood and severity. For example, subjects in vaccine trials must be enabled to demonstrate that their HIV seropositivity is due to their having been vaccinated rather than to natural infection. This may be accomplished by providing them with documents attesting to their participation in vaccine trials, or by maintaining a confidential register of trial subjects, from which information can be made available to outside agencies at a subject's request.

Confidentiality between physician and patient   Patients have the right to expect that their physicians and other health-care professionals will hold all information about them in strict confidence and disclose it only to those who need, or have a legal right to, the information, such as other attending physicians, nurses, or other health-care workers who perform tasks related to the diagnosis and treatment of patients. A treating physician should not disclose any identifying information about patients to an investigator unless each patient has given consent to such disclosure and unless an ethical review committee has approved such disclosure.

Physicians and other health care professionals record the details of their observations and interventions in medical and other records. Epidemiological studies often make use of such records. For such studies it is usually impracticable to obtain the informed consent of each identifiable patient; an ethical review committee may waive the requirement for informed consent when this is consistent with the requirements of applicable law and provided that there are secure safeguards of confidentiality. (See also Guideline 4 Commentary: *Waiver of the consent requirement.*) In institutions in which records may be used for research purposes without the informed consent of patients, it is advisable to notify patients generally of such practices; notification is usually by means of a statement in patient-information brochures. For research limited to patients' medical records, access must be approved or cleared by an ethical review committee and must be supervised by a person who is fully aware of the confidentiality requirements.

Issues of confidentiality in genetic research   An investigator who proposes to perform genetic test of known clinical or predictive value on biological samples that can be linked to an identifiable individual must obtain the informed consent of the individual or, when indicated, the permission of a legally authorized representative. Conversely, before performing a genetic test that is of known predictive value or gives reliable information about a known heritable condition, and individual consent or permission has not been obtained, investigators must see that biological samples are fully anonymized and unlinked; this ensures that no information about specific individuals can be derived from such research or passed back to them.

When biological samples are not fully anonymized and when it is anticipated that there may be valid clinical or research reasons for linking the results of genetic tests to research subjects, the investigator in seeking informed consent should assure prospective subjects that their identity will be protected by secure coding of their samples (encryption) and by restricted access to the database, and explain to them this process.

When it is clear that for medical or possibly research reasons the results of genetic tests will be reported to the subject or to the subject's physician, the subject should be informed that such disclosure will occur and that the samples to be tested will be clearly labelled.

Investigators should not disclose results of diagnostic genetic tests to relatives of subjects without the subjects' consent. In places where immediate family relatives would usually expect to be informed of such results, the research protocol, as approved or cleared by the ethical review committee, should indicate the precautions in place to prevent such disclosure of results without the subjects' consent; such plans should be clearly explained during the process of obtaining informed consent.

Guideline 19: Right of injured subjects to treatment and compensation

Investigators should ensure that research subjects who suffer injury as a result of their participation are entitled to free medical treatment for such injury and to such financial or other assistance as would compensate them equitably for any resultant impairment, disability or handicap. In the case of death as a result of their participation, their dependants are entitled to compensation. Subjects must not be asked to waive the right to compensation.

Commentary on Guideline 19

Guideline 19 is concerned with two distinct but closely related entitlements. The first is the uncontroversial entitlement to free medical treatment and compensation for accidental injury inflicted by procedures or interventions performed exclusively to accomplish the purposes of research (non-therapeutic procedures). The second is the entitlement of dependants to material compensation for death or disability occurring as a direct result of study participation. Implementing a compensation system for research-related injuries or death is likely to be complex, however.

Equitable compensation and free medical treatment Compensation is owed to research subjects who are disabled as a consequence of injury from procedures performed solely to accomplish the purposes of research. Compensation and free medical treatment are generally not owed to research subjects who suffer expected or foreseen adverse reactions to investigational therapeutic, diagnostic or preventive interventions when such reactions are not different in kind from those known to be associated with established interventions in standard medical practice. In the early stages of drug testing (Phase I and early Phase II), it is generally unreasonable to assume that an investigational drug holds out the prospect of direct benefit for the individual subject; accordingly, compensation is usually owed to individuals who become disabled as a result of serving as subjects in such studies.

The ethical review committee should determine in advance: i) the injuries for which subjects will receive free treatment and, in case of impairment, disability or handicap resulting from such injuries, be compensated; and ii) the injuries for which they will not be compensated. Prospective subjects should be informed of the committee's decisions, as part of the process of informed consent. As an ethical review committee cannot make such advance determination in respect of unexpected or unforeseen adverse reactions, such reactions must be presumed compensable and should be reported to the committee for prompt review as they occur.

Subjects must not be asked to waive their rights to compensation or required to show negligence or lack of a reasonable degree of skill on the part of the investigator in order to claim free medical treatment or compensation. The informed consent process or form should contain no words that would absolve an investigator from responsibility in the case of accidental injury, or that would imply that subjects would waive their right to seek compensation for impairment, disability or handicap. Prospective subjects should be informed that they will not need to take legal action to secure the free medical treatment or compensation for injury to which they may be entitled. They should also be told what medical service or organization or individual will provide the medical treatment and what organization will be responsible for providing compensation.

Obligation of the sponsor with regard to compensation Before the research begins, the sponsor, whether a pharmaceutical company or other organization or institution, or a government (where government insurance is not precluded by law), should agree to provide compensation for any physical injury for which subjects are entitled to compensation, or come to an agreement with the investigator concerning the circumstances in which the investigator must rely on his or her own insurance coverage (for example, for negligence or failure of the investigator to follow the protocol, or where government insurance coverage is limited to negligence). In certain circumstances it may be advisable to follow both courses. Sponsors should seek adequate insurance against risks to cover compensation, independent of proof of fault.

Guideline 20: Strengthening capacity for ethical and scientific review and biomedical research

Many countries lack the capacity to assess or ensure the scientific quality or ethical acceptability of biomedical research proposed or carried out in their jurisdictions. In externally sponsored collaborative research, sponsors and investigators have an ethical obligation to ensure that biomedical research projects for which they are responsible in such countries contribute effectively to national or local capacity to design and conduct biomedical research, and to provide scientific and ethical review and monitoring of such research.

Capacity-building may include, but is not limited to, the following activities:

- establishing and strengthening independent and competent ethical review processes/committees
- strengthening research capacity
- developing technologies appropriate to health-care and biomedical research
- training of research and health-care staff
- educating the community from which research subjects will be drawn.

Commentary on Guideline 20

External sponsors and investigators have an ethical obligation to contribute to a host country's sustainable capacity for independent scientific and ethical review and biomedical research. Before undertaking research in a host country with little or no such capacity, external sponsors and investigators should include in the research protocol a plan that specifies the contribution they will make. The amount of capacity building reasonably expected should be proportional to the magnitude of the research project. A brief epidemiological study involving only review of medical records, for example, would entail relatively little, if any, such development, whereas a considerable contribution is to be expected to an external sponsor of, for instance, a large-scale vaccine field-trial expected to last two or three years.

The specific capacity-building objectives should be determined and achieved through dialogue and negotiation between external sponsors and host-country authorities. External sponsors would be expected to employ and, if necessary, train local individuals to function as investigators, research assistants or data managers, for example, and to provide, as necessary, reasonable amounts of financial, educational and other assistance for capacity-building. To avoid conflict of interest and safeguard the independence of review committees, financial assistance should not be provided directly to them; rather, funds should be made available to appropriate authorities in the host-country government or to the host research institution.

(See also Guideline 10: *Research in populations and communities with limited resources.*)

Guideline 21: Ethical obligation of external sponsors to provide health-care services

External sponsors are ethically obliged to ensure the availability of:
– health-care services that are essential to the safe conduct of the research;
– treatment for subjects who suffer injury as a consequence of research interventions; and,
– services that are a necessary part of the commitment of a sponsor to make a beneficial intervention or product developed as a result of the research reasonably available to the population or community concerned.

Commentary on Guideline 21

Obligations of external sponsors to provide health-care services will vary with the circumstances of particular studies and the needs of host countries. The sponsors' obligations in particular studies should be clarified before the research is begun. The research protocol should specify what health-care services will be made available, during and after the research, to the subjects themselves, to the community from which the subjects are drawn, or to the host country, and for how long. The details of these arrangements should be agreed by the sponsor, officials of the host country, other

interested parties, and, when appropriate, the community from which subjects are to be drawn. The agreed arrangements should be specified in the consent process and document.

Although sponsors are, in general, not obliged to provide health-care services beyond that which is necessary for the conduct of the research, it is morally praiseworthy to do so. Such services typically include treatment for diseases contracted in the course of the study. It might, for example, be agreed to treat cases of an infectious disease contracted during a trial of a vaccine designed to provide immunity to that disease, or to provide treatment of incidental conditions unrelated to the study.

The obligation to ensure that subjects who suffer injury as a consequence of research interventions obtain medical treatment free of charge, and that compensation be provided for death or disability occurring as a consequence of such injury, is the subject of Guideline 19, on the scope and limits of such obligations.

When prospective or actual subjects are found to have diseases unrelated to the research, or cannot be enrolled in a study because they do not meet the health criteria, investigators should, as appropriate, advise them to obtain, or refer them for, medical care. In general, also, in the course of a study, sponsors should disclose to the proper health authorities information of public health concern arising from the research.

The obligation of the sponsor to make reasonably available for the benefit of the population or community concerned any intervention or product developed, or knowledge generated, as a result of the research is considered in Guideline 10: *Research in populations and communities with limited resources.*

Appendix I

Items to be included in a protocol (or associated documents) for biomedical research involving human subjects

(Include the items relevant to the study/project in question)

1. Title of the study;
2. A summary of the proposed research in lay/non-technical language.
3. A clear statement of the justification for the study, its significance in development and in meeting the needs of the country/population in which the research is carried out;

4. The investigators' views of the ethical issues and considerations raised by the study and, if appropriate, how it is proposed to deal with them;

5. Summary of all previous studies on the topic, including unpublished studies known to the investigators and sponsors, and information on previously published research on the topic, including the nature, extent and relevance of animal studies and other preclinical and clinical studies;

6. A statement that the principles set out in these Guidelines will be implemented;

7. An account of previous submissions of the protocol for ethical review and their outcome;

8. A brief description of the site(s) where the research is to be conducted, including information about the adequacy of facilities for the safe and appropriate conduct of the research, and *relevant* demographic and epidemiological information about the country or region concerned;

9. Name and address of the sponsor;

10. Names, addresses, institutional affiliations, qualifications and experience of the principal investigator and other investigators;

11. The objectives of the trial or study, its hypotheses or research questions, its assumptions, and its variables;

12. A detailed description of the design of the trial or study. In the case of controlled clinical trials the description should include, but not be limited to, whether assignment to treatment groups will be randomized (including the method of randomization), and whether the study will be blinded (single blind, double blind), or open;

13. The number of research subjects needed to achieve the study objective, and how this was statistically determined;

14. The criteria for inclusion or exclusion of potential subjects, and justification for the exclusion of any groups on the basis of age, sex, social or economic factors, or for other reasons;

15. The justification for involving as research subjects any persons with limited capacity to consent or members of vulnerable social groups, and a description of special measures to minimize risks and discomfort to such subjects;

16. The process of recruitment, e.g., advertisement, and the steps to be taken to protect privacy and confidentiality during recruitment;

17. Description and explanation of all interventions (the method of treatment administration, including route of administration, dose, dose interval and treatment period for investigational and comparator products used);

18. Plans and justification for withdrawing or withholding standard therapies in the course of the research, including any resulting risks to subjects;

19. Any other treatment that may be given or permitted, or contraindicated, during the study;

20. Clinical and laboratory tests and other tests that are to be carried out;

21. Samples of the standardized case-report forms to be used, the methods of recording therapeutic response (description and evaluation of methods and frequency of measurement), the follow-up procedures, and, if applicable, the measures proposed to determine the extent of compliance of subjects with the treatment;

22. Rules or criteria according to which subjects may be removed from the study or clinical trial, or (in a multi-centre study) a centre may be discontinued, or the study may be terminated;

23. Methods of recording and reporting adverse events or reactions, and provisions for dealing with complications;

24. The known or foreseen risks of adverse reactions, including the risks attached to each proposed intervention and to any drug, vaccine or procedure to be tested;

25. For research carrying more than minimal risk of physical injury, details of plans, including insurance coverage, to provide treatment for such injury, including the funding of treatment, and to provide compensation for research-related disability or death;

26. Provision for continuing access of subjects to the investigational treatment after the study, indicating its modalities, the individual or organization responsible for paying for it, and for how long it will continue;

27. For research on pregnant women, a plan, if appropriate, for monitoring the outcome of the pregnancy with regard to both the health of the woman and the short-term and long-term health of the child;

28. The potential benefits of the research to subjects and to others;

29. The expected benefits of the research to the population, including new knowledge that the study might generate;

30. The means proposed to obtain individual informed consent and the procedure planned to communicate information to prospective subjects, including the name and position of the person responsible for obtaining consent;

31. When a prospective subject is not capable of informed consent, satisfactory assurance that permission will be obtained from a duly authorized person, or, in the case of a child who is sufficiently mature to understand the

implications of informed consent but has not reached the legal age of consent, that knowing agreement, or assent, will be obtained, as well as the permission of a parent, or a legal guardian or other duly authorized representative;

32. An account of any economic or other inducements or incentives to prospective subjects to participate, such as offers of cash payments, gifts, or free services or facilities, and of any financial obligations assumed by the subjects, such as payment for medical services;

33. Plans and procedures, and the persons responsible, for communicating to subjects information arising from the study (on harm or benefit, for example), or from other research on the same topic, that could affect subjects' willingness to continue in the study;

34. Plans to inform subjects about the results of the study;

35. The provisions for protecting the confidentiality of personal data, and respecting the privacy of subjects, including the precautions that are in place to prevent disclosure of the results of a subject's genetic tests to immediate family relatives without the consent of the subject;

36. Information about how the code, if any, for the subjects' identity is established, where it will be kept and when, how and by whom it can be broken in the event of an emergency;

37. Any foreseen further uses of personal data or biological materials;

38. A description of the plans for statistical analysis of the study, including plans for interim analysis, if any, and criteria for prematurely terminating the study as a whole if necessary;

39. Plans for monitoring the continuing safety of drugs or other interventions administered for purposes of the study or trial and, if appropriate, the appointment for this purpose of an independent data-monitoring (data and safety monitoring) committee;

40. A list of the references cited in the protocol;

41. The source and amount of funding of the research: the organization that is sponsoring the research and a detailed account of the sponsor's financial commitments to the research institution, the investigators, the research subjects, and, when relevant, the community;

42. The arrangements for dealing with financial or other conflicts of interest that might affect the judgement of investigators or other research personnel: informing the institutional conflict-of-interest committee of such conflicts of interest; the communication by that committee of the pertinent details of the information to the ethical review committee; and the transmission by that committee to the research subjects of the parts of the information that it decides should be passed on to them;

43. The time schedule for completion of the study;

44. For research that is to be carried out in a developing country or community, the contribution that the sponsor will make to capacity-building for scientific and ethical review and for biomedical research in the host country, and an assurance that the capacity-building objectives are in keeping with the values and expectations of the subjects and their communities;

45. Particularly in the case of an industrial sponsor, a contract stipulating who possesses the right to publish the results of the study, and a mandatory obligation to prepare with, and submit to, the principal investigators the draft of the text reporting the results;

46. In the case of a negative outcome, an assurance that the results will be made available, as appropriate, through publication or by reporting to the drug registration authority;

47. Circumstances in which it might be considered inappropriate to publish findings, such as when the findings of an epidemiological, sociological or genetics study may present risks to the interests of a community or population or of a racially or ethnically defined group of people;

48. A statement that any proven evidence of falsification of data will be dealt with in accordance with the policy of the sponsor to take appropriate action against such unacceptable procedures.

66

1991 international guidelines for ethical review of epidemiological studies

Council for International Organisations of Medical Sciences

Introduction

These Guidelines are intended for investigators, health policy-makers, members of ethical review committees, and others who have to deal with ethical issues that arise in epidemiology. They may also assist in the establishment of standards for ethical review of epidemiological studies.

The Guidelines are an expression of concern to ensure that epidemiological studies observe ethical standards. These standards apply to all who undertake any of the types of activity covered by the Guidelines. Investigators must always be held responsible for the ethical integrity of their studies.

Epidemiology is defined as the study of the distribution and determinants of health-related states or events in specified populations, and the application of this study to control of health problems.

Epidemiology has greatly improved the human condition in the present century. It has clarified our understanding of many physical, biological and behavioural dangers to health. Some of the knowledge obtained has been applied to the control of environmental and biological threats to health, such as diseases due to drinking polluted water. Other epidemiological knowledge has become part of popular culture, leading to changed values and behaviour, and thus has led to improved health: examples include attitudes towards personal hygiene, tobacco smoking, diet and exercise in relation to heart disease, and the use of seat-belts to reduce the risk of traffic injury and death.

Epidemiological practice and research are based mostly on observation, and require no intervention more invasive than asking questions and carrying out routine medical examinations. Practice and research may overlap, as, for example, when both routine surveillance of cancer and

original research on cancer are conducted by professional staff of a population-based cancer registry.

Epidemiological research is of two main types: observational and experimental:

Three types of observational epidemiological research are distinguished: *cross-sectional studies* (also known as surveys), *case-control studies*, and *cohort studies*. These types of study carry minimal risk to study subjects. They involve no intervention other than asking questions, carrying out medical examinations and, sometimes, laboratory tests or x-ray examinations. The informed consent of subjects is normally required, although there are some exceptions – for example, very large cohort studies conducted exclusively by examining medical records.

A *cross-sectional* study (survey) is commonly done on a random sample of a population. Study subjects are asked questions, medically examined, or asked to submit to laboratory tests. Its aim is to assess aspects of the health of a population, or to test hypotheses about possible causes of disease or suspected risk factors.

A *case-control* study compares the past history of exposure to risk among patients who have a specified condition (cases) with the past history of exposure to this risk among persons who resemble the cases in such respects as age and sex, but do not have the specified condition (controls). Differing frequency of past exposure among cases and controls can be statistically analysed to test hypotheses about causes or risk factors. Case-control studies are the method of choice for testing hypotheses about rare conditions, because they can be done with small numbers of cases. They generally do not involve invasion of privacy or violation of confidentiality. If a case-control study requires direct contact between research workers and study subjects, informed consent to participation in the study is required; if it entails only a review of medical records, informed consent may not be required and indeed may not be feasible.

In a *cohort study*, also known as a longitudinal or prospective study, individuals with differing exposure levels to suspected risk factors are identified and observed over a period, commonly years, and the rates of occurrence of the condition of interest are measured and compared in relation to exposure levels. This is a more robust research method than a cross-sectional or case-control study, but it requires study of large numbers for a long time and is costly. Usually it requires only asking questions and routine medical examinations; sometimes it requires laboratory tests. Informed consent is normally required, but an exception to this requirement is a retrospective cohort study that uses linked medical records. In a retrospective cohort study, the initial or base-line observations may relate to exposure many years earlier to a potentially harmful agent, such as x-rays, a prescribed drug or an occupational hazard, about which details are known; the final or endpoint observations are often obtained from death certificates. Numbers of subjects may be very large, perhaps millions, so it would be impracticable to obtain their informed consent. It is essential to identify precisely every individual studied; this is achieved by methods of matching that are built into record linkage systems. After identities have been established to compile the statistical tables, all personal identifying information is obliterated, and therefore privacy and confidentiality are safeguarded.

An experiment is a study in which the investigator intentionally alters one or more factors under controlled conditions to study the effects of doing so. The usual form of epidemiological experiment is the *randomized controlled trial*, which is done to test a preventive or therapeutic regimen or diagnostic procedure. Such experiments involving human subjects should be regarded as unethical unless there is genuine uncertainty about the regimen or procedure and this uncertainty can be clarified by research.

Usually in this form of experiment, subjects are allocated at random to groups, one group to receive, the other group not to receive, the experimental regimen or procedure. The experiment compares the outcomes in the two groups. Random allocation removes the effects of bias, which would destroy the validity of comparisons between the groups. Since it is always possible that harm may be caused to at least some of the subjects, their informed consent is essential.

Epidemiology is facing new challenges and opportunities. The application of information technology to large data-files has expanded the role and capacity of epidemiological studies. The acquired immunodeficiency syndrome (AIDS) epidemic and its management have given epidemiological studies new urgency; public health authorities are using population-screening studies to establish prevalence levels of human immunodeficiency virus (HIV) infection for purposes of monitoring and restricting the spread of infection. Ahead lie entirely new challenges, such as those arising from the conjunction of molecular and population genetics.

Preamble

The general conduct of biomedical studies is guided by statements of internationally recognized principles of human rights, including the Nuremberg Code and the World Medical Association's Declaration of Helsinki, as revised (Helsinki IV). These principles also underlie the Proposed International Guidelines for Biomedical Research Involving Human Subjects, issued by the Council for International Organizations of Medical Sciences in 1982. These and similar national codes are based on the model of clinical medicine, and often address interests of "patients" or individual "subjects". Epidemiological research concerns groups of people, and the above codes do not adequately cover its special features. Proposals for epidemiological studies should be reviewed independently on ethical grounds.

Ethical issues often arise as a result of conflict among competing sets of values, such as, in the field of public health, the conflict between the rights of individuals and the needs of communities. Adherence to these guidelines will not avoid all ethical problems in epidemiological studies. Many situations require careful discussion and informed judgement on the part of investigators, ethical review committees, administrators, health-care practitioners, policy-makers, and community representatives. Externally sponsored epidemiological studies in developing countries merit special attention. A framework for the application of these guidelines is set by the laws and practices in each jurisdiction in which it is proposed to undertake studies.

The purpose of ethical review is to consider the features of a proposed study in the light of ethical principles, so as to ensure that investigators have anticipated and satisfactorily resolved possible ethical objections, and to assess their responses to ethical issues raised by the study. Not all ethical principles weigh equally. A study may be assessed as ethical even if a usual ethical expectation, such as confidentiality of data, has not been comprehensively met, provided the potential benefits clearly outweigh the risks and the investigators give assurances of minimizing risks. It may even be unethical to reject such a study, if its rejection would deny a community the benefits it offers. The challenge of ethical review is to make assessments that take into account potential risks and benefits, and to reach decisions on which members of ethical review committees may reasonably differ.

Different conclusions may result from different ethical reviews of the same issue or proposal, and each conclusion may be ethically reached, given varying circumstances of place and time; a conclusion is ethical not merely because of what has been decided but also owing to the process of conscientious reflection and assessment by which it has been reached.

General ethical principles

All research involving human subjects should be conducted in accordance with four basic ethical principles, namely *respect for persons, beneficence, non-maleficence*, and *justice*. It is usually assumed that these principles guide the conscientious preparation of proposals for scientific studies. In varying circumstances, they may be expressed differently and given different weight, and their application, in all good faith, may have different effects and lead to different decisions or courses of action. These principles have been much discussed and clarified in recent decades, and it is the aim of these Guidelines that they be applied to epidemiology.

Respect for persons incorporates at least two other fundamental ethical principles, namely:

a) *autonomy*, which requires that those who are capable of deliberation about their personal goals should be treated with respect for their capacity for self-determination; and

b) *protection of persons* with impaired or diminished autonomy, which requires that those who are dependent or vulnerable be afforded security against harm or abuse.

Beneficence is the ethical obligation to maximize possible benefits and to minimize possible harms and wrongs. This principle gives rise to norms requiring that the risks of research be reasonable in the light of the expected benefits, that the research design be sound, and that the investigators be competent both to conduct the research and to assure the well-being of the research subjects.

Non-maleficence ("Do no harm") holds a central position in the tradition of medical ethics, and guards against avoidable harm to research subjects.

Justice requires that cases considered to be alike be treated alike, and that cases considered to be different be treated in ways that acknowledge the difference. When the principle of justice is applied to dependent or vulnerable subjects, its main concern is with the rules of *distributive justice*. Studies should be designed to obtain knowledge that benefits the class of persons of which the subjects are representative: the class of persons bearing the burden should receive an appropriate benefit, and the class primarily intended to benefit should bear a fair proportion of the risks and burdens of the study.

The rules of distributive justice are applicable within and among communities. Weaker members of communities should not bear disproportionate burdens of studies from which all members of the community are intended to benefit, and more dependent communities and countries should not bear disproportionate burdens of studies from which all communities or countries are intended to benefit.

General ethical principles may be applied at individual and community levels. At the level of the individual (*microethics*), ethics governs how one person should relate to another and the moral claims of each member of a community. At the level of the community, ethics applies to how one community relates to another, and to how a community treats each of its members (including prospective members) and members of other groups with different cultural values (macroethics). Procedures that are unethical at one level cannot be justified merely because they are considered ethically acceptable at the other.

Ethical principles applied to epidemiology

Informed consent

Individual consent

1. When individuals are to be subjects of epidemiological studies, their informed consent will usually be sought. For epidemiological studies that use personally identifiable private data, the rules for informed consent vary, as discussed further below. Consent is informed when it is given by a person who understands the purpose and nature of the study, what participation in the study requires the person to do and to risk, and what benefits are intended to result from the study.

2. An investigator who proposes not to seek informed consent has the obligation to explain to an ethical review committee how the study would be ethical in its absence: it may be impractical to locate subjects whose records are to be examined, or the purpose of some studies would be frustrated – for example, prospective subjects on being informed would change the behaviour that it is proposed to study, or might feel needlessly anxious about why they were subjects or study. The investigator will provide assurances that strict safeguards will be maintained to protect confidentiality and that the study is aimed at protecting or advancing health. Another justification for not seeking informed consent may be that subjects are made

aware through public announcements that it is customary to make personal data available for epidemiological studies.

3. An ethical issue may arise when occupational records, medical records, tissue samples, etc. are used for a purpose for which consent was not given, although the study threatens no harm. Individuals or their public representatives should normally be told that their data might be used in epidemiological studies, and what means of protecting confidentiality are provided. Consent is not required for use of publicly available information, although countries and communities differ with regard to the definition of what information about citizens is regarded as public. However, when such information is to be used, it is understood that investigators will minimize disclosure of personally sensitive information.

4. Some organizations and government agencies employ epidemiologists who may be permitted by legislation or employees' contracts to have access to data without subjects' consent. These epidemiologists must then consider whether it is ethical for them, in a given case, to use this power of access to personal data. Ethically, they may still be expected either to seek the consent of the individuals concerned, or to justify their access without such consent. Access may be ethical on such grounds as minimal risk of harm to individuals, public benefit, and investigators' protection of the confidentiality of the individuals whose data they study.

Community agreement

5. When it is not possible to request informed consent from every individual to be studied, the agreement of a representative of a community or group may be sought, but the representative should be chosen according to the nature, traditions and political philosophy of the community or group. Approval given by a community representative should be consistent with general ethical principles.

When investigators work with communities, they will consider communal rights and protection as they would individual rights and protection. For communities in which collective decision-making is customary, communal leaders can express the collective will. However, the refusal of individuals to participate in a study has to be respected: a leader may express agreement on behalf of a community, but an individual's refusal of personal participation is binding.

6. When people are appointed by agencies outside a group, such as a department of government, to speak for members of the group, investigators and ethical review committees should consider how authentically these people speak for the group, and if necessary seek also the agreement of other representatives. Representatives of a community or group may sometimes be in a position to participate in designing the study and in its ethical assessment.

7. The definition of a community or group for purposes of epidemiological study may be a matter of ethical concern. When members of a community are naturally conscious of its activities as a community and feel common interests with other members, the community exists, irrespective of the study proposal. Investigators will be sensitive to how a community is constituted or defines itself, and will respect the rights of underprivileged groups.

8. For pupposes of epidemiological study, investigators may define groups that are composed of statistically, geographically or otherwise associated individuals who do not normally interact socially. When such groups are artificially created for scientific study, group members may not readily be identifiable as leaders or representatives, and individuals may not be expected to risk disadvantage for the benefit of others. Accordingly, it will be more difficult to ensure group representation, and all the more important to obtain subjects' free and informed consent to participate.

Selective disclosure of information

9. In epidemiology, an acceptable study technique involves selective disclosure of information, which seems to conflict with the principle of informed consent. For certain epidemiological studies non-disclosure is permissible, even essential, so as to not influence the spontaneous conduct under investigation, and to avoid obtaining responses that the respondent might give in order to please the questioner. Selective disclosure may be benign and ethically permissible, provided that it does not induce subjects to do what they would not otherwise consent to do. An ethical review committee may permit disclosure of only selected information when this course is justified.

Undue influence

10. Prospective subjects may not feel free to refuse requests from those who have power or influence over them. Therefore the identity of the investigator or other person assigned to invite prospective subjects to participate must be made known to them. Investigators are expected to explain to the ethical review committee how they propose to neutralize such apparent influence. It is ethically questionable whether subjects should be recruited from among groups that are unduly influenced by persons in authority over them or by community leaders, if the study can be done with subjects who are not in this category.

Inducement to participate

11. Individuals or communities should not be pressured to participate in a study. However, it can be hard to draw the line between exerting pressure or offering inappropriate inducements and creating legitimate motivation. The benefits of a study, such as increased or new knowledge, are proper inducements. However, when people or communities lack basic health services or money, the prospect of being rewarded by goods, services or cash payments can induce participation. To determine the ethical propriety of such inducements, they must be assessed in the light of the traditions of the culture.

12. Risks involved in participation should be acceptable to subjects even in the absence of inducement. It is acceptable to repay incurred expenses, such as for travel. Similarly, promises of compensation and care for damage, injury or loss of income should not be considered inducements.

Maximizing benefit

Communication of study results

13. Part of the benefit that communities, groups and individuals may reasonably expect from participating in studies is that they will be told of findings that pertain to their health. Where findings could be applied in public health measures to improve community health, they should be communicated to the health authorities. In informing individuals of the findings and their pertinence to health, their level of literacy and comprehension must be considered. Research protocols should include provision for communicating such information to communities and individuals.

Research findings and advice to communities should be publicized by whatever suitable means are available. When HIV-prevalence studies are conducted by unlinked anonymous screening, there should be, where feasible, provision for voluntary HIV-antibody testing under conditions of informed consent, with pre- and post-test counselling, and assurance of confidentiality.

Impossibility of communicating study results

14. Subjects of epidemiological studies should be advised that it may not be possible to inform them about findings that pertain to their health, but that they should not take this to mean that they are free of the disease or condition under study. Often it may not be possible to extract from pooled findings information pertaining to individuals and their families, but when findings indicate a need of health care, those concerned should be advised of means of obtaining personal diagnosis and advice.

When epidemiological data are unlinked, a disadvantage to subjects is that individuals at risk cannot be informed of useful findings pertinent to their health. When subjects cannot be advised individually to seek medical attention, the ethical duty to do good can be served by making pertinent health-care advice available to their communities.

Release of study results

15. Investigators may be unable to compel release of data held by governmental or commercial agencies, but as health professionals they have an ethical obligation to advocate the release of information that is in the public interest.

Sponsors of studies may press investigators to present their findings in ways that advance special interests, such as to show that a product or procedure is or is not harmful to health. Sponsors must not present interpretations or inferences, or theories and hypotheses, as if they were proven truths.

Health care for the community under study

16. The undertaking of an epidemiological project in a developing country may create the expectation in the community concerned that it will be provided with health care, at least while the research workers are present. Such an expectation should not be frustrated, and, where people need health care, arrangements should be made to have them treated or they should be referred to a local health service that can provide the needed care.

Training local health personnel

17. While studies are in progress, particularly in developing countries, the opportunity should be taken to train local health workers in skills and techniques that can be used to improve health services. For instance, by training them in the operation of measuring devices and calculating machines, when a study team departs it leaves something of value, such as the ability to monitor disease or mortality rates.

Minimizing harm

Causing harm and doing wrong

18. Investigators planning studies will recognize the risk of causing harm, in the sense of bringing disadvantage, and of doing wrong, in the sense of transgressing values. Harm may occur, for instance, when scarce health personnel are diverted from their routine duties to serve the needs of a study, or when, unknown to a community, its health-care priorities are changed. It is wrong to regard members of communities as only impersonal material for study, even if they are not harmed.

19. Ethical review must always assess the risk of subjects or groups suffering stigmatization, prejudice, loss of prestige or self-esteem, or economic loss as a result of taking part in a study. Investigators will inform ethical review committees and prospective subjects of perceived risks, and of proposals to prevent or mitigate them. Investigators must be able to demonstrate that the benefits outweigh the risks for both individuals and groups. There should be a thorough analysis to determine who would be at risk and who would benefit from the study. It is unethical to expose persons to avoidable risks disproportionate to the expected benefits, or to permit a known risk to remain if it can be avoided or at least minimized.

20. When a healthy person is a member of a population or sub-group at raised risk and engages in high-risk activities, it is unethical not to propose measures for protecting the population or sub-group.

Preventing harm to groups

21. Epidemiological studies may inadvertently expose groups as well as individuals to harm, such as economic loss, stigmatization, blame, or withdrawal of services. Investigators who find sensitive information that may put a group at risk of adverse criticism or treatment should be discreet in communicating and explaining their findings. When the location or circumstances of a study are important to understanding the results, the investigators will explain by what means they propose to protect the group from harm or disadvantage; such means include provisions for confidentiality and the use of language that does not imply moral criticism of subjects' behaviour.

Harmful publicity

22. Conflict may appear between, on the one hand, doing no harm and, on the other, telling the truth and openly disclosing scientific findings. Harm may be mitigated by interpreting data in a way that protects the interests of those at risk, and is at the same time consistent with scientific integrity. Investigators should, where possible, anticipate and avoid misinterpretation that might cause harm.

Respect for social mores

23. Disruption of social mores is usually regarded as harmful. Although cultural values and social mores must be respected, it may be a specific aim of an epidemiological study to stimulate change in certain customs or conventional behaviour to lead through change to healthful behaviour – for instance, with regard to diet or a hazardous occupation.

24. Although members of communities have a right not to have others impose an uninvited "good" on them, studies expected to result in health benefits are usually considered ethically acceptable and not harmful. Ethical review committees should consider a study's potential for beneficial change. However, investigators should not overstate such benefits, in case a community's agreement to participate is unduly influenced by its expectation of better health services.

Sensitivity to different cultures

25. Epidemiologists often investigate cultural groups other than their own, inside or outside their own countries, and undertake studies initiated from outside the culture, community or country in which the study is to be conducted. Sponsoring and host countries may differ in the ways in which, in their cultures, ethical values are understood and applied – for instance, with regard to autonomy of individuals.

Investigators must respect the ethical standards of their own countries and the cultural expectations of the societies in which epidemiological studies are undertaken, unless this implies a violation of a transcending moral rule. Investigators risk harming their reputation by pursuing work that host countries find acceptable but their own countries consider offensive. Similarly, they may transgress the cultural values of the host countries by uncritically conforming to the expectations of their own.

Confidentiality

26. Research may involve collecting and storing data relating to individuals and groups, and such data, if disclosed to third parties, may cause harm or distress. Consequently, investigators should make arrangements for protecting the confidentiality of such data by, for example, omitting information that might lead to the identification of individual subjects, or limiting access to the data, or by other means. It is customary in epidemiology to aggregate numbers so that individual identities are obscured. Where group confidentiality cannot be maintained or is violated, the investigators should take steps to maintain or restore a group's good name and status. Information obtained about subjects is generally divisible into:

Unlinked information, which cannot be linked, associated or connected with the person to whom it refers; as this person is not known to the investigator, confidentiality is not at stake and the question of consent does not arise.

Linked information, which may be:
- anonymous, when the information cannot be linked to the person to whom it refers except by a code or other

means known only to that person, and the investigator cannot know the identity of the person;

- non-nominal, when the information can be linked to the person by a code (not including personal identification) known to the person and the investigator; or

- nominal or nominative, when the information is linked to the person by means of personal identification, usually the name.

Epidemiologists discard personal identifying information when consolidating data for purposes of statistical analysis. Identifiable personal data will not be used when a study can be done without personal identification – for instance, in testing unlinked anonymous blood samples for HIV infection. When personal identifiers remain on records used for a study, investigators should explain to review committees why this is necessary and how confidentiality will be protected. If, with the consent of individual subjects, investigators link different sets of data regarding individuals, they normally preserve confidentiality by aggregating individual data into tables or diagrams. In government service the obligation to protect confidentiality is frequently reinforced by the practice of swearing employees to secrecy.

Conflict of interest

Identification of conflict of interest

27. It is an ethical rule that investigators should have no undisclosed conflict of interest with their study collaborators, sponsors or subjects. Investigators should disclose to the ethical review committee any potential conflict of interest. Conflict can arise when a commercial or other sponsor may wish to use study results to promote a product or service, or when it may not be politically convenient to disclose findings.

28. Epidemiological studies may be initiated, or financially or otherwise supported, by governmental or other agencies that employ investigators. In the occupational and environmental health fields, several well-defined special-interest groups may be in conflict: shareholders, management, labour, government regulatory agencies, public interest advocacy groups, and others. Epidemiological investigators may be employed by any of these groups. It can be difficult to avoid pressures resulting from such conflict of interest, and consequent distorted interpretations of study findings. Similar conflict may arise in studies of the effects of drugs and in testing medical devices.

29. Investigators and ethical review committees will be sensitive to the risk of conflict, and committees will not normally approve proposals in which conflict of interest is inherent. If, exceptionally, such a proposal is approved,

the conflict of interest should be disclosed to prospective subjects and their communities.

30. There may appear to be conflict when subjects do not want to change their behaviour and investigators believe that they ought to do so for the sake of their health. However, this may not be a true conflict of interest, as the investigators are motivated by the subjects' health interests.

Scientific objectivity and advocacy

31. Honesty and impartiality are essential in designing and conducting studies, and presenting and interpreting findings. Data will not be withheld, misrepresented or manipulated. Investigators may discover health hazards that demand correction, and become advocates of means to protect and restore health. In this event, their advocacy must be seen to rely on objective, scientific data.

Ethical review procedures

Requirement of ethical review

32. The provisions for ethical review in a society are influenced by economic and political considerations, the organization of health care and research, and the degree of independence of investigators. Whatever the circumstances, there is a responsibility to ensure that the Declaration of Helsinki and the CIOMS International Guidelines for Biomedical Research Involving Human Subjects are taken into account in epidemiological studies.

33. The requirement that proposals for epidemiological studies be submitted to independent ethical review applies irrespective of the source of the proposals – academic, governmental, health-care, commercial, or other. Sponsors should recognize the necessity of ethical review and facilitate the establishment of ethical review committees. Sponsors and investigators are expected to submit their proposals to ethical review, and this should not be overlooked even when sponsors have legal power to permit investigators access to data. An exception is justified when epidemiologists must investigate outbreaks of acute communicable diseases. Then they must proceed without delay to identify and control health risks. They cannot be expected to await the formal approval of an ethical review committee. Nevertheless, in such circumstances the investigator will, as far as possible, respect the rights of individuals, namely freedom, privacy, and confidentiality.

Ethical review committees

34. Ethical review committees may be created under the aegis of national or local health administrations, national

medical research councils, or other nationally representative health-care bodies. The authority of committees operating on a local basis may be confined to one institution or extend to all biomedical studies undertaken in a defined political jurisdiction. However committees are created, and however their jurisdiction is defined, they should establish working rules – regarding, for instance, frequency of meetings, a quorum of members, decision-making procedures, and review of decisions, and they should issue such rules to prospective investigators.

35. In a highly centralized administration, a national review committee may be constituted to review study protocols from both scientific and ethical standpoints. In countries with a decentralized administration, protocols are more effectively and conveniently reviewed at a local or regional level. Local ethical review committees have two responsibilities: – to verify that all proposed interventions have been assessed for safety by a competent expert body, and – to ensure that all other ethical issues are satisfactorily resolved.

36. Local review committees act as a panel of investigators' peers, and their composition should be such as can ensure adequate review of the study proposals referred to them. Their membership should include epidemiologists, other health practitioners, and lay persons qualified to represent a range of community, cultural and moral values. Committees should have diverse composition and include representatives of any populations specially targeted for study. The members should change periodically to prevent individuals from becoming unduly influential, and to widen the network involved in ethical review. Independence from the investigators is maintained by precluding any member with a direct interest in a proposal from participating in its assessment.

Ethical conduct of members of review committees

37. Ethical review committee members must carefully guard against any tendencies to unethical conduct on their own part. In particular, they should protect the confidentiality of review-committee documents and discussions. Also, they should not compel investigators to submit to unnecessary repetition of review.

Representation of the community

38. The community to be studied should be represented in the ethical review process. This is consistent with respect for the culture, the dignity and self-reliance of the community, and the aim of achieving community members' full understanding of the study. It should not be considered that lack of formal education disqualifies community members from joining in constructive discussion on issues relating to the study and the application of its findings.

Balancing personal and social perspectives

39. In performing reviews, committees will consider both personal and social perspectives. While, at the personal level, it is essential to ensure individual informed and free consent, such consent alone may not be sufficient to render a study ethical if the individual's community finds the study objectionable. Social values may raise broad issues that affect future populations and the physical environment. For example, in proposals for the widespread application of measures to control intermediate hosts of disease organisms, investigators will anticipate the effects of those measures on communities and the environment, and review committees will ensure that there is adequate provision for the investigators to monitor the application of the measures so as to prevent unwanted effects.

Assuring scientific soundness

40. The primary functions of ethical review are to protect human subjects against risks of harm or wrong, and to facilitate beneficial studies. Scientific review and ethical review cannot be considered separately: a study that is scientifically unsound is unethical in exposing subjects to risk or inconvenience and achieving no benefit in knowledge. Normally, therefore, ethical review committees consider both scientific and ethical aspects. An ethical review committee may refer technical aspects of scientific review to a scientifically qualified person or committee, but will reach its own decision, based on such qualified advice, on scientific soundness. If a review committee is satisfied that a proposal is scientifically sound, it will then consider whether any risk to the subject is justified by the expected benefit, and whether the proposal is satisfactory with regard to informed consent and other ethical requirements.

Assessment of safety and quality

41. All drugs and devices under investigation must meet adequate standards of safety. In this respect, many countries lack resources to undertake independent assessment of technical data. A governmental multidisciplinary committee with authority to co-opt experts is the most suitable body for assessing the safety and quality of medicines, devices and procedures. Such a committee should include clinicians, pharmacologists, statisticians and epidemiologists, among others; for epidemiological studies, epidemiologists occupy a position of obvious significance. Ethical review procedures should provide for consultation with such a committee.

Equity in the selection of subjects

42. Epidemiological studies are intended to benefit populations, but individual subjects are expected to accept any risks associated with studies. When research is intended to benefit mostly the better off or healthier members of a population, it is particularly important in selecting subjects to avoid inequity on the basis of age, socioeconomic status, disability or other variables. Potential benefits and harm should be distributed equitably within and among communities that differ on grounds of age, gender, race, or culture, or other variables.

Vulnerable and dependent groups

43. Ethical review committees should be particularly vigilant in the case of proposals involving populations primarily of children, pregnant and nursing women, persons with mental illness or handicap, members of communities unfamiliar with medical concepts, and persons with restricted freedom to make truly independent choices, such as prisoners and medical students. Similar vigilance is called for in the case of proposals for invasive research with no direct benefit to its subjects.

Control groups

44. Epidemiological studies that require control (comparison) or placebotreated (i.e., non-treated) groups are governed by the same ethical standards as those that apply to clinical trials. Important principles are that:

 (i) the control group in a study of a condition that can cause death, disability or serious distress should receive the most appropriate currently established therapy; and

 (ii) if a procedure being tested against controls is demonstrated to be superior, it should be offered promptly to members of the control group.

A study will be terminated prematurely if the outcome in one group is clearly superior to that in the other, and all subjects will be offered the better treatment. Research protocols should include "stopping rules", i.e., procedures to monitor for, and act upon, such an event. Investigators must continually bear in mind the potential benefits of the study to the control group, and the prospect of improved health care from applying the findings to the control group.

Randomization

45. Trials in which the choice of regimen or procedure is determined by random allocation should be conducted only when there is genuine uncertainty about differences in outcome of two or more regimens or procedures. Where randomization is to be used, all subjects will be informed of the uncertainty about optimum regimens or procedures, and that the reason for the trial is to determine which of two or more is in the subjects' best interests. Informing subjects about such uncertainty can in itself arouse anxiety among patients, who may already be anxious for other reasons; therefore, tact and delicacy are required in communicating the information. Ethical review committees should ascertain whether investigators refer explicitly to informing subjects about this uncertainty, and should enquire what will be done to allay subjects' anxiety about it.

Random allocation also can cause anxiety: persons chosen for, or excluded from, the experimental regimen or procedure may become anxious or concerned about the reasons for their being chosen or excluded. Investigators may have to communicate to members of the study population some basic concepts about application of the laws of chance, and reassure them that the process of random allocation is not discriminatory.

Provision for multi-centre studies

46. When participation in a multi-centre study is proposed according to a common protocol, a committee will respect different opinions of other committees, while not compromising on the application of the ethical standards that it expects investigators to observe; and it will attempt to reconcile differences so as to preserve the benefits that only a multi-centre study can achieve. One way of doing so could be to include in the common protocol the necessary procedures. Another would be for the several committees to delegate their review functions to a joint committee of the centres collaborating in the study.

Compensation for accidental injury

47. Some epidemiological studies may inadvertently cause harm. Monetary losses should be promptly repaid. Compensation is difficult when it is not appropriate to make monetary payments. Breach of confidentiality or insensitive publication of study findings, leading to loss of group prestige, or to indignity, may be difficult to remedy. When harm results from a study, the body that has sponsored or endorsed the study should be prepared to make good the injury, by public apology or reparation.

Externally sponsored studies

48. Externally sponsored studies are studies undertaken in a host country but initiated, financed, and sometimes wholly or partly carried out by an external international or national agency, with the collaboration or agreement of the authorities or the host country.

Such a study implies two ethical obligations:

The initiating agency should submit the study protocol to ethical review, in which the ethical standards should be no less exacting than they would be for a study carried out in the initiating country.

The ethical review committee in the host country should satisfy itself that the proposed study meets its own ethical requirements.

49. It is in the interest of the host country to require that proposals initiated and financed externally be submitted for ethical approval in the initiating country, and for endorsement by a responsible authority of the same country, such as a health administration, a research council, or an academy of medicine or science.

50. A secondary objective of externally sponsored studies should be the training of health personnel of the host country to carry out similar study projects independently.

51. Investigators must comply with the ethical rules of the funding country and the host country. Therefore, they must be prepared to submit study proposals to ethical review committees in each country. Alternatively, there may be agreement to the decision of a single or joint ethical review committee. Moreover, if an international agency sponsors a study, its own ethical review requirements may have to be satisfied.

Distinguishing between research and programme evaluation

52. It may at times be difficult to decide whether a particular proposal is for an epidemiological study or for evaluation of a programme on the part of a health-care institution or department. The defining attribute of research is that it is designed to produce new, generalizable knowledge, as distinct from knowledge pertaining only to a particular individual or programme.

For instance, a governmental or hospital department may want to examine patients' records to determine the safety and efficacy of a facility, unit or procedure. If the examination is for research purposes, the proposal should be submitted to the committee that considers the ethical features of research proposals. However, if it is for the purpose of programme evaluation, conducted perhaps by staff of the institution to evaluate a therapeutic programme for its effects, the proposal may not need to be submitted to ethical review; on the contrary, it could be considered poor practice and unethical not to undertake this type of quality assurance. The prospect of benefit or avoidance of harm to patients may constitute an ethical value that outweighs the risk of breaching the confidentiality of former patients whose medical records are liable to be inspected without their consent.

If if is not clear whether a proposal involves epidemiological study or routine practice, it should be submitted to the ethical review committee responsible for epidemiological protocols, for its opinion on whether the proposal falls within its mandate.

Information to be provided by investigators

53. Whatever the pattern of the procedure of ethical review, the investigator must submit a detailed protocol comprising:

- a clear statement of the objectives, having regard to the present state of knowledge, and a justification for undertaking the investigation in human subjects;
- a precise description of all proposed procedures and interventions, including intended dosages of drugs and planned duration of treatment;
- a statistical plan indicating the number of subjects to be involved;
- the criteria for terminating the study; and
- the criteria determining admission and withdrawal of individual subjects, including full details of the procedure for obtaining informed consent.

Also, the protocol should:

- include information to establish the safety of each proposed procedure and intervention, and of any drug, vaccine or device to be tested, including the results of relevant laboratory and animal research;
- specify the presumed benefits to subjects, and the possible risks of proposed procedures
- indicate the means and documents proposed to be used for eliciting informed consent, or, when such consent cannot be requested, state what approved alternative means of obtaining agreement will be used, and how it is proposed to protect the rights and assure the welfare of subjects;
- provide evidence that the investigator is properly qualified and experienced, or, when necessary, works under a competent supervisor, and that the investigator has access to adequate facilities for the safe and efficient conduct of the research; – describe the proposed means of protecting confidentiality during the processing and publication of study results; and
- refer to any other ethical considerations that may be involved, and indicate that the provisions of the Declaration of Helsinki will be respected.

Operational guidelines for ethics committees that review biomedical research

UNDP/World Bank/WHO Special Program for Research and Training in Tropical Diseases (TDR)

Final

21 February 2000, version 1.8

Comments and suggestions are invited:

Dr. Juntra Karbwang

Clinical Coordinator

Product Research and Development

TDR

World Health Organization

CH-1211 Geneva 27

Switzerland

Tel +41 22 791 3867/8

Fax +41 22 791 4854

E-mail: karbwangj@who.ch

Table of contents

Preface

The ethical and scientific standards for carrying out biomedical research on human subjects have been developed and established in international guidelines, including the Declaration of Helsinki, the CIOMS International Ethical Guidelines for Biomedical Research Involving Human Subjects, and the WHO and ICH Guidelines for Good Clinical Practice. Compliance with these guidelines helps to ensure that the dignity, rights, safety, and well-being of research participants are promoted and that the results of the investigations are credible.

All international guidelines require the ethical and scientific review of biomedical research alongside informed consent and the appropriate protection of those unable to consent as essential measures to protect the individual person and the communities who participate in research. For the purposes of these Guidelines, biomedical research includes research on pharmaceuticals, medical devices, medical radiation and imaging, surgical procedures, medical records, and biological samples, as well as epidemiological, social, and psychological investigations.

These Guidelines are intended to facilitate and support ethical review in all countries around the world. They are based on a close examination of the requirements for ethical review as established in international guidelines, as well as on an evaluation of existing practices of ethical review in countries around the world. They do not, however, purport to replace the need for national and local guidelines for the ethical review of biomedical research, nor do they intend to supersede national laws and regulations.

The majority of biomedical research has been predominantly motivated by concern for the benefit of already privileged communities. This is reflected by the fact that the WHO estimates that 90% of the resources devoted to research and development on medical problems are applied to diseases causing less than 10% of the present global suffering. The establishment of international guidelines that assist in strengthening the capacity for the ethical review of biomedical research in all countries contributes to redressing this imbalance.

1 Objective

The objective of these Guidelines is to contribute to the development of quality and consistency in the ethical review of biomedical research. The Guidelines are intended to complement existing laws, regulations, and practices, and to serve as a basis upon which ethics committees (ECs) can develop their own specific written procedures for their functions in biomedical research. In this regard, the Guidelines establish an international standard for ensuring quality in ethical review. The Guidelines should be used by national and local bodies in developing, evaluating, and progressively refining standard operating procedures for the ethical review of biomedical research.

2 The role of an EC

The purpose of an EC in reviewing biomedical research is to contribute to safeguarding the dignity, rights, safety, and well-being of all actual or potential research participants. A cardinal principle of research involving human participants is 'respect for the dignity of persons'. The goals of research, while important, should never be permitted to override the health, well-being, and care of research participants. ECs should also take into consideration the principle of justice. Justice requires that the benefits and burdens of research be distributed fairly among all groups and classes in society, taking into account age, gender, economic status, culture, and ethnic considerations.

ECs should provide independent, competent, and timely review of the ethics of proposed studies. In their composition, procedures, and decision-making, ECs need to have independence from political, institutional, professional, and market influences. They need to similarly demonstrate competence and efficiency in their work.

ECs are responsible for carrying out the review of proposed research before the commencement of the research. They also need to ensure that there is regular evaluation of the ethics of ongoing studies that received a positive decision.

ECs are responsible for acting in the full interest of potential research participants and concerned communities, taking into account the interests and needs of the researchers, and having due regard for the requirements of relevant regulatory agencies and applicable laws.

3 Establishing a system of ethical review

Countries, institutions, and communities should strive to develop ECs and ethical review systems that ensure the broadest possible coverage of protection for potential research participants and contribute to the highest attainable quality in the science and ethics of biomedical research. States should promote, as appropriate, the establishment of ECs at the national, institutional, and local levels that are independent, multi-disciplinary, multi-sectorial, and pluralistic in nature. ECs require administrative and financial support.

Procedures need to be established for relating various levels of review in order to ensure consistency and facilitate cooperation. Mechanisms for cooperation and communication need to be developed between national committees and institutional and local committees. These mechanisms should ensure clear and efficient communication. They should also promote the development of ethical review within a country as well as the ongoing education of members of ethics committees. In addition, procedures need to be established for the review of biomedical research protocols carried out at more than one site in a country or in more than one country. A network of ethical review should be established at the regional, national, and local levels that ensures the highest competence in biomedical review while also guaranteeing input from all levels of the community.

4 Constituting an EC

ECs should be constituted to ensure the competent review and evaluation of all ethical aspects of the research projects they receive and to ensure that their tasks can be executed free from bias and influence that could affect their independence.

ECs should be multidisciplinary and multi-sectorial in composition, including relevant scientific expertise, balanced age and gender distribution, and laypersons representing the interests and the concerns of the community.

ECs should be established in accordance with the applicable laws and regulations of the country and in accordance with the values and principles of the communities they serve.

ECs should establish publicly available standard operating procedures that state the authority under which the committee is established, the functions and duties of the EC, membership requirements, the terms of appointment, the conditions of appointment, the offices, the structure of the secretariat, internal procedures, and the quorum requirements. ECs should act in accordance with their written operating procedures.

It may be helpful to summarize the activities of the EC in a regular (annual) report.

4.1 Membership requirements

Clear procedures for identifying or recruiting potential EC members should be established. A statement should be drawn up of the requirements for candidacy that includes an outline of the duties and responsibilities of EC members.

Membership requirements should be established that include the following:

4.1.1 the name or description of the party responsible for making appointments;

4.1.2 the procedure for selecting members, including the method for appointing a member (e.g., by consensus, by majority vote, by direct appointment);

4.1.3 conflicts of interest should be avoided when making appointments, but where unavoidable there should be transparency with regard to such interests.

A rotation system for membership should be considered that allows for continuity, the development and maintenance of expertise within the EC, and the regular input of fresh ideas and approaches.

4.2 Terms of appointment

Terms of appointment should be established that include the following:

4.2.1 the duration of an appointment,

4.2.2 the policy for the renewal of an appointment,

4.2.3 the disqualification procedure,

4.2.4 the resignation procedure,

4.2.5 the replacement procedure.

4.3 Conditions of appointment

A statement of the conditions of appointment should be drawn up that includes the following:

4.3.1 a member should be willing to publicize his/her full name, profession, and affiliation;

4.3.2 all reimbursement for work and expenses, if any, within or related to an EC should be recorded and made available to the public upon request;

4.3.3 a member should sign a confidentiality agreement regarding meeting deliberations, applications, information on research participants, and related matters; in addition, all EC administrative staff should sign a similar confidentiality agreement.

4.4 Offices

ECs should establish clearly defined offices for the good functioning of ethical review. A statement is required of the officers within the EC (e.g., chairperson, secretary), the requirements for holding each office, the terms and conditions of each office, and the duties and responsibilities of each office (e.g., agenda, minutes, notification of decisions). Clear procedures for selecting or appointing officers should be established.

In addition to the EC officers, an EC should have adequate support staff for carrying out its responsibilities.

4.5 Quorum requirements

ECs should establish specific quorum requirements for reviewing and deciding on an application. These requirements should include the following:

4.5.1 the minimum number of members required to compose a quorum (e.g., more than half the members);

4.5.2 the professional qualifications requirements (e.g., physician, lawyer, statistician, paramedical, layperson) and the distribution of those requirements over the quorum; no quorum should consist entirely of members of one profession or one gender; a quorum should include at least one member whose primary area of expertise is in a non-scientific area, and at least one member who is independent of the institution/research site.

4.6 Independent consultants

ECs may call upon, or establish a standing list of, independent consultants who may provide special expertise to the EC on proposed research protocols. These consultants may be specialists in ethical or legal aspects, specific diseases or methodologies, or they may be representatives of communities, patients, or special interest groups. Terms of reference for independent consultants should be established.

4.7 Education for EC members

EC members have a need for initial and continued education regarding the ethics and science of biomedical research. The conditions of appointment should state the provisions available for EC members to receive introductory training in the work of an EC as well as ongoing opportunities for enhancing their capacity for ethical review. These conditions should also include the requirements or expectations regarding the initial and continuing education of EC members. This education may be linked to cooperative arrangements with other ECs in the area, the country, and the region, as well as other opportunities for the initial and continued training of EC members.

5 Submitting an application

ECs are responsible for establishing well-defined requirements for submitting an application for review of a biomedical research project. These requirements should be readily available to prospective applicants.

5.1 Application

An application for review of the ethics of proposed biomedical research should be submitted by a qualified researcher responsible for the ethical and scientific conduct of the research.

5.2 Application requirements

The requirements for the submission of a research project for ethical review should be clearly described in an application procedure. These requirements should include the following:

5.2.1 the name(s) and address(es) of the EC secretariat or member(s) to whom the application material is to be submitted;

5.2.2 the application form(s);

5.2.3 the format for submission;

5.2.4 the documentation (see 5.3);

5.2.5 the language(s) in which (core) documents are to be submitted;

5.2.6 the number of copies to be submitted;

5.2.7 the deadlines for submission of the application in relation to review dates;

5.2.8 the means by which applications will be acknowledged, including the communication of the incompleteness of an application;

5.2.9 the expected time for notification of the decision following review;

5.2.10 the time frame to be followed in cases where the EC requests supplementary information or changes to documents from the applicant;

5.2.11 the fee structure, if any, for reviewing an application;

5.2.12 the application procedure for amendments to the protocol, the recruitment material, the potential research participant information, or the informed consent form.

5.3 Documentation

All documentation required for a thorough and complete review of the ethics of proposed research should be submitted by the applicant. This may include, but is not limited to,

5.3.1 signed and dated application form;

5.3.2 the protocol of the proposed research (clearly identified and dated), together with supporting documents and annexes;

5.3.3 a summary (as far as possible in non-technical language), synopsis, or diagrammatic representation ('flowchart') of the protocol;

5.3.4 a description (usually included in the protocol) of the ethical considerations involved in the research;

5.3.5 case report forms, diary cards, and other questionnaires intended for research participants;

5.3.6 when the research involves a study product (such as a pharmaceutical or device under investigation), an adequate summary of all safety, pharmacological, pharmaceutical, and toxicological data available on the study product, together with a summary of clinical experience with the study product to date (e.g., recent investigator's brochure, published data, a summary of the product's characteristics);

5.3.7 investigator(s)'s curriculum vitae (updated, signed, and dated);

5.3.8 material to be used (including advertisements) for the recruitment of potential research participants;

5.3.9 a description of the process used to obtain and document consent;

5.3.10 written and other forms of information for potential research participants (clearly identified and dated) in the language(s) understood by the potential research participants and, when required, in other languages;

5.3.11 informed consent form (clearly identified and dated) in the language(s) understood by the potential research participants and, when required, in other languages;

5.3.12 a statement describing any compensation for study participation (including expenses and access to medical care) to be given to research participants;

5.3.13 a description of the arrangements for indemnity, if applicable;

5.3.14 a description of the arrangements for insurance coverage for research participants, if applicable;

5.3.15 a statement of agreement to comply with ethical principles set out in relevant guidelines;

5.3.16 all significant previous decisions (e.g., those leading to a negative decision or modified protocol) by other ECs or regulatory authorities for the proposed study (whether in the same location or elsewhere) and an indication of modification(s) to the protocol made on that account. The reasons for previous negative decisions should be provided.

6 Review

All properly submitted applications should be reviewed in a timely fashion and according to an established review procedure.

6.1 Meeting requirements

ECs should meet regularly on scheduled dates that are announced in advance. The meeting requirements should include the following:

6.1.1 meetings should be planned in accordance with the needs of the workload;

6.1.2 EC members should be given enough time in advance of the meeting to review the relevant documents;

6.1.3 meetings should be minuted; there should be an approval procedure for the minutes;

6.1.4 the applicant, sponsor, and/or investigator may be invited to present the proposal or elaborate on specific issues;

6.1.5 independent consultants may be invited to the meeting or to provide written comments, subject to applicable confidentiality agreements.

6.2 Elements of the review

The primary task of an EC lies in the review of research proposals and their supporting documents, with special attention given to the informed consent process, documentation, and the suitability and feasibility of the protocol. ECs need to take into account prior scientific reviews, if any, and

the requirements of applicable laws and regulations. The following should be considered, as applicable:

6.2.1 Scientific design and conduct of the study

6.2.1.1 the appropriateness of the study design in relation to the objectives of the study, the statistical methodology (including sample size calculation), and the potential for reaching sound conclusions with the smallest number of research participants;

6.2.1.2 the justification of predictable risks and inconveniences weighed against the anticipated benefits for the research participants and the concerned communities;

6.2.1.3 the justification for the use of control arms;

6.2.1.4 criteria for prematurely withdrawing research participants;

6.2.1.5 criteria for suspending or terminating the research as a whole;

6.2.1.6 the adequacy of provisions made for monitoring and auditing the conduct of the research, including the constitution of a data safety monitoring board (DSMB);

6.2.1.7 the adequacy of the site, including the supporting staff, available facilities, and emergency procedures;

6.2.1.8 the manner in which the results of the research will be reported and published;

6.2.2 Recruitment of research participants

6.2.2.1 the characteristics of the population from which the research participants will be drawn (including gender, age, literacy, culture, economic status, and ethnicity);

6.2.2.2 the means by which initial contact and recruitment is to be conducted;

6.2.2.3 the means by which full information is to be conveyed to potential research participants or their representatives;

6.2.2.4 inclusion criteria for research participants;

6.2.2.5 exclusion criteria for research participants;

6.2.3 Care and protection of research participants

6.2.3.1 the suitability of the investigator(s)'s qualifications and experience for the proposed study;

6.2.3.2 any plans to withdraw or withhold standard therapies for the purpose of the research, and the justification for such action;

6.2.3.3 the medical care to be provided to research participants during and after the course of the research;

6.2.3.4 the adequacy of medical supervision and psychosocial support for the research participants;

6.2.3.5 steps to be taken if research participants voluntarily withdraw during the course of the research;

6.2.3.6 the criteria for extended access to, the emergency use of, and/or the compassionate use of study products;

6.2.3.7 the arrangements, if appropriate, for informing the research participant's general practitioner (family doctor), including procedures for seeking the participant's consent to do so;

6.2.3.8 a description of any plans to make the study product available to the research participants following the research;

6.2.3.9 a description of any financial costs to research participants;

6.2.3.10 the rewards and compensations for research participants (including money, services, and/or gifts);

6.2.3.11 the provisions for compensation/treatment in the case of the injury/disability/death of a research participant attributable to participation in the research;

6.2.3.12 the insurance and indemnity arrangements;

6.2.4 Protection of research participant confidentiality

6.2.4.1 a description of the persons who will have access to personal data of the research participants, including medical records and biological samples;

6.2.4.2 the measures taken to ensure the confidentiality and security of personal information concerning research participants;

6.2.5 Informed consent process

6.2.5.1 a full description of the process for obtaining informed consent, including the identification of those responsible for obtaining consent;

6.2.5.2 the adequacy, completeness, and understandability of written and oral information to be given to the research participants, and, when appropriate, their legally acceptable representative(s);

6.2.5.3 clear justification for the intention to include in the research individuals who cannot consent, and a full account of the arrangements for obtaining consent or authorization for the participation of such individuals;

6.2.5.4 assurances that research participants will receive information that becomes available during the course of the research relevant to their participation (including their rights, safety, and well-being);

6.2.5.5 the provisions made for receiving and responding to queries and complaints from research participants or their representatives during the course of a research project;

6.2.6 Community considerations

6.2.6.1 the impact and relevance of the research on the local community and on the concerned communities from which the research participants are drawn;

6.2.6.2 the steps taken to consult with the concerned communities during the course of designing the research;

6.2.6.3 the influence of the community on the consent of individuals;

6.2.6.4 proposed community consultation during the course of the research;

6.2.6.5 the extent to which the research contributes to capacity building, such as the enhancement of local healthcare, research, and the ability to respond to public health needs;

6.2.6.6 a description of the availability and affordability of any successful study product to the concerned communities following the research;

6.2.6.7 the manner in which the results of the research will be made available to the research participants and the concerned communities.

6.3 Expedited review

ECs should establish procedures for the expedited review of research proposals. These procedures should specify the following:

6.3.1 the nature of the applications, amendments, and other considerations that will be eligible for expedited review;

6.3.2 the quorum requirement(s) for expedited review;

6.3.3 the status of decisions (e.g., subject to confirmation by full EC or not).

7 Decision-making

In making decisions on applications for the ethical review of biomedical research, an EC should take the following into consideration:

7.1 a member should withdraw from the meeting for the decision procedure concerning an application where there arises a conflict of interest; the conflict of interest should be indicated to the chairperson prior to the review of the application and recorded in the minutes;

7.2 a decision may only be taken when sufficient time has been allowed for review and discussion of an application in the absence of non-members (e.g., the investigator, representatives of the sponsor, independent consultants) from the meeting, with the exception of EC staff;

7.3 decisions should only be made at meetings where a quorum (as stipulated in the EC's written operating procedures) is present;

7.4 the documents required for a full review of the application should be complete and the relevant elements mentioned above (see 6.2) should be considered before a decision is made;

7.5 only members who participate in the review should participate in the decision;

7.6 there should be a predefined method for arriving at a decision (e.g., by consensus, by vote); it is recommended that decisions be arrived at through consensus, where possible; when a consensus appears unlikely, it is recommended that the EC vote;

7.7 advice that is non-binding may be appended to the decision;

7.8 in cases of conditional decisions, clear suggestions for revision and the procedure for having the application re-reviewed should be specified;

7.9 a negative decision on an application should be supported by clearly stated reasons.

8 Communicating a decision

A decision should be communicated in writing to the applicant according to EC procedures, preferably within two weeks' time of the meeting at which the decision was made. The communication of the decision should include, but is not limited to, the following:

8.1 the exact title of the research proposal reviewed;

8.2 the clear identification of the protocol of the proposed research or amendment, date and version number (if applicable). on which the decision is based;

8.3 the names and (where possible) specific identification numbers (version numbers/dates) of the documents reviewed, including the potential research participant information sheet/material and informed consent form;

8.4 the name and title of the applicant;

8.5 the name of the site(s);

8.6 the date and place of the decision;

8.7 the name of the EC taking the decision;

8.8 a clear statement of the decision reached;

8.9 any advice by the EC;

8.10 in the case of a conditional decision, any requirements by the EC, including suggestions for revision and the procedure for having the application re-reviewed;

8.11 in the case of a positive decision, a statement of the responsibilities of the applicant; for example, confirmation of the acceptance of any requirements imposed

by the EC; submission of progress report(s); the need to notify the EC in cases of protocol amendments (other than amendments involving only logistical or administrative aspects of the study); the need to notify the EC in the case of amendments to the recruitment material, the potential research participant information, or the informed consent form; the need to report serious and unexpected adverse events related to the conduct of the study; the need to report unforeseen circumstances, the termination of the study, or significant decisions by other ECs; the information the EC expects to receive in order to perform ongoing review; the final summary or final report;

8.12 the schedule/plan of ongoing review by the EC;

8.13 in the case of a negative decision, clearly stated reason(s) for the negative decision;

8.14 signature (dated) of the chairperson (or other authorized person) of the EC.

9 Follow-up

ECs should establish a follow-up procedure for following the progress of all studies for which a positive decision has been reached, from the time the decision was taken until the termination of the research. The ongoing lines of communication between the EC and the applicant should be clearly specified. The follow-up procedure should take the following into consideration:

9.1 the quorum requirements, the review procedure, and the communication procedure for follow-up reviews, which may vary from the requirements and procedures for the initial decision on an application;

9.2 the follow-up review intervals should be determined by the nature and the events of research projects, though each protocol should undergo a follow-up review at least once a year;

9.3 the following instances or events require the follow-up review of a study:

a any protocol amendment likely to affect the rights, safety, and/or well-being of the research participants or the conduct of the study;

b serious and unexpected adverse events related to the conduct of the study or study product, and the response taken by investigators, sponsors, and regulatory agencies;

c any event or new information that may affect the benefit/risk ratio of the study;

9.4 a decision of a follow-up review should be issued and communicated to the applicant, indicating a modification, suspension, or termination of the EC's original decision or confirmation that the decision is still valid;

9.5 in the case of the premature suspension/termination of a study, the applicant should notify the EC of the reasons for suspension/termination; a summary of results obtained in a study prematurely suspended/terminated should be communicated to the EC;

9.6 ECs should receive notification from the applicant at the time of the completion of a study;

9.7 ECs should receive a copy of the final summary or final report of a study.

10 Documentation and archiving

All documentation and communication of an EC should be dated, filed, and archived according to written procedures. A statement is required defining the access and retrieval procedure (including authorized persons) for the various documents, files, and archives.

It is recommended that documents be archived for a minimum period of 3 years following the completion of a study.

Documents that should be filed and archived include, but are not limited to,

10.1 the constitution, written standard operating procedures of the EC, and regular (annual) reports;

10.2 the curriculum vitae of all EC members;

10.3 a record of all income and expenses of the EC, including allowances and reimbursements made to the secretariat and EC members;

10.4 the published guidelines for submission established by the EC;

10.5 the agenda of the EC meetings;

10.6 the minutes of the EC meetings;

10.7 one copy of all materials submitted by an applicant;

10.8 the correspondence by EC members with applicants or concerned parties regarding application, decision, and follow-up;

10.9 a copy of the decision and any advice or requirements sent to an applicant;

10.10 all written documentation received during the follow-up;

10.11 the notification of the completion, premature suspension, or premature termination of a study;

10.12 the final summary or final report of the study.

Glossary

The definitions provided within this glossary apply to terms as they are used in these Guidelines. The terms may have different meanings in other contexts.

advice
Non-binding considerations adjoined to a decision intended to provide ethical assistance to those involved in the research.

applicant
A qualified researcher undertaking the scientific and ethical responsibility for a research project, either on his/her own behalf or on behalf of an organization/firm, seeking a decision from an ethics committee through formal application.

community
A community is a group of people understood as having a certain identity due to the sharing of common interests or to a shared proximity. A community may be identified as a group of people living in the same village, town, or country and, thus, sharing geographical proximity. A community may be otherwise identified as a group of people sharing a common set of values, a common set of interests, or a common disease.

conflict of interest
A conflict of interest arises when a member (or members) of the EC holds interests with respect to specific applications for review that may jeopardize his/her (their) ability to provide a free and independent evaluation of the research focused on the protection of the research participants. Conflicts of interests may arise when an EC member has financial, material, institutional, or social ties to the research.

decision
The response (either positive, conditional, or negative) by an EC to an application following the review in which the position of the EC on the ethical validity of the proposed study is stated.

investigator
A qualified scientist who undertakes scientific and ethical responsibility, either on his/her own behalf or on behalf of an organization/firm, for the ethical and scientific integrity of a research project at a specific site or group of sites. In some instances a coordinating or principal investigator may be appointed as the responsible leader of a team of subinvestigators.

protocol
A document that provides the background, rationale, and objective(s) of a biomedical research project and describes its design, methodology, and organization, including ethical and statistical considerations. Some of these considerations may be provided in other documents referred to in the protocol.

protocol amendment

A written description of a change to, or formal clarification of, a protocol.

requirements

In the context of decisions, requirements are binding elements that express ethical considerations whose implementation the ethics committee requires or views as obligatory in pursuing the research.

research participant

An individual who participates in a biomedical research project, either as the direct recipient of an intervention (e.g., study product or invasive procedure), as a control, or through observation. The individual may be a healthy person who volunteers to participate in the research, or a person with a condition unrelated to the research carried out who volunteers to participate, or a person (usually a patient) whose condition is relevant to the use of the study product or questions being investigated.

sponsor

An individual, company, institution, or organization that takes responsibility for the initiation, management, and/or financing of a research project.

SUPPORTING DOCUMENTS

Council for International Organizations of Medical Sciences (CIOMS), in collaboration with the World Health Organization (WHO). *International Ethical Guidelines for Biomedical Research Involving Human Subjects*. Geneva 1993.

Council for International Organizations of Medical Sciences (CIOMS). *International Guidelines for Ethical Review of Epidemiological Studies*. Geneva 1991.

Council of Europe. *Convention for the Protection of Human Rights and Dignity of the Human Being with Regard to the Application of Biology and Medicine: Convention on Human Rights and Biomedicine*. European Treaty Series – No. 164. Oviedo, 4 April 1997.

Department of Health, Education, and Welfare, Office of the Secretary, Protection of Human Subjects. *Belmont Report: Ethical Principles and Guidelines for the Protection of Human Subjects of Research. Report of the National Committee for the Protection of Human Subjects of Biomedical and Behavioural Research*. DHEW Publication No. (OS) 78-0013 and No. (OS) 78-0014. 18 April 1979.

International Conference on Harmonization of Technical Requirements for the Registration of Pharmaceuticals for Human Use (ICH). *Note for Guidance on Good Clinical Practice* (CPMP/ICH/135/95) 1 May 1996.

World Health Organization (WHO). Guidelines for Good Clinical Practice (GCP) for Trials on Pharmaceutical Products. Annex 3 of *The Use of*

Essential Drugs. Sixth Report of the WHO Expert Committee. Geneva: World Health Organization, 1995: 97–137.

World Medical Association, *Declaration of Helsinki: Recommendations Guiding Physicians in Biomedical Research Involving Human Subjects*. Adopted by the 18th World Medical Assembly, Helsinki, Finland, June 1964. Amended by the 29th World Medical Assembly, Tokyo, Japan, October 1975, the 35th World Medical Assembly, Venice, Italy, October 1983; the 41st World Medical Assembly, Hong Kong, September 1989; and the 48th General Assembly, Somerset West, Republic of South Africa, October 1996.

World Medical Association, *Declaration of Lisbon on the Rights of the Patient*. Adopted by the 34th World Medical Assembly, Lisbon, Portugal, September/October 1981, and amended by the 47th General Assembly, Bali, Indonesia, September 1995.

Operational guidelines for ethics committees that review biomedical research

UNDP/World/Bank/WHO
Special Programme for
Research & Training in Tropical Diseases (TDR)

Committees

International Working Party

Solomon Benatar, South Africa
Chifumbe Chintu, Zambia
Francis P. Crawley, Belgium (Chairman)
Dafna Feinholz, Mexico
Christine Grady, USA
Dirceau Greco, Brazil
Hakima Himmich, Morocco
Andrew Kitua, Tanzania
Olga Kubar, Russia
Mary Ann Lansang, Philippines
Reidar Lie, Norway
Vasantha Muthuswamy, India
Renzong Qiu, China
Judit Sándor, Hungary

Secretariat

Juntra Karbwang, TDR WHO (Project Coordinator)
Howard Engers, TDR WHO
David Griffin, WHO
Tikki Pang, WHO
Daniel Wikler, WHO
Myint Htwe, SEARO, WHO
Chen Ken, WPRO, WHO
Representative, EMRO, WHO
Representative, PAHO, WHO
Mariam Maluwa, UNAIDS

Claire Pattou, UNAIDS
John Bryant, CIOMS
Ryuichi Ida, UNESCO
Delon Human, WMA

Consultation Partners

Odette Morin Carpentier, International Federation of Pharmaceutical Manufacturers' Associations
Elaine Esber, FDA Representative to the International Conference on Harmonization
Nadia Tornieporth, SmithKline Beecham Biologics
Wen Kilama, African Malaria Vaccine Testing Network
Robert Eiss, National Institutes of Health, USA
Melody H. Lin, Office for Protection from Research Risks (OPRR), USA
Dixie Snider, Centers for Disease Control and Prevention, USA
Henry Dinsdale, National Council on Ethics in Human Research, Canada
Peteris Zilgalvis, Council of Europe
Laurence Cordier, European Commission (Frédérick Gay)
Fergus Sweeney, European Medicines Evaluation Agency
Betty Dodet, Fondation Marcel Mérieux
Tom Wilkie, Wellcome Trust, UK
Kries De Clerck, European Forum for Good Clinical Practice
Jean-Marc Husson, International Federation of Associations of Pharmaceutical Physicians
Denis Lacombe, European Organization for Research & Treatment of Cancer
Frank Wells, Faculty of Pharmaceutical Medicine, UK
Sabine Vital, Aventis Pasteur

11 Background

The *Operational Guidelines for Ethics Committees That Review Biomedical Research* is the result of a wide international consultation begun in August 1999 at A Seminar on the Ethical Review of Clinical Research in Asian & Western Pacific Countries organized by TDR WHO in Chiang Mai, Thailand. The participants at the seminar expressed a need for international guidance on the constitution and operation of ethics committees.

The first draft of these *Guidelines* was discussed at a workshop for members of African Ethical Review Committees organized by TDR WHO and the African Malaria Vaccine Testing Network in Arusha, Tanzania, on 5 November 1999. The draft was subsequently presented to an Interim Meeting of the Forum for Ethical Review Committees in the Asian &

Western Pacific Regions (FERCAP) in Bethesda, MD, USA, on 9 November 1999. It was also distributed for consultation at the Global Forum for Bioethics in Research organized by the NIH and WHO in Bethesda on 7–10 November 1999. Following these initial consultations the *Guidelines* were redrafted and widely distributed for comment.

Further development of these *Guidelines* was carried out under the auspices of a Secretariat composed of representatives from WHO, UNAIDS, CIOMS, UNESCO, and the WMA. Responsibility for drafting these *Guidelines* was given to an International Drafting Committee of 14 experts from various continents representing a wide range of disciplines in biomedical research and bioethics. The consultation process was carried out through representatives from the African Malaria Vaccine Testing Network, Council of Europe, European Commission, European Medicines Evaluation Agency, National Institutes of Health (USA), Food & Drug Administration (USA), Office for Protection from Research Risks (USA), Centers for Disease Control and Prevention (USA), National Council on Ethics in Human Research (Canada), Faculty of Pharmaceutical Medicine (United Kingdom), European Organization for Research & Treatment of Cancer, International Federation of Pharmaceutical Physicians, Foundation Marcel Mérieux, International Federation of Pharmaceutical Manufacturers' Associations, International Conference on Harmonization, and European Forum for Good Clinical Practice. In addition, the draft text was widely distributed to organizations of ethics committees in Europe and the United States as well as to experts in the field of biomedical research ethics. On 2 January 2000 a new draft was prepared and distributed to the members of the Drafting Working Party, the Secretariat, and the Consultation Partners as well as to other parties who had commented or expressed an interest.

Following on the reception of a wide range of detailed comments from around the world, the text was then widely discussed at a Meeting on Guidelines and Standard Operating Procedures for Ethical Review Committees held in Bangkok on 10–12 January 2000. Participants in this meeting were drawn from the regions of Africa, Asia, Latin America, North America, and Europe, from international organizations, (including WHO, UNAIDS, UNESCO, CIOMS, EFGCP, and IFPMA), and from universities and research institutions. A final deliberation took place at a Drafting Meeting held on 13 January 2000 in Bangkok. Following the Drafting Meeting a final set of comments were solicited and integrated into the final document.

The purpose of this wide consultative process was to ensure extensive input while fostering the sharing of knowledge from developing and developed countries alongside organizations and institutions with varying degrees of experience and expertise. This process also help to prepare for the dissemination of the final text through an international process of capacity building that would strengthen national and local infrastructures for ethical review throughout the world.

The *Operational Guidelines for Ethics Committees That Review Biomedical Research* are proposed by the WHO and CIOMS as a support for improving the organization, quality, and standards of ethical review around the world. These *Guidelines* take into account current practices while suggesting guidance for a harmonized state-of-the-art approach.

68

Registration of an institutional review board (IRB) or independent ethics committee (IEC)

Office for Human Research Protections (OHRP)

NOTE: All research that is conducted, supported, or regulated by any US Government Agency under the Federal Policy (or Common Rule) for the Protection of Human Subjects is subject to certain uniform requirements regarding IRB membership, IRB review and approval criteria, IRB operations and recordkeeping, and informed consent. In addition to the information provided on this website, review that provided at the FDA Website.

A Responsibilities of domestic IRBs and international IECs providing review and oversight of FDA-regulated research

1. The IRB should ensure that all human subject research that is regulated by the Food and Drug Administration (FDA), and for which the IRB provides review and oversight, complies with FDA regulations at Title 21 Code of Federal Regulations Parts 50 and 56 (21 CFR 50 and 56). FDA-regulated research in this case includes (a) clinical investigations overseen by domestic IRBs and regulated by FDA under sections 505(i) or 520(g) of the Federal Food, Drug, and Cosmetic Act; (b) clinical investigations overseen by domestic IRBs that support applications for research or marketing permits for FDA-regulated products (such as drugs, biological products, devices, food additives, and color additives); and (c) clinical investigations overseen by foreign IRBs that are required to comply with 21 CFR Part 56.

2. Except for research exempted or waived under Sections 56.104 or 56.105 of the FDA regulations, all research for which the IRB is responsible should be reviewed, prospectively approved, and subject to continuing oversight by the

IRB. The IRB should have the authority to approve, require modifications in, or disapprove the research for which it is responsible.

3. Except where specifically waived or altered by the IRB under sections 50.23, 50.24, or 56.109(c) of the FDA regulations, all research for which the IRB is responsible should require *written informed consent*, in nonexculpatory language understandable to the subject (or the subject's legally authorized representative), including the following basic elements per section 50.25(a) and (b) of the FDA regulations: (a) Identification as research; purposes, duration, and procedures; procedures which are experimental; (b) Reasonably foreseeable risks or discomforts; (c) Reasonably expected benefits to the subject or others; (d) Alternative procedures or treatments, if any, that might be advantageous to the subject; (e) Extent of confidentiality to be maintained; (f) Whether compensation or medical treatment are available if injury occurs (if more than minimal risk); (g) Whom to contact for answers to questions about the research, subjects' rights, and research-related injury; (h) Participation is voluntary; refusal to participate, or discontinuation of participation, will involve no penalty or loss of benefits to which subject is entitled; and (i) When appropriate, additional elements per Section 50.25(b) of the FDA regulations.

4. The IRB should establish written procedures for (a) conducting IRB initial and continuing review, approving research, and reporting IRB findings to the investigator and the institution; (b) determining which projects require review more often than annually, and which projects need verification from sources other than the investigator that no material changes have occurred; (c) ensuring that changes in approved research are reported promptly to the IRB and are not initiated without IRB approval, except when necessary to eliminate apparent immediate hazards to the

© Office for Human Research Protections.

subject; and (d) ensuring prompt reporting to the IRB, institutional officials, and the FDA, of any (i) unanticipated problems involving risks to subjects or others in any covered research; (ii) serious or continuing noncompliance with Federal, institutional, or IRB requirements; and (iii) suspension or termination of IRB approval for FDA-regulated research.

5. Information provided under this registration should be updated at least every 36 months in order to maintain active registration. Failure to update this information may result in termination of the IRB's registration with HHS.

6. Food and Drug Administration (FDA) regulations at 21 CFR 56.107 specify IRB membership requirements as follows:

a Each IRB shall have at least five members, with varying backgrounds to promote complete and adequate review of research activities commonly conducted by the entity. The IRB shall be sufficiently qualified through the experience and expertise of its members, and the diversity of the members, including consideration of race, gender, and cultural backgrounds and sensitivity to such issues as community attitudes, to promote respect for its advice and counsel in safeguarding the rights and welfare of human subjects. In addition to possessing the professional competence necessary to review specific research activities, the IRB shall be able to ascertain the acceptability of proposed research in terms of institutional commitments and regulations, applicable law, and standards of professional conduct and practice. The IRB shall therefore include persons knowledgeable in these areas. If an IRB regularly reviews research that involves a vulnerable category of subjects, such as children, prisoners, pregnant women, or handicapped or mentally disabled persons, consideration shall be given to the inclusion of one or more individuals who are knowledgeable about and experienced in working with these subjects.

b Every nondiscriminatory effort will be made to ensure that no IRB consists entirely of men or entirely of women, including the institution's consideration of qualified persons of both sexes, so long as no selection is made to the IRB on the basis of gender. No IRB may consist entirely of members of one profession.

c Each IRB shall include at least one member whose primary concerns are in scientific areas and at least one member whose primary concerns are in nonscientific areas.

d Each IRB shall include at least one member who is not otherwise affiliated with the institution and who is not part of the immediate family of a person who is affiliated with the institution.

e No IRB may have a member participate in the IRB's initial or continuing review of any project in which the member has a conflicting interest, except to provide information requested by the IRB.

f An IRB may, in its discretion, invite individuals with competence in special areas to assist in the review of issues which require expertise beyond or in addition to that available on the IRB. These individuals may not vote with the IRB.

B Responsibilities of IRBs providing review and oversight of federally-supported research: IRBs located in the United States

1. All IRB activities related to human subject research should be guided by the ethical principles in *The Belmont Report: Ethical Principles and Guidelines for the Protection of Human Subjects of Research* of the National Commission for the Protection of Human Subjects of Biomedical and Behavioral Research.

2. The IRB should ensure that all Federally-supported human subject research for which the IRB provides review and oversight complies with the Federal Policy* (Common Rule) for the Protection of Human Subjects. All human subject research supported by the Department of Health and Human Services (HHS) should comply with all Subparts of HHS regulations at Title 45 Code of Federal Regulations Part 46 (45 CFR 46). All Federally-supported human subject research should also comply with any additional human subject regulations and policies of the supporting Department or Agency. All Federally-supported human subject research should comply with any human subject regulations and policies of any relevant regulatory Department or Agency. In reviewing research that is both Federally-supported and FDA-regulated, the IRB should satisfy all of the responsibilities applicable to each.

* 7 CFR 1c	Department of Agriculture
10 CFR 745	Department of Energy
14 CFR 1230	National Aeronautics and Space Administration
15 CFR 27	Department of Commerce
16 CFR 1028	Consumer Product Safety Commission
22 CFR 225	Agency for International Development
24 CFR 60	Department of Housing and Urban Development
28 CFR 46	Department of Justice
32 CFR 219	Department of Defense
34 CFR 97	Department of Education
38 CFR 16	Department of Veterans Affairs

40 CFR 26	Environmental Protection Agency
45 CFR 46	Department of Health and Human Services
45 CFR 690	National Science Foundation
49 CFR 11	Department of Transportation
By Executive Order	Central Intelligence Agency
By Statute	Department of Agriculture

3. Except for research exempted or waived under Sections 101(b) or 101(i) of the Federal Policy, all research for which the IRB is responsible should be reviewed, prospectively approved, and subject to continuing oversight by the IRB. The IRB should have the authority to approve, require modifications in, or disapprove the research for which it is responsible.

4. Except where specifically waived or altered by the IRB under Sections 101(i), 116(c) and (d), or 117(c) of the Federal Policy all research for which the IRB is responsible should require *written informed consent*, in nonexculpatory language understandable to the subject (or the subject's legally authorized representative), including the following basic elements per Section 116(a) and (b) of the Federal Policy: (a) Identification as research; purposes, duration, and proc edures; procedures which are experimental; (b) Reasonably foreseeable risks or discomforts; (c) Reasonably expected benefits to the subject or others; (d) Alternative procedures or treatments, if any, that might be advantageous to the subject; (e) Extent of confidentiality to be maintained; (f) Whether compensation or medical treatment are available if injury occurs (if more than minimal risk); (g) Whom to contact for answers to questions about the research, subjects' rights, and research-related injury; (h) Participation is voluntary; refusal to participate, or discontinuation of participation, will involve no penalty or loss of benefits to which subject is entitled; and (i) When appropriate, additional elements per Section 116(b) of the Federal Policy.

5. The IRB should establish written procedures for (a) conducting IRB initial and continuing review, approving research, and reporting IRB findings to the investigator and the institution; (b) determining which projects require review more often than annually, and which projects need verification from sources other than the investigator that no material changes have occurred; (c) ensuring that changes in approved research are reported promptly and are not initiated without IRB approval, except when necessary to eliminate apparent immediate hazards to the subject; and (d) ensuring prompt reporting to the IRB, institutional officials, the relevant Department or Agency Head, any applicable regulatory body, and OHRP of any of any (i) unanticipated problems involving risks to subjects or others in any covered research; (ii) serious or continuing noncompliance with Federal, institutional, or IRB requirements; and (iii) suspension or termination of IRB approval for Federally-supported research.

6. The IRB should ensure that it has appropriate knowledge of the local context in which research for which it is responsible will be conducted.

7. The IRB Chairperson, IRB members, IRB staff, and human subject research investigators should complete appropriate education related to the protection of human subjects before reviewing or conducting human subject research.

8. The IRB should ensure the existence of adequate education and oversight mechanisms (appropriate to the nature and volume of the research being conducted) to verify that research investigators, IRB members and staff, and other relevant personnel maintain continuing knowledge of, and comply with, relevant Federal regulations, OHRP guidance, other applicable guidance, State and local law, and IRB determinations and policies for the protection of human subjects. The IRB should require documentation of such training from research investigators as a condition for conducting Federally-supported human subject research.

9. The IRB should endeavor to ensure that it is provided with resources, professional staff, and support staff appropriate to the nature and volume of the research for which it is responsible.

10. Information provided under this registration should be updated at least every 36 months in order to maintain active registration. Failure to update this information may result in termination of the IRB's registration with HHS.

11. The Federal Policy (Common Rule) for the Protection of Human Subjects and Department of Health and Human Services (HHS) regulations at 45 CFR 46.107 specify IRB membership requirements as follows:

a. Each IRB shall have at least five members, with varying backgrounds to promote complete and adequate review of research activities commonly conducted by the entity. The IRB shall be sufficiently qualified through the experience and expertise of its members, and the diversity of the members, including consideration of race, gender, and cultural backgrounds and sensitivity to such issues as community attitudes, to promote respect for its advice and counsel in safeguarding the rights and welfare of human subjects. In addition to possessing the professional competence necessary to review specific research activities, the IRB shall be able to ascertain the acceptability of proposed research in terms of institutional commitments and regulations, applicable law, and standards of professional conduct and practice. The IRB shall therefore include persons knowledgeable in these areas. If an IRB regularly reviews research that involves a vulnerable category of subjects, such as children, prisoners, pregnant women, or handicapped or mentally disabled persons, consideration shall be given to the inclusion of one or more individuals who are knowledgeable about and experienced in working with these subjects.

b. Every nondiscriminatory effort will be made to ensure that no IRB consists entirely of men or entirely of women, including the institution's consideration of qualified persons of both sexes, so long as no selection is made to the IRB on the basis of gender. No IRB may consist entirely of members of one profession.

c. Each IRB shall include at least one member whose primary concerns are in scientific areas and at least one member whose primary concerns are in nonscientific areas.

d. Each IRB shall include at least one member who is not otherwise affiliated with the institution and who is not part of the immediate family of a person who is affiliated with the institution.

e. No IRB may have a member participate in the IRB's initial or continuing review of any project in which the member has a conflicting interest, except to provide information requested by the IRB.

f. An IRB may, in its discretion, invite individuals with competence in special areas to assist in the review of issues which require expertise beyond or in addition to that available on the IRB. These individuals may not vote with the IRB.

C Responsibilities of IECs and IRBs providing review and oversight of federally-supported research: IECs and IRBs located outside the United States

1. All IEC/IRB activities related to human subject research should be guided either by the ethical principles in the World Medical Association's *Declaration of Helsinki (as adopted in 1996 or 2000)*, or by the ethical principles in *The Belmont Report: Ethical Principles and Guidelines for the Protection of Human Subjects of Research* of the US National Commission for the Protection of Human Subjects of Biomedical and Behavioral Research, or by other internationally recognized ethical standards.

2. The IEC/IRB should ensure that all US-supported human subject research for which the IEC/IRB provides review and oversight complies with the requirements of any applicable Federal regulatory agency as well as one of the following: (i) the US Federal Policy (Common Rule) for the Protection of Human Subjects and/or the US Department of Health and Human Services (HHS) regulations at 45 CFR 46; (ii) the May 1, 1996 International Conference on Harmonization E-6 Guidelines for Good Clinical Practice (ICH-GCP-E6) Sections 1 through 4; (iii) the 1993 Council for International Organizations of Medical Sciences (CIOMS) International Ethical Guidelines for Biomedical Research Involving Human Subjects; (iv) the 1998 Medical Research Council of Canada Tri-Council Policy Statement on Ethical Conduct for Research Involving Humans; (v) the 2000 Indian Council of Medical Research Ethical Guidelines for Research Involving Humans; or (vi) other internationally recognized standards for the protection of human subjects. In reviewing research that is both Federally-supported and FDA-regulated, the IRB should satisfy all of the responsibilities applicable to each.

3. All US-supported research for which the IEC/IRB is responsible should be reviewed, prospectively approved, and subject to continuing oversight and review at least annually by the IEC/IRB. The convened IEC/IRB, with a majority of its members present, should have authority to approve, require modifications in, or disapprove the research for which the IEC/IRB is responsible.

4. Unless authorized by the supporting US Agency, all US-supported research for which the IEC/IRB is responsible should require *written informed consent*, in nonexculpatory language understandable to the subject (or the subject's legally authorized representative), including the following basic elements: (a) Identification as research; purposes, duration, and procedures; procedures which are experimental; (b) Reasonably foreseeable risks or discomforts; (c) Expected benefits to the subject or others; (d) Alternative procedures or treatments; (e) Extent of confidentiality to be maintained; (f) Whether compensation or medical treatment are available if injury occurs (if more than minimal risk); (g) Whom to contact for answers to questions about the research, subjects' rights, and research-related injury; (h) Participation is voluntary; refusal to participate, or discontinuation of participation, will involve no penalty or loss of benefits to which subject is entitled; and (i) When appropriate, additional elements as determined by the IEC/IRB.

5. The IEC/IRB should establish written procedures for (a) verifying whether proposed activities qualify for exemption from, or waiver of, IEC/IRB review; (b) conducting initial and continuing IEC/IRB review, approving research, and reporting IEC/IRB findings to the investigator and the institution conducting the research; (c) determining appropriate continuing review intervals and oversight mechanisms for all approved research; (d) ensuring that

changes in approved research are not initiated without IEC/IRB approval, except when necessary to eliminate apparent immediate hazards to the subject; and (e) ensuring prompt reporting to the IEC/IRB, institutional officials, the relevant US Agency Head, any applicable regulatory body, and OHRP of any (i) serious or continuing noncompliance with US, institutional, or IEC/IRB requirements; (ii) unanticipated problems involving risks to subjects or others in any covered research; and (iii) suspension or termination of IEC/IRB approval for US-supported research.

6. The IEC/IRB should acknowledge that special protections are needed for vulnerable populations of subjects and should ensure the concurrence of the supporting US Agency prior to the involvement of pregnant women, prisoners, children, or fetuses in US-supported research for which the IEC/IRB is responsible.

7. The IEC/IRB Chairperson, IEC/IRB members, IEC/IRB staff, and human subject research investigators should complete appropriate education and training before reviewing or conducting human subject research. Educational modules available on the OHRP website may be used for such training, or the IEC/IRB may utilize other appropriate educational materials of its own choosing.

8. The IEC/IRB should ensure the existence of adequate education and oversight mechanisms (appropriate to the nature and volume of the research being conducted) to verify that research investigators, IEC/IRB members and staff, and other relevant personnel maintain continuing knowledge of, and comply with, relevant policies and procedures for the protection of human subjects. The IEC/IRB should require documentation of such training from research investigators as a condition for conducting US-supported human subject research.

9. The IEC/IRB should endeavor to ensure that it is provided with resources, professional staff, and support staff appropriate to the nature and volume of the research for which it is responsible.

10. Information provided under this registration should be updated at least every 36 months in order to maintain active status. Failure to update this information may result in termination of the IRB's registration with HHS.

11. The IEC/IRB should observe the following membership guidelines:
a. Each IEC/IRB should have at least five members, with varying backgrounds to promote complete and adequate review of research activities commonly conducted by the institution. The IEC/IRB should be sufficiently qualified through the experience and expertise of its members, and the diversity of the members, including consideration of race, gender, and cultural backgrounds and sensitivity to such issues as community attitudes, to promote respect for its advice and counsel in safeguarding the rights and welfare of human subjects. In addition to possessing the professional competence necessary to review specific research activities, the IEC/IRB should be able to ascertain the acceptability of proposed research in terms of institutional commitments and regulations, applicable law, and standards of professional conduct and practice. The IEC/IRB should therefore include persons knowledgeable in these areas. If an IEC/IRB regularly reviews research that involves a vulnerable category of subjects, such as children, prisoners, pregnant women, or handicapped or mentally disabled persons, consideration should be given to the inclusion of one or more individuals who are knowledgeable about and experienced in working with these subjects.
b. Every nondiscriminatory effort should be made to ensure that no IEC/IRB consists entirely of men or entirely of women, including consideration of qualified persons of both sexes, so long as no selection is made to the IEC/IRB on the basis of gender. No IEC/IRB should consist entirely of members of one profession.
c. Each IEC/IRB should include at least one member whose primary concerns are in scientific areas and at least one member whose primary concerns are in nonscientific areas.
d. Each IEC/IRB should include at least one member who is not otherwise affiliated with the entity and who is not part of the immediate family of a person who is affiliated with the entity.
e. No IEC/IRB should have a member participate in the IEC's/IRB's initial or continuing review of any project in which the member has a conflicting interest, except to provide information requested by the IEC/IRB.
f. An IEC/IRB may, in its discretion, invite individuals with competence in special areas to assist in the review of issues which require expertise beyond or in addition to that available on the IEC/IRB. These individuals should not vote with the IEC/IRB.

If you have questions about human subject research, click *ohrp@osophs.dhhs.gov*

69

International guidelines on bioethics
(informal listing of selected international codes, declarations, guidelines, etc. on medical ethics/bioethics/health care ethics/human rights aspects of health)

European Forum for Good Clinical Practice/Council for International
Organisations of Medical Sciences

3rd Edition

Supplement to *The EFGCP News*, Autumn 2000

Salve 2
European Forum for Good Clinical Practice

Author: Sev S. Fluss

Special Adviser
Council for International Organizations of
Medical Sciences (CIOMS)

This listing is published as a Supplement to *The EFGCP News*, Autumn 2000. It is the second revised edition of the same listing published as a Supplement to *The EFGCP News*, September 1998 and December 1999. The copyright remains with the original author. For copies and other information on EFGCP publications, contact FP Crawley, Editor, *The EFGCP News*, Schoolbergenstraat 47, B-3010 Kessel-Lo, Belgium; Fax +32 16 35 03 69; E-mail: fpc@pandora.be. Suggested additions or revisions may be sent to FP Crawley and/or SS Fluss.

This listing, which does not purport to be comprehensive, was largely initiated by Ms. Abeer Khoury de Bellet (Amman/Geneva), Intern, Office of the Executive Administrator for Health Policy in Development, WHO (November 1995–January 1996). The kind assistance of Ms. Isabel Monreal (Clermont-Ferrand, France), an Intern in the same Office during the period July–October 1996, in preparing this update is gratefully acknowledged, as is that of Ms. Emma Fitzpatrick (Melbourne, Australia), an Intern during the period June–July 1997. Also acknowledged, with appreciation, is the assistance provided by Dr. Hooman Peimani, a Canadian specialist in international relations, during the

period November–December 1997. The date of adoption of the particular text is indicated in brackets; where there are two dates, the second indicates the year of the most recent revision of which the compilers are aware. Persons using or consulting this list are invited to communicate any additional information that may contribute to its improvement to Mr. S. S. Fluss, c/o CIOMS, WHO, 1211 Geneva 27: Tel.: +41 (22) 791.22.02; Fax: +41 (22) 791.31.11; E-mail: "flusss@who.ch" or "sfluss@vtx.ch" any additional information that may contribute to its improvement.

Intergovernmental organizations

Council of Europe

Committee of Ministers
- Resolution on Harmonisation of Legislations of Member States Relating to Removal of Human Tissues and Organs for Therapeutic Purposes (1978)
- Recommendation on Regulations for Automated Medical Data Banks (1981)
- Recommendation Concerning the Legal Protection of Persons Suffering from Mental Disorders Placed as Involuntary Patients (1983)
- Recommendation on the European Prison Rules (1987)
- Recommendation to Member States Concerning a Common European Public Health Policy to Fight the Acquired Immunodeficiency Syndrome (AIDS) (1987)
- Final Text of the 3rd Conference of European Ministers for Health on Organ Transplantation (Paris, 16–17 November 1987), Revision of Resolution (78) 29 (1978)
- Recommendation on the Collection of Epidemiological Data on Primary Health Care (1989)
- Recommendation to Member States on the Ethical Issues of HIV Infection in the Health Care and Social Settings (1989)

- Recommendation on Prenatal Genetic Screening, Prenatal Genetic Diagnosis and Associated Genetic Counselling (1990)
- Recommendation Concerning Medical Research on Human Beings (1990)
- Recommendation on Genetic Testing and Screening for Health Care Purposes (1992)
- Recommendation on Screening as a Tool of Preventive Medicine (1994)
- Final Text of the 5th Conference of European Health Ministers on "Social Challenge to Health: Equity and Patients' Rights in the Context of Health Reforms" (Warsaw, 7–8 November 1996)
- Convention on Human Rights and Biomedicine (1997)
- Recommendation on the Protection of Medical Data (1997)
- Additional Protocol on the Prohibition of Cloning Human Beings (1997)
- Recommendation on Liver Transplantation from Living Donors (1997)
- Recommendation on Xenotransplantation (1997)
- Recommendation Concerning the Ethical and Organisational Aspects of Health Care in Prison (1998)
- Protocol on the Prohibition of Cloning Human Beings (1998)
- Protocol on Organ Transplant (1999)
- Recommendation on Xenotransplantation (1999)
- Revised European Social Charter (1999)
- Recommendation on Principles Concerning the Legal Protection of Incapable Adults (1999)

Second summit (Strasbourg, 10–11 October 1997)
- Action Plan adopted on 11 October 1997 (para. 4, on "Prohibition of the cloning of human beings")

Parliamentary Assembly
- Recommendation and Resolution on the Rights of the Sick and Dying (1976)
- Recommendation on the Situation of the Mentally Ill (1977)
- Recommendation on Genetic Engineering (1982)
- Recommendation on the Supply and Utilisation of Human Blood and Blood Products (1984)
- Recommendation on the Use of Human Embryos and Foetuses for Diagnostic, Therapeutic, Scientific, Industrial and Commercial Purposes (1986)
- Recommendation on a Co-ordinated European Health Policy to Fight the Acquired Immunodeficiency Syndrome in Prisons (1988)
- Recommendation on the Use of Human Embryos and Foetuses for Research Purposes (1989)

- Recommendation on the Preparation of a Convention on Bioethics (1991)
- Recommendation on the Medical and Welfare Rights of the Elderly: Ethics and Policies (1994)
- Order No. 534 (1997) on Research and the Cloning of Human Beings (1997)
- Opinion No. 202 (1997) on the Draft Additional Protocol to the Convention on Human Rights and Biomedicine on the Prohibition of Cloning Human Beings (1997)
- Recommendation on Fighting Social Exclusion and Strengthening Social Cohesion in Europe (1998)
- Recommendation on Xenotransplantation (1999)
- Recommendation on the Human Rights and Dignity of the Terminally Ill and the Dying (1999)

Ad Hoc Committee of Experts on Bioethics
- Principles in the Field of Human Artificial Procreation (1989)

Steering Committee on Bioethics (CDBI) (Documents in preparation)
- Protocol on Organ Transplantation (finalised by the CDBI in December 1999)
- Draft Protocol on Biomedical Research (2001?)
- Draft Protocol on the Protection of the Human Embryo and the Foetus (2002?)
- Draft Protocol on Problems Relating to Human Genetics (2002?)

European Union

European Council
- European Council Declaration on Banning the Cloning of Human Beings (1997)

European Commission
- Good Clinical Practice in the Conduct of Clinical Trials on Medicinal Products for Human Use (1991)

European Parliament
- Resolution on a Charter on the Rights of Women in Childbirth (1988)
- Resolution on European Harmonisation of Medicoethical Questions (1988)
- Resolution on the Ethical and Legal Problems of Genetic Engineering (1989)
- Resolution on Artificial Insemination in Vivo and in Vitro (1989)
- Resolution on Abortion (1990)
- Resolution on Women and Health Care (1990)

- Resolution on Prohibiting Trade in Transplant Organs (1993)
- Resolution on Cloning of the Human Embryo (1993)
- Resolution on Cloning (1997)
- Resolution on Human Cloning (1998)
- Resolution on International Women's Day and the Violation of Women's Rights (1998)
- Resolution on the Development of Public Health Policy in the European Community (1999)

Group of Advisers on the Ethical Implications of Biotechnology

- Opinion on Ethical Questions Arising from the Commission Proposal for a Council Directive on Legal Protection for Biotechnological Inventions (1993)
- Opinion on Products Derived from Human Blood or Blood Plasma (1993)
- Opinion on the Ethical Implications of Gene Therapy (1994)
- Opinion on Ethical Aspects of the Labelling of Foods Derived from Modern Biotechnology (1995)
- Opinion on Ethical Aspects of Prenatal Diagnosis (1996)
- Opinion on Ethical Aspects of Patenting Inventions Involving Elements of Human Origin (1996)
- Opinion on Ethical Aspects of Cloning Techniques (1997)
- Opinion on the Ethical Aspects of the 5th Research Framework Programme (1997)

European Group on Ethics in Science and New Technologies

- Ethical Aspects of Human Tissue Banking (1998)
- Ethical Aspects of Research Involving the Use of the Human Embryo in the Context of the Fifth Framework Programme (1998)
- Ethical Issues of Healthcare in the Information Society (1999)

International conference on harmonisation of technical requirements for registration of pharmaceuticals for human use (ICH)

- Guideline for Good Clinical Practice (ICH Harmonised Tripartite Guideline) (1997)

International Labour Organisation

- Technical and Ethical Guidelines for Workers' Health Surveillance (1999)

Nordic Council on Medicines

- Nordic Guidelines on Good Clinical Trial Practice (1989)

Organization of African Unity

- Resolution on Bioethics (1996)

UNAIDS (Joint United Nations Programme on HIV/AIDS)

- Guidance Document on Ethical Considerations in HIV Preventive Vaccine Research (2000)
- International Guidelines on HIV/AIDS and Human Rights (with the Office of the United Nations High Commissioner for Human Rights) (1998)

United Nations

- Resolution XI (Human rights and scientific and technological developments), adopted on 12 May 1968 by the International Conference on Human Rights (Teheran, 22 April – 13 May 1968)
- The Vienna Declaration and Programme of Action, adopted by the World Conference on Human Rights (14–28 June 1993) (paras. 11 and 58) (1993)
- The Programme of Action adopted at the International Conference on Population and Development (Cairo, 5–13 September 1994) (para. 7.17) (1994)
- The Beijing Declaration and Platform for Action, adopted at the Fourth World Conference on Women (Beijing, 4–15 September 1995) and endorsed by the United Nations General Assembly on 22 December 1995 (paras. 106 (g) and 109 (h) and (l)) (1995)

General Assembly

- International Covenant on Civil and Political Rights (Article 7) (1966)
- Resolution 2450 (XXIII) on "Human rights and scientific and technological Developments", adopted on 19 December 1968
- Declaration on the Rights of Mentally Retarded Persons (1971)
- Principles of Medical Ethics Relevant to the Role of Health Personnel, Particularly Physicians, in the Protection of Prisoners and Detainees Against Torture and Other Cruel, Inhuman or Degrading Treatment or Punishment (1982)
- Declaration on the Human Rights of Individuals Who are not Nationals of the Country in Which They Live (Article 6) (1985)
- Principles for the Protection of Persons with Mental Illness and for the Improvement of Mental Health Care (1991)
- Resolution 53/152 on "The Human Genome and Human Rights" (1998)

Commission on Human Rights

- Resolution on Non-Discrimination in the Field of Health (1989)
- Resolution on Human Rights and Bioethics (1993)
- Resolution on Human Rights and Bioethics (1997)
- Decision on Human Rights and Scientific and Technological Developments (1998)
- Resolution on the Rights of the Child (1998)
- Resolution on Human Rights and Forensic Medicine (1998)
- Resolution on Human Rights and Bioethics (1999)
- Resolution on Human Rights and HIV/AIDS (1999)
- Resolution on Human Rights and Forensic Science (2000)
- Resolution on Traffic in Women and Girls (2000)
- Resolution on Elimination of Violence against Women (2000)
- Resolution on Human Rights of Migrants (2000)
- Resolution on Human Rights of Persons with Disabilities (2000)
- Resolution on the Adverse Effects of the Illicit Movement and Dumping of Toxic and Dangerous Products and Wastes on the Enjoyment of Human Rights (2000)
- Resolution on the Rights of the Child (2000)
- Resolution on the Right to Food (2000)

Committee on Economic, Social and Cultural Rights

- General Comment No. 12 on the Right to Adequate Food (1999)
- General Comment No. 14 on the Right to the Highest Attainable Standard of Health (2000)

UNESCO

- Recommendation on the Status of Scientific Researchers (1974)
- Malta Recommendations on Human Rights Teaching, Information and Documentation (Section 8) (1987)
- Universal Declaration on the Human Genome and Human Rights (adopted on 11 November 1997)
- Guidelines for the Implementation of the Universal Declaration on the Human Genome and Human Rights (1999)
- Declaration on Science and the Use of Scientific Knowledge; and Science-Agenda-Framework for Action. Adopted at the World Conference on Science (Budapest, 26 June – 1 July 1999)
- Resolution on Bioethics and the Rights of the Child (2000)

United Nations Population Fund (UNFPA)

- Declaration of Ethical Principles, adopted by the Roundtable on Ethics, Population and Reproductive Health (New York, 8–10 March 1994)

World Health Organization

- Ethical Criteria for Medicinal Drug Promotion (1988)
- Ethical Guidelines for Epidemiological Investigations (issued by the Scientific Working Group on Epidemiology of the Special Programme for Research and
- Training in Tropical Diseases) (1989)
- Guiding Principles on Human Organ Transplantation (1991)
- Recommendations of the WHO Scientific Group on Recent Advances in Medically Assisted Conception (1992)
- Research Guidelines for Evaluating the Safety and Efficacy of Herbal Medicines (Regional Office for the Western Pacific, 1993)
- Declaration on the Promotion of Patients' Rights in Europe (WHO Regional Office for Europe) (1994)
- Guidelines for the Establishment of Scientific and Ethical Review Bodies (issued by the UNDP/UNFPA /WHO/ World Bank Special Programme of Research, Development and Research Training in Human Reproduction) (1994)
- Guidelines for Research on Reproductive Health Involving Adolescents (issued by the UNDP/UNFPA/ WHO/World Bank Special Programme of Research, Development and Research Training in Human Reproduction) (1994)
- Guidelines for Good Clinical Practice for Trials on Pharmaceutical Products (1995)
- Guidelines for Clinical Research on Acupuncture (WHO Regional Office for the Western Pacific) (1995)
- Mental Health Care Law: Ten Basic Principles (1996)
- Guidelines for the Promotion of Human Rights of Persons with Mental Disorders (1996)
- Resolution on Cloning in Human Reproduction (adopted by the Fiftieth World Health Assembly) (1997)
- Statement of WHO Expert Advisory Group on Ethical Issues in Medical Genetics (1998)
- Resolution on Ethical, Scientific and Social Implications of Cloning in Human Health (adopted by the Fifty-first World Health Assembly) (1998)
- Proposed International Guidelines on Ethical Issues in Medical Genetics and Genetic Services (1998)
- Operational Guidelines for Ethics Committees That Review Biomedical Research (2000)

Non-Governmental Organizations

Amnesty International

- Declaration on the Participation of Health Personnel in the Death Penalty (1981; 1988)

- Declaration on the Role of Health Professionals in the Exposure of Torture and Ill-Treatment (1996)
- Principles for the Medical Investigation of Torture and Other Cruel, Inhuman or Degrading Treatment (1996)
- Plan of Action Against Torture. Adopted by the International Conference on Torture (Stockholm, 4–6 October 1996)

Commonwealth Medical Association

- Ethical Code (1974)
- Guiding Principles on Medical Ethics and Human Rights (1995)
- Declaration on the Role of Medical Ethics and a Woman's Right to Health, Including Sexual and Reproductive Health (1997)

Conference internationale des ordres et des organismes d'attributions similaires

- Principles of Medical Ethics (1987)

Council for International Organizations of Medical Sciences (CIOMS)

- Principles of Medical Ethics Relating to Prisoners and Detainees (1983)
- The Declaration of Inuyama on Human Genome Mapping, Genetic Screening and Gene Therapy (1990)
- International Guidelines for Ethical Review of Epidemiological Studies (1991)
- International Ethical Guidelines for Biomedical Research Involving Human Subjects (1993)
- The Declaration of Ixtapa: A Global Agenda for Bioethics (1994)

European Alliance of Genetic Support Groups

- Ethical Code (1996)
- Briefing Paper on Cloning (1997)

European Association for Bioindustries (EUROPABIO)

- Core Ethical Values (1998)
- Information Paper on Ethical, Social and Public Awareness Issues in Gene Therapy (2000)

European Association of Tissue Banks

- Ethical Code (1994)

European Dialysis and Transplant Association-European Renal Association

- Statement on Safeguards for Live Kidney Donors (1986)

European Forum for Good Clinical Practice

- Guidelines and Recommendations for European Ethics Committees (1995; 1997)

European Medical Research Councils

- Recommendations on Human In-Vitro Fertilisation and Embryo Transfer (1983)
- Recommendations on Gene Therapy in Man (1988)

European Network of GCP Auditors and Other GCP Experts (ENGAGE)

- Optional Guideline for Good Clinical Practice Compliance and Quality Systems Auditing (the ENGAGE Guideline) (1997)

European Society of Human Reproduction and Embryology

- Declaration (Voluntary Moratorium on Cloning Human Beings) (1998)

FIGO (International Federation of Gynecology and Obstetrics) Committee for the Study of Ethical Aspects of Human Reproduction

- Statement on Surrogate Motherhood (1989)
- Recommendations on Sex Selection (1988; 1994)
- Statement on Anencephaly and Organ Transplantation (1989)
- Recommendations on Ethical Considerations in Sterilization (1990)
- Recommendations on Research on Pre-embryos (1990)
- Recommendations on Selective Reduction of Multiple Pregnancy (1990)
- Recommendations on Ethical Issues Concerning Prenatal Diagnosis of Disease in the Conceptus (1991)
- Guidelines for the Use of Embryonic or Fetal Tissue for Therapeutic Clinical Applications (1992)
- Recommendations on Ethical Aspects of Newborn Care (1992)
- Recommendations on Donation of Genetic Material for Human Reproduction (1994)

- Recommendations on the Ethical Framework for Gynaecologic and Obstetric Care (1994)
- Recommendations on Ethical Considerations Concerning the Use of Anti-progestins (1994)
- Recommendation on the Donation of Genetic Material for Human Reproduction (1994)
- Recommendations on Guidelines Regarding Informed Consent (1997)
- Recommendations on Ethical Aspects of the Management of Severely Malformed Newborn Infants (1997)
- Recommendations on Ethical Guidelines Regarding Altering Genes in Humans (1997)
- Recommendations on Ethical Aspects of HIV Infection and Reproduction (1997)
- Recommendations on Ethical Aspects of the Introduction of Contraceptive Methods for Women (1997)
- Recommendations on Ethical Guidelines on the Sale of Gametes and Embryos (1997)
- Recommendations on the Ethical Aspects of Sexual and Reproductive Rights (1997)
- Recommendations on Ethical Aspects in the Management of Newborn Infants at the Threshold of Viability (1997)
- Recommendations on Some Ethical Issues in the Doctor/Patient Relationship (1997)
- Recommendations on Patenting Human Genes (1997)
- Recommendations on Cloning in Human Reproduction (1997)
- Resolution on Violence Against Women. Adopted by the FIGO General Assembly in Copenhagen on 5 August 1997 (1997)

Human Genome Organisation (HUGO)

- Statement on the Principled Conduct of Genetics Research (1996)
- Statement on DNA Sampling Control and Access (1998)
- Statement on Cloning (1999)

HUGO Ethics Committee
- Statement on Benefit Sharing (2000)

International Advisory Board of the III World Congress on in Vitro Fertilization and Embryo Transfer

- Helsinki Statement on Human in Vitro Fertilization (1985)

International Commission on Medical Neutrality

- Charter of Medical Neutrality (1991)

International Commission on Occupational Health

- International Code of Ethics for Occupational Health Professionals (1991)

International Committee of the Red Cross

- Geneva Conventions I (Article 12), II (Article 12), III (Article 13), IV (Article 32) (1949). Protocol I of the Additional Protocols (Articles 11 and 16) (1977)

International Confederation of Midwives

- International Code of Ethics for Midwives (1993)

International Council of Nurses

- Code for Nurses (1973; 1989)
- Statement on the Nurse's Role in the Care of Detainees and Prisoners (1975)
- Statement on the Nurse's Role in Safeguarding Human Rights (1983)
- Statement on Nurses and Torture (1989; reviewed in 1991)
- Statement on the Death Penalty and Participation by Nurses in Executions (1989; reviewed in 1991)
- Statement on Mental Health/Psychiatric Nursing (1995)
- Code of Ethics for Nurses (2000)

International Council of Prison Medical Services

- The Oath of Athens (1979)

International Federation of Pharmaceutical Manufacturers Associations (IFPMA)

- IFPMA Code of Pharmaceutical Marketing Practices (1981; 1999)

International Federation of Red Cross and Red Crescent Societies

- Statement on the Ethics of Voluntary, Non-Remunerated Blood Donation (the Hanover Statement) (1990)
- Decision on Voluntary, Non-Remunerated Blood Donation (1991)

International Medical Parliamentarians Organization

- London Statement on Medical Ethics and Human Rights (1995)

International Organization for Standardization (ISO)

- Clinical Investigation of Medical Devices: International Standard (1996)

International Planned Parenthood Federation

- IPPF Charter on Sexual and Reproductive Rights (1996)
- Statement of Copenhagen Round Table Meeting on the IPPF Charter on Sexual and Reproductive Rights (1996)

International Society of Blood Transfusion

- Code of Ethics for Blood Donation and Transfusion (1981)

International Union of Psychological Science

- Statement of the IUPsyS [on professional standards of ethics in the practice of psychology] (1996)

Inter-Parliamentary Union

- Resolution on Bioethics and its Implications Worldwide for Human Rights Protection (1995)

Islamic Organization for Medical Sciences

- Islamic Code of Medical Ethics (1981)

Medical Women's International Association

- Resolutions on ethics and statements on diverse ethical issues adopted by the MWIA Congresses between 1929 and 2000
- Resolution on Cancer (1992; 1998)
- Statements on Health As a Basic Human Right (1993; 1999)
- Statement on Female Genital Mutilation and Other Harmful Traditional Practices (1994)
- Statement on Reproductive Health (1996)
- Resolution on Oncology (1998)
- Resolution on Reproductive Technologies (1998)
- Resolution on Healthcare Policy (1998)
- Resolution on HIV and AIDS (1998)
- Resolution on Violence against Women (1998)

Network for European CNS Transplantation and Restoration (NECTAR)

- Ethical Guidelines for the Use of Human Embryonic or Fetal Tissue for Experimental and Clinical Neurotransplantation and Research (1994)

Standing Committee of European Doctors (CP)

- First Statement on Storage of Medical Data in Computer Banks (1982)
- Statement on Medical Secrecy in Community Law (1984)
- Motion on Withdrawal of Services (1985)
- Recommendations on Ethical Problems Concerning Artificial Insemination (1985)
- Declaration of Madrid on aid to the dying (1987)
- Recommendations concerning AIDS (1989)
- Statement of Madrid on doctors, ethics, and torture (1989)
- Analysis of the human genome (1989)
- Recommendations on teaching medical ethics (1993)
- Trade in organ transplantation (1993)
- Statement on living wills/advance directives (1993)
- Statement on limitation of health resources and medical ethics (1993)
- Information on ethical and economic consequences of the limitation of resources for health care (1994)

Transplantation Society

- Statement (on policy and ethical aspects of organ transplantation) (1970)
- Guidelines for the Distribution and the Use of Organs from Cadaver Sources and from Living Unrelated Donors (1985)
- Recommendations on Ethical and Policy Issues (1994)

World Confederation for Physical Therapy

- Guidelines Concerning Torture and Other Cruel, Inhuman and Degrading Treatment (1995)
- Resolution in Support of Victims of Torture (1999)

World Federation for Mental Health

- Declaration of Human Rights and Mental Health (1989)

World Medical Association

- Declaration of Geneva (physician's oath) (1948; 1994)
- International Code of Medical Ethics (1949; 1983)
- Regulations in Time of Armed Conflict (1956; 1983)
- Twelve Principles of Provision of Health Care in Any National Health Care System (1963; 1983)
- Declaration of Helsinki: Recommendations Guiding Physicians in Biomedical Research Involving Human Subjects (1964; 1975; 1983; 1989; 1996)
- Statement on Genetic Counselling and Genetic Engineering (1987)

- Recommendations Concerning Medical Care in Rural Areas (1964; 1983)
- Statement on Family Planning (1969; 1983)
- Declaration of Sydney (on death) (1968; 1983)
- Declaration of Oslo (on therapeutic abortion) (1970; 1983)
- Statement on the Use of Computer [*sic*] in Medicine (1973; 1983)
- Declaration of Tokyo (guidelines for medical doctors on non-involvement in torture or other maltreatment of prisoners) (1975)
- Statement on Body Searches of Prisoners (1993)
- Statement on the Use and Misuse of Psychotropic Drugs (1975; 1983)
- Resolution on Physician Participation in Capital Punishment (1981)
- Declaration on Principles of Health Care for Sports Medicine (1981; 1993)
- Declaration of Lisbon on the Rights of the Patient (1981; 1995)
- Declaration of Venice on Terminal Illness (1983)
- Statement of Policy on the Care of Patients with Severe Chronic Pain in Terminal Illness (1990)
- Statement on Medical Manpower I (1983; 1986)
- Statement on Child Abuse and Neglect (1984; 1995)
- Declaration on Human Rights and Individual Freedom of Medical Practitioners (1985)
- Statement on Live Organ Trade (1985)
- Declaration on Physician Independence and Professional Freedom (1986)
- Declaration of Madrid on Professional Autonomy and Self-Regulation (1987)
- Statement on In-Vitro Fertilization and Embryo Transplantation (1987)
- Declaration on Euthanasia (1987)
- Declaration on Human Organ Transplantation (1987)
- Statement on Access to Health Care (1988)
- Statement on the Professional Responsibility of Physicians in Treating AIDS Patients (1988)
- Statement on Economic Sanctions or Boycotts (1988)
- Resolution on Medical Group Practice (1988)
- Statement on Fetal Tissue Transplantation (1989)
- Statement on Persistent Vegetative State (1989)
- Declaration of Hong Kong on the Abuse of the Elderly (1989; 1990)
- Declaration on Medical Education (1991)
- Declaration on Hunger Strikers (1991; 1992)
- Statement on Issues Raised by the HIV Epidemic (1992)
- Declaration on the Human Genome Project (1992)
- Statement on Physician-Assisted Suicide (1992)
- Statement on Home Medical Monitoring, "Tele-Medicine" and Medical Ethics (1992)

- Statement on Medical Malpractice (1992)
- Statement on Medical Ethics in the Event of Disasters (1994)
- Resolution on Physicians' Conduct Concerning Human Organ Transplantation (1994)
- Statement on Ethical Aspects of Embryonic Reduction (1995)
- Statement on Health Promotion (1995)
- Statement on Ethical Issues Concerning Patients with Mental Illness (1995)
- Resolution on Human Rights (1990; 1995)
- Statement on Patient Advocacy and Confidentiality (1993)
- Declaration on Family Violence (1996)
- Statement on Weapons and their Relation to Life and Health (1996)
- Statement on Professional Responsibility for Standards of Medical Care (1996)
- Statement on Family Planning and the Right of a Woman to Contraception (1996)
- Resolution on Cloning (1997)
- Statement on the Health Hazards of Tobacco Products (1997)
- Declaration with Guidelines for Continuous Quality Improvement in Health Care (1997)
- Declaration of Hamburg on Support for Medical Doctors Refusing to Participate in, or to Condone, the Use of Torture or Other Forms of Cruel, Inhuman, or Degrading Treatment (1997)
- Proposal for a United Nations Rapporteur on the Independence and Integrity of Health Professionals (1997)
- Resolution on the Prohibition of Access of Women to Health Care and the Prohibition of Practice by Female Doctors in Afghanistan (1997)
- Resolution on Economic Embargoes and Health (1997)
- Declaration of Ottawa on the Right of the Child to Health Care (1998)
- Resolution on The Hague Appeal for Peace (1998)
- Resolution on the Medical Workforce (1998)
- Resolution on Medical Care for Refugees (1998)
- Declaration on Nuclear Weapons (1998)
- Resolution Supporting the Ottawa Convention (1998)
- Resolution on the Inclusion of Medical Ethics and Human Rights in the Curriculum of Medical Schools World-Wide (1999)
- Statement on Medical Process Patents (1999)
- Statement on the Working Relationship between Physicians and Pharmacists in Medicinal Therapy (1999)
- Statement on Accountability, Responsibilities and Ethical Guidelines in the Practice of Telemedicine (1999)

World Psychiatric Association

- Declaration of Hawaii (1977)
- Declaration of Hawaii II (1983)
- Statement and Viewpoints on the Rights and Legal Safeguards of the Mentally Ill (1989)
- Declaration on the Participation of Psychiatrists in the Death Penalty (1989)
- Declaration of Madrid (1996)
- Guidelines Concerning Specific Situations [euthanasia, torture, death penalty, selection of sex, organ transplantation] (1996)

Governmental Entity

Holy See

- Declaration on Euthanasia (1980)
- Encyclical Letter on the Value and Inviolability of Human Life (Evangelium Vitae) (1995)

Congregation for the Doctrine of the Faith

- Instruction on Respect for Human Life in Its Origin and on the Dignity of Procreation (Donum Vitae) (1987)

Pontifical Academy for Life

- Reflections on Cloning (1997)

Pontifical Academy of Sciences

- Declaration on the Artificial Prolongation of Life and Determining Exactly the Moment of Death (1989)

Pontifical Council for Pastoral Assistance to Health Care Workers

- Charter for Health Care Workers (1995)

Miscellaneous International Texts

- Nuremberg Code (adopted by the US Tribunal on 19 July 1947)
- Conclusions and Recommendations of the International Symposium on the Effects on Human Rights of Recent Advances in Science and Technology (Barcelona, 25–28 March 1985). Organized by UNESCO and the International Social Sciences Council
- Summary Report of the International Summit Conference on Bioethics (Ottawa) (1987)
- Ethical Guidelines for Human Reproduction Research in the Muslim World (1992)
- Bilbao Declaration. Adopted by the International Workshop on Legal Aspects of the Human Genome Project (Bilbao, Spain, 24–26 May 1993)
- Fukui Statement on International Bioethics. Adopted at the Third International Bioethics Seminar (Fukui, Japan, 19–21 November 1993)
- Common Position on Ethics of Biomedical Research and the Biopharmaceutical Industry of the Representatives of the European Patients' Organizations (Brussels, 10 January 1994)
- Statement on Human Gene Therapy adopted by the International Symposium on Human Gene Therapy (Inuyama and Nagoya, Japan, 1995)
- Seoul Declaration on Brain Death. Adopted by the 4th Congress of the Asian Society of Transplantation (Seoul, 28 August 1995)
- Statement on the Promotion of Patients' Rights. Adopted by the European Forum of Medical Associations and WHO (Stockholm, 1–2 February 1996)
- Model Ethical Code for Psychiatrists (draft version developed by a Working Group of the Network of Reformers in Psychiatry at its Fourth Meeting, Madrid, 29–31 August 1996)
- Kampala Declaration on Prison Conditions in Africa. Adopted by the Pan African Seminar on Prison Conditions in Africa (Kampala, Uganda, 19–21 September 1996)
- Declaration of Manzanillo. Adopted by the 1st Latin American Meeting on Bioethics and the Human Genome (Manzanillo (Colima State), Mexico, 9–12 October 1996)
- Melbourne Declaration on Physician-Assisted Dying. Adopted by the 11th International Conference of the World Federation of Right to Die Societies (Melbourne, 15–18 October 1996)
- Health on the Net Foundation Code (HONcode) (1996; 1997)
- Proposed Model Ethical Protocol for Collecting DNA Samples. Prepared by the North American Regional Committee of the Human Genome Diversity Project (1998?)
- New Delhi Charter on Global Drugs Law. Adopted by the International Conference on Global Drugs Law (New Delhi, 28 February–3 March 1997)
- Recommendations (notably on human cloning) of the 9th Fiqh [Islamic Jurisprudence] – Medical Seminar, organised jointly by the Islamic Organization for Medical Sciences, WHO (Eastern Mediterranean Regional Office), the Arab Educational, Scientific and Cultural Organization, and the Fiqh Academy of the Organization of the Islamic Conference (Casablanca, 14–17 June 1997)

- Communiqué of the Denver Summit of the Eight (22 June 1997) (para. 47 on "Human Cloning")
- The Nuremberg Code of 1997. Adopted by the Nuremberg Regional Group of International Physicians Against Nuclear War on 20 August 1997
- The Uganda Declaration of 1997. Adopted on 31 August 1997 at the 1st International Federation of Medical Students' Associations Training Workshop on Human Rights and Medicine (Kampala and Mbarara, Uganda, 23 August–1 September 1997)
- The Right to Health Declaration. Adopted by the 1st International Federation of Medical Students' Associations Training Workshop on Human Rights and Medicine in Kampala on 31 August 1997 by the above-mentioned Workshop
- The Dakar Declaration. Adopted at the 4th Regional Conference/General Assembly of the Inter-African Committee (IAC), organised jointly by WHO and IAC (Dakar, 17–21 November 1997)
- The Calicut Declaration: Principles of Ethics in Health Care. Adopted by a meeting organised by the Pain and Palliative Care Society in Calicut, Kerala, India, on 22–23 November 1997
- The New Delhi Declaration. Adopted by the International Conference on Global Health Law (New Delhi, 5–7 December 1997)
- Declaration in Defence of Cloning and the Integrity of Scientific Research. Signed by Humanist Laureates of the International Academy of Humanism (1997)
- Forging the Link Between Health and Human Rights. Statement of the Consortium for Health and Human Rights (François-Xavier Bagnoud Center for Health and Human Rights; Global Lawyers and Physicians; International Physicians for the Prevention of Nuclear War; and Physicians for Human Rights), issued to mark the 50th Anniversary of the Universal Declaration of Human Rights (1998)
- Deontology and Good Practices in Epidemiology. Recommendations of the Association of French-speaking Epidemiologists (ADELF) (1998)
- The Barcelona Declaration on Policy Proposals to the European Commission on Basic Ethical Principles in Bioethics and Biolaw (adopted in November 1998 by Partners in the BIOMED II Project)
- Resolution No. 1 of the European Conference of National Ethics Committees (adopted at the 4th Conference, Oporto, 9–10 November 1998)
- Tokyo Communiqué, International Summit of National Bioethics Commissions (1998)
- The Ethical Duties of Psychiatrists. Adopted by the Network of Reformers in Psychiatry (in the CCEE/NIS countries, April 1998)
- Bangalore Communiqué on Science and Society. Adopted at the International Symposium on Science and Society (Bangalore, 27–29 January 1999)
- Statement on Physicians' Autonomy. Adopted by the European Forum of Medical Associations and WHO (Tel Aviv, 7–9 March 1999)
- Declaration on Human Cloning. Adopted by the participants at the Journées Internationales de Bioéthique (Yaoundé, Cameroon, 8–10 March 1999)
- Amsterdam Statement on Access to Medicines. Adopted at the Conference on Increasing Access to Essential Drugs in a Globalized Economy: Working towards Solutions (Amsterdam, 25–26 November 1999)
- Statement on Patenting of the Human Genome. Adopted by the European Forum of Medical Associations and WHO (Warsaw, 17–19 March 2000)
- The Monaco Statement on Considerations on Bioethics and the Rights of the Child. Adopted at the International Symposium on Bioethics and the Rights of the Child (Monaco, 28–30 April 2000)
- The eHealth Code of Ethics. Issued by the eHealth Ethics Initiative (2000)

Index